MASSIMO **SIMION**

CLINICAL OSSEOINTEGRATION
AND BONE REGENERATION

To Lorenzo, who wishes to enjoy himself as a free man
in life and profession
as I have done and am doing

One book, one tree: In support of reforestation worldwide and to address the climate crisis, for every book sold Quintessence Publishing will plant a tree (https://onetreeplanted.org/).

First published as OSTEOINTEGRAZIONE CLINICA E RIGENERAZIONE OSSEA in Italian in 2022 by Quintessenza Edizioni, Italy.

How do you read a QR code?
Inside this book, you will find QR codes linked to the relevant videos. To access these videos, you will need to scan the QR code with the camera of your mobile device. Frame the QR code with the camera of your smartphone or tablet, and follow the prompts to view the video.

A CIP record for this book is available from the British Library.
ISBN 978-1-78698-141-7

QUINTESSENCE PUBLISHING DEUTSCHLAND

Quintessenz Verlags-GmbH
Ifenpfad 2–4
12107 Berlin
Germany
www.quintessence-publishing.com

Quintessence Publishing Co Ltd
Grafton Road, New Malden
Surrey KT3 3AB
United Kingdom
www.quintessence-publishing.com

Translation: Alexandra Rendon, Bologna, Italy
Editing, Layout, Production and Reproduction: Quintessenz Verlags-GmbH, Berlin, Germany

Printed and bound in Croatia by Graficki zavod Hrvatske d.o.o.

MASSIMO **SIMION**

CLINICAL OSSEOINTEGRATION AND BONE REGENERATION

COAUTHORS:
FABIANA **ALLEVI**
MARIO **BERETTA**
FABIO **BERNARDELLO**
FEDERICO **BIGLIOLI**
PAOLO **BOZZOLI**
ELENA **CANCIANI**
CHRISTER **DAHLIN**
DANIELE **DE SANTIS**
CLAUDIA **DELLAVIA**
LUCA **FERRANTINO**
FILIPPO **FONTANA**

ELEONORA **IDOTTA**
MICHELE **MAGLIONE**
CARLO **MAIORANA**
MARCO **MORRA**
MYRON **NEVINS**
PIER FRANCESCO **NOCINI**
RICCARDO **NOCINI**
STEFANO **PIERONI**
ALBERTO **PISPERO**
ROBERTO **PISTILLI**
ALESSANDRA **SIRONI**
GIOVANNI **ZUCCHELLI**

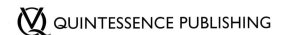 QUINTESSENCE PUBLISHING

Berlin | Chicago | Tokyo
Barcelona | London | Milan | Paris | Prague | Seoul | Warsaw
Beijing | Istanbul | Sao Paulo | Zagreb

CONTENTS

CONTENTS

CONTENTS

CONTENTS

CONTENTS

CONTENTS

PRESENTATION

This timely text presents clinicians with significant, interesting, and new information in the field of implant dentistry. Osseointegrated implants, introduced by P.I. Brånemark, allowed for predictable dental implant therapy and changed the scope of treatment for the replacement of teeth in edentulous patients.

This comprehensive textbook is a concerted endeavor to explore the clinical efforts of all dental implant surgeons. It brings to light the improvements and progress made by clinicians over a period of more than 30 years.

The editor has engaged surgical and restorative experts for the solutions they have found for their patient's problems.

Massimo Simion and I discovered one another in 1990, when he invited me to Milan as a keynote speaker at the first Italian Academy of Osseointegration. He shared his early clinical cases on guided bone regeneration, and I invited him to join our research and clinical courses at the Institute for Advanced Dental Studies and to present his significant findings at the International Symposium in Boston. We have continued to share our research results, including at the 2022 International Symposium, where we introduced new techniques and biomaterials for augmenting the alveolar process to successfully support osseointegrated implants. Successful implant therapy depends upon proper diagnosis and treatment planning to support osseointegration.

These chapters describe the relevant anatomy and surgical techniques for the treatment of both partially and completely edentulous patients. Long-term cases provide examples of the careful decisions around diagnosis and treatment planning, as well as how to engage patient understanding and cooperation.

The text also explores the developments in implant dentistry. Immediate implant placement has expanded into immediate implant loading. Guided implant surgery opens the door to future possibilities. Finally, no leading surgeon can avoid all complications. This text covers the management of complications, including the practical resolution of peri-implantitis.

Every dental team that performs bone augmentation procedures and/or implant rehabilitation should have this text in their library and become familiar with its wisdom on patient care before, during, and after treatment. It is a fabulously complete work, and I congratulate the editor, Massimo Simion, as well as the contributors.

Myron Nevins

INTRODUCTION

My collaboration with Quintessence Publishing began in the early 1990s. In those days, world dentistry was living extraordinary years: Osseo-integration techniques according to the Bråne-mark system were spreading like wildfire in all continents, radically reshaping the therapeutic approach to partially and completely edentulous patients, and guided tissue regeneration was rapidly extending from periodontal applications to peri-implant bone regeneration.

I was fortunate to be able to participate in the development of these two extraordinary world-changing events at a very young age. My first publication on guided bone regeneration (GBR) was published in the International Journal of Periodontics and Restorative Dentistry in 1994, and since then, I have consistently collaborated with Quintessence Publishing, both to publish scientific articles and to participate as a speaker at every Symposium on Periodontics and Restorative Dentistry in Boston, chaired by Myron Nevins. For over 20 years, we have been discussing the idea of a book on osseointegration and bone regeneration, but only now did I finally tackle the project. My hesitation stemmed from the fact that writing such a far-reaching book would require an immense amount of work, with the danger of the writing never ending. The greatest risk was that once the book was finally finished and published, it would already be overtaken by the rapid evolution of scientific knowledge. I didn't want to write a book and, once finished, wish that I had done it differently.

Today, the speed at which knowledge is being acquired has slowed considerably compared to the first 20 pioneering years. Of course, we learn to use new digital technologies on a daily basis, which makes our work easier and more precise, but the biologic principles and surgical techniques of osseointegration and GBR are essentially equivalent to those developed between the 1980s and 1990s. In the end, I felt that writing this book was finally feasible based on the wealth of information that is now available and, presumably, its stable application for a long time, or perhaps forever.

My aim was to produce a work available to everyone—one that could be used as a textbook by students of dentistry and by those approaching osseointegrated implantology techniques for the first time but also useful for experts wanting to refine their techniques for bone regeneration and the treatment of peri-implant soft tissue in even the most complex esthetic cases. To accomplish this, I have faithfully followed the syllabus of my university course for students and the annual course that I have been holding for implant dentists for more than 20 years. All the concepts and clinical cases illustrated during these courses are presented here.

As Myron Nevins says, *"No one can be an expert in all subjects. Only presumptuous ignoramuses consider themselves such."* For this reason, I have drawn on the help of the researchers and clinicians with whom I have collaborated most closely over the past 30 years.

These voices are joined by some emerging young people of great talent, and certainly bright futures. To all of them goes my heartfelt thanks. I also want to thank all the staff at Quintessence Publishing Italia for their patience and dedication during the production of this book.

Massimo Simion

CURRICULA

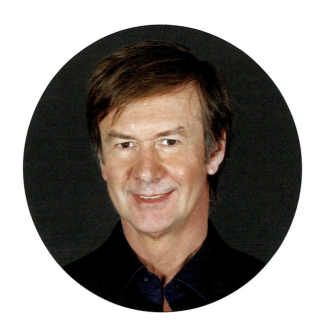

MASSIMO SIMION

Degree in Medicine and Surgery at the University of Milan in 1979. Specialized in Dentistry and Dental Prosthetics at the same University in 1981. Associate Professor for the teaching of Periodontology and Implantology at the University of Milan.

Member of the Board of the European Association for Osseointegration (EAO) from 1998 to 2005, President of the EAO from 2001 to 2003 and Immediate Past-President for the years 2004–2005.

EAO Council Member 2005–2011.

Founder of the Italian Academy of Osseointegration.

Active Member and Vice-President of the Italian Society of Periodontology and Implantology (SidP) for the years 2003–2005. President 2023–2024 of the Italian Academy of Osseointegration (IAO).

Referee of the International Journal of Periodontics and Restorative Dentistry.

He has published numerous articles in scientific journals and is an international speaker on the subject of periodontology, osseointegration and bone regeneration.

CURRICULA

FABIANA ALLEVI • Degree in Medicine in 2010, specialized in Maxillofacial Surgery in 2016 at the University of Milan. In 2019, she obtained her PhD in Odontostomatological Sciences at the same university. Currently works as a Medical Consultant at the UO of Maxillofacial Surgery of ASST Santi Paolo e Carlo, Presidio San Paolo (Milan).

MARIO BERETTA • Degree in Dentistry and Dental Prosthetics from the University of Milan in 1999. Specialist in Oral Surgery. PhD in Implantology and Innovative Techniques in Implant Prosthetics at the University of Milan. Adjunct Professor at the School of Specialization in Oral Surgery at the University of Milan. Awarded national qualification as second-rank professor in 2017. Tutor at the Reference Centre for the treatment of edentulous and severe maxillary atrophies (Dir. Prof. C Maiorana). UOC Maxillofacial Surgery and Odontostomatology (Dir. Prof. AB Gianni) (IRCCS Fondazione Policlinico-Cà Granda Milano). His activity is mainly focused on Implantology, Advanced Osseointegration and Periodontology. He is author of numerous publications in national and international journals and speaker at national and international congresses.

FABIO BERNARDELLO • Graduated in Medicine and Surgery in 1990. Specialized in Pathological Anatomy and Histology in 1994 at the University of Verona. He was Adjunct Professor for the teaching of Oral Surgery (University "Alma Mater Studiorum" of Bologna and University "Aldo Moro" of Bari). Active member and currently advisor in the IPA (International Piezoelectric Surgery Academy) Board of Directors. He is author or co-author of about 30 scientific articles published in international peer-reviewed journals.

FEDERICO BIGLIOLI • Degree in Medicine and Surgery in 1992 from the University of Milan and subsequent specialization in Maxillofacial Surgery and Microsurgery at the same University. After directing the UO of Maxillofacial Surgery at the IRCCS Galeazzi in Milan (2010-2012), he assumed the role he still holds today as Director of the UO of Maxillofacial Surgery at the ASST Santi Paolo e Carlo. Currently Full Professor and Director of the School of Specialization in Maxillofacial Surgery at the University of Milan. Author of 119 scientific publications, most of them in international journals, and co-author of 11 scientific textbooks, 8 of which are in English. He deals with the various fields into which maxillofacial surgery is divided, concentrating his interest on surgery of facial and trigeminal nerve lesions, reconstructive head-neck microsurgery, and oncological surgery of the oral cavity and face.

PAOLO BOZZOLI • Degree in Dentistry and Dental Prosthetics from the University of Milan in 1991. Active SICOI member. Has obtained: Certificate in Mobile prosthetics and diagnosis and therapy of myoarthropathies (Prof. Palla University of Zurich), Diploma in Clinical Periodontology (Prof. J. Linde University of Gothenburg), Certificate in Oral Rehabilitation by means of implants (Prof. J. Linde J. Wennstrom, University of Gothenburg), Certificate in Fixed and removable prosthodontics (Prof. N.P. Lang University of Berne), Certificate in Evidence-Based-Treatment Planning (Prof. J. Linde Prof. T. Berglund), Attending member of the Continuous Education in Dentistry of the Ariminum Research & Dental Education Center with title of Senator. Master in Implantology and Oral Rehabilitation at New York University. Speaker at theoretical-practical courses in basic and advanced implantology. Speaker at national congresses. Lecturer at the Post-Graduate Course in Implantology at the University of Modena and Bologna. Lecturer at the 2nd Level Master in Digital Dentistry at the University of Insubria. Scientific Tutor at the Zimmer Institute in Winterthur Zurich. Author and co-author of scientific articles in international journals. Particularly involved in research on regenerative techniques of sinus lift and immediate loading. Trainer ZFX digital project (optical impression and digital workflow).

ELENA CANCIANI • Graduated cum laude in Medical and Pharmaceutical Biotechnology with a focus on tissue engineering and PhD in Morphological Sciences at the University of Milan (Unimi). A Research Fellow at the Department of Biomedical, Surgical and Dental Sciences (DISBIOC) of Unimi, she works at the Thin Sections Laboratory (Dir. Prof. Dellavia), conducting research in the following areas: microscopic anatomy, cell and organotypic cultures, molecular and histological analyses of dental and periodontal tissues under physiological conditions or in the presence of biomaterials and metal prostheses. He participates in research and development projects on new biomaterials, scaffolds and medical devices for the regeneration and treatment of periodontal tissues and bone tissue in particular, collaborating with numerous national and international

CURRICULA

companies and laboratories in the dental and orthopedic field. He has attended numerous national and international research institutes to learn and deepen his knowledge of the new technologies available for the preparation, observation and interpretation of the morphological data obtained. He has also participated in projects that have received funding from the Novara and Milan Community Foundations and non-profit associations. The results of his research activities have been presented at both national and international congresses and are documented by publications indexed on PubMed.

CHRISTER DAHLIN • Dr Christer Dahlin is a Professor in Guided Tissue Regeneration and Oral Surgery at Department of Biomaterials, University of Gothenburg, Sweden. He is the President-elect and a member of the Executive board for the Osteology Foundation. Professor Dahlin is considered one of the pioneers in the development of the concept of Guided Bone Regeneration. He has over thirty years of experience in this field as well as on implant treatment and related research. He has published numerous articles and textbooks on these topics. He frequently travels worldwide to lecture, conduct research and teach on this and other implant-related topics.

DANIELE DE SANTIS • Degree in Medicine and Surgery in 1989 from the University of Verona. Specialized in Odontostomatology and Maxillofacial Surgery at the University of Verona, he graduated in Dental Implantology at the Université Sophia Antipolis of Nice in France. Since 1992 to date Medical Director at the Dental and Maxillofacial Surgery Clinic (Dir. Prof. Pier Francesco Nocini) of the Verona Hospital. Member and scientific director from 2001 to date of the "University Master's Degree Programme in Oral Surgery and Implantology" at Verona University. Visiting Professor at the Christian Albrechts Universität in Kiel (Germany) in 2003 and, since 2006, Associate Professor in Dental Materials Science at the Degree Course in Dentistry and Dental Prosthetics at the same university. Instructor in a training program in oral surgery on anatomical preparation at the Medizinische Universität Graz (Austria). Court-appointed technical consultant for the Court of Verona. In 2018 he obtained the qualification as Full Professor (ASN announcement D.D. 1532/2016 concurrency sector 06/F1). Referee since 2021 of the Doctorate in Odontostomatological Sciences. He has published in the most important international journals. Author of the books: 'Treatise on pre-prosthetic surgery' (Martina, 2005) and 'New perspectives in implant prosthetics and regenerative surgery' (Quintessenza Edizioni 2010). He is co-author of 'Materials and technologies in dentistry' (Ariesdue ed., 2011). Member of the editorial board of: International Journal of Implant Dentistry, Journal of Indian Society of Periodontology and Quintessence International.

CLAUDIA DELLAVIA • Degree with honors in Dentistry and Dental Prosthetics (OPD) and PhD in Morphological Sciences at the University of Milan (Unimi). Full Professor of Human Anatomy at the Department of Biomedical, Surgical and Dental Sciences (DISBIOC) of Unimi with teaching tenure for numerous three-year degree courses at the Faculty of Medicine and Surgery, for the single-cycle degree courses in OPD and in Medicine and Surgery (international course), and for the Schools of Specialization in Dental Surgery, Pediatric Dentistry and Orthodontics. Member of the board of teachers for the PhD in Clinical Research at Unimi. She carries out her research activities in the field of macroscopic, microscopic and functional anatomy of the stomatognathic apparatus in the Thin Sections Laboratory she directs at DISBIOC. Author of more than 90 publications in international journals indexed in PubMed. She has scientific collaborations with national and international teaching and research centres belonging to Italian, European, US and African universities.

LUCA FERRANTINO • Degree in Dentistry from the University of Milan in 2009. Scholarship SIdP (Italian Society of Periodontology and Implantology) for the two-year period 2010-2011. Master in Oral Sciences at the University Complutense of Madrid in Spain in 2012, and in 2015 PhD in Bone Regeneration at the University of Milan and at the University Complutense of Madrid. Tutor in Periodontology at the University Dental Clinic of Milan 2012-2018. Since 2013 he has been following Prof. Massimo Simion in his teaching and research activities, and with him he has published several articles on implantology and regenerative techniques of hard and soft oral tissues. Since 2019, he is Adjunct Professor for the Degree Course in Dentistry at the University of Milan.

CURRICULA

FILIPPO FONTANA • FILIPPO FONTANA - Degree in Dentistry and Dental Prosthetics with 110/110 cum laude from the University of Milan. Specialized in Dental Surgery at the same university with 70/70 cum laude. In 2017 he obtained the national scientific qualification (ASN) as Associate Professor. Adjunct Professor at the School of Specialization in Oral Surgery at the University of Milan 2012-2016. Active member of the Italian Academy of Osseointegration (IAO). From 2000 to 2017 he was attending physician at the Implantology Department of the Cà Granda Foundation Dental Clinic (Dir. Prof. C Maiorana). Winner of a scholarship for further training abroad in 2002, he spent the period September 2002 – June 2003 at the Department of Oral Medicine, Infection and Immunity - Harvard School of Dental Medicine - Boston (Dir. JP Fiorellini) as a clinical assistant and researcher. He was a clinical and research consultant at the Institute for Dental Research and Education (IDRE) (Dir. Prof. M Simion). Author of national and international publications, he focuses his clinical activity on periodontology and implantology with a special emphasis on bone regeneration.

ELEONORA IDOTTA • Degree in Dentistry and Dental Prosthetics with 110 cum laude in 2006, from the University of Messina. Intern at the Department of Odontostomatology, AOU G. Martino, Messina. From 2007 to 2010 she carried out clinical-assistance activities at the UOS of Odontostomatology of the G. Martino Hospital of Messina with particular reference to: Odontostomatological Surgery, diagnosis and treatment of Osteonecrosis of the Maxillary Biphosphonates. From 2007 to 2010 tutor of the 2nd level Master's Degree Course in Oral Implantology and Prosthetic Rehabilitation. University of Messina. In 2010 he obtained his PhD in Implant-Prosthetic Technologies in Dentistry at the University of Messina. In 2012, she completed her specialization in Dental Surgery at the University of Milan. Author of scientific papers and a textbook on peri-implantitis with Prof. M. Simion.

MICHELE MAGLIONE • MICHELE MAGLIONE - Graduated with honors in Medicine and Surgery from the University of Milan in 1992, and specialized with honors in Odontostomatology in 1995 at the same University. Author of publications in national and international journals on the subject of implants, and speaker at national and international congresses and courses. Active member of the Italian Academy of Prosthetic Dentistry (AIOP), and member of the European Academy of Osseointegration (EAO). He practices as a dentist in Canegrate (MI) and in Milan in collaboration with Prof. Massimo Simion.

CARLO MAIORANA • Full Professor of Oral Diseases. Professor of Oral Surgery, University of Milan. Director of the School of Specialization in Oral Surgery, University of Milan. Medical Director UOC Maxillofacial Surgery and Odontostomatology Policlinic Foundation, Director of the Implantology Centre for edentulism and maxillary atrophies, IRCCS Policlinic Cà Granda Foundation. Author of 160 publications in international journals. Reviewer and Board Member of numerous international journals.

MARCO MORRA • Degree in Chemistry from the Faculty of Science at the University of Turin in 1986. His professional activity has always focused on the study, characterization and modification of the surface properties of materials. After gaining experience in research centers on the surface properties of materials used in optical communications and of polymeric and biomedical materials Co-founder of Nobil Bio Ricerche in 1994, where he delved into the surface treatment and analysis of titanium implant screws. Co-author of a couple of texts, more than one hundred publications and about twenty patents on different aspects of material surfaces, with an H-index of 48.

MYRON NEVINS • DDS, is the Editor of the International Journal of Periodontics & Restorative Dentistry and Associate Clinical Professor of Periodontology at the Harvard School of Dental Medicine. Dr. Nevins is the former Director and President of the Academy of Osseointegration Foundation Board. Dr. Nevins is a past President of the American Academy of Periodontology and a former Director and Chairman of the American Board of Periodontology where his contributions have been recognized with the Gold Medal and the Master Clinician Awards. He was previously Director at the Institute for Advanced Studies, and a former director at the American Academy of Periodontology Foundation. He is an adjunct Professor at the University of Michigan School of Dentistry. Dr. Nevins was also a Diplomate for the American Board of Periodontology. He maintains a private practice limited to Periodontics and Implantology in Swampscott, Massachusetts. Dr. Nevins is the founder and President of Perio Imp Research, Inc.

CURRICULA

 PIER FRANCESCO NOCINI • Degree in Medicine and Surgery, University of Pavia in 1981. Postgraduate diploma in Odontostomatology, University of Verona in 1985. Postgraduate diploma in Maxillofacial Surgery, University of Verona in 1990. Magnificent Rector of the University of Verona, Director of the UOC Maxillofacial Surgery and Dentistry and Member of the Interdepartmental Management Board and of the AOUI Verona Health Council. 2012–2013: Member of the Commission for National Scientific Qualification of the Ministry of Education, University and Research for Competition Sector 06/E3 Neurosurgery and Maxillofacial Surgery. 2017–2019: Past-President of the Italian Society of Maxillofacial Surgery. From 2020 to present President of the College of Maxillofacial Surgery Lecturers. Has participated as a speaker at countless national and international scientific congresses. He is the author of 250 articles. He has also edited numerous books, treatise chapters and monographs with international circulation. In the course of his decades-long university career, he has held numerous teaching posts in the degree courses in Medicine and Surgery, Dentistry and Dental Prosthetics, the degree course in Dental Hygiene, specialization schools and university masters courses. He has also been invited as Visiting Professor in Degree Courses, Masters and training seminars at prestigious national and international universities.

 RICCARDO NOCINI • Degree in Medicine and Surgery with 110 cum laude from the University of Verona in 2017. From 1 November 2019 to date Doctor in specialist training, School of Specialization in Otolaryngology, Azienda Ospedaliera Universitaria Integrata (AOUI) of Verona. Fields of interest: oncologic head and neck surgery, endoscopic nasal surgery, endoscopic ear surgery, reconstructive microsurgery, laser surgery of the larynx, facial plastic surgery and aesthetic medicine.Participation in the scientific organization of the courses of Anatomic Dissection of the Head and Neck (Cadaver Lab) with U.O.C of Otolaryngology (AOUI Verona). He has published in the most important international journals. Member of the editorial board of national and international scientific journals, such as: Frontiers in Dental Medicine, Journal of Applied Sciences (MDPI), Journal of Clinical Medicine (MDPI) and Section Editor for the journal Annals of Maxillofacial Surgery. Active Member Italian Society of Microsurgery (SIM).

 STEFANO PIERONI • Degree in Dentistry and Specialization in Oral Surgery Odontostomatology at the University of Milan. 2010-2017 frequenter of the implantology department at the Dental Clinic in via della Commenda at the University of Milan. Since 2013 he has been working with Prof. Massimo Simion as second operator during the Advanced Surgery and Immediate Loading courses, as well as during the annual course. Author of publications in national and international journals, he focuses his clinical and research activity on topics such as bone regeneration, peri-implant soft tissue and aesthetic prosthetics. Since 2014, he has been a speaker at national and international congresses and courses. He practices his profession in Milan, devoting himself mainly to prosthetic rehabilitations on natural teeth and implants. Ordinary member of the Italian Academy of Osseointegration and the Italian Academy of Esthetic Dentistry.

 ALBERTO PISPERO • Degree in Dentistry and Dental Prosthetics in 2006. Specialization in Odontostomatological Surgery in 2009 with full marks and honors at the University of Milan. Since 2019 he has been a PhD in Odontostomatological Sciences. Since 2010 medical consultant and tutor for students of the degree course in Dentistry at the Dental Clinic of ASST Santi Paolo e Carlo in Milan. Since 2017 winner of a teaching contract at the University of Milan for the Degree Course in Dentistry and Dental Prosthetics and the specialization course in Odontostomatological Surgery. Lecturer at specialization courses in Oral Pathology and Surgery. Founder with Prof. G Lodi and Dr R Franchini of the non-profit organization ACAPO (Association for the fight against cancer and oral pathologies). Active member of the International Academy of Osseointegration (IAO) and has been its secretary since 2019. Member of the International Team for Implantology (ITI), member of the Italian Society of Oral Pathology and Medicine (SIPMO), author of articles and posters presented in national and international congresses.

CURRICULA

ROBERTO PISTILLI • Degree in Medicine and Surgery from the University of Rome in 1983. Specialist in Maxillofacial Surgery since 1988; manager maxillofacial surgeon at the ACO S. Camillo in Rome from 1989 to 1994, at the ACO S. Giovanni Addolorata in Rome (1994-1999) and at the ACO S. Filippo Neri in Rome (1999-07/2015) with high professionalism (P1) and at the ACO S. Camillo in Rome from August 2015 to date with the same appointment. Director of the Annual Postgraduate Course in Oral Surgery and Implantology at ACO San Filippo Neri in Rome (2001-2015). Director of the Annual Course in Rational Dissection of the Anatomical Loggias of the Neck and Oral Cavity held at the University Miguel Hernandez de Helche, S. Juan de Alicante (Spain). Adjunct Professor at the Universities of Bologna and Genoa. Author of the book Anatomy and Surgery of the Oral Cavity (EditaliaMedica). Contributor to other textbooks in the field of Dentistry and Maxillofacial Surgery. Active Member I.A.O. Member of the Scientific Committee of the International Journal of Osseointegration. Member of the Editorial Board of the European Journal of Oral Implantology. Director CAO Rome from 01-01-2012 to 31-12-2017. Currently President of the Cultural Commission CAO Rome. President of SIRIO Roma ARCOI (Roman Academy of Oral Surgery and Implantology) from 2012 to date. President of the GISOS Society from 2019 to date. President of the Inthema Society from 2020 to present. Author of publications in national and international indexed scientific journals. Speaker at numerous courses and congresses in Italy and abroad.

ALESSANDRA SIRONI • Graduated with honors in Dental Hygiene from the University of Milan in 2011. She has attended numerous refresher courses in Italy and abroad, including: theoretical-practical course on osseointegration, regeneration and peri-implantitis held by Prof. M Simion, theoretical-practical course on the treatment of the periodontal patient, held by Dr. Ghezzi and Dr. Masiero. Theoretical module of Surgical Periodontology for Hygienists held by Prof. G Zucchelli. Clinical course in Periodontology at the University Clinics Folktandvarden in Gothenburg, Sweden, held by Prof. Berglund, Prof. Cassel and Dr. Koch. Theoretical-practical course in non-surgical periodontal therapy held by Prof. Graziani, Prof. Tomasi and Dr. Suvan. Specialization in the treatment of peri-implantitis and complex periodontal cases, has been working with Studio Simion since 2012.

GIOVANNI ZUCCHELLI • Degree in Dentistry and Dental Prosthetics with honors in 1998. PhD in "Medical Biotechnology", specializing in "Biomedical Technologies" at the University of Bologna. Full Professor of Periodontology at the University of Bologna. Director of the Department of Periodontology and Dental Hygiene at the University of Bologna. Coordinator of the Degree Course in Dental Hygiene at the University of Bologna. Honorary Member of the American Academy of Periodontology (AAP). President of the Italian Academy of Osseointegration (IAO). Member of the Editorial Board of the International Journal of Periodontics and Restorative Dentistry, and member of the Editorial Board of the Journal of Periodontology and International Journal Oral Implanatology. Associate Editor of the International Journal of Esthetic Dentistry. Active member of EAED (European Academy of Esthetic Dentistry), SIdP (Italian Society of Periodontology and Implantology) and IAO (Italian Academy of Osseointegration); member of EFP (European Federation of Periodontology). Author of more than 130 publications impacted in the periodontal and implant field. Winner of awards for scientific research in periodontology in Italy, Europe and the United States. Speaker at the most important national and international congresses in the field of Periodontology and Implantology. Co-author of two textbooks on periodontal plastic surgery (Ed. Martina) and Co-author of the chapter "Mucogingival Therapy-Periodontal Plastic Surgery" in the book "Clinical Periodontology and Implant Dentistry" (Lindhe J, Lang NP, Karring T [eds], Wiley-Blackwell. Author of the books "Mucogingival Aesthetic Surgery" and "Mucogingival Aesthetic Surgery on Implants" published by Quintessence Publishing Italy.

HISTOLOGICAL FEATURES OF OSSEOUS TISSUE

CHAPTER 1

Edited by Claudia Dellavia and Elena Canciani

INTRODUCTION

The alveolar bone is a vital, mineralized connective tissue of ectomesenchymal origin. It consists of a network of protein fiber bundles arranged in layers and is permeated by dense mineral deposits. The protein fibers provide strength and flexibility to the bone tissue, while the mineral deposits impart hardness and rigidity. Bone cells adapt to mechanical stresses to maintain this tissue architecture. They also assist in maintaining homeostasis in plasma calcium levels via bone remodeling processes. Alveolar bone contains more extracellular matrix (ECM) than cellular matrix. The ECM consists of an organic component (about 33%) and an inorganic component (about 67%). The inorganic component is responsible for providing mechanical support and maintaining the calcium homeostasis of the body. The outer layer of bone is covered by the periosteum, which is divided into three layers: the germinative layer, the nutritious/sensory layer, and the fibrous layer. The inner aspect of bone is covered by the endosteum, a thin connective membrane comprising a single layer of cells with osteogenic potential.

The deepest layer of the periosteum is the germinative layer, which is rich in osteoblasts and their precursors.

The intermediate nutritious layer provides vascularization for 15% to 20% of the cortical bone and is characterized by blood vessels immersed in the matrix and mixed with fibroblasts, which maintain tissue texture.

Finally, the fibrous layer is formed by bundles of collagen fibers that keep it nonelastic and fixed to the bone surface.

Knowledge of histology is a basic requirement for performing high-level clinical work. It helps clinicians select the correct clinical protocols and surgical techniques. Thus, this chapter and chapter 3, on the biologic principles of osteointegration, are the most important in the entire book.

Massimo Simion

The main functions of the periosteum are:

- to resist tractional and torsional forces applied to bone (mechanical function);
- to supply required nutrients for cell turnover of bone tissue, which is extremely vital (trophic function);
- to provide proprioceptive and nociceptive information and activate repair, modeling, and remodeling processes with its reservoir of osteoprogenitor cells (sensory function).

TYPES OF BONE TISSUE

There are two types of alveolar bone, nonlamellar bone and lamellar bone. Nonlamellar bone consists of a network of collagen fibers delimiting large cavities filled with vessels. The collagen fibers first form an osteoid matrix, which then organizes to form a woven fiber structure (woven bone). This type of immature bone is present in all cases of neodeposition.

The formative process of nonlamellar woven bone involves several steps. First, osteoblasts must process osteoid, which is a nonmineralized substance made of collagen fibers and a matrix containing glycoproteins and proteoglycans. Continuous apposition of new osteoid matrix causes the previously deposited matrix to mineralize, advancing the mineralization front. Osteoid undergoes calcification via the deposition of minerals such as calcium and phosphates, which are then transformed into hydroxyapatite.

The maturation process, understood as organization and mineralization, leads osteoid to arrange itself into a weave of fibers that evolve into woven bone. At this stage, some osteoblasts become trapped in the matrix of calcified bone tissue in the form of osteocytes. These trapped osteocytes are lodged in irregularly dispersed lacunae in the calcified matrix and remain connected to one other though bone canaliculi that contain their cytoplasmic extensions.

Numerous anastomoses in the canalicular system ensure a network for signaling.[1]

Lamellar bone represents the mature form of human bone tissue. It is organized in layers of lamellae, among which the lacunae containing the osteocytes are found. The lamellae are connected by canaliculi that pass through their entire thicknesses. Lamellar bone is less cellular than nonlamellar bone and presents as either compact bone or spongy bone.

Compact lamellar bone is characterized by osteons (or Haversian systems). Osteons are functional units with a cylindrical shape made up of groups of between 1 and 20 concentric lamellae that leave a cavity (Haversian canal) in the center, through which blood/lymphatic vessels and myelinated nerve fibers run (**Fig 1**). Volkmann's canals are smaller-caliber neurovascular canals that cross the bone transversely or obliquely to its major axis, connecting Haversian canals to each other and opening onto the periosteal and endosteal surfaces of the bone (**Fig 2**).

In the osteon, the innermost lamellae are those that have been most recently deposited. The osteocytes are confined to the bone lacunae and are arranged in concentric rings within the lamellae. Numerous canaliculi radiate from the lacunae in all directions. The osteocytes communicate with each other via gap junctions between the cytoplasmic extensions. The osteocyte cell body and its extensions are separated from the walls of the lacunae and canaliculi by a thin layer of osteoid. Even in mature bone, the lacunae and canaliculi form a continuous system of cavities to allow metabolic and gaseous exchanges between the blood and osteocytes.[1] Bone undergoes continuous remodeling with the destruction of old osteons, whose remnants are left behind as irregular, interstitial lamellae systems. On the outermost aspect of the compact bone, osteons are delimited by a system of concentric lamellae of dense cortical bone called circumferential or external limiting lamellae.

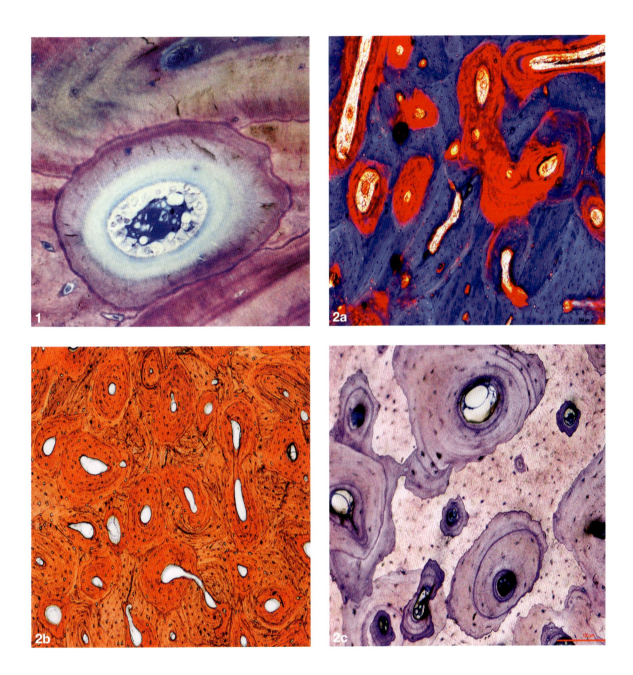

Fig 1 The lamellae are not yet well delineated around the neurovascular canal of Havers, where oste-oblastic cells, vessels, and nerve fibers can be seen. Toluidine blue and Pyronin yellow staining; ×400 magnification. *Fig 2* Cortical bone in three colors to highlight different aspects of mineralization (×200 magnification). (a) The bone stained with Goldner's trichrome modified for hard tissue shows less-mineralized and more recently deposited lamellae in red and bone with a high degree of mineralization in blue. (b) Red Alizarin staining makes it possible to observe the entire mineralized matrix without defining the levels of mineralization, which are evident with the Toluidine blue and Pyronine yellow staining. (c) Toluidine blue and Pyronine yellow staining highlights the shape of the newly formed osteons undergoing remodeling and immersed in a matrix with a high level of mineralization.

Spongy lamellar bone is composed of thin laminae called trabeculae, which are formed by irregular bone lamellae that branch and anastomose into a 3D network containing bone marrow within its lattice (medullary cavities).

Osteocytes are contained in the lacunae, and their extensions are contained in the canaliculi that open into the medullary cavities[1] **(Fig 3)**.

THE COMPOSITION OF BONE TISSUE

Bone tissue is a connective tissue characterized by an abundant ECM that consists of fibers, an amorphous substance of glycoprotein origin, and an inorganic component in which numerous cells are dispersed.

ECM

The inorganic portion of the ECM is made up of mostly hydroxyapatite crystals, calcium carbonate, calcium fluoride, and magnesium phosphate. The hydroxyapatite crystals are deposited among the Type I collagen fibers of the organic portion, which are themselves immersed in an amorphous substance consisting mainly of noncollagenous proteins and adhesion proteins **(Fig 4)**. The noncollagenous proteins include phosphoproteins, osteocalcin, matrix Gla protein (MGP), lipids, lipoproteins, and alkaline phosphatase. The adhesion proteins include osteopontin, osteonectin, fibronectin, thrombospondin, and sialoproteins.[2]

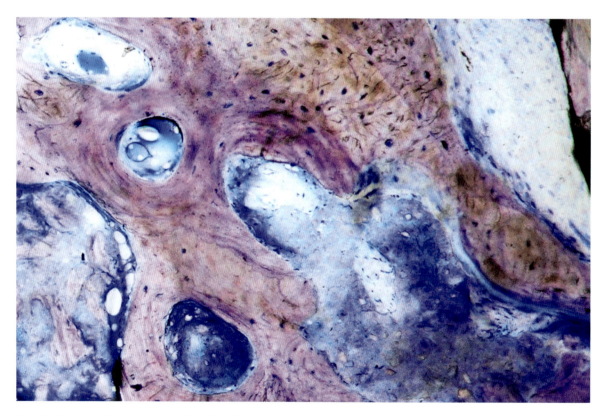

Fig 3 Spongy alveolar bone. The thick bone trabeculae are surrounded by matrix of varying degrees of mineralization that is undergoing remodeling. Areas of newly deposited osteoid matrix are depicted in blue, areas of mineralizing tissue (woven bone) are seen in purple, and areas with a high degree of mineralization are shown in brown. Toluidine blue and Pyronin yellow staining; ×400 magnification.

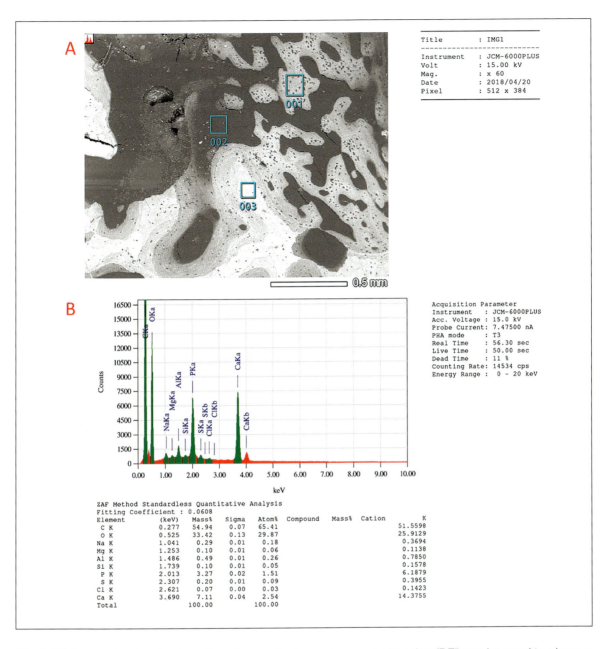

Fig 4 (A) *A scanning in a backscattered scan electron microscope imaging (BEI) can be used to observe the density of the matrix based on the atomic number of the elements it is composed of in different shades of gray. The lighter area is more mineralized than the darker one. (B) In relation to image a, the areas in the blue box can be further analyzed by defining the element analysis using a detector to identify the characteristic X-rays of each element present in the sample under analysis. This information is then processed by dedicated software that generates the spectrum and indicates the percentage mass of the most-represented chemical elements. Certain elements can then be analyzed to make comparisons between samples, for example, by calculating the ratio between the amount of calcium and phosphate contained in different samples to better understand the degree of mineralization of regenerated tissue.*

Noncollagenous proteins

The role of noncollagenous proteins is still being studied, but they seem to be involved in the mineralization processes of bone tissue.

Phosphoproteins are proteins conjugated to phosphoric acid residues.

They have the characteristic of binding calcium and thus act as mineral nucleators.[3] Proteoglycans, on the other hand, inhibit calcification by masking sites on collagen fiber, which reduces chemical interactions and limits the sequestration of calcium ions and calcium phosphate complexes.[4]

Osteocalcin is produced by osteoblasts and is the most abundant noncollagenous protein in bone, accounting for about 20% of the noncollagenous matrix proteins.[5,6] It contains three calcium-binding Gla (gamma-carboxyglutamic acid) residues and is dependent on vitamin K. Its physiologic role is to regulate mineralization by facilitating the formation of mineralized nodules.[7] Like alkaline phosphatase, osteocalcin is used clinically as a marker of osteoblastic activity, and serum osteocalcin is used as a marker of bone turnover.[8]

Adhesion proteins

Adhesion proteins are located on the cell surface and have the function of creating bonds with other cells and/or the ECM.

Osteopontin is a relatively abundant noncollagenous sialoprotein produced by osteoblasts. According to the literature, it functions as a chemoattractant for osteoclasts.

It binds with these osteoclasts thanks to the RGD (arginylglycylaspartic acid) sequence that increases intracellular calcium by activating the phospholipase C pathway in the osteoclast. Osteopontin also has binding sites for hydroxyapatite crystals. It is regulated by vitamin D, which promotes its secretion and therefore the formation of inorganic bone matrix.[2,9]

Osteonectin is an acidic glycoprotein that supports bone remodeling and maintains bone mass in vertebrates. It is synthesized by osteoclasts, as well as by fibroblasts, tendon cells, and odontoblasts. Osteonectin binds to collagen and hydroxyapatite and assists in the subsequent formation of the ECM and the promotion of the nucleation of mineral groups.[2,5]

Fibronectin is a ubiquitous cell adhesion protein produced by cells in the bone both locally and nonlocally. Nonlocal fibronectin is transported via the circulatory stream. Although not fully understood, fibronectin's function in bone seems to be coordinating the migration, interactions, and differentiation of osteoblast precursors.[10]

The role of thrombospondin in bone tissue is still unknown. This protein is known to have calcium-binding sites and the RGD sequence.[4]

Bone sialoprotein (BSP), like osteopontin, is a sialoprotein found exclusively in the skeleton. In addition to promoting cell adhesion by activating osteoclasts, it is thought to be a hydroxyapatite nucleator, although its sensitivity to vitamin D is still unknown.[6]

The cellular elements of bone

The cells that make up bone are osteoblasts, osteocytes, and osteoclasts.

Osteoblasts are the main cells responsible for bone formation. They synthesize the components of the extracellular organic matrix (especially collagen Type I, proteoglycans, and glycoproteins) and control matrix mineralization. Osteoblasts are round, mononucleated cells derived from osteoprogenitor cells residing in the periosteum and endosteum. They are located on bone surfaces that show active matrix deposition.

Osteoblasts can eventually differentiate into either lining cells or osteocytes. Osteoblast morphology varies in the active deposition phase, during which they present as either large cubic or tapered cells. In the inactive phase, they appear as thinned fusiform cells[1] **(Fig 5)**.

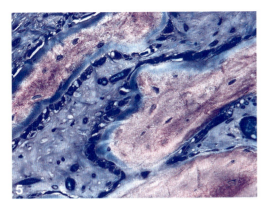 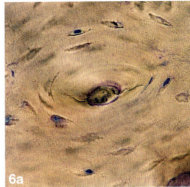 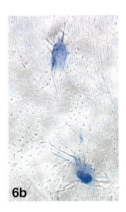

Fig 5 *Osteoblasts cords in the vicinity of newly formed bone trabeculae in an active deposition phase. Toluidine blue and Pyronin yellow staining; ×400 magnification.* *Fig 6* *Osteocytes lodged in osteocyte lacunae. (a) Several osteocytes can be seen residing in compact bone tissue with a high degree of mineralization. Toluidine blue and Pyronin yellow staining; ×600 magnification. (b) Two osteocytes characterized by cytoplasmic processes that reside in the osteocyte canaliculi. Toluidine blue and Pyronin yellow staining; ×1,000 magnification.*

Osteoblasts produce an enzyme called alkaline phosphatase, which is very important in the early stages of mineralization. Alkaline phosphatase is considered an early marker of osteogenesis because it is produced by differentiated osteoblasts in the first days of the bone matrix deposition process. In in vitro studies, the activity of this important marker is usually studied 7 and 14 days after the seeding of cells ready to deposit new mineralized matrix.[11]

Osteocytes are star-shaped cells that remain in the mineralized bone matrix during the matrix deposition phase, residing in the osteocyte lacunae. They are osteoblasts that have entered a state of quiescence, and once trapped in the already formed bone, they can participate in bone remodeling **(Fig 6a)**. They are unable to carry out mitotic division and remain inside the lacunae, where they renew and maintain the ECM by communicating with each other through cytoplasmic extensions that run through channels between the lacunae (osteocytic canaliculi)[1] **(Fig 6b)**.

Osteoclasts are very large, phagocytic, multinucleated cells of monocyte-macrophage lineage that can develop and adhere to the bone matrix and subsequently secrete lytic enzymes capable of degrading and breaking down the organic and mineral components of bone. The matrix degradation process results in the formation of specialized extracellular compartments known as Howship's lacunae **(Fig 7)**. One of the enzymes that osteoclasts produce is TRAP (tartrate-resistant acid phosphatase), which plays a very important role in many biologic processes, including collagen synthesis and degradation, macrophage recruitment, and the regulation of bone mineralization.

TRAP has been observed in the ECM at remodeling fronts, and in fact, it is customary to use anti-TRAP stain to identify osteoclasts in areas of bone undergoing resorption.[13]

The correct balance of osteoblastic deposition activity and osteoclastic resorption activity regulates bone remodeling by maintaining calcium-phosphate homeostasis and tissue morphology.[1,11] Osteocytes are mechanosensors that are capable of perceiving loads applied to the bone and subsequently coordinating bone remodeling by activating or inhibiting the activity of effector cells.[14] Thus, mechanical forces can induce changes in bone microarchitecture and density, which is of clinical relevance for the design of implant-supported restorations.[15,16]

Another characteristic of osteocytes is that they modify their biologic and biochemical activities according to homeostatic principles, secreting cytokines and growth factors that regulate tissue repair during fracture healing processes.[17] Osteocytes activate bone modeling and remodeling based on the need to adapt to tension and/or damage.[17]

Activation seems to depend on signaling resulting from forces imparted on the bone that radiate into the lacuna-canalicular system containing interstitial fluid.[17,18]

The alveolar bone has a faster remodeling rate at both cortical (minor changes) and trabecular (major changes) levels compared to other bones because it is subjected to continuous stimulation from various directions. The mandible typically exhibits continuous and rapid changes in the orientation, thickness, connectivity, and spacing of its trabeculae.[17]

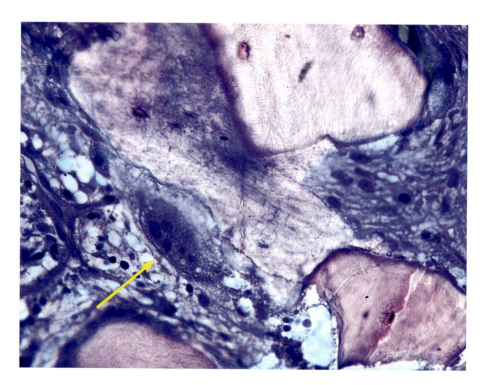

Fig 7 *An osteoclast in an active resorption process. The cell is lodged on the edge of a bony trabecula in a Howship's lacuna that has just been formed by lytic enzymes released to degrade the bone matrix. Toluidine blue and Pyronin yellow staining; ×600 magnification.*

MICROSCOPIC STRUCTURE OF THE ALVEOLAR BONE

The alveolar bone is the part of the alveolar process that rests on top of the basal component of the mandible and maxilla. It shares a close relationship with the dentition, and its shape, position, and volume change in response to the functional life of the teeth. In both the maxilla and mandible, the diploe structure involves two compact bone plates that enclose a spongy or trabecular part **(Fig 8)**. Two parts of the alveolar bone can be distinguished: the alveolar bone "proper," which comprises the wall of the alveolus where the teeth roots are housed, and the "supporting" alveolar bone, which surrounds the proper alveolar bone. The inner surface of the alveolus consists of a layer of specialized compact bone tissue called bundle bone. Bundle bone is characterized by the insertion of periodontal ligament (PDL) collagen fibers, known as Sharpey's fibers. Radiographically, this layer presents as a radiopaque band about 1.2 mm thick, and it is clinically referred to as lamina dura. At the crestal level, the lamina dura continues with the compact lingual bone plate, whereas on the vestibular side, the bundle bone forms the bone crest in continuity with the vestibular compact bone plate more apically.

The trabecular pattern of the alveolar bone varies according to location within the arches. In portions of the arches that undergo less masticatory load, the trabecular composition is thin and dense, whereas in areas subjected to more stress, trabeculae are thick and more widely spaced, arranged according to the direction of the forces.[19] The pattern of trabeculae in jaw bones differs from that

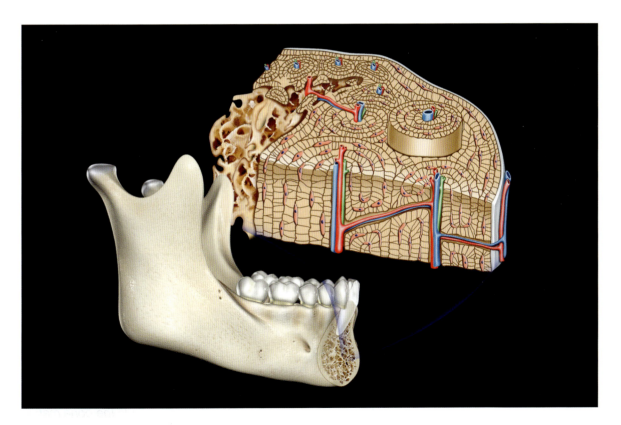

Fig 8 *Structure of the mandibular bone.*

in long bones, as found in micro CT studies.[20] In the femur, for example, the trabeculae of the bone resemble scattered rods in the medullary spaces, whereas in the alveolar bone, the trabeculae are characterized by a greater thickness and width, resulting in reduced medullary space. Histomorphometric analyses have also shown that mineral density, bone volume fractions, and trabecular thickness in the alveolar bone are also higher than in the femur.

Compared to the maxilla, the mandible appears to undergo more pronounced bone remodeling and has higher mineral density and better bone quality, which is understood by Lekholm and Zarb to be represented by the ratio of cortical to trabecular bone tissue.[21,22] Microstructural changes in the jaw bones can be caused by edentulism, changes in masticatory loading, hormonal conditions, and age. It has been observed that the mandible and anterior maxilla show microstructural changes that are more pronounced in patients of advanced age, resulting in bone that is predominantly cortical in composition. Furthermore, von Wowern and Stoltze showed that mandibular cortical porosity increases with age without interfering with trabecular bone mass, which was not found to correlate with aging.[23]

BONE SHAPING AND REMODELING

Once the bone is formed, the new mineralized tissue begins to be remodeled by resorption and deposition processes. These phenomena of resorption and tissue matrix deposition occur simultaneously and lead to the cyclic replacement and regeneration of the biologic components of the tissue, according to systemic and local functional needs (dental load and eruptive phenomena). The combination of these processes allows the bone to change morphologically in accordance with physical stimulations and to reach configurations that are appropriate for supporting the loads placed on

it.[24] The metabolic mediation conducted by bone tissue (ie, functioning as a calcium and phosphate reserve) is controlled and connected to remodeling phenomena, as well as being driven by hormonal mechanisms.

Bone modeling is considered a distinct process from bone remodeling.[19] Bone modeling is the process of modifying/constituting the initial bone architecture. It has been suggested that external stimuli (ie, load variations) on the bone tissue trigger neoapposition phenomena and subsequent bone modeling in response to changes in the support required from the bone segment. Remodeling, on the other hand, refers to a change that occurs within the mineralized bone structure, without concomitant change in the architecture of the segment in which it occurs. Bone remodeling includes bone matrix renewal processes, changes to meet metabolic demands, and the replacement of immature primary bone with lamellar bone during bone formation. Bone remodeling is made possible by the constant presence of bone multicellular units (BMUs) in the tissue. A BMU is composed of an osteoclastic front on the bone surface undergoing resorption (ie, the resorption front), a compartment containing blood vessels and pericytes, and a layer of osteoblasts at the newly formed organic matrix (ie, the apposition front). Pericytes are undifferentiated mesenchymal cells that partially surround the endothelial cells of capillaries and venules. They can differentiate into osteoblasts given the appropriate stimulation by osteoinductive and/or osteopromoting growth factors.

Cutting cones are the main mechanism of bone modeling in the healing phase, particularly following fractures. They are characterized by an osteoclastic resorption front followed by a string of osteoblastic cells that lay down new bone matrix **(Fig 9a)**. The cutting cone passes through the fracture site, which is healed by the formation of numerous secondary osteons **(Figs 9b to 9d)**. This process is very slow and can take months or years.[25,26]

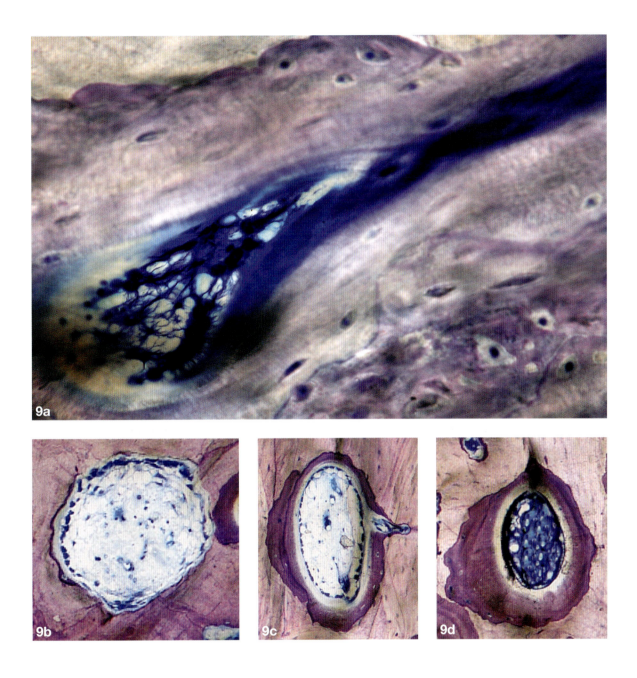

Fig 9 (a) *A cutting cone. The process of bone resorption sometimes takes place in channels dug longitudinally into the tissue, which results in the formation of cavities called cutting cones. Toluidine blue and Pyronin yellow staining; ×600 magnification. (b to d) Stages of new matrix deposition by the osteoblast chordae until the formation of a secondary osteon. Toluidine blue and Pyronin yellow staining; ×400 magnification.*

Recent studies[16] describe the viscoelastic properties of bone that vary as the tension to which the tissue is subjected changes. Following an increase in the load affecting it, Young's modulus of elasticity increases, expressing the propensity of a tissue to lengthen or shorten as a result of a loading force. To renew itself, repair itself, and adapt to continuous functional demands, stimuli, and loads, bone tissue undergoes constant remodeling, which enables it to preserve its strength or increase its rigidity.

Biochemical aspects

The remodeling process is cyclic and involves a complex series of phenomena that are finely regulated by systemic factors, such as hormones involved in both the regulation of skeletal growth and calcium metabolism (parathormone [PTH], growth hormone, leptin, and calcitonin) and local factors, such as cytokines, prostaglandins, and certain proteins, that are responsible for the interaction between osteoblasts and osteoclasts.[12,27,28] Communication between osteoblasts and osteoclasts can occur directly via cell-to-cell contacts through ligand-receptor interactions or indirectly via the secretion of soluble molecules such as cytokines, hormones, and growth factors.[27–29]

Biomechanical aspects

When microdamage accumulates in the interstitial bone tissue, microfractures present as discontinuities in the calcium-rich matrix, reflecting cracks and fractures in the mineral component that can evolve into a macrofracture due to continuous cyclic fatigue.[29] When microfractures occur at a slow rate, the bone has the opportunity to repair itself, a response that is referred to as targeted remodeling. Osteons can act as barriers to prevent the coalescence of microfractures and prevent breakage. In fact, dispersed microfractures have a higher energy absorption potential than coalescing ones. The mechanical behavior of compact bone is related to its hierarchical microstructure in terms of content, fiber direction, and the arrangement of osteons along the load axis. The more mineralized and less collagen-rich primary osteons develop more dispersed microfractures than secondary osteons derived from bone remodeling. Strength, energy-absorbing capacity, and modulus of elasticity appear to decrease with increasing percentage of the total bone surface occupied by osteons.[30]

There are many physiologic, pathologic, and pharmacologic systemic conditions that can affect cortical/trabecular thickness, mineralization, collagen content (bone tissue structure), and bone metabolism, thus modifying mechanical properties such as strength, rigidity, and fragility. With aging, bone trabeculae become thinner and are associated with significantly more highly mineralized trabeculae,[31] ultimately resulting in osteoporosis, which is characterized by reduced strength and increased bone fragility due to reduced osteoblastic activity, bone matrix formation, and mineralization.

FORMATION OF THE JAW BONES

Bone growth, function, and structure are biologically dependent on each other. The bone's growth program involves not only the bone tissue itself but also the soft tissues that cover it, such as muscles, the mucous membrane, and the vascular and nerve formations. The bones of the skull develop in relation to the central and peripheral nervous system. In fact, during development and growth, the dura mater regulates the sutures of the cranial vault and apparently also the synchondroses of the base, thanks to the continuous expression of regulatory genes.

When the encephalon expands, it compresses the dura mater, which comes into direct contact with the cranial bones, thus stimulating the pathway of signals for the development of the skull.

The bones of the splanchnocranium and some of the neurocranium originate from the embryonic connective tissue derived from the neural crests, while the remainder of the neurocranium originates from the mesodermal connective tissue of the somites in analogy to that of the long bones.

The embryonic derivation of the jaw bones is different than that of most bones of the skeleton, and the results are reflected in differing osteoclastogenic potentials, meaning the bones are affected differently by diseases of the skeletal system.[32] For example, the alteration of physiologic microarchitecture and systemic bone loss observed in osteoporotic experimental animals are site-specific, with the reduction in bone mineral density generally being lower in the cranial bones and jaw bones than in the long bones, lumbar vertebrae, and ileum.[33]

The mode of ossification of the different skeletal components of the skull also has some specificities. Bone formation in the skull occurs via two main mechanisms: intramembranous (direct) ossification and endochondral (indirect) ossification.

Intramembranous ossification leads to bone formation without intermediate processes. This is accomplished through deposition from primitive connective tissue mesenchymal cells with rich vascular support at the site of future bone deposition. After cellular differentiation, osteoblasts initiate the interstitial deposition of collagen-rich osteoid matrix, developing ossification centers characterized by small bundles of packed collagen fibers that gradually mineralize through the deposition of calcium salts in the intercellular spaces and adjacent osteoid **(Fig 10)**. All the flat bones that make up the vault of the skull and most of the maxillofacial complex are membranous bones, as are some parts of the bones that make up the base of the skull, for example, the squama and tympanic portion of the temporal bone. Intramembranous ossification genetically predetermines which bones will be subject to growth by traction during embryonic development.

A particular form of direct ossification is mantle ossification, typical of the mandible, which is characterized by the direct deposition of bone within the mesenchyme surrounding Meckel's cartilage (first pharyngeal arch) as a biomechanical scaffold. The body of the mandible and most of the mandibular ramus originate from this type of ossification. The remaining part of the ramus, including the condylar and coronoid processes, develop from secondary cartilage cores that undergo indirect ossification. At the end of ossification, Meckel's cartilage is completely resorbed, while the connective tissue that interposes at the median level between the two cartilages (right and left) differentiates into chin fibrocartilage (symphysis).[34,35]

Endochondral (indirect) ossification leads to the formation of bone from a primitive hyaline cartilage model. From the cartilaginous template, there is cell hypertrophy leading to calcification of the intracellular matrix, with subsequent degeneration of the chondrocytes. The cartilage matrix is then invaded by blood vessels and osteoblasts, reabsorbed, and replaced with osteoid **(Fig 11)**. This mechanism is responsible for the formation of all the long bones of the skeleton and can also be found in some bones of the skull base, such as the occipital bone (not intraparietal), temporal bone (petrous and mastoid portions, hearing ossicles, and styloid process), sphenoid (body, small wings, large wings), and ethmoid.

The endochondral ossification genetically predetermines bones that will be subject to high pressures during embryonic development.[36]

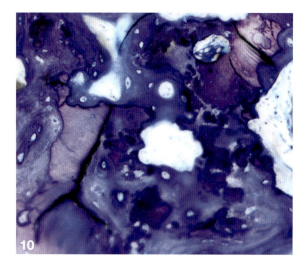 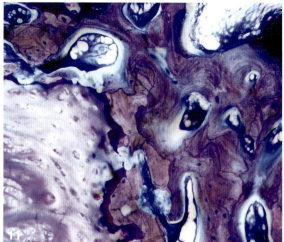

Fig 10 *Process of intramembranous bone formation. In purple, mineralized islands surrounded by connective matrix are observed. Toluidine blue and Pyronin yellow staining; ×400 magnification.* **Fig 11** *Process of endochondral bone formation. Cartilage can be seen on the left of the image, which is progressively replaced by bone tissue (right). Toluidine blue and Pyronin yellow staining; ×400 magnification.*

REFERENCES

1. Dellavia C, Gagliano N, Orlando F. I colori e le forme della ricerca in odontoiatria. Atlante di istologia orale. Quintessenza Italy, 2011.

2. Al-Qtaitat AI, Aldalaen SM. A review of noncollagenous proteins; their role in bone. Am J Life Sci 2014;2: 351–355.

3. Mundy GR. Bone Remodeling and its Disorders. Martin Dunitz, 1995.

4. Nudelman F, Lausch AJ, Sommerdijk NAJM, Sone ED. In vitro models of collagen biomineralization. J Struct Biol 2013;183:258–269.

5. George A, Veis A. Phosphorylated proteins and control over apatite nucleation, crystal growth, and inhibition. Chem Rev 2008;108:4670–4693.

6. Massaro EJ, Rogers JM. The Skeleton: Biochemical, Genetic, and Molecular Interactions in Development and Homeostasis. Humana Press, 2004.

7. Nakamura A, Dohi Y, Akahane M, et al. Osteocalcin secretion as an early marker of in vitro osteogenic differentiation of rat mesenchymal stem cells. Tissue Eng Part C Methods 2009;15:169–180.

8. Wanby P, Nobin R, Von S-P, Brudin L, Carlsson M. Serum levels of the bone turnover markers dickkopf-1, sclerostin, osteoprotegerin, osteopontin, osteocalcin and 25-hydroxyvitamin D in Swedish geriatric patients aged 75 years or older with a fresh hip fracture and in healthy controls. J Endocrinol Invest 2016;39: 855–863.

9. Carmagnola D, Botticelli D, Canciani E, Rossi F, Milani S, Dellavia C. Histologic and immunohistochemical description of early healing at marginal defects around implants. Int J Periodontics Restorative Dent 2014;34:e50–e57.

10. Tang CH, Yang RS, Huang TH, Liu SH, Fu WM. Enhancement of fibronectin fibrillogenesis and bone formation by basic fibroblast growth factor via protein kinase C-dependent pathway in rat osteoblasts. Mol Pharmacol 2004;66:440–449.

11. Varoni E, Canciani E, Palazzo B, et al. Effect of Poly-L-Lysine coating on titanium osseointegration: From characterization to in vivo studies. J Oral Implantol 2015;41:626–631.

12. Canciani E, Dellavia C, Marazzi MG, et al. RNA isolation from alveolar bone and gene expression analysis of RANK, RANKL and OPG: A new tool to monitor bone remodeling and healing in different bone substitutes used for prosthetic rehabilitation. Arch Oral Biol 2017;80:56–61.

13. Hayman AR. Tartrate-resistant acid phosphatase (TRAP) and the osteoclast/immune cell dichotomy. Autoimmunity 2008;41:218–223.

14. Klein-Nulend J, van Oers RF, Bakker AD, Bacabac RG. Nitric oxide signaling in mechanical adaptation of bone. Osteoporos Int 2014;25:1427–1437.

15. Frost HM. A 2003 update of bone physiology and Wolff's Law for clinicians. Angle Orthod 2004;74:3–15.

16. Berglundh T, Abrahamsson I, Lindhe J. Bone reactions to longstanding functional load at implants: An experimental study in dogs. J Clin Periodontol 2005;32:925–932.

17. Pellegrini G, Toma M, Francetti L, Cavalli N, Carmagnola D, Dellavia C. Implant placement in sites with adverse anatomical and biomechanical conditions: Critical review. Dental Cadmos 2018;86;9–23.

18. Heino TJ, Kurata K, Higaki H, Väänänen HK. Evidence for the role of osteocytes in the initiation of targeted remodeling. Technol Health Care 2009;17:49–56.

19. Lindhe J, Lang NP, Karring T. Clinical Periodontology and Oral Implantology, ed 4. Blackwell, 2010.

20. Zhou S, Yang Y, Ha N, et al. The specific morphological features of alveolar bone. J Craniofac Surg 2018;29:1216–1219.

21. Lekholm U, Zarb G. Patient selection and preparation. In: Brånemark PI, Zarb G, Albrektsson T (eds). Tissue-Integrated Prostheses: Osseointegration in Clinical Dentistry. Quintessence, 1985:199–209.

22. Devlin H, Horner K, Ledgerton D. A comparison of maxillary and mandibular bone mineral densities. J Prosthet Dent. 1998;79:323–7.

23. von Wowern N, Stoltze K. Pattern of age related bone loss in mandibles. Scand J Dent Res 1980;88:134–146.

24. Hollinger JO, Srinivasan A, Alvarez-Urena P, et al. Bone tissue engineering: Growth factors and cytokines. Elsevier 2011;5:281–300.

25. Pazzaglia UE, Zarattini G, Giacomini D, Rodella L, Menti AM, Feltrin G. Morphometric analysis of the canal system of cortical bone: An experimental study in the rabbit femur carried out with standard histology and micro-CT. Anat Histol Embryol 2010;39:17–26.

26. Marsell R, Einhorn TA. The biology of fracture healing. Injury 2011;42:551–555.

27. Raisz LG. Physiology and pathophysiology of bone remodeling. Clin Chem 1999;45:1353–1358.

28. Matsuo K, Irie N. Osteoclast-osteoblast communication. Arch Biochem Biophys 2008;473:201–209.

29. Goldring SR. Inflammatory mediators as essential elements in bone remodeling. Calcif Tissue Int 2003;73:97–100.

30. Greenstein G, Cavallaro J, Tarnow D. Assessing bone's adaptive capacity around dental implants: A literature review. J Am Dent Assoc 2013;144:362–368.

31. Zhang W, Tekalur SA, Baumann M, McCabe LR. The effects of damage accumulation on the tensile strength and toughness of compact bovine bone. J Biomech 2013;46:964–972.

32. Koehne T, Vettorazzi E, Küsters N, et al. Trends in trabecular architecture and bone mineral density distribution in 152 individuals aged 30-90 years. Bone 2014;66:31–38.

33. Chaichanasakul T, Kang B, Bezouglaia O, Aghaloo TL, Tetradis S. Diverse osteoclastogenesis of bone marrow from mandible versus long bone. J Periodontol 2014;85:829–836.

34. Liu XL, Li CL, Lu WW, Cai WX, Zheng LW. Skeletal site-specific response to ovariectomy in a rat model: Change in bone density and microarchitecture. Clin Oral Implants Res 2015;26:392–398.

35. Dellavia C. Compendio di anatomia oro-facciale per l'attività clinica odontostomatologica. Edises, 2016.

36. Mjör IA, Fejerkov O. Embriologia e istologia del cavo orale. Edi-Ermes, 1988.

SURGICAL ANATOMY OF THE MAXILLA AND MANDIBLE

CHAPTER 2

Edited by Filippo Fontana and Roberto Pistilli

INTRODUCTION

The purpose of this chapter is to provide clear and concise information on the main anatomical structures of interest to the oral surgeon.

The anatomical analysis is organized with the oral cavity divided into four areas: the mandibular symphysis, the posterior mandible (mandibular body), the anterior maxilla, and the posterior maxilla. Each area is further subdivided into the lingual aspect, the bone plane, and the buccal aspect.

This subdivision allows for easy and immediate identification of the relevant anatomical structures in each area where surgery is performed.

CHIN SYMPHYSIS AND INTRAFORAMINAL AREA

The mandibular symphysis is the portion of the mandible that lies between the two mental foramina. It is a strategically significant area because it is the site of many implant-supported restorations. This area encompasses several anatomical structures.

Buccal aspect

Mental nerve

The mental nerve is an anatomical structure of great significance for oral surgeons because many surgical procedures are performed in its proximity.

Successful implant therapy and the prevention of surgical complications depend on a thorough knowledge of the topographic anatomy of the jaw bones and surrounding anatomical structures.

Massimo Simion

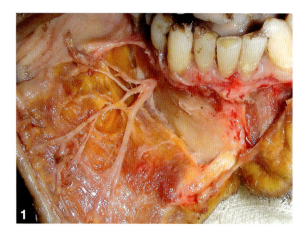 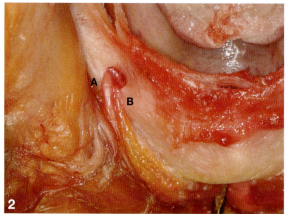

Fig 1 *Course and branches of the neurovascular bundle and the mental artery from the mental foramen to the submucosa of the lip.* *Fig 2* *Evidence of the mental foramen in the body of the mandible, where the neurovascular complex of the same name emerges. A: mental nerve; B: mental artery.*

Together with the incisive nerve, it is one of the terminal branches of the inferior alveolar nerve. It exits the body of the mandible through the mental foramen and branches out into the submucosa of the lower lip. It normally divides into three branches. One branch turns forward and downward to innervate the skin of the chin, and the other two turn anteriorly and upward to innervate the skin and mucosa of the lower lip and the mucosa of the inferior alveolar surface **(Fig 1)**.

Mental artery

The mental artery is the most voluminous of the terminal branches of the inferior alveolar artery. It emerges from the bony compartment at the level of the mental foramen to perfuse the soft tissues of the chin and lower lip. It anastomoses with branches of the inferior labial artery.

Mental foramen

The mental foramen is an opening in the mandibular canal at the lateral surface of the body of the mandible from which the mental neurovascular bundle emerges **(Fig 2)**. The mental foramen is frequently located between the first and second premolars or sometimes even inferior to the second premolar. On average, it lies at the midpoint between the inferior border of the mandible and the upper alveolar margin. It is important to note that the mandibular canal does not reach the mental foramen perpendicularly. It frequently turns externally upward and backward, forming a sort of knee bend. It is very important to know this anatomical feature to avoid damaging the neurovascular bundle. In edentulous patients, the mental foramen becomes more superficial occlusally with advancing bone atrophy. Radiographic and clinical identification of the mental foramen is fundamental in all oral surgical procedures.

Bone plane

Incisive nerve

The incisive nerve is one of the two terminal branches of the inferior alveolar nerve. It forms at the level of the premolar region after the other terminal branch (the mental nerve) leaves the body of the mandible through the mental foramen. The incisive nerve is smaller than the mental nerve and runs inside the body of the mandibular symphysis. It supplies dental, interdental, and interalveolar branches to the mandibular anterior teeth and the

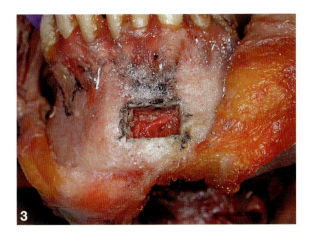

Fig 3 *The incisive nerve and its artery in the body of the mandible running in the direction of the mandibular symphysis.*

corresponding periodontal complex. Clinical and radiographic identification of the incisive nerve is challenging.

Incisive artery

The incisive artery follows the course of the incisive nerve to form a neurovascular bundle. It is the terminal, smaller branch of the bifurcation of the inferior alveolar artery. It runs inside the mandible until reaching the midline and anastomosing with the contralateral artery **(Fig 3)**.

Lingual aspect

Sublingual artery

At the lingual aspect of the mandibular symphysis, it is important to check for the presence of terminal perforating branches of the anastomosis between the sublingual artery (a branch of the lingual artery) and the submental arteries (branches of the facial artery). Careful analysis with CBCT can be used to provide precise indications of the presence and location of these vessels. In the event of incorrect implant site preparation with perforation of the lingual cortical, a lesion of this anastomosis can occur with consequent and potentially dangerous extraosseous bleeding **(Fig 4)**.

MANDIBULAR BODY

The posterior mandible is an area of enormous anatomical interest to the dentist and oral surgeon because it is the site of numerous surgical procedures, ranging from simple tooth extraction to extensive bone regeneration for implant placement purposes. This area is characterized by the presence of many structures on its lingual and buccal aspects, as well as structures inside the body of the bone.

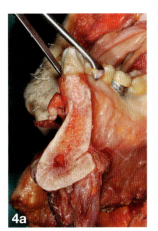
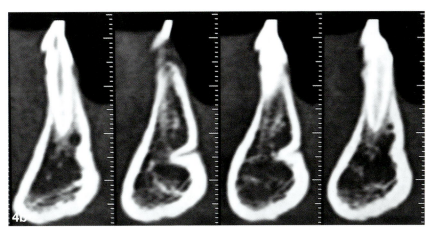

Fig 4 *Image and corresponding CT sections of a perforating branch from an anastomosis between the sublingual artery and submental artery at the lingual aspect of the mandibular symphysis.*

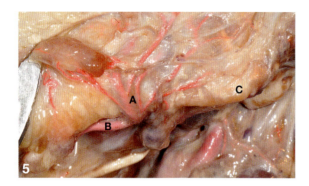 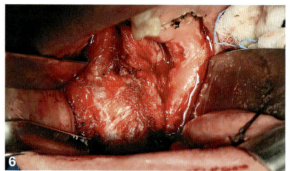

Fig 5 *A: facial artery; B: submental artery; C: angle of the mandible.* **Fig 6** *The buccal nerve running buccal to the third molar along the external oblique line.*

Buccal aspect

Facial artery

The facial artery is one of the anterior branches of the external carotid artery. It may be of significance for oral surgery in its course from the submandibular triangle to the lateral margin of the nose **(Fig 5)**. In fact, this artery reaches the inferior border of the mandible in front of the anterior limit of the masseter muscle to turn around the mandibular body and thus pass into the facial tissues in the direction of the labial commissure.

At the level of the mandibular molars, this vessel can be reached from the oral cavity by incising the buccal mucosa and the buccinator and passing through the underlying adipose tissue.

It is possible to damage the facial artery in the process of performing partial-thickness flap elevation. Therefore, whenever possible, it is important to perform a subperiosteal elevation and prevent the flap from rotating and protect it from sharp instruments.

Buccal nerve

The buccal nerve is a sensory nerve that is distributed to the mucosal surface of the cheek, the gingiva of the mandibular molars, and the skin near the labial commissure. It is a branch of the mandibular nerve, which itself is the third branch of the

trigeminal nerve, and crosses the submucosa at the level of the retromolar trigone **(Fig 6)**.

Bone plane

Inferior alveolar nerve

Many oral surgical procedures are performed in proximity to the inferior alveolar nerve. It is the intermediate branch of the mandibular nerve and runs lateral to the lingual nerve between the pterygoid muscles. It is a sensory nerve that enters the body of the mandible through the mandibular foramen at the level of the lingula (ie, Spix spine) and then runs entirely inside the mandibular canal to end in its two final branches, the incisive and mental nerves. Before entering the body of the mandible, the inferior alveolar nerve first emits the lingual nerve and then the mylohyoid nerve. During its course through the canal, the inferior alveolar nerve emits the lower dental branches destined for the posterior mandibular teeth and the corresponding periodontal complex.

Inferior alveolar artery

The inferior alveolar artery is a branch of the first (mandibular) segment of the maxillary artery. It follows the same course as the nerve of the same name in the mandibular canal, issuing dental and alveolar branches.

Mandibular canal

The endosseous mandibular canal represents a very useful radiographic marker for dentists and oral surgeons because it can be used to identify the course of the inferior alveolar neurovascular (plexus) bundle. It begins at the mandibular foramen, descends downward along the ramus, and then folds forward with a horizontal course inferior to the roots of the mandibular molars. At the premolar region, it divides into two canals: the narrower incisive canal, which continues the course of the mandibular canal, and the mental canal, which bends laterally upward and backward to open into the mental foramen **(Fig 7)**.

Lingual aspect

Mylohyoid nerve

The mylohyoid nerve is separated from the inferior alveolar nerve before its entry into the body of the mandible. It turns downward, running into the mylohyoid line of the mandible, and then heads toward the floor of the oral cavity **(Fig 8)**. It sends branches to the mylohyoid muscle and the anterior belly of the digastric muscle. In 10% of cases, a sensory branch of this nerve penetrates the mandible at the level of the mandibular symphysis and participates in the innervation of the mandibular incisors. This anatomical variant can be very important for providing local anesthesia.

Lingual nerve

The lingual nerve is a sensory branch of the mandibular nerve that carries fibers for general sensitivity (touch, pressure, pain, temperature) to the tongue and sublingual region. On its way, it also receives visceral effector and gustatory fibers of the facial nerve via the tympanic cord. It initially runs close to the inferior alveolar nerve and then passes more medial and anterior, running lateral to the internal pterygoid muscle. In the posterior part of the oral cavity, at the lingual surface of the mandible at the level of the second and third molars, this nerve can be very superficial, just below the mucosa, which is of importance when performing surgery in the retromolar space, especially when extracting mandibular third molars **(Fig 9)**.

Mylohyoid artery

The mylohyoid artery originates from the inferior alveolar artery before it enters the mandibular canal. It follows the course of the mylohyoid nerve along the mylohyoid line **(Fig 10)**. The mylohyoid artery can be lacerated if implant site preparations

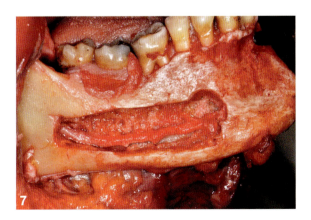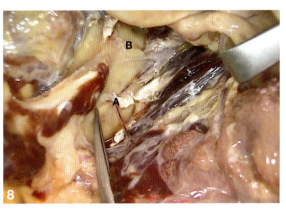

Fig 7 *Evidence of the mandibular canal and the course of the inferior alveolar nerve bundle.* **Fig 8** *Course of the mylohyoid nerve on the lingual aspect of the mandibular body anterior to the mandibular lingula. A: mylohyoid nerve; B: mandibular lingula.*

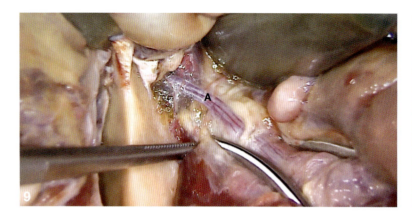
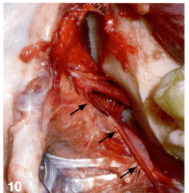
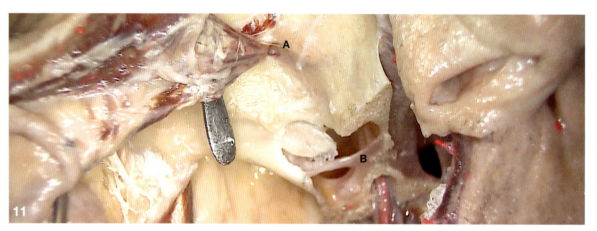

Fig 9 *Course of the lingual nerve near the body of the mandible at the level of the molars. A: lingual nerve.* Fig 10 *Origin and course of the mylohyoid artery on the lingual aspect of the mandible.* Fig 11 *The infraorbital neurovascular bundle emerging from the homonymous foramen and the descending palatine artery. A: infraorbital neurovascular bundle; B: descending palatine artery.*

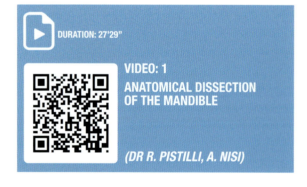

DURATION: 27'29"

VIDEO: 1
ANATOMICAL DISSECTION
OF THE MANDIBLE

(DR R. PISTILLI, A. NISI)

puncture the lingual cortical, which can result in significant bleeding. Special attention must be given to the location of the mylohyoid artery in patients where the body of the mandible presents with an undercut at the level of the molars. The anatomical situation must be identified during surgical planning, both by palpating the lingual surface of the mandible and by performing a CBCT examination.

ANTERIOR MAXILLA

The anterior maxilla is delimited by the maxillary canines and is the site of many dental surgeries, many of which aim to improve esthetics.

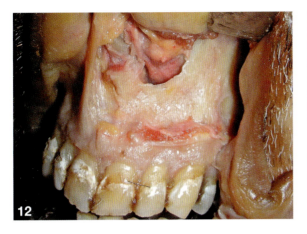 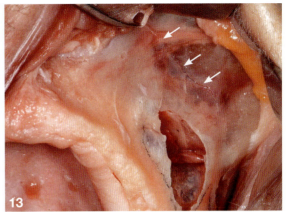

Fig 12 *Pyriform aperture at the level of the anterior maxilla.* ***Fig 13*** *Course of the canalis sinuosus.*

Buccal aspect

Infraorbital nerve

The infraorbital nerve is the intermediate branch of the maxillary nerve, which is the second branch of the trigeminal nerve. It enters the oral cavity through the infraorbital foramen before fanning out into its terminal segments. Its branches innervate a very large area that encompasses the lower eyelid, the wing of the nose and nasal pyramid, and the mucosa and skin of the upper lip. In its bony course, it also emits alveolar branches directed to the maxillary teeth and the corresponding periodontium **(Fig 11)**.

Infraorbital foramen

The infraorbital foramen is the opening of the infraorbital canal and is located approximately 5 to 8 mm inferior to the midpoint of the inferior orbital rim and 4 to 5 mm medial to a vertical line passing through the center of the pupil. It is the exit point of the infraorbital neurovascular bundle. The infraorbital foramen serves as an anatomical landmark of clinical relevance in procedures involving extensive bone regeneration or the insertion of zygomatic implants, as well as when performing extractions or the enucleation of cystic lesions in nearby teeth.

Bone plane

Nasal floor

The nasal cavities are located superior to the anterior maxilla.

The anterior portion of the nasal floor consists of the maxillary palatine process, which is crossed at the midline by the incisive or nasopalatine canal. Especially in cases of extensive resorption of the anterior superior maxilla, it is possible to identify the pyriform aperture (ie, the common anterior orifice of the nasal cavities) by elevating the vestibular flap, which will give the perception that the nasal floor is inferior to the pyriform aperture **(Fig 12)**.

Canalis sinuosus

The canalis sinuosus is a neurovascular canal branching from the infraorbital canal. The anterior alveolar nerve runs through the canalis sinuosus, directed mesially in the canine region of the anterior maxilla.

The canalis sinuosus runs between the nasal cavity and the anterior margin of the sinus cavity. If this canal is disturbed during an implant placement procedure, discomfort and/or pain may result in the anterior maxilla **(Fig 13)**.

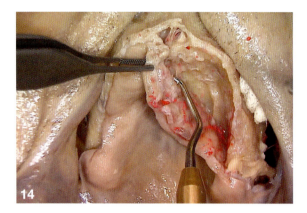
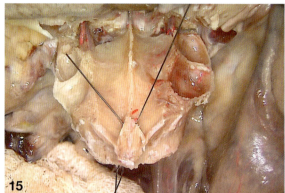
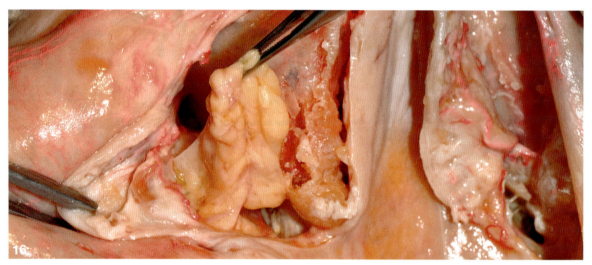

Fig 14 *The nasopalatine nerve emergence from the anterior palatine foramen.* **Fig 15** *The incisive canal at the level of the anterior maxilla is highlighted by the insertion of a wire.* **Fig 16** *Bichat's fat pad in the vestibular flap.*

Palatal aspect

Nasopalatine nerve

The nasopalatine nerve (Scarpa's nerve) is a nerve trunk that originates from the pterygopalatine nerve, which is an internal branch of the maxillary nerve (the second branch of the trigeminal nerve) **(Fig 14)**. The nasopalatine nerve is a particularly long medial branch that runs along the nasal septum to enter the buccal cavity palatal to the maxillary incisors via the incisive canal. It innervates a small area of the anterior palatine mucosa. It is important to identify this nerve during the surgical

phase, though injury to the nerve does not pose problems for the patient. In some cases, intentional resection of this structure is performed for better passivation of the palatal flap.

Anterior palatal foramen

The anterior palatal foramen is the opening of the incisive canal at the level of the anterior maxilla **(Fig 15)** through which the nasopalatine vascular bundle reaches the buccal cavity. It is located on the midline posterior to the maxillary central incisors. In the case of advanced anterior maxillary atrophy, this foramen can be emptied of its neurovascular component and filled in for the purpose of bone regeneration.

POSTERIOR MAXILLA

The posterior maxilla encompasses the entire area posterior to the canines up to the pterygopalatine fossae. It is affected by several neighboring anatomical structures.

Vestibular aspect

Buccal fat bad
The buccal fat pad (Bichat's fat pad) is a collection of adipose tissue located in the cheek in the area of the maxillary molars. It lies in the space between the masseter and buccinator muscles and can be reached, either intentionally or accidentally, when incising the periosteum for the release of the vestibular flap **(Fig 16)**.

Bone plane

Maxillary sinus
The maxillary sinus is a structure of enormous clinical interest to dental implantologists, both as the upper limit for implant placement and in cases involving bone grafting. The maxillary sinus is the largest paranasal cavity and occupies a large part of the posterior maxillary body. It has a triangular pyramid shape. The base is the vertical lateral wall of the nasal cavity, and the apex is oriented in the direction of the zygomatic process. The roof or upper wall of the maxillary sinus forms the floor of the orbit, the posterior wall is the tuberosity of the maxilla, and the anterior wall is at the canine fossa. This antrum communicates with the nasal cavities via the semilunar hiatus, which is located near the roof of the sinus. The size and extension of this structure are very variable and influenced by several factors. After tooth loss, this structure may extend into the alveolar process. The maxillary sinus is lined on the inside with a bilaminar sinus membrane, also called Schneider's membrane, which is characterized by a ciliated epithelium.

Posterior superior alveolar artery
The posterior superior alveolar artery is a voluminous vessel that originates at the maxillary tuberosity. It is a branch of the maxillary segment of the maxillary artery. In its course, it emits many branches destined for the posterior superior dental elements. The terminal part of this artery supplies the buccal surface of the alveolar process. It is of clinical interest to implantologists not so much because of its area of origin, which is far from dental surgical procedures, but because it contributes to the formation of the alveolar antral artery, which can be injured during sinus elevation procedures.

Alveolo antral artery
The alveolar antral artery originates from the anastomosis of the posterior superior alveolar artery with branches of the infraorbital artery. It normally runs within the bony lateral sinus wall at variable heights that sometimes coincide with the sites chosen for the antrostomy during sinus floor elevation. The diameter of the alveolar antral artery is also very variable, and in some cases, its size is such that it represents a risk factor to be analyzed during the presurgical planning phase.
Lacerating this vessel can result in intraoperative hemorrhages, which although rarely severe, can complicate the operation by interfering with visibility and lead to the appearance of diffuse hematomas and potential pathologic syndromes like hemosinus **(Fig 17)**.

Pterygo-palatine fossa
The pterygopalatine fossa is an anatomical space posterior to the maxillary tuberosity that includes some important anatomical structures, including

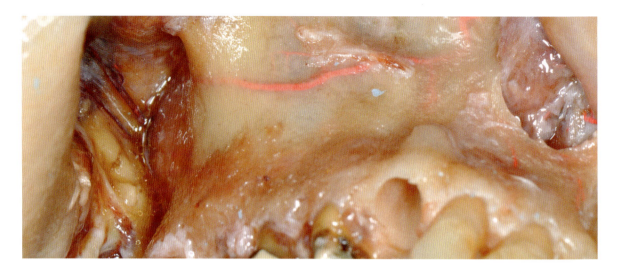

Fig 17 *Course of the alveolar antral artery in the lateral sinus wall.*

the maxillary nerve, the internal maxillary artery, and the pterygoid venous plexus. These anatomical structures are not usually affected by oral procedures, but they may be disturbed by careless anesthetic maneuvers or during tooth extraction.

Palatal aspect

Greater palatine foramen

The greater palatine foramen is the exit of the palatine canal at the level of the oral cavity through which the palatine neurovascular bundle passes. It is located at the level of the hard palate at the second and third maxillary molars, frequently at the transition between the horizontal plane of the hard palate and the vertical plane of the maxillary alveolar process.

It is important to identify this anatomical landmark to avoid injuring the neurovascular bundle during palatal flap elevation or free/pedicle graft harvesting procedures (**Fig 18**).

Greater palatine artery

The greater palatine artery is the main branch of the descending palatine artery, which is a branch of the maxillary artery. It enters the oral cavity through the greater palatine foramen.

Emerging from the latter, it turns anteriorly and runs within the submucosa of the palate, frequently resting inside a groove between the hard palate and the alveolar process. Its terminal branch reaches the incisive foramen to anastomose with the branches of the nasopalatine artery. It

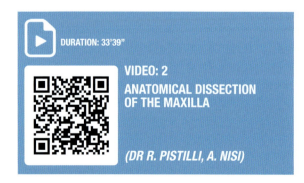

DURATION: 33'39"

VIDEO: 2
ANATOMICAL DISSECTION OF THE MAXILLA

(DR R. PISTILLI, A. NISI)

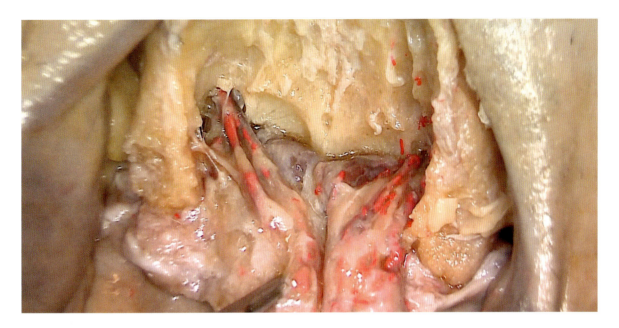

Fig 18 *The major palatine foramina and the emergence of the neurovascular bundle.*

vascularizes the mucosa of the hard palate and the gingiva on the palatal aspect.

Anterior palatine nerve

The anterior palatine nerve originates from the pterygopalatine nerve, which is a branch of the maxillary nerve. It runs in the palatine canal between the maxillary tuberosity and the pterygoid process of the sphenoid bone, exiting through the greater palatine foramen to enter the palate. It follows the course of the greater palatine artery to innervate a large portion of the ipsilateral palate and the gingiva of the palatal aspect of the alveolar process.

RECOMMENDED READINGS

Du Brul LE. Anatomia Orale di Sicher. Milano: Edi Ermes, 1982.

Netter FH. Atlante di anatomia umana. Milano: Edra, 1989.

Pistilli R, Felice P. Anatomia e chirurgia del cavo orale - Mandibola e Pavimento Orale. Pescara: Editalia Medica, 2018.

BIOLOGIC FOUNDATIONS OF OSSEOINTEGRATION

CHAPTER 3

Edited by Massimo Simion

INTRODUCTION

It all started in the early 1960s. In those days, implantology was considered the black sheep of dentistry. Many so-called "implantologists" were self-taught practitioners who improvised and used implants made without the slightest quality control, causing major disasters for unsuspecting patients who underwent treatment. In none of the world's universities did implantology constitute a teaching subject, and clinicians who practiced it were often ashamed of it and did not talk about it with their colleagues. In the early 1950s, Professor Per Ingvar Brånemark worked as an orthopedist at Lund University in Sweden, performing in vivo studies on the physiology and microcirculation of bone tissue.[1] To perform these studies, he invented titanium chambers shaped like hollow screws **(Figs 1 and 2)**.

These were implanted in the diaphyses of rabbit long bones.[2] A microscope was placed at the upper end of the chamber with a light at the lower end to observe the behavior of vital, regenerating bone tissue subjected to various physical and chemical stimuli.

In the research protocol, the titanium chambers were to be removed after a few months to be reused in other animals. It was discovered, however, that the rabbits' bones had contracted such an intimate relationship with the titanium chambers

As with histology, in-depth knowledge of the biologic phenomena underlying bone regeneration and osseointegration is indispensable for performing high-level clinical work. By complementing natural biologic processes, we increase success rates; by counteracting them, we create disasters.

Massimo Simion

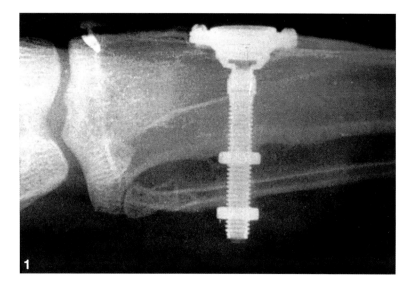 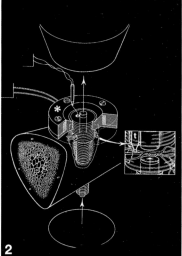

Fig 1 *Radiograph showing the titanium chamber that Brånemark and his team used in the 1960s for the in vivo study of blood microcirculation.* **Fig 2** *The microscopic apparatus for using the titanium chamber.*

that it was impossible to remove them. Brånemark termed this phenomenon osseointegration. From this chance discovery, the idea of creating a new implant system for the extra- and intraoral rehabilitation of patients was born.

In the early 1960s, Brånemark moved to the University of Gothenburg and began a series of clinical studies on the use of titanium for the construction of different implant forms, ranging from hollow-basket designs to threaded cylindric screws.

He treated a number of patients with various disabilities, as well as some volunteers from his circle of collaborators.[3]

After 15 years of studies and clinical experience, the scientific, biomechanical, and clinical aspects of osseointegrated implantology were well understood and defined.

But in the early days, Brånemark encountered skepticism from the scientific community, which was prejudiced due to the bad reputation of implantology. In 1965, the first longitudinal study with a large number of subjects on the treatment of completely edentulous patients began, and the concept of osseointegration was widely validated and universally accepted after a longitudinal study with data on a huge number of patients with follow-ups of up to 15 years was published in 1981.[4]

In 1982, George Zarb of the University of Toronto organized the Toronto Conference on Osseointegration in Clinical Dentistry.

From that moment, Brånemark's discovery not only radically transformed the image of implantology worldwide but, in fact, completely revolutionized the therapeutic choices and treatment plans for all of dentistry.

In the following years, the availability of a scientifically validated and reliable implant method made it possible to treat both partially and fully edentulous patients worldwide with high success rates.

DEFINITION OF OSSEOINTEGRATION

In 1967, Brånemark defined the concept of osseointegration as "direct and functional contact between vital bone and the surface of an implant."[5] This definition emphasizes the fundamental histologic characteristic peculiar to titanium and very few other metals of contracting extremely intimate relationships with bone tissue without the interposition of any other tissue, particularly connective or epithelial tissue (Fig 3).

This characteristic of titanium substantially differentiates osseointegrated implants from older-generation implants—so-called "osseofibrointegrated implants," which were characterized by the interposition of a thin layer of connective tissue between the bone and the implant surface.

The definition of osseointegration was later modified by Albrektsson and Sennerby,[6] who added the concept of "implant under load." This was in response to criticism that direct bone contact with the implant was a purely histologic finding and was objectifiable only before implants were subjected to functional loading. Critics believe that the connective tissue would still be interposed between the implant and the bone once loading took place.

The definitions of both Brånemark and Albrektsson have been validated by countless publications that have histologically demonstrated the stability of bone-to-implant (BIC) contact throughout the duration of implant function. The limitation of these definitions is that they are purely histologic and not applicable to everyday clinical practice, so in 1986 one of Brånemark's closest collaborators, Tomas Albrektsson, coined the clinical criteria for implant success,[7] which are discussed later in the chapter.

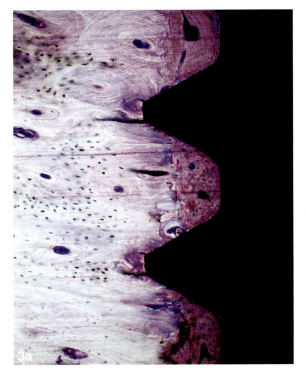 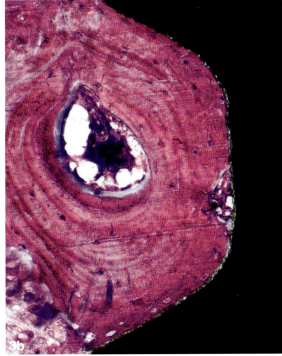

Fig 3 Histologic image of the interface between bone and an osseointegrated titanium implant. Under the light microscope, the direct contact between the bone and titanium is evident. There is no interposition of any other tissue. Toluidine blue/Pyronin G staining; ×10 magnification (a), ×40 magnification (b).

HISTOLOGIC AND FUNCTIONAL DIFFERENCES BETWEEN NATURAL TEETH AND OSSEOINTEGRATED IMPLANTS

(With Dr Eleonora Idotta)

Surrounding osseointegrated implants are the peri-implant tissues, represented by the mucosa and bone tissue, which differ substantially from the periodontal tissues at both the deep and superficial levels.

Periodontal and peri-implant soft tissues

The periodontium is a complex anatomical structure consisting of the gingiva, root cementum, periodontal ligament (PDL), and alveolar bone **(Fig 4a)**.
Proceeding from the free gingival margin in the apical direction is the keratinized gingiva on the outer aspect, divided into the free gingiva and attached gingiva, separated from the poorly keratinized alveolar mucosa by the mucogingival junction. On the inner aspect, facing the tooth, the gingiva is lined by the sulcular and junctional epithelium. More deeply, the gingival connective tissue is present.

The gingiva is connected to the dentition via the periodontal attachment, which in turn, consists of an epithelial attachment and a connective attachment. The epithelial attachment is mediated by hemidesmosomes, which make the junctional epithelium adhere to the tooth's enamel or root dentin.

The connective attachment is a more complex and efficient structure, isolating the deep periodontium from the oral environment, which is rich in bacteria and other pathogens. The connective attachment consists of a set of collagen fibers organized and oriented in different directions:

- **Vertical fibers** run from the attached gingiva to the marginal gingiva.
- **Longitudinal fibers** are arranged along the gingival connective tissue on the buccal and lingual sides.
- **Circular fibers are** located in the lamina propria of the gingiva and surround the collar of the tooth.
- **Transseptal fibers** are arranged above the interdental septum, crossing the interdental papillae and connecting adjacent teeth.
- **Dentogingival fibers** are arranged radially and run from the root cementum to the gingival lamina propria.
- **Dentoperiosteal fibers** run from the root cementum to the alveolar periosteum.

An inherent characteristic of transseptal, dentogingival, and dentoperiosteal fibers is that they are arranged perpendicular to the root surface and insert firmly into the root cementum by means of Sharpey's fibers. The peri-implant soft tissues constitute a simpler and less efficient structure for isolating deep peri-implant tissues from the contaminants of the oral cavity **(Fig 4b)**.

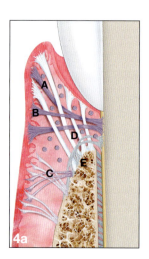
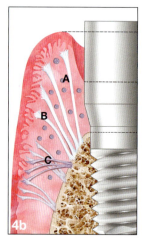

Fig 4 *Differences between the periodontal* (a) *and peri-implant attachment apparatus* (b). *A: vertical fibers; B: longitudinal fibers; C: circular fibers and transseptal fibers; D: dentogingival fibers; E: dentoperiosteal fibers.*

Although it is possible to observe a peri-implant sulcus marginally, a junctional epithelium, and an epithelial attachment mediated by hemidesmosomes, more deeply, the connective attachment differs substantially from the periodontal attachment. In fact, it is not really an attachment at all because the collagen fibers run parallel to the surface of the implant or prosthetic abutment and do not attach to the root cementum, which is absent. Thus, only vertical, longitudinal, and circular fibers are present. The absence of a true connective attachment makes the peri-implant marginal tissue less resistant to chemical, physical, and biologic insults, as well as to probing maneuvers.

At the level of the peri-implant mucosa, the distance between the free margin and the bone crest is an average of 3 to 4 mm, of which approximately 2 mm are occupied by the epithelial attachment and 1 to 1.5 mm are occupied by the connective attachment.

These measurements are similar to the periodontal biologic width.[8]

Around an implant, however, there is no standard biologic width as there would be around a natural tooth because the width of the implant's transmucosal path essentially depends on how far apically the implant is placed relative to the bone crest and the thickness of the crestal mucosa at the time of its placement.

Histologic studies in animals have shown that there are also differences between the composition of periodontal and peri-implant marginal tissues. The gingival connective tissue, which surrounds the natural tooth, is composed of two distinct compartments: the more superficial one adjacent to the junctional epithelium and the deeper one adjacent to the connective attachment. The connective tissue of the former consists of 63% collagen fibers, 16% fibroblasts, 7% vessels, 2% inflammatory cells, and 12% residual tissue. The second compartment consists of 76% collagen fibers, 5% fibroblasts, 3% vessels, 0.5% inflammatory cells, and 15% residual tissue. Peri-implant mucosa, on the other hand, presents a more uniform and more scar-like tissue structure, with more collagen fibers (87%), fewer fibroblasts (0.8%), few vessels (6%) and little residual tissue (4.8%) **(Fig 5)**.[8,9]

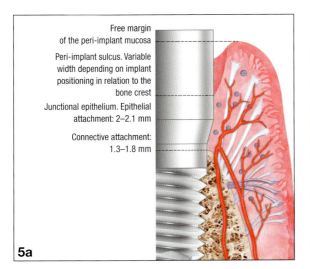
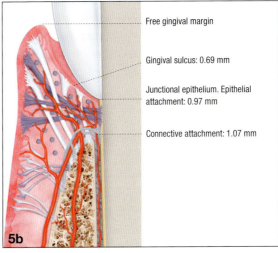

Fig 5 *Dimensional differences between peri-implant and periodontal soft tissue.* (a) *Implant.* (b) *Natural tooth. The vascularization at the level of the periodontal tissues is greater due to the vessels from the PDL.*

The epithelial and connective seals that serve as important barriers against the external environment around the implant are formed within a very short time (1–2 weeks) after the insertion of a transmucosal implant or the reopening of a submerged implant.

The epithelial seal is already mature after 6 to 8 weeks, and the connective seal is mature after 6 to 12 weeks.[8]

The outer surface of the implant mucosa is normally lined with keratinized epithelium, but it can also be lined with nonkeratinized epithelium, depending on the palatal/lingual position of the implant and whether masticatory mucosa is present on the edentulous ridge prior to implant insertion.

Numerous studies have demonstrated the importance of a sufficient band of keratinized mucosa to maintain the health of peri-implant tissues in the long term.[10]

Periodontal and peri-implant supporting bone tissue

The most significant anatomical differences between natural teeth and implants are found at the level of the supporting bone tissue. The relationship between the root of a natural tooth and the alveolar bone is mediated by a real articulation, a gomphosis.

The fibers of the PDL run in various directions, from perpendicular to oblique, from the root cementum to the alveolar bone, and are inserted via Sharpey's fibers.

This structural organization, together with the vascularization and fluid present in the periodontal space, makes it possible to evenly distribute and cushion the forces transmitted to the bone by the occlusal load during static and dynamic jaw activity and mastication.

Peri-implant bone tissue, on the other hand, does not have such a sophisticated structure.

The relationship between the implant and the bone is more akin to ankylosis, with direct contact between the bone and implant surfaces without the interposition of other tissues. In fact, there is a space at the interface between implant surfaces and bone.

This space has been measured with scanning electron microscopy (SEM) to be between 200 and 300 angstroms. This almost virtual space is occupied by only proteoglycans. In such a structure, occlusal forces are transmitted directly to the bone without any cushioning.

Additionally, whereas the PDLs of natural teeth lend them a certain degree of mobility depending on root length and the width of the periodontal space, osseointegrated implants are practically immobile.

PDLs give natural teeth the ability to migrate within the alveolar process.

When subjected to lateral forces, such as orthodontic forces or light premature occlusal contacts, a tooth is able to move in the direction of the force vector.

On the side where the root exerts pressure against the alveolar process, osteoclast activation leads to progressive bone resorption, while on the opposite side, the traction exerted by the PDL leads to osteoblast activation and consequent bone neoapposition.

Thus, teeth "escape" traumatic forces by progressively changing position. Without a PDL, implants are unable to move within the bone and, if subjected to occlusal trauma, can remain stable only so long as the peri-implant bone is able to withstand the magnitude of the traumatic forces. Beyond that limit, the bone fractures, and the implant loses osseointegration.

This characteristic of not being able to move within the alveolar process is taken advantage of in the orthodontic field by using implants as a maximum anchorage point to move entire sectors of natural teeth.

PERIODONTAL AND PERI-IMPLANT SUPPORTING BONE TISSUE

Brånemark's implant system was based on the use of threaded cylindric root form implants made of commercially pure titanium (CPT) with machined, almost smooth, untreated surfaces that were only decontaminated and sterilized. The surgical protocol involved the complete submersion of the implants under the mucosa for a period of 3 months in the mandible and 6 months in the maxilla to allow for osseointegration without loading or bacterial and/or epithelial interference.

The most widely used criteria for evaluating the success of an individual implant are still those proposed by Albrektsson et al in 1986:[7]

- The individually tested implant must be clinically immobile.
- No peri-implant bone radiolucency should be present upon radiographic examination.
- After the first year of prosthetic loading, marginal bone resorption must not exceed 0.2 mm per year.
- There must be no painful neurologic symptoms or infections.

These criteria define implant success rates, which are distinct and vary widely from the implant survival rates that are often reported in the literature. Conflating these terms can lead to enormous confusion. Implant survival rates account for all implants still present in the oral cavity, regardless of the presence of pathology of any kind, meaning that implants that might be expelled due to peri-implantitis a few days after the examination are included among the surviving implants.

The first longitudinal study on the long-term success of osseointegrated implants began in 1965 and was published in 1981 by Adell et al.[4] The study included 650 totally edentulous patients in whom 4,100 implants were placed and followed for a period of up to 15 years.

The first patients, treated at the beginning of the learning curve of the surgical technique and with follow-ups up to 10 years, showed success rates of 81% in the maxilla and 95% in the mandible, with corresponding values for the success of prosthetic restoration of 89 and 100%, respectively. The most recently treated group of patients, with follow-ups of only 5 years, showed significantly higher success rates: 95% in the maxilla and 99% in the mandible, with corresponding success rates for prosthetic restoration of 96% and 100%, respectively.

Adell's study represents a true milestone in the field of osseointegrated implantology and described the behavior of implants and contiguous bone tissue from the moment of insertion and throughout the subsequent years.

Adell et al noted that most implant failures occurred during the first year of prosthetic loading, leading to the conclusion that "a predictable prognosis can only be made for an individual patient after the first year of loading."

Thus, if an implant was still stable and asymptomatic after 1 year of function, it could be assumed that it would continue to function for the rest of the patient's life. This statement was valid for Brånemark implants with a machined surface, whereas the function of more modern, rough-surface implants can become impaired by infections of the peri-implant tissues even after a number of years.

The second observation made by Adell at all, which is still valid today, concerns the small (about 1.5 mm) cone of resorption that forms around the implant platform during the first year of prosthetic loading. In subsequent years and under normal conditions, resorption tends to slow, with an average progression of 0.1 mm per year **(Figs 6 and 7)**. Albrektsson and Zarb.[11] attributed this initial bone loss to the natural phenomenon of bone remodeling and the surgical trauma that results from the mucous membrane being dislodged.

Animal studies[12,13] instead attribute this initial loss to the presence of bacteria in the microgap that exists between an implant and its abutment. They have shown that by positioning this interface close to the bone crest, it is possible to amplify or minimize the amount of initial crestal bone loss. Platform switching, which entails using a prosthetic abutment with a smaller diameter than the implant platform, is now proposed by many manufacturers, and in some cases, it has been shown to minimize initial peri-implant bone resorption.[14] In daily clinical practice, small angular defects around the implant head are an occasional finding even in the presence of platform switching and other more modern prosthetic connection solutions. As of yet, there is no definitive explanation for the initial small resorption that occurs following implant placement, and it is likely that multiple factors influence its formation and extent. From the data in the literature with long-term studies, it does not appear that this initial resorption adversely affects the health or esthetics of implant rehabilitations.

Since publication of the study by Adell et al,[4] many other long-term studies have demonstrated the predictability of machined Brånemark implants, with evaluations of more than 6,000 implants with follow-ups between 10 and 32 years and implant survival rates between 91 and 100%. **Table 1** shows the results of studies with follow-ups of more than 10 years.[15–25]

The long-term studies published on machined surface implants have demonstrated a very low susceptibility of these implants to the modern plague of implantology—peri-implantitis. In fact, a very small percentage of implants were found

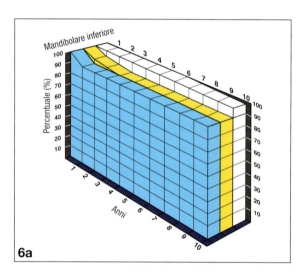

6a

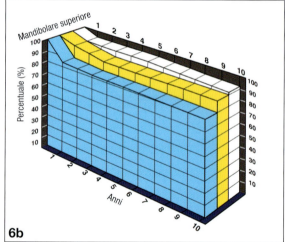

6b

Fig 6 *Marginal bone levels (y) over the years (x) in the study by Adell et al.[4] After an initial resorption of about 1.5 mm, the bone level tends to stabilize.* *Fig 7* *Periapical radiograph showing the small angular defect of approximately 1.5 mm that occurs after the first year of prosthetic loading in osseointegrated implants.*

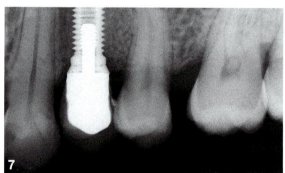

7

Table 1 Review of studies on machined Brånemark-type implants placed in native bone.

Study	Implant survival rate	No. of implants	No. of patients	Follow-up	Average MBL (SD)
Lindquist et al (1996)[15]	98.9%	273	47	15 y	1.2 mm
Ekelund et al (2003)[16]	98.9%	Same population of Lindquist et al (1996)[15]		20 y	1.6 (0.90) mm
Jemt and Johansson (2006)[17]	90.9%	450	76	15 y	2.1 (0.58) mm
Lekholm et al (2006)[18]	91%	69	27	20 y	1 mm
Jemt (2008)[19]	100%	47	38	15 y	N/A
Astrand et al (2008) [20]	99.2%	123	21	20 yi	2.33 mm
Jemt (2009)[21]	100%	41	35	10 y	0.26 (0.66) mm
Dierens et al (2013)[22]	91.5%	118	97	18.4 y	1.7 (0.88) mm
Bergenblock et al (2012)[23]	96.8%	53	40	18.4 y	0.9 (0.76) mm
Simion et al (2015)[24]	93.2%	59	29	12 y	0.78 (0.88) mm
Simion et al (2018)[25]	97.7%	382	105	20.7 y	1.9 (0.9) mm

MBL = Marginal bone loss; N/A: Not applicable.

to suffer from progressive bone loss. In a recent retrospective study, Simion et al[25] analyzed all available patients treated with machined implants between 1985 and 2001, with follow-ups between 13 and 32 years. A total of 105 partially or fully edentulous patients, 43 men and 62 women, ranging between 18 and 72 years old, were treated with a total of 382 machined implants placed in both the maxilla and mandible.

The cumulative survival rate was 97.7%, and the success rate was found to be 92.7%.

The average marginal bone loss was found to be 1.9 ± 0.9 mm, and only 7 (1.8%) of the 382 implants showed signs of peri-implantitis after a period of function between 13 and 32 years.

It should be considered, however, that the surgical protocol for placing most of the implants consisted of two surgical phases with periods of complete implant submersion for between 3 and 6 months.

THE PROCESS OF OSSEOINTEGRATION

According to Brånemark,[26] the life of an implant can be divided into three distinct and overlapping periods: the healing period, the remodeling period, and the equilibrium period. The moment an implant is inserted into the bone, the osseointegration process begins. The bone, which has been injured by the surgical preparation of the implant site, begins to heal and regenerate until it comes into contact with the surface of the implant. This healing process is characterized by a series of well-defined events that occur over a period of 3 to 6 months.

A recent histologic and histomorphometric preclinical study by Simion et al[27] described the events that occur in the first 3 months of an implant's life. A total of 36 block sections, including implants, were prepared for light microscope examination at different time intervals: immediately after insertion (T0), 1 day after insertion (T1), 7 days after insertion

(T7), 15 days after insertion (T15), 30 days after insertion (T30), and 90 days after insertion (T90).

At T0 (immediately after insertion), the implants showed an extremely low percentage of direct BIC of between 23 and 25%, and BIC was generally limited to the most coronal portion of the implant in contact with the mandibular cortical. Spaces without contact were filled with blood clots and residual bone particles from site preparation and implant placement **(Figs 8 and 9)**.

After 1 day, the histologic features were identical to those of the previous day.

There was very low BIC (12.9–16.9%) and no signs of cellular activity directed toward bone regeneration **(Figs 10 and 11)**.

After 7 days, intense resorption of residual bone particles was observed with simultaneous adjacent bone neoapposition. Near the particles, intense osteoblastic activity with osteoid tissue formation could be observed. When the particles were in the vicinity of the implant surface, bone neoformation was evident directly in contact with the implant. In areas lacking particles, bone regeneration was poor. The BIC was still very low (23.5–24.9%) **(Figs 12 and 13)**.

After 15 days, osteoblastic activity appeared intensified in all samples.

The bone particles were almost completely resorbed and replaced by new bone consisting of islands of woven bone surrounded by osteoid tissue and the osteoblastic rim. The newly formed bone was often in contact with the implant surface. The BIC was still very low in all samples (24.9–26.9%) **(Figs 14 and 15)**.

After 30 days, a large amount of new woven bone associated with intense osteoblastic activity was evident in all samples, especially at the level of the cutting cones or bone remodeling units (BRU), a sign of maturation of the woven bone into lamellar bone. The BIC values were also increased to between 38.9 and 42.5% **(Figs 16 and 17)**.

After 90 days, mature lamellar bone in direct contact with the implant surface could be observed in all samples.

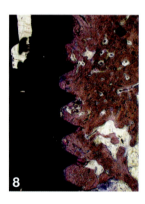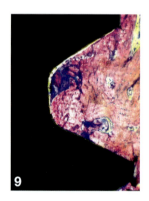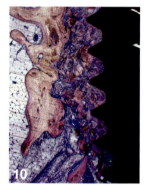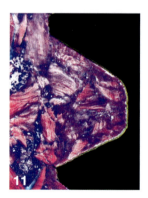

Fig 8 *Histologic image of a sample at day 0. Toluidine blue/Pyronin G staining; ×4 magnification.*
Fig 9 *Immediately after implant placement, the spaces between threads were filled with blood clots and bone particles left over from site preparation. Toluidine blue/Pyronin G staining; ×20 magnification.*
Fig 10 *Day 1: The histologic features are identical to the previous day. Toluidine blue/Pyronin G staining; ×4 magnification.* **Fig 11** *Histologic image on day 1 at higher magnification. The residual bone particles and the blood clot occupying the spaces between the implant threads are evident. Toluidine blue/Pyronin G staining; ×20 magnification.*

Osteoproliferative activity appeared to be strongly reduced, and numerous primary osteons were present in the regenerated bone.

The BIC had increased to between 41.7 and 48.6% **(Figs 18 and 19)**.

The osseointegration process just described can be divided into *(1)* the hemostatic phase, *(2)* the inflammatory phase, *(3)* the proliferative phase, and *(4)* the remodeling phase.

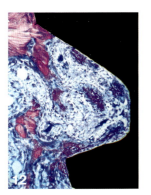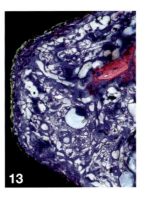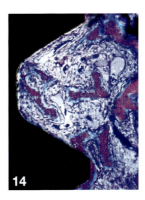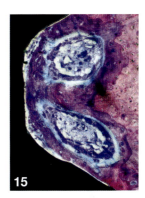

Fig 12 *Day 7: Intense resorption activity of residual bone particles and adjacent bone neoapposition is evident. Toluidine blue/Pyronin G staining; ×20 magnification.* *Fig 13* *At higher magnification, bone neoformation in direct contact with the implant is evident on day 7. Toluidine Blue/Pyronin G staining; ×40 magnification.* *Fig 14* *Day 15: The bone particles are almost completely resorbed and replaced by new interlaced fiber bone. Toluidine blue/Pyronin G staining; ×20 magnification.* *Fig 15* *At higher magnification, the newly formed bone is visibly in contact with the implant surface on day 15. Toluidine blue/Pyronin G staining; ×40 magnification.*

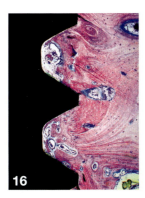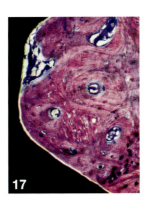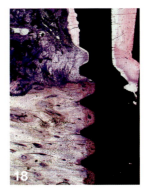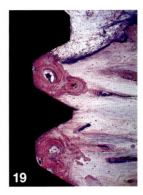

Fig 16 *Day 30: a large amount of new interlaced fiber bone associated with intense osteoblastic activity is evident, especially at the level of the cutting cones. Toluidine blue/Pyronin G staining; ×10 magnification.* *Fig 17* *At higher magnification, new osteons in contact with the implant are evident on day 30. Toluidine Blue/Pyronin G staining; ×40 magnification.* *Fig 18* *After 90 days, mature lamellar bone in direct contact with the implant surface was observed in all samples. Toluidine blue/Pyronin G staining; ×4 magnification.* *Fig 19* *At higher magnification, the newly formed secondary osteons in contact with the implant surface are evident at 90 days. Toluidine blue/Pyronin G staining; ×10 magnification.*

Hemostatic phase

Immediately after implant insertion, the empty spaces between the implant surface and the native bone are filled with blood, and the hemostatic phase begins. Hemostasis involves the aggregation and activation of platelets that release growth factors such as platelet-derived growth factor (PDGF) and transforming growth factor beta (TGF-ß), which promote vascular and fibroblast proliferation. Activated platelets also stimulate the conversion of fibrinogen into fibrin and thus the formation of the blood clot. Fibrin adheres to the surfaces of native bone, implants, and residual bone particles.

Inflammatory phase

The anaerobic peri-implant environment leads to the diapedesis of polymorphonuclear leukocytes that cross the vascular wall and enter the clot with ameboid movement. They begin to phagocytize the bacteria and release granules containing defensins that perforate the bacterial cell walls and also secrete cytokines that amplify inflammation. Macrophages rush in and clean the area of bacteria and necrotic bone debris. When the bacterial load decreases, macrophages begin to stimulate bone neoformation, promoting angiogenesis and the resolution of inflammation. They secrete hypoxia-inducible factor (HIF) and angiogenic and fibrogenic growth factors such as PDGF and fibroblast growth factor (FGF) to initiate the proliferative phase.

Proliferative phase

The first event of the proliferative phase is the formation of new vessels for the supply of oxygen, and bone neoformation occurs in the vicinity of new capillaries. Pericytes and endothelial cells play key roles in this phase.

Pericytes detach from the vascular wall, and endothelial cells begin to proliferate. New capillaries are thus formed, stabilized by the pericytes, which invade the space while actively regenerating. This phase is called angiogenesis and is fundamental for bone regeneration. Stimulated by PDGF and FGF secreted by macrophages, fibroblasts arrive and deposit a collagen matrix to form granulation tissue.

Pericytes detach from the vascular surface and migrate into the peri-vascular spaces to become osteoblast progenitor cells. They multiply under the influence of growth factors and form cell aggregates, then adhere to the surface of native bone, residual bone chips, and the implant. Under the stimulus of bone morphogenetic proteins (BMPs), TGF-ß, and Wnts, pericytes transform into osteoblasts.

Osteoblasts begin to synthesize a Type I organic collagen matrix that is accelerated by the presence of autologous bone chips, resulting in the formation of osteoid tissue.

Osteoid tissue mineralizes with the deposition of calcium and phosphate crystals, and osteoblasts simultaneously become trapped in the new bone tissue and transform into osteocytes. This is how woven bone, an immature bone consisting of disordered fibers and numerous osteocytes, is formed (Fig 20).

Remodeling phase

The remodeling phase begins with the formation of cutting cones. A vascular loop is formed in the vicinity of the bone to be replaced. From the apex of the loop, monocytes emerge from the vessel by diapedesis and adhere to the bone, transforming into osteoclasts. They begin to reabsorb the bone using acidic substances and proteases.

The vascular loop grows in the resulting tunnel, forming the Haversian canal. At the same time, pericytes detach from the vascular wall, attach

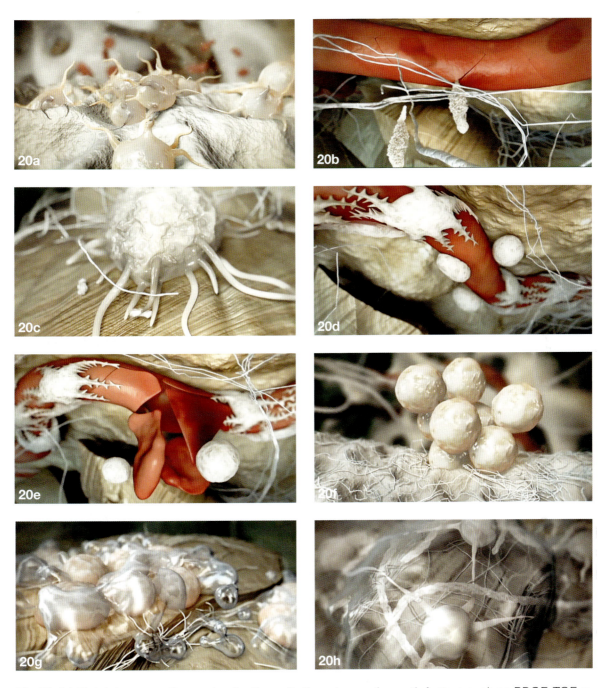

Fig 20 (a) *Platelet aggregation and activation with the release of growth factors such as PDGF, TGF-α, and TGF-ß. (b) Polymorphonuclear leukocytes cross the vascular wall and migrate into the clot. (c) Macrophages help remove bacteria and debris and secrete growth factors. (d) Pericytes detach from the vascular wall. (e) Endothelial cells begin to proliferate, forming new vessels. (f) Pericytes migrate into the perivascular spaces and turn into preosteoblasts and then osteoblasts. (g) Osteoblasts begin to secrete collagen Type I matrix and form osteoid tissue. (h) The osteoid tissue mineralizes, and the osteoblasts become trapped and transform into osteocytes, forming woven bone. (Courtesy of Geistlich Biomaterials.)*

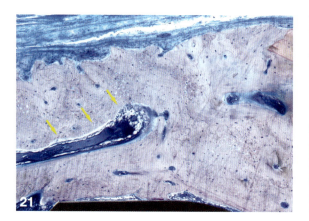 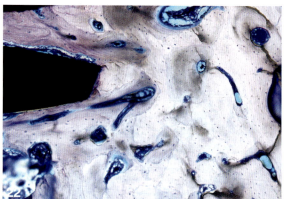

Fig 21 Cutting cone replacing immature woven bone near the surface of an implant. Toluidine blue staining; ×40 magnification. (Reprinted with permission from Int J Periodontics Restorative Dent 2016;26: 415–443.) *Fig 22* Peri-implant bone tissue 3 months after implant placement. The intense remodeling activity of the cutting cones is evident. Toluidine blue staining; ×20 magnification. (Reprinted with permission from Int J Periodontics Restorative Dent 2016;26:415–423.)

themselves to the tunnel wall, transform into osteoblasts, and deposit concentric layers of lamellar bone. This is the formation process of osteons that make up mature lamellar bone **(Figs 21 and 22)**. Whereas woven bone is poorly mineralized and not very resistant to loading, lamellar bone is very dense and load resistant. The remodeling process is complete after a period of between 3 and 6 months, depending on the quality of the native bone tissue and the age and regenerative protential of the patient. Smoking, alcohol consumption, certain systemic diseases, and the consumption of bisphosphonates, which block osteoclastic activity, adversely affect the process of osseointegration and bone maturation.

At the end of remodeling, an indefinite period of equilibrium begins, in which peri-implant bone turnover returns to normal levels. Cutting cone activity is reduced, and structural changes in the bone are minimal, although still present, as the peri-implant bone is able to adapt to the new loads transmitted by the prosthesis.

BONE ADAPTATION TO MECHANICAL STRESS

The ability of bone to adapt to different mechanical stress situations has been known for many years and is described by Wolff's Law.[28] Mechanical stress, expressed as microstrain (a unit of measurement that expresses the deformation of biologic tissues), has been applied to bone with increasing intensity to determine its effects.[29] Under mechanical stress with values below 200 microstrain, bone tends to atrophy.

It demineralizes, with the diameter of long bones decreasing and the lumen of the medullary canal becoming wider.

This situation is comparable to the muscle atrophy that occurs when patients are confined to bed by long debilitating illnesses or when astronauts live in space for long periods without gravity.

Under mechanical stress values between 200 and 2,500 microstrain, an equilibrium situation is established, in which the tendency toward

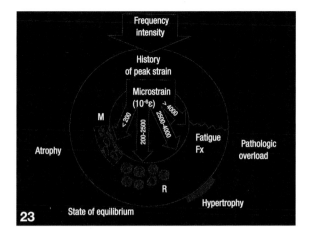
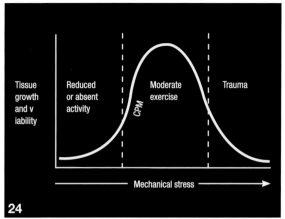

Fig 23 Adaptation of bone tissue to different mechanical stresses. Bone atrophy results from low loads. With the application of increasing mechanical stresses, bone will first enter a state of equilibrium, then hypertrophy, and eventually pathologic overload. **Fig 24** Sinusoidal curve expressing Wolff's Law. The abscissae represents the mechanical stress, with the bone trophism in ordinates.

demineralization is equal to the rate of new bone apposition. If the stress increases to values between 2,500 and 4,000 microstrain, the bone goes into hypertrophy.

Mineralization and bone volume increase, and the lumen of the medullary canal is reduced. This situation can be compared to the somatic changes that occur in body builders, in whom not only muscle mass increases but also the size of the skeletal structure to withstand the increased mechanical stress of lifting weights. When mechanical stress exceeds 4,000 microstrain, the bones undergo fatigue atrophy, leading to pathologic fracture **(Fig 23)**.

Wolff's Law can be represented graphically by a sinusoidal curve **(Fig 24)**, in which the x-axis shows the mechanical stress and the y-axis shows the trophism of the bone: at low stress values the bone atrophies, as the stress increases the bone adapts, hypertrophying and mineralizing until it reaches a maximum threshold beyond which stress becomes traumatic and the bone

atrophies. The adaptability of bone tissue is very obvious in the masticatory apparatus of patients. The progressive atrophy of the jaws of partially and totally edentulous patients is a well-known phenomenon, and atrophy can be halted and even regress when appropriate mastication forces are restored via implant-supported prostheses. The resulting masticatory function and physiologic mechanical stress induce an increase in mineralization and bone volume **(Figs 25 and 26)**.

The ability of the bone tissue to progressively adapt to loading is very important from a clinical point of view for determining when prosthetic loads should be applied to osseointegrated implants. In the presence of very dense, highly mineralized bone, such as in the mandible, loading is indicated immediately after implant placement. On the other hand, in the presence of poorly mineralized bone without a large medullary and cortical component, as in the lateral sectors of the maxilla, progressive loading is indicated, in which the implant is left unloaded for a submerged

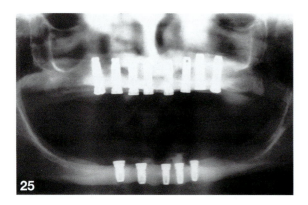 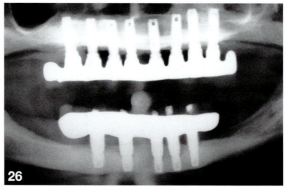

Fig 25 *A panoramic radiograph showing the rehabilitation of an extremely atrophic mandible with five implants.* **Fig 26** *After 7 years, the increased trophism of the bone, again under physiologic loads, is evident.*

integration period of 6 to 8 months and then loaded with a provisional prosthesis in subocclusion for 3 months and finally a definitive prosthesis with adequate occlusion. Progressive loading is particularly important following sinus elevation procedures, where the regenerated bone often has reduced mechanical stress resistance characteristics. Progressive loading allows the peri-implant bone to gradually adapt to the increased mechanical stresses from occlusion and mastication.

BIOLOGIC PRINCIPLES OF OSSEOINTEGRATION

According to Tomas Albrektsson et al,[30] it is essential that certain biologic principles and rules are observed for an implant to osseointegrate and be successful in the long term. The following factors are all important for success:

- Biocompatibility of the implant material
- Microstructure of the implant
- Macrostructure of the implant
- Biomechanics
- Surgical protocol
- Prosthetic Protocol
- Follow-up

Biocompatibility of the implant material

In general, materials that are sufficiently biocompatible to allow direct contact between implants and bone are ceramics (ie, oxides of certain metals). Although many metals, including gold, platinum, silver, and surgical steel, are biocompatible and can be used in the human body, their biocompatibility is not sufficient to achieve osseointegration. The most widely used material for osseointegration is titanium, which oxidizes quickly when exposed to air and is coated with the ceramic titanium dioxide.

Titanium is a very reactive material that interacts rapidly with the external environment. Its rapid oxidation once exposed to air (for as little as a few milliseconds) provides a protective coat that makes it extremely inert and biocompatible. Pure titanium, however, is a rather soft metal that is unsuitable for fine machining and unable to withstand prolonged stress.

Therefore, CPT is used because it has traces of impurities from other metals that can significantly increase its mechanical properties. Traces of nitrogen, carbon, hydrogen, iron, and oxygen are all present in the four grades of CPT, which decrease in purity but improve in mechanical properties. In the original Brånemark system, Grade 2 CPT implants were used, which were extremely biocompatible and corrosion resistant but rather brittle and, in rare cases, prone to fracture. Today, Grade 4 CPT is used because it is stronger and equally biocompatible.

In some cases, the titanium alloy Ti_6Al_4V, improperly referred to as "Grade 5 titanium," is used. This alloy, which contains 90% titanium, 6% aluminum, and 4% vanadium, has high mechanical strength and good biocompatibility characteristics, but its ability to achieve integration with the bone equal to CPT is questionable. For this reason, the Ti_6Al_4V alloy is currently used only for the construction of abutments and prosthetic fixation screws.

In the past, other ceramics have been proposed for implant construction, including alumina, tricalcium phosphate, and calcium hydroxyapatite (HA). Alumina (Al_2O_3) has the advantage of being white and translucent, making it suitable for use in esthetic areas, where it is desirable to avoid the dark appearance of titanium through tissues. But its excessive rigidity and brittleness pose high risks of fractures.

Tricalcium phosphate was once used as a coating for titanium or alloy implants due to its affinity to bone and its very high biocompatibility, but its tendency for rapid resorption led to high implant failure rates. For the same reasons, HA was widely used in the early 1990s as an implant coating, but its excessive roughness favored bacterial adhesion, leading to high rates of peri-implantitis.[31,32] One ceramic that has been intensively studied in the implant field in recent years is zirconia (ZrO_2). Zirconia is now the material of choice for the construction of partial dentures and crowns in esthetic areas due to its high strength, white color, and high biocompatibility. Some studies[33,34] have shown its ability to integrate effectively with bone even if surface treatment is more difficult than with titanium. Further clinical studies with long-term follow-ups are needed to determine the predictability of this material for implant construction.

At the interface between the oxide and bone biomolecules, certain physical and chemical bonds take place that can be grouped into three categories:[35] van der Waals bonds, hydrogen bonds, and covalent and ionic chemical bonds.

The first two types of bonds are extremely weak, whereas chemical bonds are stronger but less extensive.

Due to the scarcity of cohesive forces between the implant surface and the bone, the microstructure and macrostructure of the implant are of paramount importance for mechanical stability within the bone.

Microstructure of the implant
(With Dr Morra)

The microstructural characteristics of an implant surface are defined by its roughness and porosity. Surface roughness is traditionally expressed with the parameters Ra and Sa, measures that express the arithmetic mean value of the deviations of the actual surface profile from the mean line in microns. This description, however, does not provide a complete indication of surface roughness. Porosity, which is an important risk factor for peri-implantitis, may also be present or absent.

Clarity is needed for evaluating implant surface roughness. The combination of a seemingly easy and intuitive measurement and marketing pressure have led to great confusion, both among clinicians and researchers working at an academic level. In 2009, Wennerberg and Albrektsson[36] wrote, "Unfortunately, the standards for surface metrology in articles published today vary so much in quality that any attempt at a systematic review of the importance of surface roughness in bone healing has inevitable limitations; what might otherwise be considered a good scientific article may have unacceptable standards for describing surface metrology. In other words, what is defined as 'rough' in one article may be considered 'smooth' in another, and conclusions are therefore difficult." Factors affecting the measurement of implant surface characteristics are described in the following sections.

Measurements for linear roughness (R) and area roughness (S)

In the early days of implantology, roughness was measured exclusively via contact systems. A tip was placed in contact with the surface and passed along a path of predefined length, according to the height profile that was recorded. **Figure 27** illustrates a roughness profile measured on a machined surface.

The maximum peak-to-valley distance is just over 2 μm (thousandths of a millimeter), meaning the surface is essentially smooth, hence the shiny, reflective appearance of the machined portions of implants. This profile was obtained along a linear path and is therefore referred to as 2D or linear roughness.

From the profile values, the various linear roughness parameters are calculated, indicated by a capital R and followed by a lowercase letter.

Over the years, technologic developments have led to the spread of non-contact roughness measurement techniques. All modern approaches exploit the acquisition of surface images and their processing into a 3D structure.

The subsequent roughness calculation is no longer limited to a line but can be performed over the entire image area or in select areas. Modern techniques therefore provide 3D (ie, area) roughness measurements. **Figure 28** illustrates the 3D processing of the same machined surface whose roughness profile was shown in **Fig 36**. In this case, the measurement of surface roughness was obtained using the stereo SEM technique. In practice, by exploiting the principle of stereoscopic

vision, two images of the same field were acquired from slightly different angles of observation. The combination of the two images allows the field of observation to be developed three-dimensionally, generating the image in **Fig 37**, and the software processes the 3D data of the chosen area.

The parameters thus obtained are referred to as area roughness, indicated by a capital S and followed by a lowercase letter.

In general, measuring area roughness provides more consistent and reliable data than a linear measurement because a larger area is analyzed and the measurement is not influenced by, for example, the direction of the measurement, which could lead to artifacts in surfaces with preferentially oriented roughness. Beyond these observations, Ra and Sa parameters, although two representations of a similar physical variable, rest on different foundations and cannot be directly compared.

The use of these values has the following further limitations:

1. Use of a single parameter to describe roughness. The roughness of a surface is almost always expressed solely by the value of Ra or the area analogue Sa. These parameters essentially indicate the arithmetic mean of the absolute height values along the profile or in the selected area. However, the height profile of a route or area consisting of a few very big ups and downs can present the same Ra (or Sa) value as a route of the same length with much smaller but more numerous ups and downs. Thus, Ra/Sa values do not fully describe the nature of implant surface roughness.

2. Dependence of roughness parameters on often overlooked variables. The mathematical formulas for calculating some of the main roughness parameters depend on the length of the path (or area) being measured. In other words, the value measured on the same surface and with the same instrument is generally different if it is measured on a path of, say, 100 μm or 1 mm.

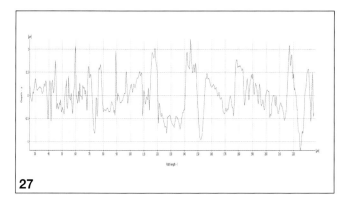

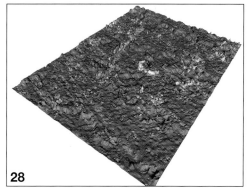

Fig 27 *Typical line roughness profile obtained by contact measurement on a machined surface.*
Fig 28 *3D processing of a machined surface, obtained by image acquisition and basis for calculation of area roughness parameters.*

Based on these premises, we follow the recommendations of Wennerberg and Albrektsson for reconciling the descriptive rigor and practicality of surface roughness presentation. They suggest describing the topography of implant surfaces by means of a pair of area roughness parameters: Sa and Sdr. Sdr represents the ratio between the real area of a surface and its geometric area (which is, for example, 100 μm² in the case of a field that is 10 μm in length).

It thus indicates how much the surface morphology amplifies the contact area between an implant and the host tissue. It is expressed as a percentage and is a function of both the height of the peaks and their density.

Evolution of implant microstructure

Sdr is particularly suitable for describing the evolution of implant surfaces. For the sake of consistency for comparison, all the data cited in the following discussion are homogeneous, having been obtained using the SEM stereo technique from pairs of images taken at ×2,000 magnification over areas of 80 × 110 μm.

The microstructure of the original Brånemark implants involved poorly rough surfaces, with Sa values of around 0.40 μm and Sdr values of around 25%. These implants were nonporous and machined, with no further modification after coming out of the turning tool except for decontamination and sterilization **(Figs 29 and 30)**. Between 1965 and 2000, millions of implants with this surface type were placed worldwide, with high success rates over 30 years.

At the same time, another much rougher and more porous surface treatment (Sa 2.3 μm) called titanium plasma spray (TPS) was available, obtained by spraying molten titanium powders at a high temperature onto the implant surface **(Figs 31 and 32)**.

This surface treatment had the advantage of significantly increasing the contact surface between bone and implant, as evidenced by the Sa value of 6 μm and the Sdr value of 72%, but the combination of the considerable height of the roughness peaks and the high surface area caused excessive bacterial deposition and a higher incidence of peri-implantitis.

After the year 2000, all companies abandoned the original machined surfaces and produced "active" surfaces, which were surfaces roughened by acid etching or air-borne particle abrasion and acid etching.

The modulation of osteogenesis at the cellular level by controlling implant surface topography has been described in a large number of studies, the most representative of which are probably those of Boyan[37,38] and Davies.[39,40] Davies also pointed out that high surface area and microroughness also lead to a strong implant interaction with blood at the implant site and a significant platelet activation effect, resulting in the release of chemokines and cytokines that rapidly trigger the healing process. In fact, this type of topography is extremely procoagulant, so much so that the surfaces of titanium medical devices used in cardiovascular applications are carefully polished precisely to prevent any residual roughness from causing clotting phenomena.

The practical translation of these concepts has led to the clinical introduction of SLA (sandblasted, large-grit, and acid-etched; Straumann) **(Figs 34 and 35)** and DAE (double acid-etched) implant surfaces **(see Figs 33, 36, and 37)**.

SLA surface treatment involves an initial air-borne particle abrasion phase with coarse-grained

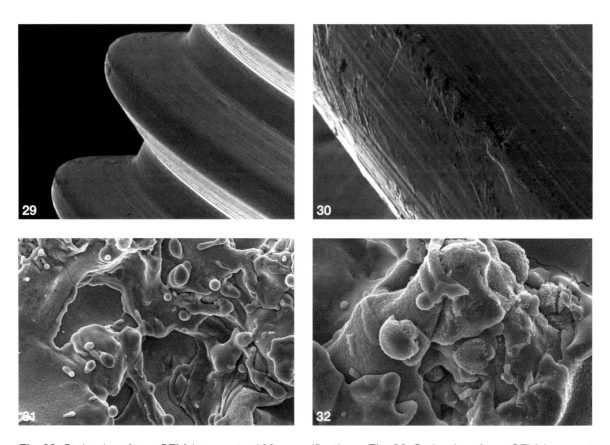

Fig 29 Stained surface. SEM image at ×100 magnification. **Fig 30** Stained surface. SEM image at ×500 magnification. **Fig 31** TPS surface. SEM image at ×5,000 magnification. **Fig 32** TPS surface. SEM image at ×10,000 magnification.

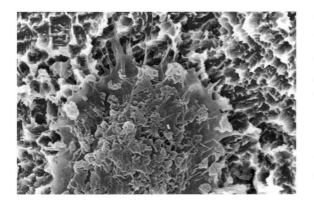

Fig 33 Osteoblastic cell cultured in vitro on a surface obtained by double acid etching. Note the relative size of the cell body and the distance between roughness peaks. SEM image at ×10,000 magnification.

alumina (400–500 µm), followed by double acid etching. The result is bimodal roughness, clearly visible in **Fig 35**, in which larger craters from airborne particle abrasion coexist within the microroughness caused by double acid etching. This surface has an Sa value of about 1.75 µm and an Sdr of 90%, which is the most significant aspect of this process. The DAE surface is also produced with double acid etching but is not preceded by air-borne particle abrasion.

Although DAE surfaces have a much lower Sa value (about 0.45 µm) because they lack the high peaks caused by air-borne particle abrasion, their microroughness structure ensures an Sdr value of around 80%.

SLA and DAE surface treatments represented a big step forward compared to TPS surfaces. In fact, with lower vertical roughness (as shown by the Sa values) and thus reduced propensity compared to TPS for bacterial deposition, they ensure a much higher contact surface and peak density (as indicated by Sdr).

The concepts introduced with SLA and DAE underpin many of the implant surfaces in clinical use today.

Alongside these technologies, it is important to mention the alternative surface treatments that have been widely used. TiOBlast (Astra Tech) and Osseospeed (Astra Tech) surfaces are obtained via an air-borne particle abrasion process with titanium oxides to avoid the permanence of foreign particle residues on the implant surface.

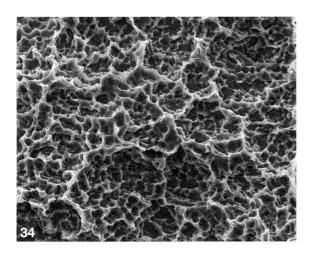

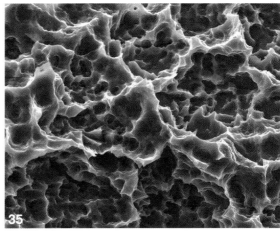

Fig 34 SLA surface. SEM image at ×5,000 magnification. *Fig 35* SLA surface. SEM image at ×10,000 magnification.

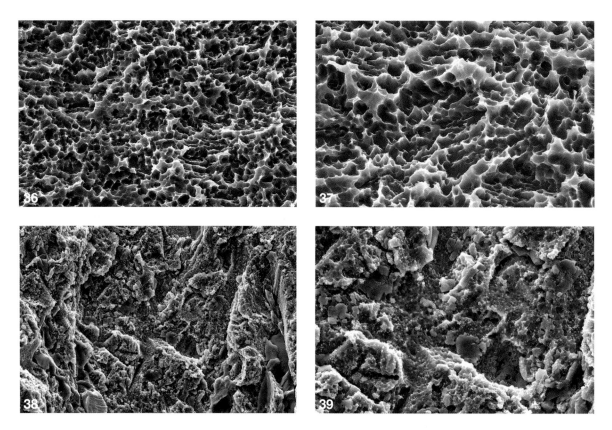

Fig 36 *DAE surface. SEM image at ×5,000 magnification.* **Fig 37** *DAE surface. SEM image at ×10,000 magnification.* **Fig 38** *Osseospeed surface. SEM image at ×5,000 magnification.* **Fig 39** *Osseospeed surface. SEM image at ×10,000 magnification.*

In the case of Osseospeed surface treatment, airborne particle abrasion is followed by a phase of surface enrichment in fluorine.

The resulting surface **(Figs 38 and 39)** has an Sa value of 1.27 μm and an Sdr values of about 50%. A completely different technique is used to create the TiUnite (Nobel Biocare) implant surface. An electrochemical process in an aqueous solution causes the surface oxide layer to grow and release hydrogen, which "erupts" from the surface and generates a small volcano–like structure with craters up to a few μm in diameter **(Figs 40 and 41)**.

This surface differs from the others in its porosity and has an Sa value of 1.1 μm and an Sdr value of 50%. The rationale behind the use of rougher surfaces lies in the fact that some research[39,40] seems to show that they may support remote osseointegration. Remote osseointegration represents the concept that bone could form directly on the surface of the implant before migrating from the pre-existing bone to the edges of the preparation (ie, contact osseointegration).

This would reduce osseointegration time. In fact, as shown in a recent histologic study,[27] the

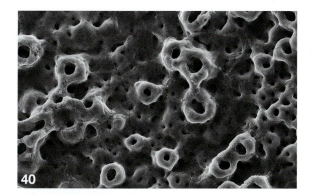

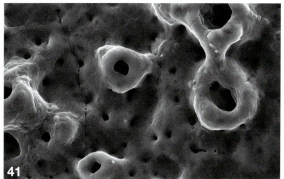

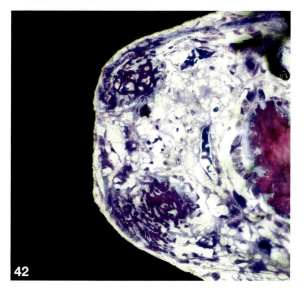

Fig 40 *TiUnite surface. SEM image at ×5,000 magnification.* **Fig 41** *TiUnite surface. SEM image at ×10,000 magnification.* **Fig 42** *Histologic image of a machined surface implant 2 weeks after insertion. Bone neoformation in direct contact with the implant surface is evident. Toluidine blue/Thyronine G staining; ×40 magnification.*

possibility of achieving contact osseointegration depends more on the presence of residual bone particles than on the roughness of the implant surface **(Fig 42)**.

Clinical experience seems to indicate a certain advantage to using moderately rough implant surfaces in the presence of soft bone and low insertion torque (20–25 Ncm). For this reason, there is a tendency to choose implants that have a rough surface in the apical 50% and a machined surface in the coronal 50% to exploit the potential advantages of surface roughness in the deeper portions

of the bone, far from bacterial colonization, and to maintain a smoother surface in the more superficial areas to reduce the risk of peri-implantitis. Hybrid systems **(Figs 43 and 44)** have been devised to fulfill these requirements and currently offer the best compromise.[41] Today, there are new trends resulting from technologic development.

Following several decades of intensive studies, the last few years have witnessed the debut of implant surface nanoengineering in the clinical field. With the implants described previously, surfaces owe their activity to a physical variable (roughness), but intensive research has explored the stimulation of cell behavior at the tissue/implant interface by coating the titanium surface with biologic molecules including proteins, peptides, and glycosaminoglycans. With appropriate techniques, it is possible to bind nanolayers (ie, layers a few nanometers thick) of biologic molecules to titanium surfaces in a stable manner, preventing them from dissolving in the implant site and exploiting their properties to stimulate healing processes.

A specific technique that has already entered the clinical field involves coating implant surfaces with hyaluronic acid.[42]

This molecule is involved in many tissue regeneration processes and is also extremely hydrophilic, imparting considerable surface wettability. The coating is only a few billionths of a meter thick (for comparison, the hydroxyapatite ceramic coatings of the past were about a thousand times thicker), and the hyaluronic acid molecules are bound to the surface by chemical bonding. Due to the very limited thickness, it is difficult to visualize these nanostructures with traditional electron microscopy, though it is possible to do so with typical nanotechnology instruments, such as the atomic force microscope (AFM).

This process is clinically used with hybrid implants to impart activity to the machined portion that is no longer related to topography but to biochemical stimulation.

Figure 45 compares AFM images obtained from a machined surface and the same surface subjected to the hyaluronic acid coating process. Note how the vertical scale is only 80 nm and how the exceptional vertical resolution of the measuring instrument allows the morphology developed by the molecular layer of hyaluronic acid on the machined surface to be appreciated.

Implant macrostructure

The macrostructure of the implant design plays a fundamental role in osseointegration. An implant's ability to integrate depends on its primary stability

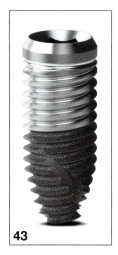
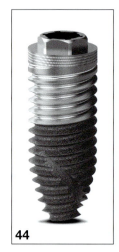
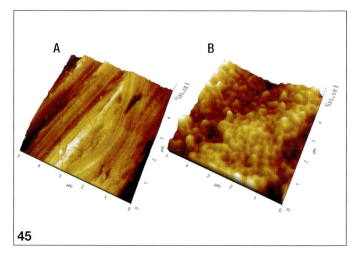

Fig 43 iMax hybrid system (iRES) with internal hexagonal connection. *Fig 44* iMax hybrid system with external hexagonal connection. *Fig 45* AFM images of (A) a stained surface and (B) the same surface with hyaluronic acid coating.

at the time of insertion, which in turn, is highly dependent on its shape.

Osseointegrated implants are generically referred to as root form implants because they are shaped like the roots of natural teeth.

They are cylindric and conical to various degrees. The original Brånemark implants were single threaded with a perfectly cylindric shape and an unthreaded apex.

Implants of this shape can be inserted into the alveolar bone without prior tapping, so they were very suitable for the treatment of edentulous mandibular ridges, where the bone is highly mineralized. In the soft maxillary bone, however, the impossibility of underpreparing and the need to tap the recipient site can compromise primary implant stability. This explains the different rates of osseointegration observed in the maxilla and the mandible, with the latter having significantly higher values.

In modern implants, this problem has been solved by slightly conical and very tapered implants with threaded apices with diameters well below the implant diameter **(Fig 46)**.

This self-tapping feature and the ability to exert an expansive force against the wall of the recipient site greatly increased the possibility of successfully inserting implants, even in soft bone.

A very accentuated taper, however, while presenting considerable advantages for use in soft bone, is very risky to use in mandibular cortical bone, where the excessive pressure on the lateral walls of the site, made up of hard, rigid bone, may cause microfractures and ischaemia,[43–45] potentially resulting in partial bone resorption or even implant failure.

Another feature common to many new-generation implants is the presence of double threading. Instead of having a single thread extending from the head to the apex of the implant, there are two threads that run parallel to one another. In this way, the inclination of the threads is greater, and the progression of the implant insertion into the recipient site is greater, resulting in better visual control during progression and greater insertion torque in soft bone **(Fig 47)**.

Implant design is also of fundamental importance for the distribution of occlusal and masticatory loads from the implant to the bone.

The greater the surface area orthogonally opposed to the vector of a given force, the less pressure is applied at any single point on the surface. Older-generation implants, very often in the shape of a blade, pointed helicoid, or needle, had a very small surface area that could oppose the load perpendicularly, especially when compared to the width of the root surface of the teeth they were replacing.

Thus, the occlusal forces were concentrated directly on the apex of the implant and therefore on the bone, resulting in lytic phenomena and mobilization of the implant **(Fig 48)**.

Modern implants benefit from the presence of a thread along the entire interface with the bone and a slightly conical shape, which allow forces applied in the apicocoronal direction to be broken down and distributed throughout the implant body **(Fig 49)**.

Lateral or oblique and rotational forces, however, tend to be concentrated at the level of the head and apex of the implant and are less tolerated **(Fig 50)**. In the case of significant oblique forces, implants of the greatest possible length should be selected.

Implant biomechanics
(With Dr Michele Maglione)

Implant-supported prosthetic rehabilitation treatment planning requires the evaluation of numerous clinical aspects, including the consideration of functional biomechanical risk.

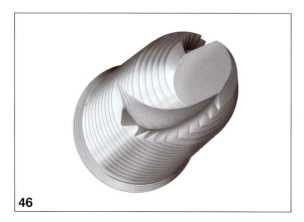

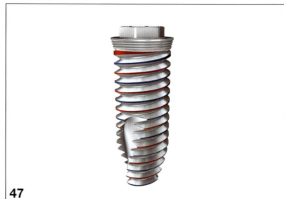

Fig 46 New generation implant with a slight taper (6 degrees) and a tapered, self-tapping apex. *Fig 47* Double threading of an iMAX implant. The two threads (red and blue) run parallel to one another along the entire length of the implant. *Fig 48* Older, blade-type implant concentrating all axial occlusal forces at the apex, creating an osteolysis overload phenomena.

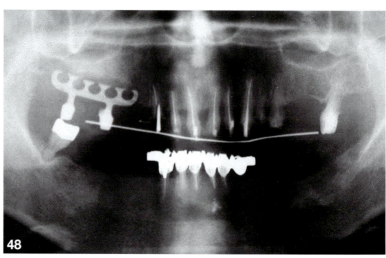

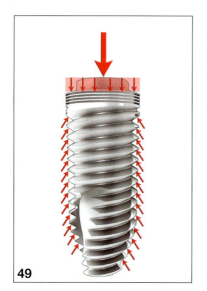

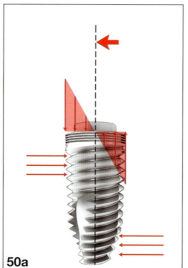

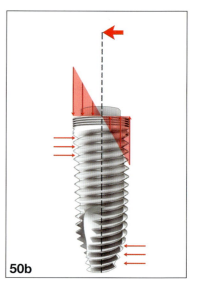

Fig 49 New generation implant. Axial forces are reduced by the presence of the thread along the entire implant surface. *Fig 50* (a) Lateral and oblique forces tend to be concentrated at the head and apex of an implant and are less tolerated. (b) A longer implant has greater resistance to oblique forces.

Geometric risk factors

When designing implant-supported restorations, geometric risk factors must be considered to optimize the distribution of mechanical stresses on the bone-implant-prosthesis complex. Each of the following points must be considered:

- The number of implants being placed and the number of root units being replaced
- Implant tripod arrangement
- The presence of natural dentition
- Implants not connected to natural teeth
- Position of the implants in relation to the prosthetic center
- Crown-root ratio
- Use of large-diameter implants
- Dimensions and morphology of the occlusal surface

Renouard and Rangert set up an experimental model to assess the biomechanical stresses to which implant-supported prostheses are subjected during function [46] **(Fig 51)**.

Starting from a configuration with one mesial and one distal abutment supporting an intermediate element, they evaluated the mechanical stress on the abutments when subjected to a known stress and assigned it a value of 100%. Inserting an intermediate implant in the same model in line with the previous ones and applying the same stress, they measured a mechanical stress of 67% (ie, a reduction of 33%).

On the basis of this experimental model, it may be considered useful to place a number of implants that is equal to the number of missing teeth. Clinically, however, this is true only when replaced two or three teeth.

In more extensive rehabilitations, the number of implants may be significantly lower depending on the patient's anatomical characteristics and the number of teeth to be replaced.

There is, in fact, a vast literature supporting the possibility of using only six implants for maxillary rehabilitation and only four implants for mandibular rehabilitation[4,25,26,47] for achieving high long-term success rates. Bo Rangert's experimental model was also able to demonstrate how a tripod arrangement of three implants **(Figs 52 and 53)** can lead to a reduction in mechanical stress of up to 33%, while the use of only two implants with one element in extension causes an increase in load of up to 200%.

The tripod arrangement allows greater resistance to the oblique and rotational forces to which a prosthetic structure with implants arranged on the same axis is susceptible **(Fig 54)**.

This concept is valid not only for partial prosthetic restorations but also for complete prosthetic restorations because placing implants on the widest circumferential arc possible allows for a better distribution of functional stresses and a considerable reduction in biomechanical risk **(Figs 55 to 57)**.

In a restoration for a totally edentulous arch, the axis joining the two most distal implants is called the axis of rotation, and the axis joining the two most mesial implants is called the axis of resistance. From a clinical point of view, the greater the distance between these two axes, the greater the distal extensions of the overdenture can be. Indeed, this distance is taken empirically as a reference point for the construction of the distal extensions: the distal overhang of the extensions should not be greater than the distance between the axis of rotation and the axis of resistance. Although this rule is empirical and not supported by scientific evidence, it has been successfully used in daily clinical practice for years.

Elements in extension in restorations of three teeth lead to a 200% increase in stress. They are therefore strongly discouraged, especially in molar areas, where the masticatory forces are greatest.

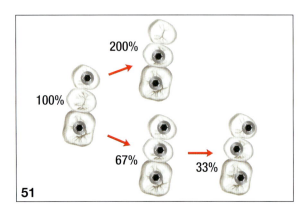

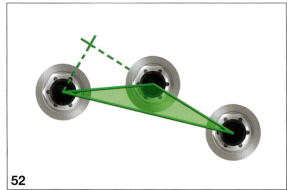

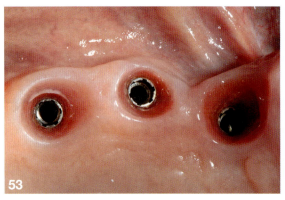

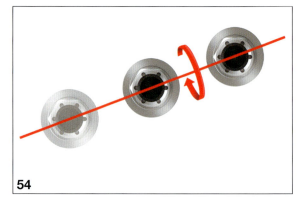

Fig 51 Rangert's diagram of the biomechanical stresses to which the implant-supported prosthesis is subjected during function. *Fig 52* A tripod arrangement of three implants can lead to a reduction in mechanical stress of up to 33%. *Fig 53* Clinical image of three implants with a tripod arrangement. *Fig 54* Three in-line implants are arranged on a single axis of rotation and are therefore more susceptible to oblique and rotational forces.

A discussion that has been going on for years concerns the splinting of natural teeth to implants in the mistaken belief that it helps the latter to support the occlusal load.

Although there is no evidence in the literature against performing this procedure, one must consider the natural mobility of the tooth in relation to the relative rigidity of the implant. Once subjected to loading, the natural tooth tends to move, to intrude slightly, thanks to the periradicular dimensional tolerance allowed by the presence of the PDL. The implant, on the other hand, comparable to a tooth in ankylosis, does not move **(Fig 38)**.

Therefore in an implant-natural tooth structure, the occlusal loads are concentrated on the implant, almost as if the natural tooth were simply an element in extension **(Figs 59a and 59b)**. For this same reason, implant and natural tooth bridge structures, where the unfavorable lever arm becomes even longer, are strongly discouraged **(Fig 59c)**.

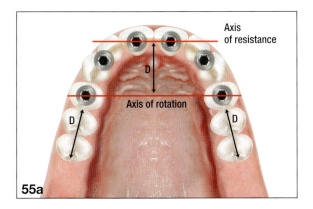
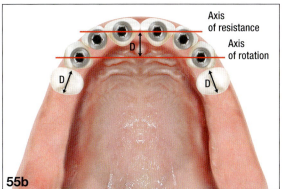

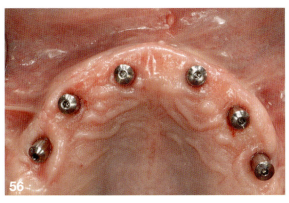
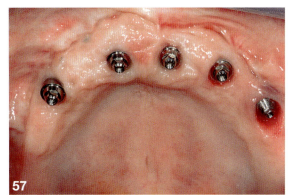

Fig 55 *The size of the distal extensions should be equal to the distance between the axis of rotation and the axis of resistance. (a) Implants over a wide arc. (b) Implants almost in line.* **Fig 56** *Clinical example of implants with widely spaced axes of rotation and resistance, creating a biomechanically favorable situation.* **Fig 57** *Implants placed in a near-line, creating a biomechanically unfavorable situation.*

A rather common clinical condition among completely edentulous patients is a discrepancy in the sagittal plane between the maxillary and mandibular residual alveolar process. This discrepancy, which usually results in a skeletal Class III condition, may be due to centripetal bone resorption of the maxilla and centrifugal bone resorption of the mandible, whether associated or not with a pre-existing skeletal Class III relationship. In consequent implant rehabilitation, the axes of the prosthetic elements may be significantly more buccal than those of the implants, introducing significant oblique and rotational forces that pose a serious biomechanical risk. In these cases, it is necessary, where possible, to compensate for the increased biomechanical risk with a greater number of implants with longer lengths and larger diameters **(Figs 60 and 61)**. The latter strategy should also be used in cases of severe alveolar resorption treated with short implants and an unfavorable crown/implant ratio.

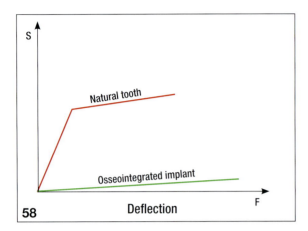
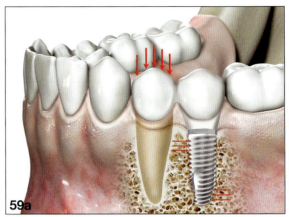
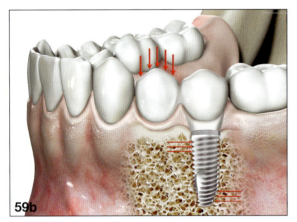
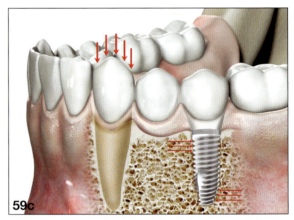

Fig 58 *Comparison of the biomechanical behavior of a natural tooth and an osseointegrated implant (green line). The application of a force of equal intensity produces different effects. In the natural tooth (red line), there is an initial deflection (which is about 80 µm) related to the presence of the PDL, whereas in the implant there is no spatial change.* **Fig 59** *(a and b) Natural tooth-implant structure. (c) Natural tooth-bridge-implant structure.*

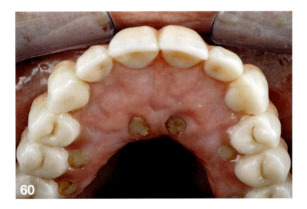
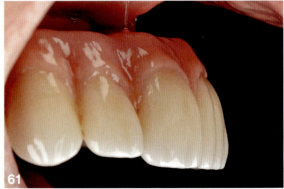

Fig 60 *Clinical image of a complete maxillary rehabilitation. The Class III skeletal relationship involves a significant discrepancy between the implant axis (more palatal) and the dental axis (more buccal).* **Fig 61** *From a lateral view, the considerable buccal extension is evident.*

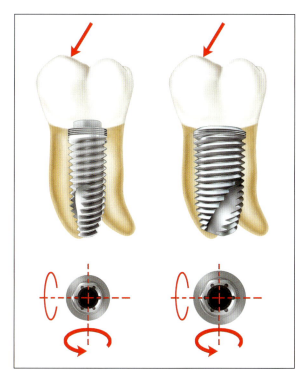

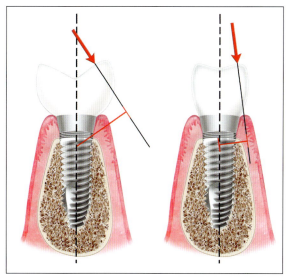

Fig 63 *The use of larger-diameter implants (about 5 mm) reduces the biomechanical risk.*

Fig 62 *Size discrepancies between molar crowns and implant diameters can introduce oblique forces.*

The rehabilitation of single molars can also result in oblique or rotational occlusal forces due to the difference in diameter between the implant and the tooth. For this reason, there is a tendency to use larger diameter implants whenever possible, around 5 mm, to reduce the crown/root ratio in the horizontal plane **(Fig 62)**. For the same reason, it is necessary to model crowns with smaller buccolingual dimensions and with less inclined cusp slopes than the natural teeth. In this way, the results of the forces applied on the oblique cusp slopes fall closer to the long axis of the tooth, reducing the rotational component **(Fig 63)**.

REFERENCES

1. Brånemark PI. Experimental investigation of microcirculation in bone marrow. Angiology. 1961;12:293–305.
2. Brånemark PI. Intravital microscopy: Its present status and its potentialities. Med Biol. 1966;16:100–108.
3. Brånemark PI, Zarb G, Albrektsson T. Tissue-Integrated Prosthesis. Lombard, Illinois: Quintessence Publishing, 1987.
4. Adell R, Lekholm U, Rockler B, Brånemark PI. A 15-year study of osseointegrated implants in the treatment of the edentulous jaw. Int J Oral Surg. 1981;10:387–416.

5. Brånemark PI, Adell R, Breine U, Hansson BO, Lindström J, Ohlsson A. Intra-osseous anchorage of dental prostheses. I. Experimental studies. Scand J Plast Reconstr Surg. 1969;3:81–100.

6. Albrektsson T, Sennerby L. State of the art in oral implants. J Clin Periodontol. 1991;18:474–481.

7. Albrektsson T, Zarb G, Worthington P, Eriksson AR. The long-term efficacy of currently used dental implants: a review and proposed criteria of success. Int J Oral Maxillofac Implants. 1986;1:11–25.

8. Berglundh T, Lindhe J. Dimension of the periimplant mucosa. Biological width revisited. J Clin Periodontol. 1996;23:971–973.

9. Araujo MG, Lindhe J. Peri-implant health. J Periodontol. 2018; 89(Suppl 1): 249–256.

10. Brito C, Tenenbaum HC, Wong BKC, Schmitt C, Nogueira Filho G. Is keratinized mucosa indispensable to maintain peri-implant healt? A systematic review of the literature. J Biomed Mater Res B Appl Biomater. 2014 Apr;102(3):643–650.

11. Albrektsson T. Zarb GA. Current interpretation of the osteointegrated response: clinical significance. Int J Prosthodont. 1993;6:95–105.

12. Cochran DL, Mau LP, Higginbottom FL, Wilson TG, Bosshardt DD, Schoolfield J, Jones AA. Soft and hard tissue histologic dimensions around dental implants in the canine restored with smaller-diameter abutments: A paradigm shift in peri-implant biology. Int J Oral Maxillofac Implants. 2013;28:494– 502.

13. Broggini N, McManus LM, Hermann JS, Medina R, Schenk RK, Buser D, Cochran DL. Peri-implant inflammation defined by the implant-abutment interface. J Dent Res. 2006;85:473–478.

14. Lazzara RJ, Porter SS, Platform Switching: a new concept in implant dentistry for controlling postrestorative crestal bone levels, Int J Periodontics Restorative Dent. 2006; 26:9–17.

15. Lindquist LW, Carlsson GE, Jemt T. A prospective 15-year follow-up study of mandibular fixed prostheses supported by osseointegrated implants. Clinical results and marginal bone loss. Clin Oral Implants Res. 1996;7:329–336.

16. Ekelund JA, Lindquist LW, Carlsson GE, Jemt T. Implant treatment in the edentulous mandible: a prospective study on Brånemark system implants over more than 20 years. Int J Prosthodont. 2003;1:602–608.

17. Jemt T, Johansson J. Implant treatment in the edentulous maxillae: a 15-year follow-up study on 76 consecutive patients provided with fixed prostheses. Clin Implant Dent Relat Res. 2006;8:61–69.

18. Lekholm U, Gröndahl K, Jemt T. Outcome of oral implant treatment in partially edentulous jaws followed 20 years in clinical function. Clin Implant Dent Relat Res. 2006;8:178–186.

19. Jemt T. Single implants in the anterior maxilla after 15 years of follow-up: comparison with central implants in the edentulous maxilla. Int J Prosthodont. 2008;21:400–408.

20. Astrand P, Ahlqvist J, Gunne J, Nilson H. Implant treatment of patients with edentulous jaws: a 20-year follow-up. Clin Implant Dent Relat Res. 2008;10: 207–217.

21. Jemt T. Cemented CeraOne and porcelain fused to TiAdapt abutment single-implant crown restorations: a 10-year comparative follow-up study. Clin Implant Dent Relat Res. 2009;11:303–310.

22. Dierens M, Vandeweghe S, Kisch J, Persson GR, Cosyn J, De Bruyn H. Long-term follow-up of turned single implants placed in periodontally healthy patients after 16 to 22 years: microbiologic outcome. J Periodontol. 2013;84:880–894.

23. Bergenblock S, Andersson B, Fürst B, Jemt T. Long-term follow-up of CeraOne™ single-implant restorations: an 18-year follow-up study based on a prospective patient cohort. Clin Implant Dent Relat Res. 2012;14:471–479.

24. Simion M, Gionso L, Grossi GB, Briguglio F, Fontana F. Twelve-Year Retrospective Follow-Up of Machined Implants in the Posterior Maxilla: Radiographic and Peri-Implant Outcome. Clin Implant Dent Relat Res. 2015;17 Suppl 2: 343–351.

25. Simion M, Nevins M, Rasperini G, Tironi F. A 13- to 32-Year Retrospective Study of Bone Stability for Machined Dental Implants. Int J Periodontics Restorative Dent. 2018;38:489–493.

26. Brånemark PI, Hansson BO, Adell R, Breine U, Lindström J, Hallén O, Ohman A. Osseointegrated implants in the treatment of the edentulous jaw. Experience from a 10-year period. Scand J Plast Reconstr Surg Suppl. 1977;16:1–132.

27. Simion M, Benigni M, Al-Hezaimi K, Kim DM. Early bone formation adjacent to oxidized and machined implant surfaces: a histologic study. Int J Periodontics Restorative Dent. 2015;35:9–17.

28. Wolff J. Das gesetz der tansformation der knochen. Berlin: Hirshwalk, 1892.

29. Hart NH, Nimphius S, Rantalainen T, Ireland A, Siafarikas A, Newton RU. Mechanical basis of bone strength: influence of bone material, bone structure and muscle action. J Musculoskelet Neuronal Interact. 2017;17:114–439.

30. Albrektsson T, Brånemark PI, Hansson HA, Lindström J. Osseointegrated implants. Requirements for ensuring a long-lasting, direct bone-to-implant anchorage in man. Acta Orthp Scand. 1981;52:155–170.

31. Ichikawa T, Hirota K, Kanitani H, Miyake Y, Matsumoto N. In vitro adherence of Streptococcus constellatus to dense hydroxyapatite and titanium. J Oral Rehabil. 1998;25:125–127.

32. Ichikawa T, Hirota K, Kanitani H, Wigianto R, Kawamoto N, Matsumoto N, Miyake Y. Rapid bone resorption adjacent to hydroxyapatite-coated implants. J Oral Implantol. 1996;22:232–235.

33. Rocchietta I, Fontana F, Addis A, Schupbach P, Simion M. Surface-modified zirconia implants: tissue response in rabbits. Clin Oral Implants Res. 2009;20:844-50.

34. Pieralli S, Kohal RJ, Jung RE, Vach K, Spies BC. Clinical Outcomes of Zirconia Dental Implants: A Systematic Review J Dent Res. 2017;96:38–46.

35. Kasemo B. Biocompatibility of titanium implants: surface science aspects. J Prosthet Dent. 1983;49:832–837.

36. Wennerberg, A, Albrektsson T. On implant surfaces: a review of current knowledge and opinions. Int J Oral Maxillofac Implants. 2010;25:63–74.

37. Boyan BD, Lossdörfer S, Wang L, Zhao G, Lohmann CH. Osteoblasts generate an osteogenic microenvironment when grown on surfaces with rough microtopographies. Eur Cell Mater. 2003;6:22–27.

38. Boyan BD, Schwartz Z. Modulation of osteogenesis via implant surface design, in: Davies J E editor. Bone Engineering. Toronto: em squared, 2000;232–239.

39. Davies JE, Housseini MM, Histodynamics of endosseous wound healing, in: Davies JE editor. Bone Engineering, Toronto: em squared, 2000;1–14.

40. Davies JE. Understanding peri-implant endosseous healing. J Dent Educ. 2003;67:932–949.

41. Tarnow D. Dental implants in periodontal care. Opin Periodontol. 1993;157–162.

42. Morra M, Cassinelli C, Torre E, Iviglia G. Permanent wettability of a novel, nanoengineered, clinically available, hyaluronan-coated dental implant. Clin Exp Dent Res. 2018;4:196–205.

43. Cha JY, Pereira MD, Smith AA, Houschyar KS, Yin X, Mouraret S, Brunski JB, Helms JA. Multiscale analysis of the bone-implant interface. J Dent Res. 2015;3:482–490.

44. Coyac BR, Leahy B, Salvi G, Hoffman W, JB, Helms JA. A preclinical model links osseo-densification due to misfit and osseo-destruction due to stress/strain. Clin Oral Impl Res. 201;12:1238–1249.

45. Nevins M, Nevins M, Schupbach P, Fiorellini J, Lin Z, Kim D. The impact of bone compression on bone-to-implant contact of an osseointegrated implant: a canine study. Int J Periodontics Restorative Dent. 2012;32:637–645.

46. Renouard F, Rangert B. Risk factor in implant dentistry. Simplified clinical analysis for predictable treatment. Quintessence Publishing Co, Inc. 1999.

47. Maló P, Rangert B, Nobre M. "All-on-Four" immediate-function concept with Brånemark System implants for completely edentulous mandibles: a retrospective clinical study. Clin Implant Dent Relat Res. 2003;5 Suppl 1:2–9.

SURGICAL TECHNIQUES FOR ACHIEVING OSSEOINTEGRATION

CHAPTER 4

Edited by Massimo Simion

GENERAL PRINCIPLES

It is commonly believed that the success rates of an implant system depend essentially on the surface characteristics and design of the implant; in reality, these characteristics, while important, only partially affect the clinical outcome. As with all surgical procedures, the most important variables of implant surgery are, without doubt, the knowledge, experience, and manual dexterity of the surgeon. The probability that an implant will osseointegrate is intimately related to the surgical technique that is used, the type of bone present, and the subsequent loading strategy.

Good surgical protocol entails meeting the following basic goals:
- Minimal surgical trauma
- Primary implant stability
- Adequate healing and appropriate loading times for submerged and nonsubmerged implants
- Secondary implant stability

Correct surgical technique complements the biologic phenomena that regulate bone and soft tissue regeneration.

Massimo Simion

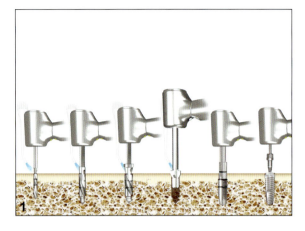 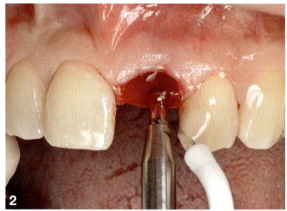

Fig 1 *Rules to be observed for correct implant site preparation.* **Fig 2** *Irrigation with sterile saline solution during implant site preparation.*

MINIMAL SURGICAL TRAUMA

The surgical act of placing an implant inevitably involves trauma to the bone and surrounding soft tissues.

The chances of achieving osseointegration increase with reduced trauma to these tissues.

One of the major risks encountered during the preparation of an implant recipient site is excessive heating of the bone. While studying the behavior of bone tissue subjected to various physicochemical stimuli in the 1970s for his PhD thesis, Dr Anders Eriksson performed an in-depth study on the effect of heat on bone.[1] Using the titanium chambers described in chapter 3 for *in vivo* microscopic examination, he observed the healing processes of bone subjected to increasing temperature gradients in rabbit diaphyses.

These studies showed that if bone is heated above 47°C, protein coagulation and microthrombosis phenomena occur within the vascular microcirculation, along with subsequent healing through the formation of scar connective tissue in the absence of newly formed bone.

In fact, overheating the bone by only 10°C above basal body temperature leads to necrosis of the bone margins of the recipient site, which prevents subsequent osseointegration.

For this reason, continuous cooling during preparation of the implant site with the drills is essential, and the following guidelines must be observed **(Figs 1 and 2)**:

- Always use sharp drills.
- Drill with reduced rotation speeds between 800 and 1,800 rpm.
- Provide abundant irrigation with sterile saline.
- Use a back-and-forth movement with the drills, without exerting excessive pressure, to allow the saline solution to cool the apex as well.
- Use a sequence of burs with increasing diameters to remove a minimal amount of bone as each bur passes.
- A speed of around 15 rpm is appropriate for performing tapping and implant insertion.

PRIMARY IMPLANT STABILITY

Primary implant stability is defined as the absence of implant mobility at the time of insertion. Bone tissue can only regenerate on completely immobile surfaces, so it is essential for osseointegration that the implant is fully stable after its insertion.

In the literature,[2–4] the maximum mobility that still allows osseointegration to occur ranges between 10 and 150 μm. Generally, primary implant stability is achieved through contact between the apex of the threads and the cortical bone at the recipient site, while the core of the implant is rarely in contact with the bone **(Figs 3 and 4)**.[5]

In the presence of poorly compacted bone, the bone particles remaining from site preparation and implant insertion are compressed at the interface between the bone and the implant and contribute to stability. However, this is only an initial effect as these particles undergo osteoclastic resorption in the following days, resulting in a temporary decrease in stability **(Fig 5)**.

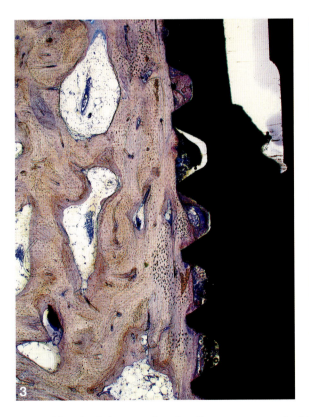
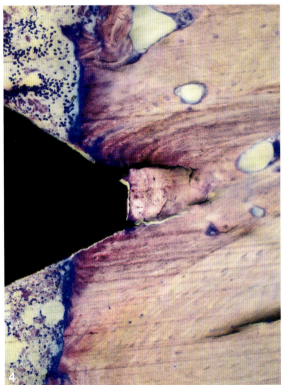

Fig 3 Histologic image showing the engagement of the apex of the implant coils with the walls of the implant site, a determiner of primary stability. Toluidine Blue/Pyronin G staining; ×4 magnification. (Reprinted with permission from Int J Periodontics Restorative Dent 2015;35:9–17.) *Fig 4* At higher magnification, it can be seen that there is no bone contact between one thread and the other and that the space is filled with a blood clot. Toluidine blue/Pyronin G staining; ×40 magnification. (Reprinted with permission from Int J Periodontics Restorative Dent 2015;35:9–17.)

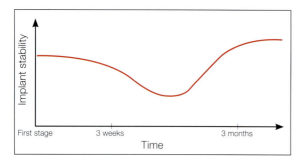

Fig 5 *The trend of implant stability in the first months after insertion. Primary stability tends to decrease after week 3 and then increases to its maximum value after 3 months (secondary stability).*

Primary stability depends mainly on four factors:
1. The amount of bone tissue.
2. The quality of bone tissue.
3. The shape of the implant.
4. The surgical insertion technique.

Bone tissue quantity and quality were classified by Zarb and Lekholm in 1985.[6] The alveolar bone is divided into five classes, from A to E, depending on its quantity in both the maxilla and the mandible.

The authors, however, do not define precise parameters and measurements **(Fig 6)**:
- **Class A** is defined as alveolar bone with the least possible atrophy after nontraumatic tooth loss without loss of bone support. It can be likened to the situation of a patient who has been edentulous for only a few months.

Class A bone generally allows for implants to be placed correctly without performing regenerative techniques.

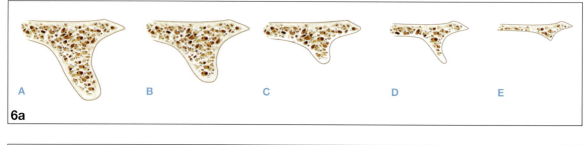

6a

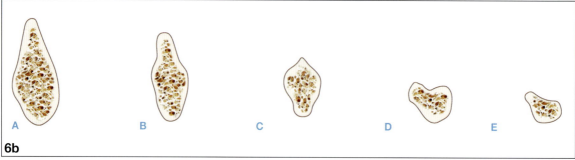

6b

Fig 6 *Zarb and Lekholm's 1985 classification of the amount of bone tissue. (a) Maxilla. (b) Mandible.*[6]

- **Class B** atrophy can be found in patients who have been edentulous for some time but who have alveolar bone with a minimum vertical dimension of at least 10 mm and a thickness of 5 to 6 mm. Implants can be placed without additional techniques.
- **Class C** is considered advanced atrophy with a vertical bone dimension of at least 10 mm but with insufficient thickness. This class allows implants to be placed only in association with regenerative techniques or bone grafts.
- **Classes D** to E represent the most severe forms of atrophy and, in the maxilla, implant treatment is possible only after performing maxillofacial surgery, such as Le Fort 1–type interpositional grafting.

The quality of the alveolar bone is categorized into four types, from 1 to 4, according to its density **(Fig 7)**:

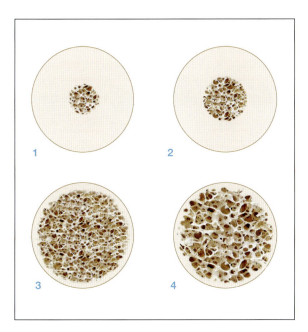

Fig 7 Zarb and Lekholm's 1985 classification of bone tissue quality.[6]

- **Type D1** is highly mineralized bone with a very thick cortical and a dense medullare bone. It is a bone type characteristic of the body of the mandible medial to the mental foramina.
- **Type D2** bone is characterized by a well-represented cortical and medulla with dense trabeculae.
  This type of bone is generally found in both the anterior and posterolateral sectors of the mandible.
- **Type D3** bone has a thin cortical and a spongiosa with dense trabeculae. This type of bone is typical of the anterior maxilla medial to the maxillary sinuses.
- **Type D4** is the bone with the worst mechanical qualities, with an absent cortical and a poorly mineralized spongiosa with widely spaced trabeculae.
  It is generally found in the posterolateral sectors of the maxilla, as well as in other sectors in patients with osteoporosis.

The method for determining the class of bone quality is entirely clinical, based on what the clinician feels during preparation of the implant recipient site, and is therefore characterized by enormous individual variability.

Radiographic methods to determine bone quality class are based on the radiopacity of CT or CBCT images and are generally indicative only and cannot be used to determine the bone class of a given site precisely.

Naturally, the greater the quantity and quality of bone tissue are, the greater the chances are of achieving adequate primary implant stability. The mechanical characteristics of the bone are of much greater importance because excellent stability can be achieved in well-mineralized bone (Class 1 or 2) even if there is a limited amount, whereas the placement of implants in abundant but poorly mineralized bone (Class 4) can be problematic.

There are three methods for assessing primary stability after implant placement:

1. Insertion torque
2. Evaluating the sound after percussion
3. Resonance frequency analysis (RFA) to determine the implant stability quotient (ISQ)

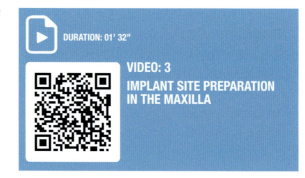

DURATION: 01' 32"

VIDEO: 3
IMPLANT SITE PREPARATION IN THE MAXILLA

Insertion torque

As previously mentioned, primary implant stability depends, in part, on the implant design. A slightly conical shape and a very tapered and self-tapping apex allow for the insertion of implants in underprepared sites (ie, sites prepared with drills of a smaller diameter than the implant) to compress the preparation walls and increase insertion torque and implant stability **(Fig 8)**. On the other hand, the use of conical implants in Class 1 and 2 bone increases the risk of too high insertion torque and excessive lateral pressures, with consequent damage to the peri-implant bone and/or the prosthetic connection structures of the implant head. In these cases, it is always necessary to carry out prior tapping of the site to avoid exceeding insertion torque values of 50 Ncm.

An experimental study by Nevins et al[7] in the compact bone of the canine mandible involved histologic and histomorphometric comparison of three groups of implants placed with three different degrees of compression (low, medium, and high) on the lateral walls of the site. Compression was obtained by preparation and tapping (low compression), underpreparation with a self-tapping implant (medium compression), and underpreparation with a non-self-tapping implant (high compression).

The sites that performed best in every respect were those with medium compression.

These results were confirmed by an experimental study[8] that showed that the insertion of high-torque implants causes microfractures and

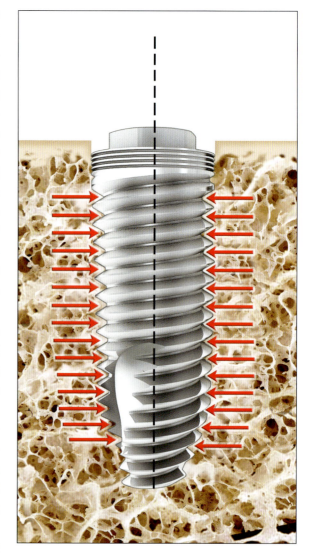

Fig 8 *With slightly tapered implants and self-tapping apexes, underpreparation allows some compression to be exerted on the preparation walls, increasing insertion torque and implant stability.*

ischemia of the peri-implant bone, resulting in increased resorption and reduced bone neoformation. In another study, Coyac et al[9] showed that an excessive discrepancy in diameter between the preparation and the implant leads to immediate osseodensification and subsequent osteodestruction from excessive mechanical stress.

The insertion torque is not synonymous with primary implant stability as it expresses the rotational force that is required to insert the implant to the bottom of the preparation.

Nonetheless, it is fairly accurate as an expression of the stability achieved by the implant once in its final position.

The ideal insertion torque ranges between 30 and 50 Ncm. Insertion torques below 30 Ncm are associated with more implant failures, and insertion torques above 50 Ncm can be significantly detrimental. Evaluation of the insertion torque is carried out using micromotors equipped with torque controllers and manual ratchets with a torque wrench (Fig 9).

Sound evaluation after percussion

The evaluation of sound after striking the implant with a metal instrument is an empirical but simple and effective method.[10] Normally, the handle of a dental mirror is used to strike the implant head either directly or after screwing in a healing abutment. A bright sound indicates good implant stability, whereas a dull sound is an indication of insufficient stability (Fig 10). An implant that shows mobility at the time of its insertion has no chance of integrating with the bone.

RFA

One method for objectively and precisely measuring primary implant stability is RFA.[11,12] A small

DURATION: 04' 04"

VIDEO: 4
IMPLANT SITE PREPARATION
IN THE MANDIBLE

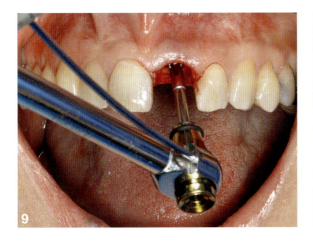
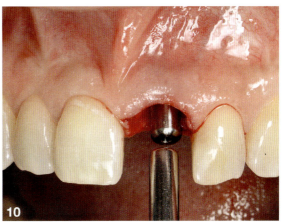

Fig 9 Evaluation of insertion torque with a dynamometric ratchet wrench. *Fig 10* Clinical evaluation of stability by percussion of the implant with a metal instrument.

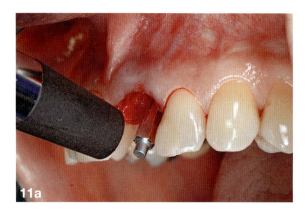
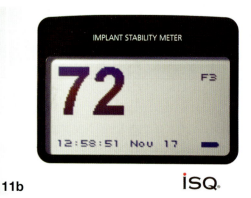

Fig 11 *Assessment of primary implant stability by determining the ISQ value. (a) Positioning the probe near the SmartPeg screwed to the implant. (b) ISQ value indicated by the display.*

metal pin (SmartPeg [Osstell] or MulTipeg [Penguin]) is screwed onto the internal thread of the implant. The measuring instrument stimulates the metal pin by emitting magnetic pulsations via a pen handpiece **(Fig 11)**. The pin then resonates at a certain frequency depending on the stability of the implant. The resonance frequency is recorded as the ISQ value.

ISQ values above 70 indicate optimum implant stability, values between 60 and 70 indicate average stability, and values below 60 indicate poor stability.

HEALING TIMES AND LOADING FOR SUBMERGED AND NONSUBMERGED IMPLANTS

According to Brånemark's original protocol for implant placement, during the osseointegration period, the implant must remain submerged under the oral mucosa without being loaded for a period of 6 months in the maxilla and 3 months in the mandible.[13–15] The rationale for this two-stage surgical protocol is based on the histologic finding of complete neoformation and maturation in lamellar bone 3 to 6 months after the surgical act of implant placement.

The two-stage technique entails innumerable advantages and still constitutes the safest approach today because it reduces the risk of infection by bacteria from the oral cavity, prevents the penetration of epithelium at the interface between the bone and the not-yet-osseointegrated implant, and guarantees a total absence of premature loading by masticatory acts or mucosa-supported mobile provisional prostheses **(Fig 12)**. When performing staged implant placement in D1-, D2-, and D3-quality bone, there is a tendency to reduce the waiting time to 4 months in the maxilla, while maintaining the 3-month healing period in the mandible. In D1-, D2-, and, in some cases, D3-quality bone, there is a tendency to perform an immediate loading procedure. Some clinical studies[16–18] have shown that osseointegration can occur even if the implant is in a transmucosal position because epithelial attachment to the healing abutment or transmucosal portion of the implant occurs within a few days.

The advantage of this one-stage approach, which is now used extensively, is that it avoids a second surgery to connect the healing abutment **(Fig 13)**. The transmucosal approach does, however, expose the implant to more to bacterial contamination in the early stages of healing and to uncontrolled loading with complete dentures in totally edentulous patients.

SECONDARY IMPLANT STABILITY

Secondary implant stability refers to the absence of implant mobility after the soft tissue healing period and maturation of the bone tissue **(Figs 14 and 15)**.

Although osseointegration can be confirmed only after several months of prosthetic loading, the

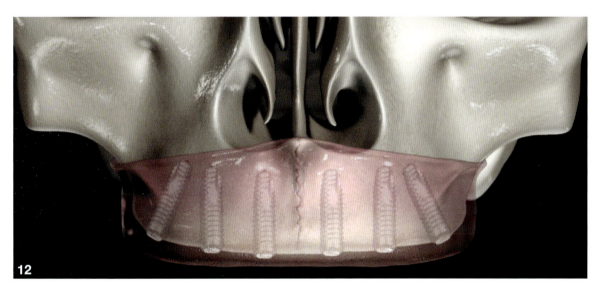

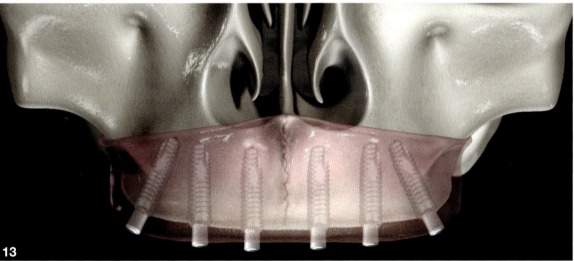

Fig 12 The position of submerged implants. *Fig 13* The position of transmucosal implants.

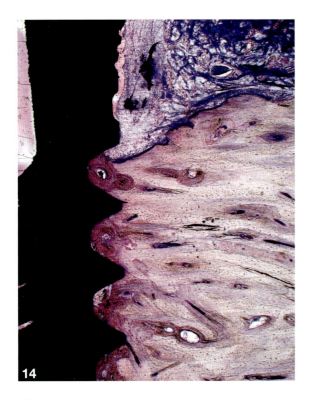 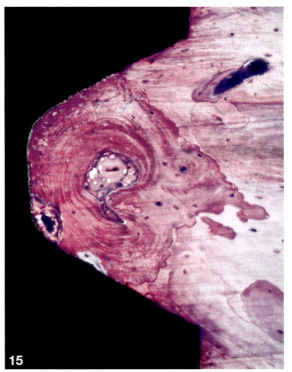

Fig 14 Histologic preparation showing the successful integration of an implant. The spaces between the threads, originally filled with only coagulum, are now occupied by lamellar bone, which determines the secondary stability. Toluidine blue/Pyronine G staining; ×4 magnification. (Reprinted with permission from Int J Periodontics Restorative Dent 2015;35:9–17.) *Fig 15* At higher magnification, a secondary osteon can be seen in contact with the implant surface. Toluidine blue/Pyronin G staining; ×20 magnification. (Reprinted with permission from Int J Periodontics Restorative Dent 2015;35:9–17.)

presence of secondary implant stability at the time of the second surgical stage is a strong indication that the implant has integrated with the bone.

The process for assessing secondary implant stability is like that for evaluating primary stability. It can be determined via clinical evaluation of implant percussion sound and RFA.

Radiographic examination by means of periapical radiographs, although always necessary, cannot provide conclusive evidence of osseointegration because the resolving power of an X-ray is not sufficient to detect slight interpositioning of connective tissue at the bone-implant interface.

SURGICAL TECHNIQUE
Patient preparation

Every surgery performed in the oral cavity carries the risk of infection. Patients must be adequately prepared for surgery to reduce the bacterial load as much as possible. The care taken to prepare patients for implant surgery differentiates clinicians who practice a noble art from those who work with a farrier's mentality.

Patient motivation and verification of patient compliance are indispensable, not only to avoid intraoperative infectious complications but to prevent peri-implant tissue infections throughout the course of the patient's life. A motivated patient who is well educated in home oral hygiene techniques is far less likely to contract peri-implantitis in later years.

In periodontal patients, it is essential to carry out comprehensive causal therapy prior to implant placement. In addition to being fully motivated, these patients must undergo full-mouth disinfection and a maintenance period of at least 3 months.

The following protocol should be prescribed to patients prior to surgery:

- Rinses with 0.2% chlorhexidine twice a day, starting 3 days before surgery and continuing for 15 days afterward
- Oral administration of antibiotic therapy with amoxicillin and clavulanic acid 1 g (or alternatives), 1 tablet every 8 or 12 hours administered 1 hour before surgery and for 5 to 7 days afterward. It is advisable to combine milk enzymes and gastroprotective supplements
- Anti-inflammatory therapy with ketoprofen 50 mg (or alternatives), 1 tablet every 12 hours administered 30 minutes before surgery and for 3 to 4 days afterward
- Diazepam 5 mg/ml, 15 to 20 drops administered 30 minutes before surgery
- Octatropine methylbromide 20 mg and diazepam 2.5 mg (Valpinax), 2 tablets 30 minutes before surgery
- Dexamethasone 4 mg (eg, Soldesam, Lab Farmacologico Milanese), only in the most complex cases, a single intramuscular injection at the end of surgery

Preparation of the surgical room

The surgical environment must be prepared to guarantee adequate asepsis.

Sterile drapes are used to isolate the patient and the instrument table, the perioral skin is thoroughly cleansed with a gauze soaked in 0.2% chlorhexidine, and the patient must wear shoe covers and a surgical cap. The medical team, after adequately washing their hands and forearms with antiseptic detergents, must wear shoe covers, surgical caps and gowns, and sterile gloves (**Fig 16**).

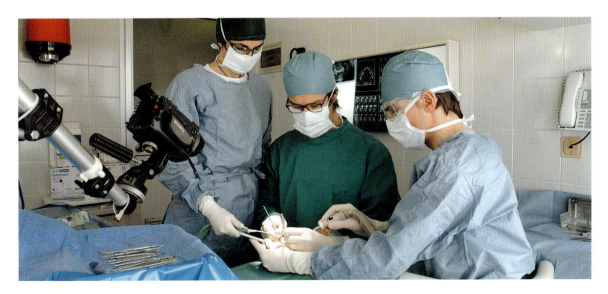

Fig 16 *Operating room set-up for implant surgery or guided bone regeneration (GBR). Aseptic conditions must be strictly observed.*

Instrumentation

There are multiple kits available for preparing the implant recipient site, and the surgical instrumentation varies according to the clinician's preference. In general, delicate and small instruments should be used. Implant surgery is closer to periodontal surgery than to maxillofacial surgery. The following is a description of a toolkit that the author has been using for many years and which allows most interventions to be performed **(Fig 17):**

- **Bard-Parker round section scalpel handle with a 15 C blade.** The round section handle allows the instrument to be easily rotated during incisions.
- **DeBakey tweezers, 15 cm with multiple tungsten carbide teeth.** DeBakey tweezers are atraumatic for tissues and allow for safe gripping of flaps even in the most distal areas thanks to their length.
- **Back-action chisel/fine chisel.** With a single instrument it is possible to perform flap detachment, bone curettage, and root planing.
- **Prichard periosteal** elevator for elevating the strong palatal flaps and retracting and protecting the flaps.
- **Columbia 4R/4L and Prichard SPR1/2 curettes.** Universal curettes for intraoperative root planing.
- **Miller CM long-shaft alveolar spoons** for removing granulation tissue from postextraction socket and deep bone defects.
- **UNC 15 periodontal probe** for all periodontal and bone defect measurements.
- **Probe calibrated** to the length of the implants.

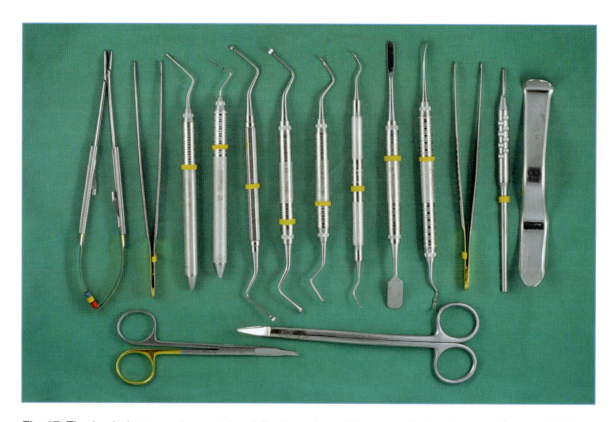

Fig 17 The basic instruments must be delicate and small because implant surgery is very similar to periodontal surgery.

- **15-cm anatomical tweezers with tungsten carbide tips** for bending and positioning guided bone regeneration (GBR) membranes without damaging them.
- **17-cm Castroviejo needle holders with tungsten carbide** terminals to allows 4-0 sutures to be used without damaging the terminals.
- **Goldman-Fox scissors** with serrated blades for trimming soft tissues without them slipping.
- **Dean scissors for cutting threads during suturing.**
- **Minnesota CRM retractor** for retracting and protecting large flaps.

Flap design

Traditional implant surgery involves incising the mucosal tissues and elevating a full-thickness flap to expose the alveolar ridge receiving the implant. More recently, flapless techniques have been developed, which involve preparing the site and inserting the implant through the mucosal tissue without elevating it.

These techniques have the advantage of being minimally invasive and are characterized by a postoperative period that is free of substantial patient discomfort.

The flapless approach, however, involves considerable risks due to the impossibility of directly assessing the size and shape of the alveolar ridge and should only be used when properly indicated and with guided surgery software.

Flapless techniques and guided surgery are described in chapter 6.

Flap design differs depending on the number of implants being placed, on whether the patient is fully or partially edentulous, and on whether hard and/or soft tissue augmentation techniques are required. These flap techniques are described in later chapters.

Flap design for single or multiple implants surrounded by natural teeth

A full-thickness incision is made in the center of the edentulous ridge, extending intrasulcularly at the level of the adjacent teeth. The extension should reach the zenith of the gingival parabolas both buccally and palatally/lingually. Vertical releasing incisions that could result in residual scarring should be avoided **(Figs 18 and 19)**. A full-thickness flap is then elevated gently with a fine periosteal elevator, both buccally and palatally/lingually. It is important to extend the flap in the apical direction to visualize any concavities that may result in exposure of the apical part of the implant outside the bone crest. After elevation, thorough root planing of the adjacent elements is performed, sparing the periodontal attachment fibers.

Flap design for single or multiple distal implants

A full-thickness incision is made in the center of the edentulous ridge, extending intrasulcularly at the level of the adjacent mesial implant. The extension must reach the zenith of the gingival parabola both buccally and palatally/lingually. A distal vertical releasing incision is made. In this case, it is also advisable to elevate a wide area to identify possible undercuts, especially in the posterolateral areas of the mandible in the lingual aspect **(Figs 20 and 21)**.

Flap design for completely edentulous maxillae

Flaps to treat completely edentulous ridges must be wide and extend beyond the most distal implants. In the maxilla, the incision is crestal and extends from an area approximately 10 mm distal to the mesial wall of the maxillary sinus to the corresponding contralateral area. Two oblique releasing

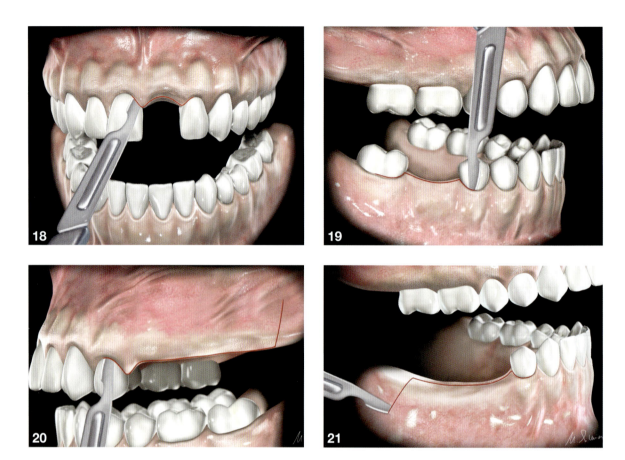

Fig 18 *Flap design for the insertion of a single implant in an anterior edentulous site.* **Fig 19** *Flap design for single implant placement in a posterolateral site missing a tooth.* **Fig 20** *Flap design for implant placement in a superior distal site with multiple missing teeth.* **Fig 21** *Flap design for implant placement in an inferior distal site with multiple missing teeth.*

incisions are indicated at the distal limits of the incision **(Fig 22)**. The full-thickness flap must be elevated both buccally and palatally to reveal any bony defects or undercuts.

Flap design for completely edentulous mandibles

In most cases of complete mandibular edentulism, the implants are placed in the horizontal branch mesial to the mental foramen, for which a ridge incision is made in the center of the keratinized mucosa extending at least 10 mm distal to the mental foramen. At the distal limits of the incision, two releasing incisions are made well beyond the foramen to avoid injuring the inferior alveolar nerve **(Fig 23)**. Great care must be taken in patients with severe mandibular atrophy because the mental foramen may be in the upper margin of the ridge. Again, the full-thickness flap must be elevated until the emergence of the inferior alveolar nerve is revealed.

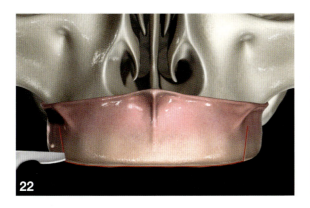 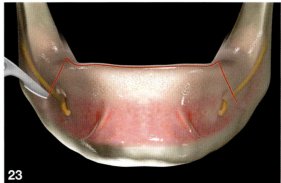

Fig 22 Flap design for implant placement in a completely edentulous maxilla. *Fig 23* Flap design for implant placement in a completely edentulous mandible.

Site preparation and implant placement

Although site preparation must be performed according to the implant placement protocol indicated by implant manufacturers, it is essential that the surgery is adapted to the quality of the patient's bone to achieve optimal insertion torque and primary implant stability.

Regardless of the quantity and quality of the bone, the insertion torque required to seat the implant to the bottom of the preparation should be between 40 and 50 Ncm.

Preparation strategies naturally depend on the design of the implant being used, but in general, the following suggestions should be considered for the various bone types.

Type D1 bone site preparation

Type D1 bone has a very thick and mineralized cortical. It always allows for optimal primary implant stability, but there is a high risk of overheating the bone and reaching an excessive torque resulting in excessive lateral pressure on the peri-implant bone. For this reason, particular caution during preparation with the drills is required, including abundant cooling with saline solution and a preparation diameter that does not deviate excessively from the implant diameter.

For example, for an implant with a diameter of 3.75 mm, the diameter of the last drill should be 3.15 mm. It is essential to always perform a complete pre-tapping of the site and a countersink to relieve compression on the bone walls near the crestal margin.

Type D2 bone site preparation

Type D2 bone also has a thick cortical and dense medullary space, so the same precautions as for Type D1 bone apply, although in some cases, only partial tapping may be recommended.

Type D3 bone site preparation

Type D3 bone is characterized by a thin cortical and a dense medullary space. It is generally present in the anterior areas of the maxilla.

There is a tendency to underprepare Type D3 bone sites to achieve adequate primary implant stability.

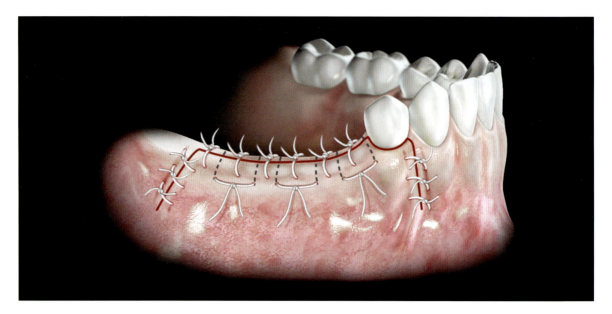

Fig 24 *Suturing technique with horizontal mattress sutures alternating with simple sutures.*

For example, for an implant with a diameter of 3.75 mm, the diameter of the final drill should be between 2.8 and 3 mm. Countersinking is performed, but tapping is rarely necessary.

Type D4 bone site preparation

Type D4 bone is the bone with the worst mechanical strength qualities and is characteristic of the posterolateral areas of the maxilla. It is essential to underprepare the implant recipient site and perform neither pretapping nor countersinking to maximize lateral pressures on the soft peri-implant bone and improve primary implant stability. For example, for a 3.75-mm-diameter implant, the final drill should have a diameter of 2 to 2.8 mm. In Types D3 and D4 bone, the use of slightly conical, double-threaded implants with a very tapered, self-tapping apex is of paramount importance.

REFERENCES

1. Eriksson A R. Heat-induced bone tissue injury. An in vivo investigation of heat tolerance of bone tissue and temperature rise in the drilling of cortical bone. Gotheborg: Thesis, 1984.

2. Brånemark PI, Zarb G, Albrektsson T. Tissue-Integrated Prosthesis. Lombard, Illinois: Quintessence Publishing, 1987.

3. Pilliar RM, Lee JM, Maniatopoulos C. Observations on the effect of movement on bone ingrowth into porous-surfaced implants. Clin Orthop Relat Res. 1986;208: 108–113.

4. Søballe K, Hansen ES, B-Rasmussen H, Jørgensen PH, Bünger C. Tissue ingrowth into titanium and hydroxyapatite-coated implants during stable and unstable mechanical conditions. J Orthop Res. 1992;10:285–299.

5. Simion M, Benigni M, Al-Hezaimi K, Kim DM. Early bone formation adjacent to oxidized and machined implant surfaces: a histologic study. Int J Periodontics Restorative Dent. 2015;35:9–17.

6. Lekholm U, Zarb GA. Patient selection and preparation. In Brånemark P-I. Zarb GA, Albrektsson T, editors. Tissue integrated protheses: Osseintegration in clinical denistry. Chicago: Quintessence Publishing, 1985.

7. Nevins M, Nevins M, Schupbach P, Fiorellini J, Lin Z, Kim D. The impact of bone compression on bone-to-implant contact of an osseointegrated implant: a canine study. J Periodontics Restorative Dent. 2012;32: 637–645.

8. Cha JY, Pereira MD, Smith AA, Houschyar KS, Yin X, Mouraret S, Brunski JB, Helms JA. Multiscale analysis of the bone-implant interface. J Dent Res. 2015;3: 482–490.

9. Coyac BR, Leahy B, Salvi G, Hoffman W, Brunski JB, Helms JA. A preclinical model links osseo-densification due to misfit and osseo-destruction due to stress/strain. Clin Oral Impl Res. 2019 ;30:1238–1249.

10. Triches DF, Alonso FR, Mezzomo LA, Schneider DR, Villarinho EA, Rockenbach MI, Teixeira ER, Shinkai RS. Relation between insertion torque and tactile, visual, and rescaled gray value measures of bone quality: a cross-sectional clinical study with short implants. Int J Implant Dent. 2019;5:9.

11. Becker W, Hujoel P, Becker BE. Resonance frequency analysis: Comparing two clinical instruments. Clin Implant Dent Relat Res. 2018;20:308–312.

12. Herrero-Climent M, Falcão A, López-Jarana P, Díaz-Castro CM, Ríos-Carrasco B, Ríos-Santos JV In vitro comparative analysis of two resonance frequency measurement devices: Osstell implant stability coefficient and Penguin resonance frequency analysis. Clin Implant Dent Relat Res. 2019;21:1124–1131.

13. Adell R, Lekholm U, Rockler B, Brånemark PI. A 15-year study of osseointegrated implants in the treatment of the edentulous jaw. Int J Oral Surg. 1981;10:387-416.

14. Brånemark PI, Adell R, Breine U, Hansson BO, Lindström J, Ohlsson A. Intra-osseous anchorage of dental prostheses. I. Experimental studies. Scand J Plast Reconstr Surg. 1969;3:81–100.

15. Albrektsson T, Sennerby L. State of the art in oral implants. J Clin Periodontol. 1991;18:474–481.

16. Buser D, Weber HP, Lang NP. Tissue integration of non-submerged implants. 1-year results of a prospective study with 100 ITI hollow-cylinder and hollow-screw implants. Clin Oral Implants Res. 1990;1:33–40.

17. Buser D, Mericske-Stern R, Bernard JP, Behneke A, Behneke N, Hirt HP, Belser UC, Lang NP. Long-term evaluation of non-submerged ITI implants. Part 1: 8-year life table analysis of a prospective multi-center study with 2359 implants. Clin Oral Implants Res. 1997;8:161–172.

18. Becker W, Becker BE, Israelson H, Lucchini JP, Handelsman M, Ammons W, Rosenberg E, Rose L, Tucker LM, Lekholm U. One-step surgical placement of Brånemark implants: a prospective multicenter clinical study. Int J Oral Maxillofac Implants. 1997;12: 454–462.

TREATMENT PLANNING AND THERAPY FOR COMPLETELY AND PARTIALLY EDENTULOUS PATIENTS

CHAPTER 5

Edited by Massimo Simion, Michele Maglione and Paolo Bozzoli

INTRODUCTION

A proper implant-supported restoration requires adequate diagnosis and treatment planning based on the information gathered from the anamnesis, oral examination, and radiographic evaluation. Most treatment failures in implantology are secondary to inadequate treatment planning. When considering a patient as a candidate for implant therapy, a precise, step-by-step treatment plan must be drafted.

DIAGNOSIS

The first fundamental step in diagnosis is the collection of anamnestic data. The best way to do this is to invite the patient to complete a questionnaire collecting all the necessary information **(Fig 1)**. The key things to consider include the presence of systemic diseases that contraindicate oral surgery and the consumption of medications or substances that may predispose the patient to complications (eg, bisphosphonates and smoking). Once the questionnaire has been completed, further questions need to be asked to expand on the relevant information that has emerged. Clinicians should bear in mind that the patient may be unaware of the implications that certain diseases or drugs may have on implant therapy.

With the oral examination, the patient is immediately placed into a classification based on complete or partial edentulism in the esthetic areas and posterolateral areas. Bi-digital inspection and palpation can provide information about the trophism of the bone in the edentulous ridges and the quality of the soft tissue. The examination should include a thorough evaluation of periodontal health, oral hygiene, the occlusal situation, and the presence of parafunctional habits, such as bruxism and clenching.

> *To assign individual patients to a classification is always reductive, as are the classifications themselves. The variables in each clinical case are infinite, and only the practitioner's experience and knowledge can lead to the correct treatment choices.*
>
> *Massimo Simion*

Anamnestic questionnaire

Last name

First name

Home address

ZIP code	**City**	**State**
Date of birth	**City**	**State**

Home phone number	**Office phone number**
Cell phone number	**Profession**

e-mail

Referred by

MEDICAL QUESTIONNAIRE
The answers to the following questionnaire are strictly confidential. Any untruthful response presents a risk to the patient, the doctor, and the practice staff and hinders the best results of any therapy.
Do you take drugs?

Do you take drugs? If yes, which ones?	☐ Yes	☐ No	☐ Don't know
Do you take anticoagulants?	☐ Yes	☐ No	☐ Don't know
Do you take steroids?	☐ Yes	☐ No	☐ Don't know
Do you suffer from diseases of the nervous system?	☐ Yes	☐ No	☐ Don't know
Do you take psychotropic drugs?	☐ Yes	☐ No	☐ Don't know
Do you suffer from osteoporosis?	☐ Yes	☐ No	☐ Don't know
Are you taking or have you taken medication for osteoporosis?	☐ Yes	☐ No	☐ Don't know
Do you suffer or have you suffered from asthma or other allergic diseases? If yes, which ones?	☐ Yes	☐ No	☐ Don't know
Have you ever had allergic reactions to the use of local anesthetics, antibiotics, or other substances? If yes, which ones?	☐ Yes	☐ No	☐ Don't know
Have you ever had any accidents during general or local anesthesia?	☐ Yes	☐ No	☐ Don't know
Do you suffer or have you suffered from changes in blood pressure? Pressure values	☐ Yes	☐ No	☐ Don't know
Do you suffer or have you suffered from diabetes mellitus?	☐ Yes	☐ No	☐ Don't know
Do you take insulin?	☐ Yes	☐ No	☐ Don't know
Do you suffer or have you suffered from heart disease? If yes, which ones?	☐ Yes	☐ No	☐ Don't know
Do you suffer or have you suffered from blood diseases?	☐ Yes	☐ No	☐ Don't know
Do you suffer from hemorrhagic diseases?	☐ Yes	☐ No	☐ Don't know
Have you had transfusions?	☐ Yes	☐ No	☐ Don't know

Fig 1 *Anamnestic questionnaire.*

Continued

Do you suffer or have you suffered from ear complaints?	☐ Yes	☐ No	☐ Don't know
SofDo you suffer or have you suffered from rheumatic diseases?	☐ Yes	☐ No	☐ Don't know
Do you suffer from digestive tract diseases? If yes, which ones?	☐ Yes	☐ No	☐ Don't know
Do you suffer or have you suffered from kidney disease?	☐ Yes	☐ No	☐ Don't know
Do you suffer or have you suffered from eye diseases?	☐ Yes	☐ No	☐ Don't know
Do you suffer or have you suffered from thyroid disease?	☐ Yes	☐ No	☐ Don't know
Are you a smoker? If yes, how many cigarettes per day?	☐ Yes	☐ No	☐ Don't know
Are you HIV positive?	☐ Yes	☐ No	☐ Don't know
Do you suffer or have you suffered from infectious diseases?	☐ Yes	☐ No	☐ Don't know
Do you use or have you used drugs?	☐ Yes	☐ No	☐ Don't know
Have you ever fallen ill with viral hepatitis type A, B, or C?	☐ Yes	☐ No	☐ Don't know
Are you a healthy carrier of hepatitis?	☐ Yes	☐ No	☐ Don't know
Suspected pregnancy?	☐ Yes	☐ No	☐ Don't know
Do you take birth control pills?	☐ Yes	☐ No	☐ Don't know
Have you been hospitalized in recent years?	☐ Yes	☐ No	☐ Don't know
Have you suffered from a serious illness in the last 3 years?	☐ Yes	☐ No	☐ Don't know
Have you undergone radiation therapy?	☐ Yes	☐ No	☐ Don't know
Do you suffer or have you suffered from epilepsy?	☐ Yes	☐ No	☐ Don't know
Do you suffer or have you suffered from headaches?	☐ Yes	☐ No	☐ Don't know
Do you suffer from skin diseases?			
Do you have any other illnesses not mentioned? / Do you have any other information to report?			
When was your last visit to a dentist?			

Patient's signature

Date ....

Fig 1 *(Continued)*

M. Simion • M. Maglione • P. Bozzoli

Radiographic examination naturally plays a key role in the 3D assessment of bone tissue. In the early days of osseointegrated implants, 2D periapical radiography was the most widely used tool for examination, but it has now been completely replaced by CBCT, which allows for the evaluation of both the vertical dimension and the thickness of the alveolar bone.

CLASSIFICATION OF TOTALLY EDENTULOUS RIDGES AND CORRESPONDING TREATMENT PLANNING

Despite their limitations, classifications do provide general guidelines that can assist clinicians in drafting the treatment plan. Since the advent of osseointegrated implants in the 1980s, numerous classifications have been proposed based on the trophism of the edentulous alveolar ridges.[1–3] Here, we refer to the 1985 classification of Lekholm and Zarb[3] for its clarity and simplicity **(Fig 2)** (see chapter 4). The indications for implant treatment are different in the maxilla and mandible because of the differences in anatomy and bone quality between the two structures.

Maxilla: therapeutic indications

1. In Class A and B maxillae, both the vertical dimension and the thickness of the bone allow for the placement of implants with standard techniques.[4,5] Subsequent prosthetic rehabilitation will take the form of a screw-retained fixed prosthesis with or without a gingival flange. Depending on the quality of the bone and the judgement of the clinician, either immediate prosthetic loading[6,7] (see chapter 8) or delayed prosthetic loading[4,5] with or without guided surgery (see chapter 6) may be performed.[8–12]

2. In Class C maxillae, the quantity of residual bone does not allow for implants to be inserted without exposing part of the threaded implant surface outside the bone structure. Therefore, it is always necessary to use regenerative techniques to treat dehiscences, fenestrations, or peri-implant bone defects (see chapters 14 to 18). More advanced cases of atrophy may require a two-stage treatment involving bone regeneration before implant placement.

3. Class D and E maxillae require major Le Fort I surgery with interpositional grafts taken from the iliac crest.[13,14]

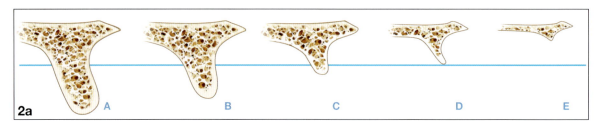

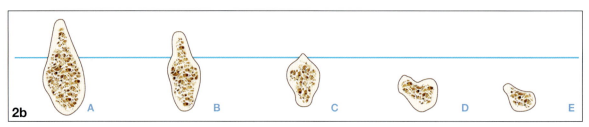

Fig 2 *Representation of the edentulous jaws according to Lekholm and Zarb's 1985 classification. (a) Maxilla. (b) Mandible.[3]*

CLINICAL CASE 1

Rehabilitation of a Class A/B maxilla with implants without prosthetic replacement of the gingival tissues

A 70-year-old patient who was formerly a smoker and was undergoing treatment with antihypertensives, presented with several edentulous sites in the maxilla and mandible. The remaining teeth were affected by numerous endodontic and structural problems related to both the coronal and radicular tissues **(Figs 3 and 4)**. In accordance with the patient's requests, the decision was made to provide an implant-supported restoration for the entire maxilla. All the remaining maxillary teeth were extracted in the same session, and the sockets were filled with deproteinized bovine bone mineral (DBBM; Bio-Oss, Geistlich Biomaterials) **(Fig 5)**. After 4 months of healing, six implants were placed medial to the mesial walls of the maxillary sinuses, and an immediate load was applied by means of a provisional prosthesis without a gingival flange because of the complete preservation of the alveolar process. After 4 months of soft tissue conditioning with the provisional **(Figs 6 and 7)**, the final ceramic prosthesis was fabricated, also without a gingival flange **(Figs 8 to 10)**.

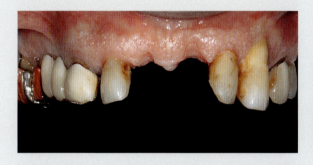

Fig 3 Clinical image of the maxilla. Several teeth are missing, and the remaining teeth are affected by multiple root caries beneath old prosthetic restorations.

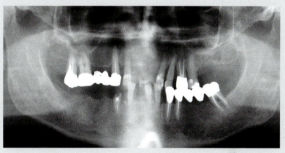

Fig 4 A panoramic radiograph shows numerous endodontic and root structural problems.

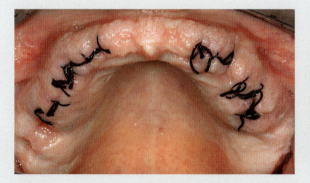

Fig 5 The state of mucosal healing 15 days after tooth extraction and grafting with Bio-Oss.

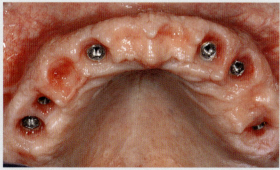

Fig 6 Six implants were placed in locations 15, 14, 12, 22, 23, and 25, with placement of the provisional after 48 hours.

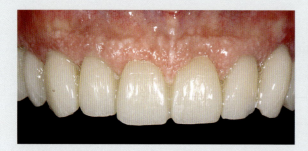 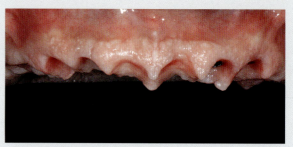

Figs 7 *(a)* Clinical image of the provisional after conditioning and tissue maturation after 4 months of function. The presence of interdental papillae and the correct shape of the gingival margin parabolas can be seen. *(b)* Clinical appearance of the mucosa upon removal of the provisional denture after 4 months. The gingival contours affected by the use of the provisional denture can be seen.

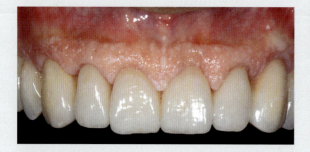 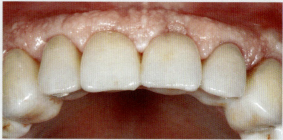

Fig 8 Final zirconia and ceramic prosthesis after 6 months of function. The absence of a gingival flange and the maturation of the natural mucosa can be seen.

Fig 9 Appearance of the buccal mucosa from an occlusal view. The considerable thickness of the keratinized mucosa can be seen.

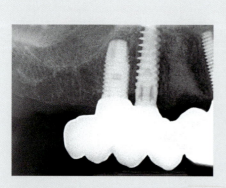 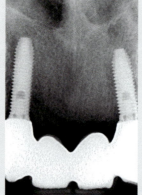 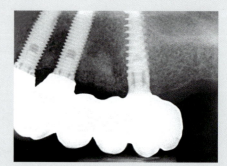

Fig 10 Follow-up with periapical radiographs of the implants after 1 year of prosthetic loading.

CLINICAL CASE 2

Rehabilitation of a maxilla with Class C atrophy with an implant-supported restoration after bone regeneration and sinus elevation procedures

A 38-year-old, nonsmoking patient presented with an extensive edentulous span in the maxilla. Teeth 17, 15, 27, and 28 (FDI tooth numbering system) were present and were temporarily maintained to support a provisional prosthesis **(Fig 11)**. Panoramic radiographs and CT scans showed Class C bone atrophy associated with bilateral expansion of the maxillary sinuses **(Figs 12 and 13)**. The residual basal bone was 10 mm in a vertical dimension and 3 mm thick in the anterior sector and 2 to 4 mm in vertical dimension by 1 to 2 mm in thickness in the posterolateral sectors.
It was decided to perform horizontal guided bone regeneration (GBR) combined with bilateral elevation of the maxillary sinuses and the floor of the nasal fossae.

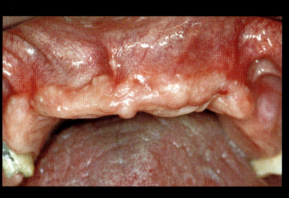

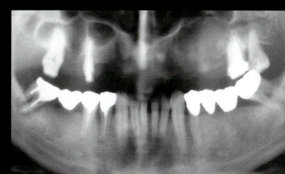

Fig 11 Clinical image of the edentulous atrophic alveolar ridge.

Fig 12 Panoramic radiograph showing the considerable expansion of the maxillary sinuses and the reduced vertical dimension of the alveolar bone at the nasal fossae.

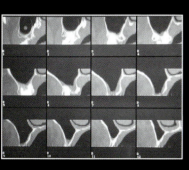
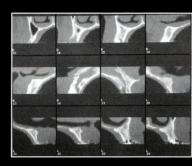
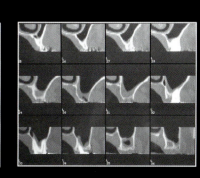

Fig 13 Axial CT cross sections showing the limited thickness of the residual alveolar ridge.

Two full-thickness flaps, one buccal and one palatal, were elevated from tooth 17 to 27, exposing the maxillary sinuses and pyriform aperture (Fig 14).

After harvesting bone from the chin with an 8-mm trephine bur, two bone blocks were placed inside the nasal floor (Fig 15), and two onlay blocks were placed at the buccal aspect of the incisor area (Fig 16). The maxillary sinuses and the spaces around the blocks were filled with freeze-dried bone allograft (FDBA). The sinus osteotomies and buccal bone blocks were covered with a titanium-reinforced extended polytetrafluorethylene (e-PTFE) membrane (Fig 17).

The healing period lasted 6 months and was free of complications. The membranes were then removed (Fig 18), and seven machined implants were placed, remaining submerged for an additional 6 months (Fig 19).

After uncovering the implants, teeth 27 and 28 were extracted, and the provisional denture was placed. The patient was finally rehabilitated with a removable fixed prosthesis (Fig 20).

In the following years, tooth 15 and some mandibular teeth were also replaced with implants (Fig 21), and the definitive zirconia and ceramic prosthesis was replaced (Fig 22).

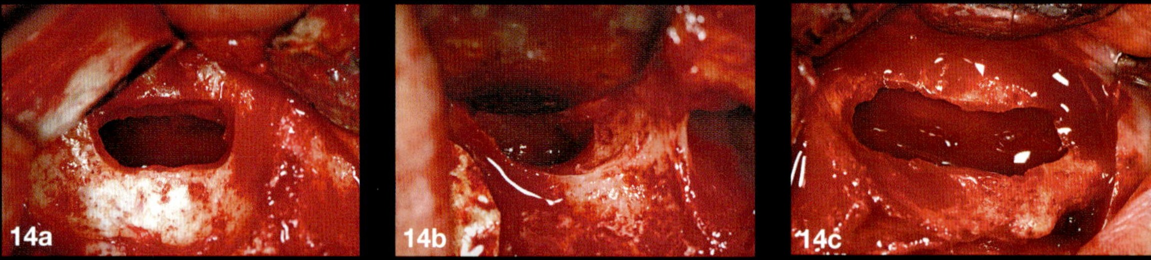

Fig 14 A wide full-thickness flap extending from tooth 17 to 27 was elevated, and osteotomies of the lateral walls of the maxillary sinuses (a and c) and the exposed nasal fossae (b) were performed.

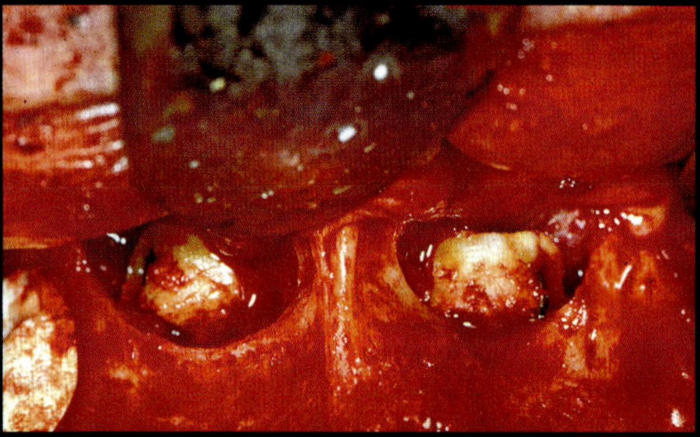

Fig 15 Two block grafts taken from the chin were placed in the floor of the nose and fixed to the septum with two osteosynthesis screws.

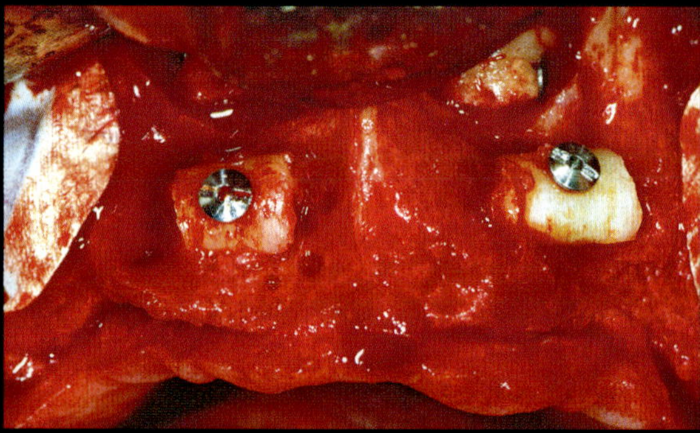

Fig 16 The maxillary sinuses were filled with FDBA, and two block grafts were attached on the buccal aspect of the ridge.

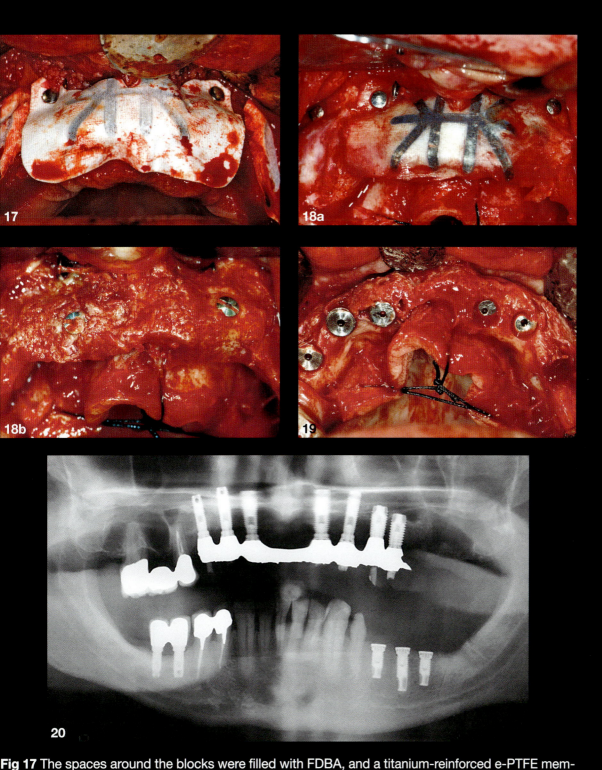

Fig 17 The spaces around the blocks were filled with FDBA, and a titanium-reinforced e-PTFE membrane was applied. **Fig 18** (a) After 6 months of submerged healing, the membranes were exposed and removed, showing (b) the new regenerated bone covering the blocks of autologous bone. **Fig 19** Seven machined implants were inserted and left to integrate in a submerged position for 6 months. **Fig 20** Panoramic radiograph of the prosthesis after 5 years of function.

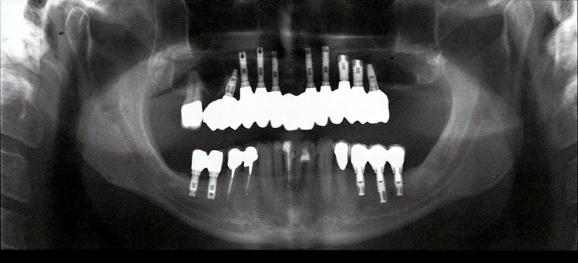

Fig 21 Control panoramic radiograph 24 years after the first operation. Teeth 15 and 25 were extracted and replaced with new implants, and the removable fixed prosthesis was replaced.

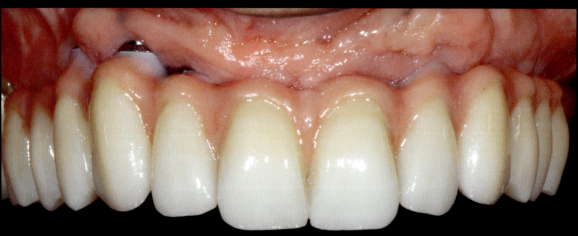

Fig 22 Clinical image of the new fixed ceramic prosthesis.

CLINICAL CASE 3

Rehabilitation of a Class D/E maxilla with an implant-supported restoration after Le Fort I surgery with interpositional bone grafting

A 52-year-old nonsmoking patient in good systemic health presented with Class D atrophy in a completely edentulous maxilla **(Fig 23)**. Centripetal resorption of the maxilla resulted in a Class III maxillomandibular relationship with pronounced mandibular protrusion **(Fig 24)**.

Le Fort I surgery with interpositional bone grafting was performed to simultaneously correct the vertical dimension of the residual bone and the maxillomandibular relationship. In the mandible, four implants (and subsequently two more) were placed in the first phase to support a fixed restoration.

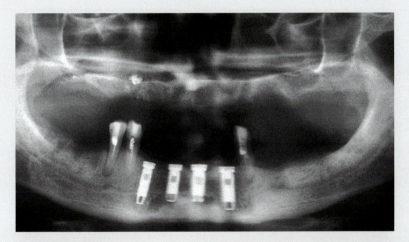

Fig 23 Panoramic radiograph showing the extremely reduced vertical dimension of the basal bone. Four implants have already been placed in the mandible, and some natural teeth have been temporarily retained to stabilize a provisional prosthesis.

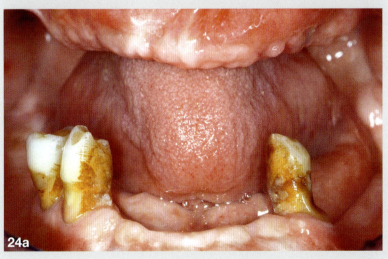
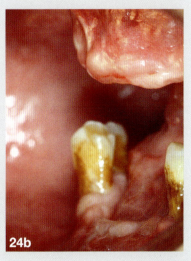

Fig 24 Clinical image of the atrophic Class D maxillary alveolar ridge. The severe sagittal plane discrepancy between the jaws in a Class III relationship is evident. *(a)* Frontal view. *(b)* Lateral view.

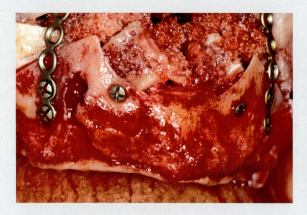

Fig 25 Osteotomy of the maxilla using the Le Fort I technique. The maxilla was advanced forward and downward to correct the maxillomandibular relationship, and blocks of bone harvested from the iliac crest were inserted to increase the vertical dimension.

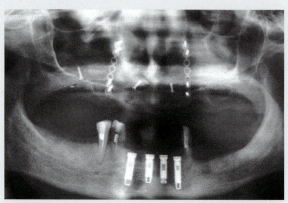

Fig 26 Control panoramic radiograph after surgery. The osteosynthesis plates used to stabilize the maxilla are visible.

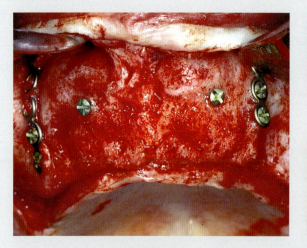

Fig 27 After 4 months of healing, the bone grafts appear perfectly integrated.

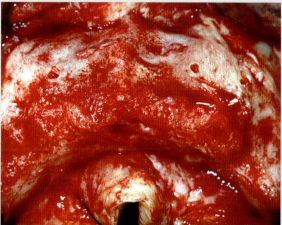

Fig 28 The osteosynthesis plates were removed together with the graft fixation screws.

The Le Fort I operation involved performing an incision in the fornix from tooth sites 17 to 27, an osteotomy of the lateral wall of the maxillary sinuses up to the nasal fossae, and an osteotomy of the nasal septum, the lateral pillars, and the pterygoid processes.

Bone blocks were harvested from the iliac crest and fixed to the floor of the maxillary sinuses and nose. The maxilla was then fixed in a protruded position with osteosynthesis plates to correct the skeletal Class III relationship **(Figs 25 and 26)**.

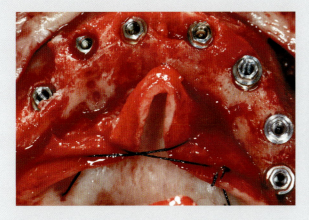

Fig 29 Seven implants with a length of 15 mm and a diameter of 3.75 mm were placed.

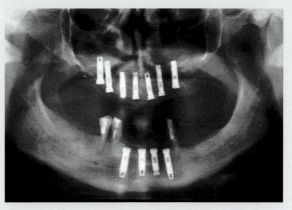

Fig 30 Postoperative panoramic radiograph.

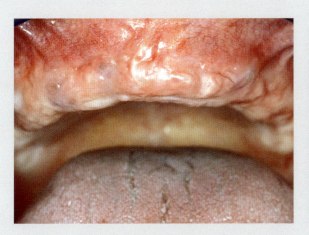

Fig 31 Healing occurred without any adverse events, and the implants remained submerged for 6 months.

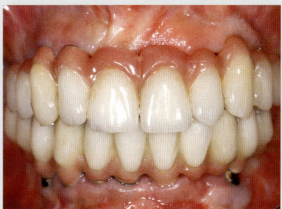

Fig 32 Two additional implants were placed in the mandible in positions 34 and 44, and the patient was rehabilitated with fixed removable dentures.

After 4 months of healing, the osteosynthesis plates were removed (**Figs 27 and 28**), and seven Brånemark-type implants, 15 mm in length by 3.75 mm in diameter, were inserted (**Figs 29 and 30**). After 6 months of submerged healing, the prosthetic abutments and a removable fixed prosthesis were connected (**Figs 31 and 32**).

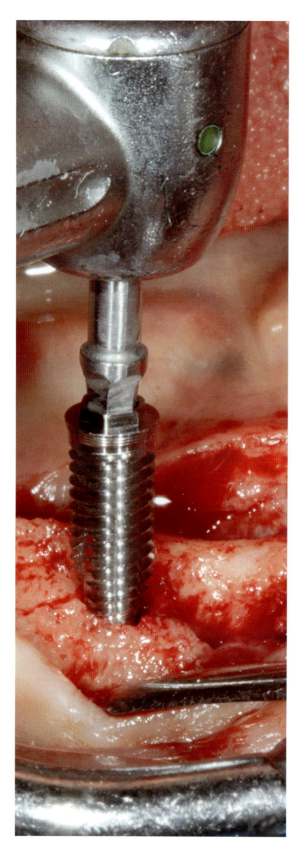

Mandible: therapeutic indications

- In Class A and B mandibles, the amount of bone available medial to the mental foramen is still very abundant and allows for the placement of implants with standard techniques. In most cases, immediate prosthetic loading is the treatment of choice, and in some cases, guided implant surgery is indicated.

- In Class C mandibles, the vertical dimension of the mandibular body is still sufficient (> 10 mm), although the thickness of its coronal portion may be very limited. If the crestal portion is limited to a few millimeters, an ostectomy can be used until sufficient thickness (4–5 mm) is obtained for implant positioning with standard techniques, but if almost the entire mandibular body is limited in thickness, it is necessary to resort to single- or two-stage GBR techniques (see chapter 16).

- In Class D mandibles, the vertical bone dimension is very limited (< 10 mm) and can be as short as 6 mm, but generally, at the level of the mandibular body medial to the mental foramina, the thickness is considerable (up to 10 mm). Therefore, due to the high quality of the bone, which is composed exclusively of cortical bone, it is possible to place short implants using standard techniques.[15] In these cases, a two-stage procedure with submerged implant healing for 3 months and delayed loading is recommended.

- Class E atrophy in the mandible is extremely rare. In fact, muscle function alone is usually sufficient to prevent the bone from atrophying beyond class D. In Class E mandibles, bone height is less than 8 mm, and its thickness is less than 3 mm. In these rare cases, it is always necessary to perform horizontal augmentation of the basal bone first and place the implants at a later stage. Generally, no more than four implants are placed so as not to weaken the mandibular body, and delayed loading is performed after 3 months of submerged implant osseointegration.

CLINICAL CASE 4

Rehabilitation of a mandible with Class A atrophy with guided implant surgery and immediate loading

A 69-year-old, nonsmoking, systemically healthy patient presented with severe periodontitis. In the maxilla, only teeth 13, 12, 11, 21, 22, and 23 were present, and 22 and 23 showed severe loss of bone support **(Fig 33)**. In the mandible, all remaining teeth appeared hopelessly compromised by periodontitis. The treatment plan included the extraction of teeth 22 and 23 and the placement of a provisional removable prosthesis in the maxilla and the extraction of all remaining teeth in the mandible for subsequent treatment with an implant-supported fixed prosthesis **(Fig 34)**.

The high amount of bone support in the jaw and the presence of an adequate band of keratinized mucosa led to a preference for treatment via flapless guided surgery. After 2.5 months of healing from the extractions, CBCT was performed with a radiographic stent for digital image matching **(Fig 35)**. The CBCT images were imported into software, and implant position planning was based on the digital diagnostic wax-up, the amount and location of the remaining mandibular bone, and soft tissue thickness **(Fig 36)**. Consequently, a surgical guide and a provisional prosthesis were constructed to be relined and passivated in the mouth after surgery.

At the time of surgery, a silicone positioner was used to aid in the fixation of the surgical template to the edentulous mandible with three endosseous pins **(Figs 37 and 38)**. The four implant sites were prepared under copious irrigation with saline solution in locations 36, 33, 43, and 46 according to the drill sequence of the guided surgery kit **(Fig 39)**. The implants were also inserted with the surgical guide **(Figs 40 and 41)**.

Once the surgical guide was removed, the implants were connected to the multiunit abutments (MUAs) **(Fig 42)** and titanium abutments **(Fig 43)** to receive the provisional prosthesis.

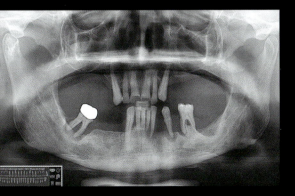

Fig 33 Initial panoramic radiograph. Teeth 22, 23, and all the mandibular teeth appear irreparably compromised by periodontitis.

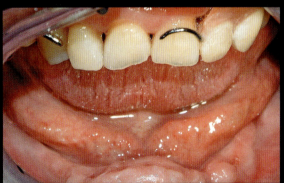

Fig 34 The maxilla was rehabilitated with a provisional removable prosthesis, and all the remaining mandibular teeth were extracted.

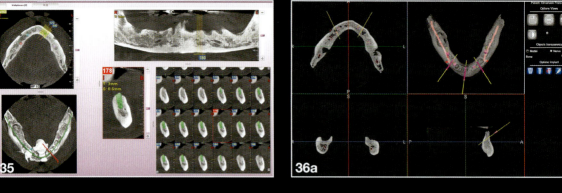

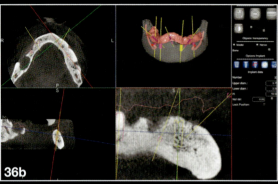

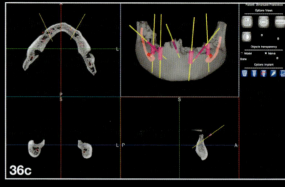

Fig 35 CBCT imaging with a radiographic stent was performed and imported into guided surgery software. **Fig 36** *(a)* Planning the correct positioning of the four implants and the three fixation pins. View of axial images. *(b)* Buccal view showing the soft tissues. *(c)* Implant positioning based on the diagnostic wax-up and residual bone volume.

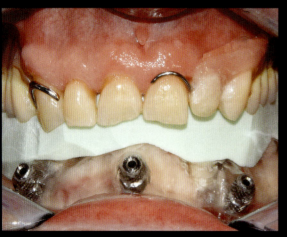

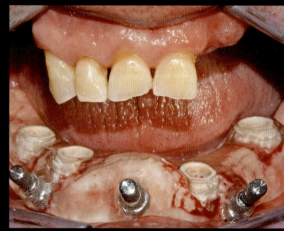

Fig 37 Surgical guide positioned in the mouth with the help of a silicone guide.

Fig 38 The surgical guide fixed with three endosseous pins.

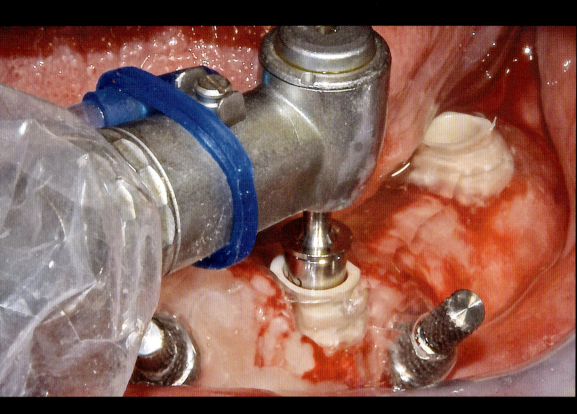

Fig 39 Implant sites 36, 33, 43, and 46 were prepared with calibrated drills and the surgical guide.

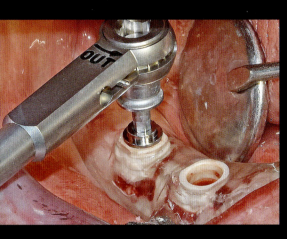

Fig 40 Insertion of the implant in position 46 with a dynamometric ratchet. The insertion torque must not exceed 45 Ncm.

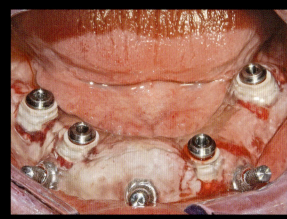

Fig 41 The implants have been placed in their locations.

The previously prepared prosthesis was placed in the mouth, with the central endosseous pin used to establish the correct position **(Fig 44)**, and connected passively by adding resin around the titanium abutments **(Fig 45)**.

After complete polymerization of the resin, the prosthesis was removed, finished, polished, and screwed back into the mouth **(Figs 46 and 47)**.

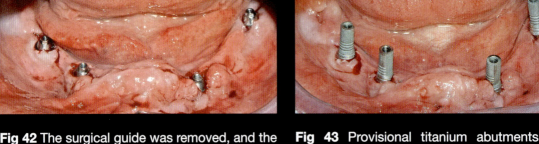

Fig 42 The surgical guide was removed, and the MUA abutments fitted.

Fig 43 Provisional titanium abutments were mounted on the MUAs.

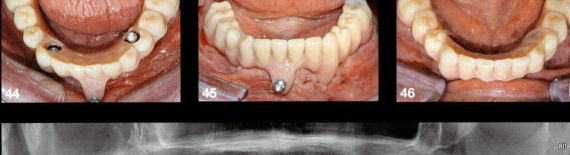

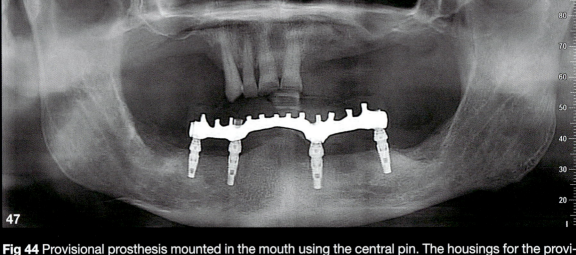

Fig 44 Provisional prosthesis mounted in the mouth using the central pin. The housings for the provisional abutments are countersunk to allow relining with resin without tension. **Fig 45** The prosthesis was passively fixed to the abutments with resin in the correct position. **Fig 46** The provisional denture was screwed back into the mouth, and the fixation holes were sealed with resin and finished. **Fig 47** Final panoramic radiograph.

CLINICAL CASE 5

Rehabilitation of a mandible with Class B atrophy with implants and early loading

A patient with a maxillary implant-supported restoration and a mandibular complete denture expressed the wish for a fixed prosthesis in the mandible as well (**Fig 48**). Panoramic radiograph imaging showed vertical bone atrophy in the posterolateral sectors but a remarkably well-preserved vertical dimension of bone in the body of the mandible (**Fig 49**), allowing for the placement of five implants mesial to the mental foramen.

A full-thickness flap was elevated, and implant site preparations were made. The two distal preparations were made slightly apart (**Fig 50**). After tapping and countersinking, five iMAX (iRES) machined surface implants were inserted (**Figs 51 and 52**). Before suturing, provisional healing abutments were placed (**Fig 53**). The provisional prosthesis was placed after 48 hours (**Figs 54 and 55**), and after 3 months of function and soft tissue maturation, an impression was taken (**Figs 56 and 57**) for the definitive prosthesis in titanium with preformed resin teeth (**Figs 58 and 59**).

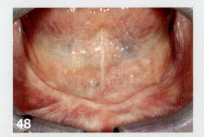
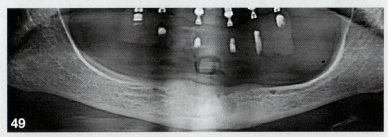

Fig 48 Clinical image of the edentulous mandible. Note the modest atrophy and the scarcity of keratinized mucosa. **Fig 49** Panoramic radiograph showing the considerable vertical dimension of the intraforaminal bone.

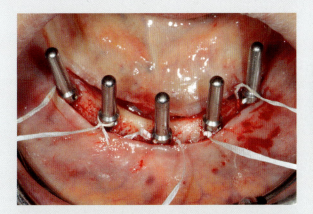
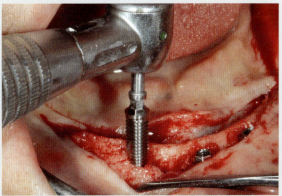

Fig 50 After full-thickness flap elevation, the implant sites were prepared. Notice that the distal parallel pins are slightly divergent.

Fig 51 After tapping and countersinking, iMAX implants with fully machined surfaces were inserted.

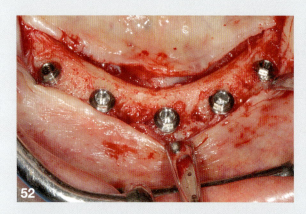
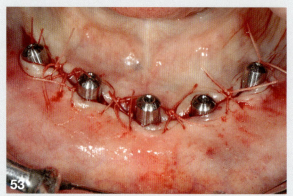

Fig 52 The implant heads were placed slightly below the alveolar ridge. **Fig 53** Healing abutments were placed, and Laurell-Gottlow sutures were placed in the peri-implant spaces.

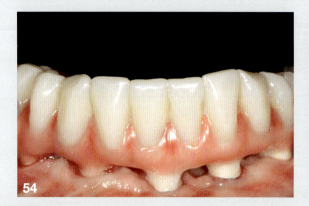
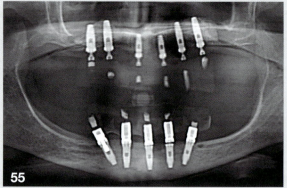

Fig 54 The provisional resin prosthesis was fitted and maintained for 6 months. **Fig 55** Radiographic image of the implants after 6 months of function.

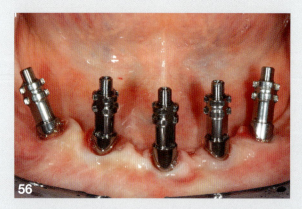
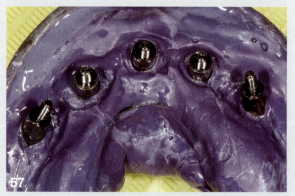

Fig 56 Impression coping abutment positioned at the time of fabrication of the definitive prosthesis. **Fig 57** Impression with personalized polyether impression tray with transfers in place.

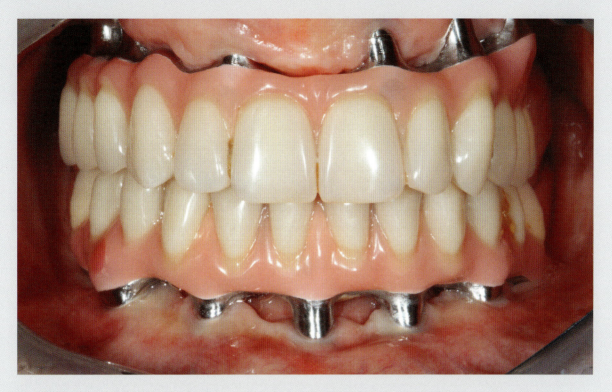

Fig 58 Definitive titanium prosthesis and prefabricated teeth delivered after 6 months of function.

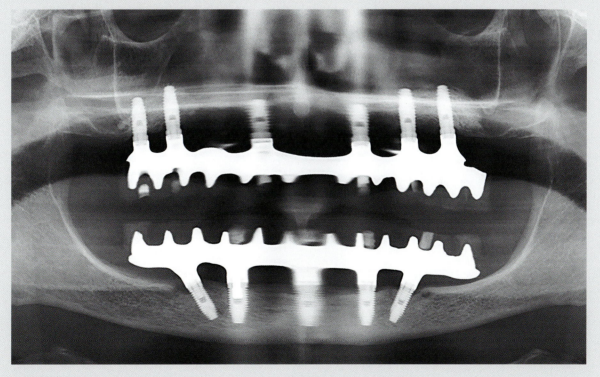

Fig 59 Panoramic radiograph after 6 months of function.

A 68-year-old, completely edentulous, nonsmoking woman in good health presented with indications for a fixed mandibular restoration. The intraoral clinical examination **(Fig 60)** and CBCT imaging showed severe vertical bone atrophy in the posterolateral sectors of the mandible and considerable horizontal bone resorption in the symphyseal region medial to the mental foramina **(Fig 61)**.

Because the thickness of the alveolar bone was incompatible with the placement of implants, the treatment plan involved horizontal ridge augmentation with resorbable collagen membrane and particulate bone graft and the subsequent placement of four implants 6 months later.

A full-thickness flap was elevated from tooth sites 16 to 26, taking care not to sever the inferior alveolar nerve, which had a supraosseous crestal path due to bone atrophy **(Fig 62)**. A resorbable porcine collagen membrane (CellGro, Orthocell) was fixed to the lower margin of the mandible with titanium pins, and a particulate graft composed of 70% autologous bone and 30% DBBM (BioOss) was placed buccal to the body of the mandible **(Fig 63)**.

The membrane was then repositioned over the graft and fixed securely to the ridge with four titanium pins **(Fig 64)**.

Healing occurred without any adverse phenomena **(Fig 65)**. After 6 months, CBCT imaging showed an increase in the thickness of the mandibular body sufficient for implant placement **(Fig 66)**. A new flap was elevated **(Fig 67)**, the crestal fixation pins were removed, and four hybrid iMAX implants (3.75 x 11 mm) were placed **(Figs 68 and 69)**.

The implants were submerged for 4 months to wait for complete osseointegration **(Fig 70)**, then the connection of the provisional abutments was performed, keeping half of the residual keratinized mucosa in a buccal position and half in a lingual position **(Fig 71)**. The final rehabilitation was performed with a removable fixed prosthesis **(Figs 72 and 73)**.

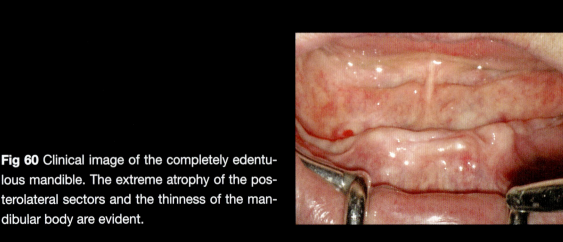

Fig 60 Clinical image of the completely edentulous mandible. The extreme atrophy of the posterolateral sectors and the thinness of the mandibular body are evident.

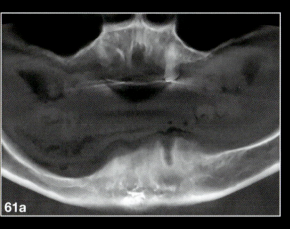
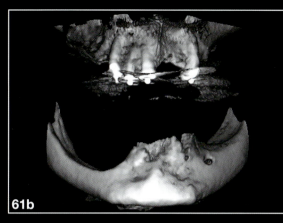
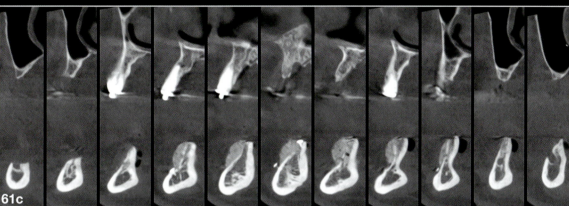

Fig 61 CBCT imaging confirmed the clinical examination. Panoramic *(a)*, 3D *(b)*, and cross-sectional (c) views.

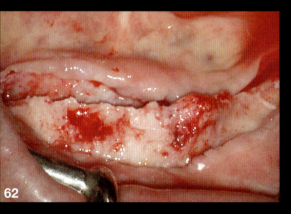
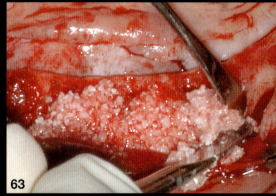

Fig 62 A full-thickness incision was made up to the areas distal to the mental foramen, taking care not to sever the inferior alveolar nerve at its emergence in the alveolar ridge. The buccal and lingual full-thickness flaps were gently elevated. **Fig 63** The upper portion of the extremely thin ridge was re-shaped with bone rongeur forceps and, after performing cortical perforations, a collagen membrane (CellGro) was applied to the lower margin of the defect. A particulate bone graft with 70% autologous bone and 30% DBBM (Bio-Oss) was placed on the buccal aspect.

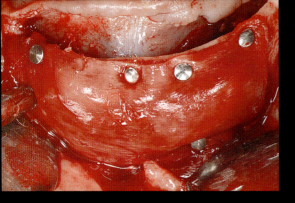

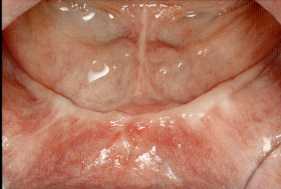

Fig 64 The membrane was tightly secured with four titanium pins to hold and stabilize the bone graft.

Fig 65 Appearance of the mucosa after 6 months of healing.

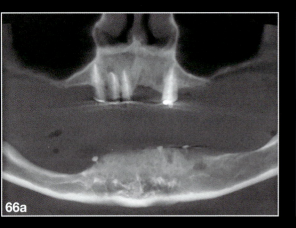

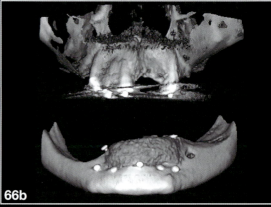

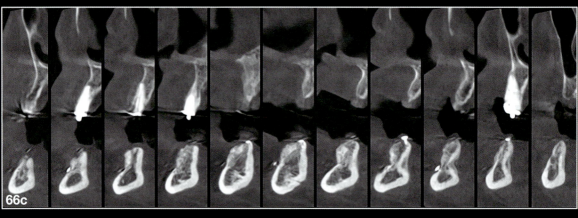

Fig 66 CBCT showing the horizontal augmentation obtained medial to the mental foramen after 6 months of healing. *(a)* Panoramic, *(b)* 3D, and *(c)* cross-sectional views.

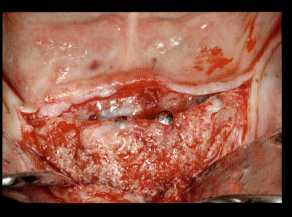

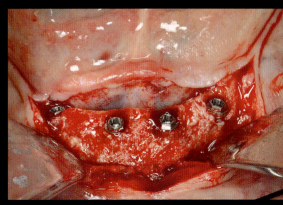

Fig 67 After 6 months of healing, a flap was elevated to expose the regenerated bone and remove the fixation pins.

Fig 68 Four iMAX hybrid implants were placed medial to the mental foramen.

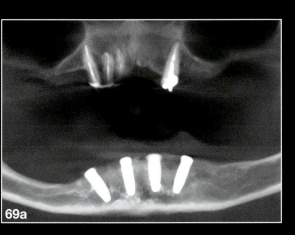

69a

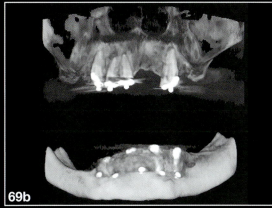

69b

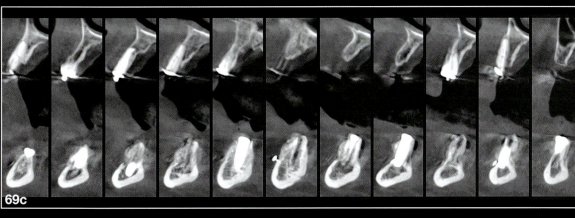

69c

Fig 69 CBCT highlighting the positioning of the implants within the regenerated bone. *(a)* Panoramic, *(b)* 3D, and *(c)* cross-sectional views.

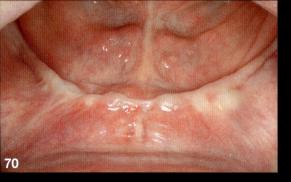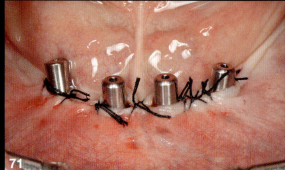

Fig 70 The implants remained submerged for another 4 months. **Fig 71** The connection of the provisional abutments was performed with a partial-thickness incision in the center of the residual keratinized mucosa, keeping half of the mucosa lingual and half of it buccal.

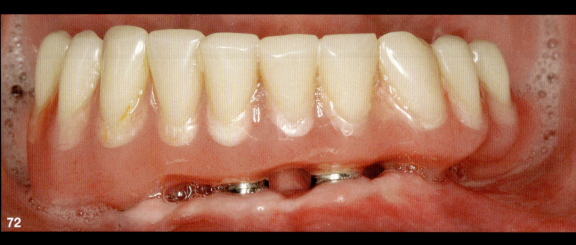

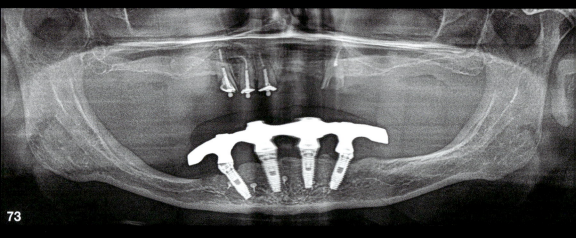

Fig 72 Toronto-type definitive prosthesis in function. Sufficient keratinized mucosa and the excellent health of the peri-implant soft tissues are evident. **Fig 73** Control panoramic radiograph after 6 months of prosthetic loading. The crestal bone margin remained stable at the first thread loop where the countersink was performed.

CLINICAL CASE 7

Rehabilitation of a mandible with Class D atrophy with short implants without regenerative

A 40-year-old patient who had been edentulous for a long time was unable to wear removable total dentures due to extreme maxillary atrophy (**Fig 74**). Panoramic radiograph (**Fig 75**), laterolateral teleradiograph (**Fig 76**), and CBCT imaging (**Fig 77**) showed Class D mandibular atrophy, with bone dimensions being 6 mm vertically and 12 mm horizontally. The maxilla, also with Class D atrophy, was rehabilitated with a Le Fort I–type procedure with an interpositional graft harvested from the iliac crest (**Fig 78**) and eight machined Brånemark implants (**Fig 79**). In the mandible, five machined Nobel Biocare implants with diameters of 3.75 mm and lengths of 7 mm were placed without the performance of any regenerative interventions. Preparation of the implant sites in the body of the mandible medial to the mental foramen (which is extremely well-mineralized bone) was performed using the entire available vertical dimension of the bone from the upper to the lower margin. Careful tapping was performed to avoid excessive expansive forces during implant placement (**Fig 80**).

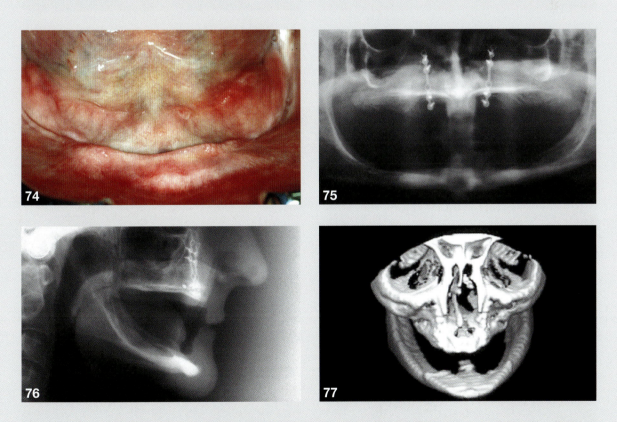

Fig 74 Clinical image of a mandible with Class D atrophy. **Fig 75** Panoramic radiograph showing a vertical dimension of 6 mm in the body of the mandible. In the maxilla, a Le Fort I–type operation with an interpositional graft harvested from the iliac crest has already been performed. **Fig 76** Laterolateral teleradiograph showing extreme mandibular atrophy. **Fig 77** On the CT scan in 3D view, the considerable horizontal dimension of the residual basal bone is visible.

The implants were inserted without excessive torque (< 40 Ncm), with the implant heads and cover screws left protruding above the bone crest **(Figs 81 and 82)**. Submerged osseointegration was allowed for 6 months in the maxilla and for 3 months in the mandible. After reopening, the patient was rehabilitated with two removable fixed Toronto-type prostheses **(Figs 83 and 84)**. After 7 years, an increase in mandibular bone volume following the restoration of masticatory function was visible **(Fig 85)**.

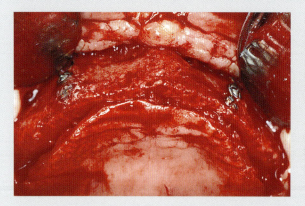

Fig 78 After 4 months of healing from the Le Fort I operation, the osteosynthesis plates were removed.

Fig 79 Eight implants (13 mm in length and 3.75 mm in diameter) were inserted.

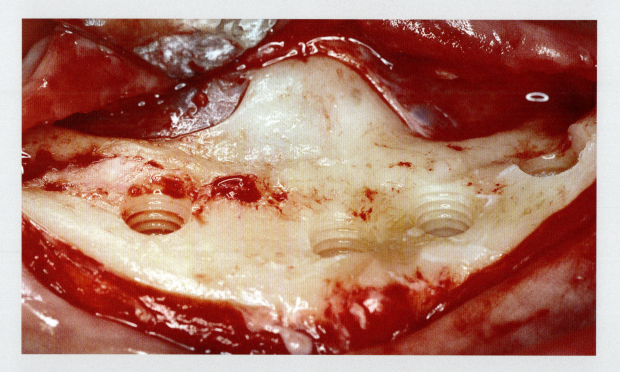

Fig 80 Preparation of the implant sites in the mandible. The basal bone appears to consist exclusively of cortical bone. The precise tapping of each site to avoid excessive expansive forces during implant placement is evident.

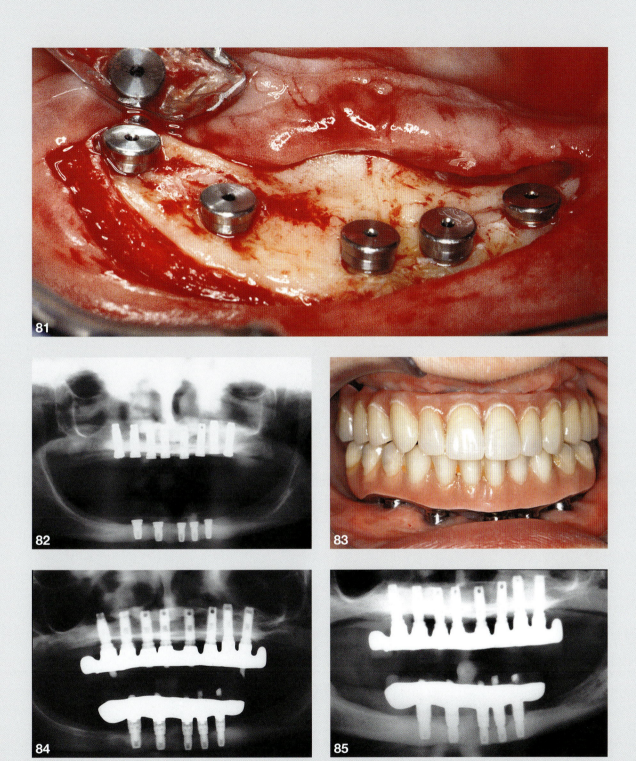

Fig 81 Five implants (7 mm in length and 3.75 mm in diameter) were inserted, leaving the heads and cover screws protruding above the crestal surface. **Fig 82** Control panoramic radiograph. **Fig 83** The patient was rehabilitated with two removable fixed prostheses. **Fig 84** Panoramic radiograph after delivery of the definitive restoration. **Fig 85** Panoramic radiograph at the 7-year follow-up. The increase in bone volume following the restoration of masticatory function is evident.

CLINICAL CASE 8

Rehabilitation of a mandible with Class E atrophy with horizontal bone regeneration

A 46-year-old completely edentulous patient had stopped wearing her mandibular complete denture for years due to its complete instability. The clinical examination **(Fig 86)**, panoramic radiograph **(Fig 87)**, and CT imaging revealed very severe Class E mandibular atrophy with a vertical dimension of 8 mm in the symphysis and a thickness of 2 to 3 mm **(Fig 88)**. Because the diameter of the implants to be placed exceeded the thickness of the available bone, the preparation of the recipient sites would

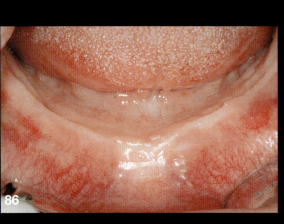
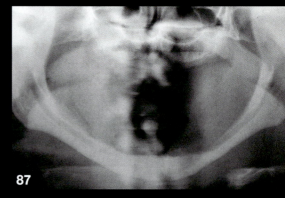

Fig 86 Extremely atrophic edentulous mandibular alveolar ridge in a 46-year-old woman. **Fig 87** The panoramic radiograph shows a vertical dimension of 8 mm in the body of the mandible. The mental foramina are in the vicinity of the upper margin of the ridge.

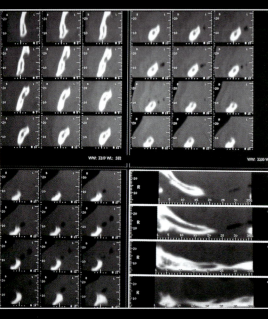
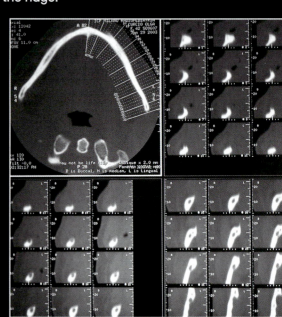

Fig 88 On the CT scan, the thinness of the entire extension of the jaw can be seen, with values ranging from 2 to 3 mm.

have interrupted the continuity of the mandible. Therefore a regenerative technique was necessary. After elevating a full-thickness flap and identifying the mental foramina **(Figs 89 and 90)**, four oblique screws were placed in the body of the mandible to establish the thickness of bone to be obtained with the GBR technique **(Fig 91)**.

Several perforations were performed in the cortical bone **(Fig 92)**, and two e-PTFE membranes were secured to the lower margin of the mandible with titanium pins. Because no intraoral sites were available for autologous bone harvesting, a particulate graft composed of a mixture of autologous bone, obtained from the cortical perforations, and demineralized freeze-dried bone allograft (DFDBA) (Regenaform) was used.

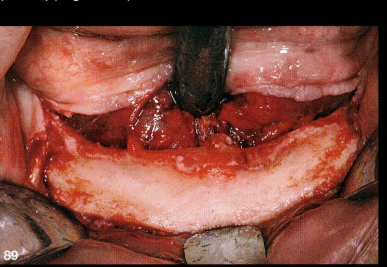 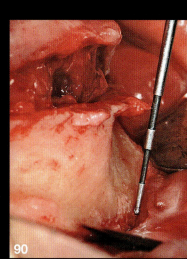

Fig 89 Two full-thickness flaps, one buccal and one lingual, exposing the inferior alveolar nerves bilaterally. **Fig 90** The vertical dimension is 8 mm, and the half-moon shape of the mandible results in a limited thickness of 2 to 3 mm.

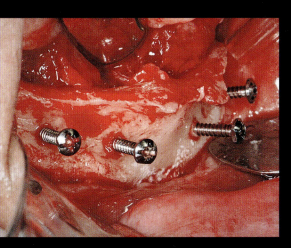 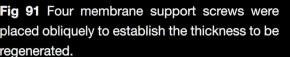 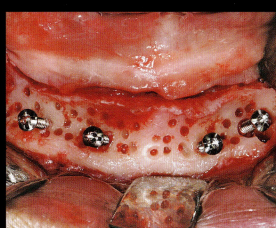

Fig 91 Four membrane support screws were placed obliquely to establish the thickness to be regenerated.

Fig 92 The cortical was abundantly perforated, and the bone particles were harvested to be used as a graft.

The graft was applied buccally around the supporting screws (Fig 93), and the membranes were re-positioned and fixed lingually (Figs 94 and 95). The flaps were released via periosteal incision and closed with horizontal mattress sutures and alternating simple sutures.

After 6 months of healing without complications, the membranes were removed, showing complete regeneration of the bone tissue (Fig 96). The bone thickness was sufficient for the placement of four machined implants 10 mm in length and 3.75 mm in diameter (Fig 97). After 3 months of submerged healing, healing abutments were placed (Fig 98), and the patient was rehabilitated with a removable fixed prosthesis (Figs 99 and 100).

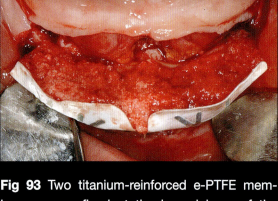

Fig 93 Two titanium-reinforced e-PTFE membranes were fixed at the buccal base of the mandible, and a mixture of autologous bone, obtained from cortical perforations, and DFDBA was placed around the supporting screws.

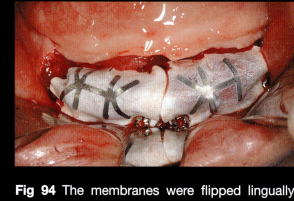

Fig 94 The membranes were flipped lingually and fixed on the mandibular crest with titanium tacks. The flaps were then released and sutured without tension.

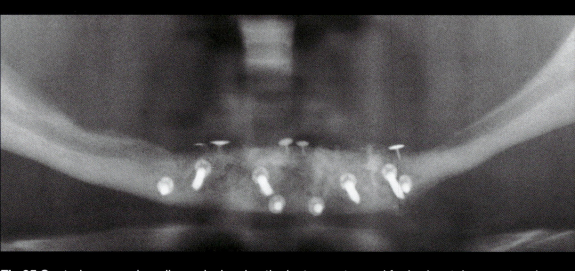

Fig 95 Control panoramic radiograph showing the instruments used for horizontal support and membrane fixation.

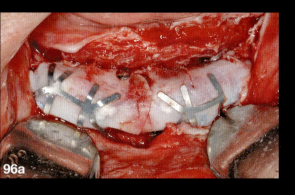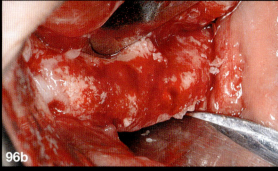

Fig 96 After 6 months of submerged healing *(a)*, the membranes were removed, revealing the newly formed bone *(b)*.

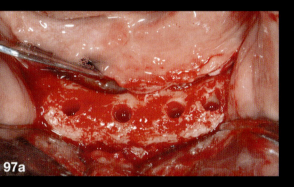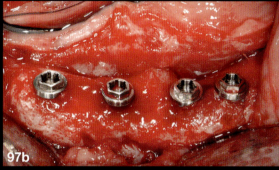

Fig 97 *(a)* It was possible to prepare four implant sites in sufficiently thick bone. *(b)* Four implants 8 mm in length and 3.75 mm in diameter were placed.

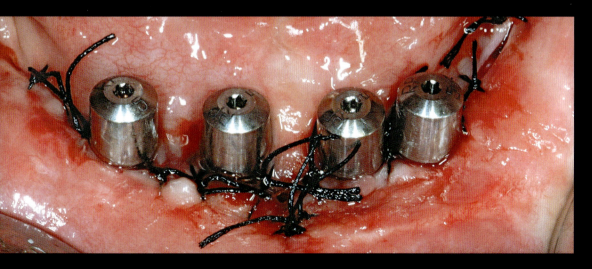

Fig 98 After 3 months of submerged healing, the second surgical phase of implant surgery was performed to connect the temporary abutments.

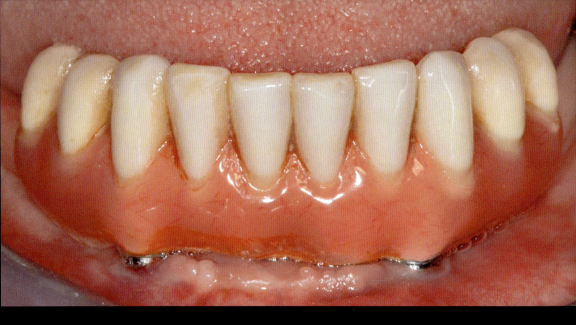

Fig 99 The patient was rehabilitated with fixed removable dentures.

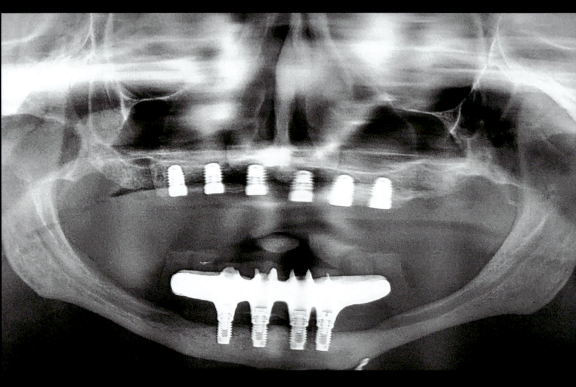

Fig 100 Control panoramic radiograph after 10 years.

TREATMENT PLANNING FOR PARTIALLY EDENTULOUS RIDGES

Posterior areas of the maxilla

The maxillary sinuses frequently limit the vertical dimension of alveolar bone available for implant placement in posterior areas of the maxilla. It is commonplace to think that the only option for treating vertical deficits in this area is sinus floor elevation. However, there are at least four distinct clinical situations, and each needs to be addressed with a different treatment approach. (Procedures in the posterior maxilla are presented in chapters 15 to 18 and 21.)

Class A

Distal edentulous maxillary ridges with minimal bone resorption and modest maxillary sinus expansion belong to Class A.

The edentulous span of the ridge is in line with the crestal margin of the adjacent teeth (ie, it is about 3 mm apical to their cementoenamel junction [CEJ]), the interarch distance is less than or equal to 10 mm, and the vertical dimension of the residual bone is greater than or equal to 8 mm (**Figs 101**).

The therapeutic indication is the simple insertion of implants with the standard technique (**Figs 102 and 103**).

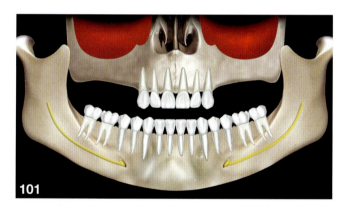

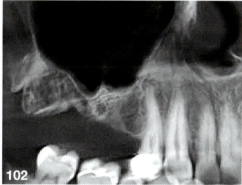

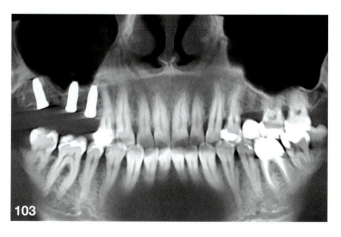

Fig 101 Class A characteristics of the posterior areas of the maxilla. The vertical dimension of the residual bone is greater than or equal to 8 mm, the distance of the ridge is approximately 3 mm from the CEJ of the remaining teeth, and the interarch distance is less than or equal to 10 mm. **Fig 102** CBCT of a Class A edentulous ridge. **Fig 103** Three iMAX hybrid implants placed according to standard protocol.

Class B

Class B edentulous maxillary alveolar ridges have not undergone major resorption, but the maxillary sinuses are very expanded. Like in class A, the edentulous ridge is in line with the crestal margin of the adjacent teeth, about 3 mm from the CEJ, and the interarch distance is less than or equal to 10 mm. However, due to the expansion of the maxillary sinuses, the vertical dimension of the residual bone is less than 8 mm **(Fig 103)**. The therapeutic indication is sinus elevation with either immediate or delayed implant placement, depending on the quantity and quality of the residual bone **(Figs 104 to 107)** (see chapter 21).

Class C

Distal edentulous maxillary ridges with minimal bone resorption and modest maxillary sinus expansion belong to Class A. The edentulous span of the ridge is in line with the crestal margin of the adjacent teeth (ie, it is about 3 mm apical to their

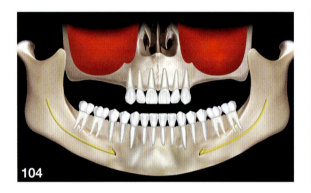
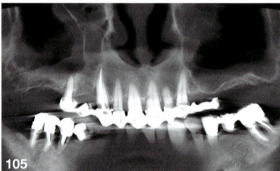

*Fig 104 Class B characteristics of the posterior areas of the maxilla. The vertical dimension of the residual bone is less than 8 mm, the distance of the ridge is approximately 3 mm from the CEJ of the remaining teeth, and the interarch distance is less than or equal to 10 mm. **Fig 105** CBCT of a Class B edentulous ridge. The extensive expansion of the maxillary sinus is evident.*

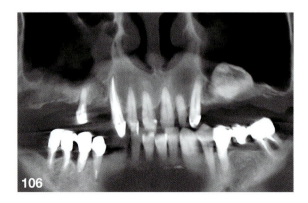
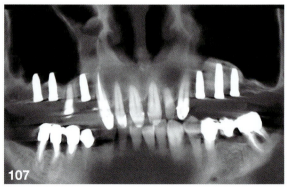

*Fig 106 A two-stage sinus elevation procedure was performed. **Fig 107** After 8 months, three hybrid iMAX implants were inserted.*

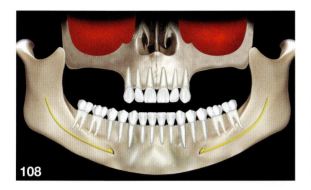

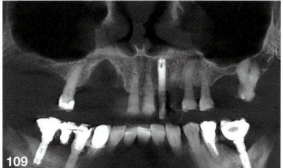

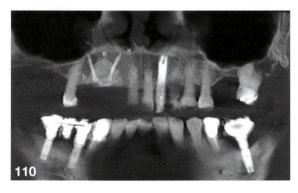

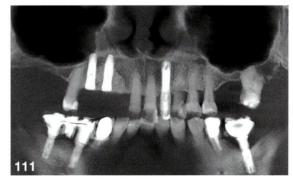

Fig 108 Class C characteristics of the posterior areas of the maxilla. The vertical dimension of the residual bone is greater than or equal to 6 to 7 mm, the distance from the ridge to the CEJ of the remaining teeth is greater than 3 mm, and the interarch distance is greater than 10 mm. *Fig 109* CBCT of a Class C ridge. Severe vertical bone resorption and reduced sinus size are evident. *Fig 110* Vertical ridge augmentation was performed using GBR. *Fig 111* After 8 months, two 13-mm machined iMAX implants were inserted.

cementoenamel junction [CEJ]), the interarch distance is less than or equal to 10 mm, and the vertical dimension of the residual bone is greater than or equal to 8 mm **(Fig 101)**.

The therapeutic indication is the simple insertion of implants with the standard technique **(Figs 102 and 103)**.

Class D

A D classification of the posterior maxilla is encountered rather frequently and occurs when a vertically resorbed alveolar ridge is associated with an expanded maxillary sinus. In this situation, the amount of residual bone is very limited, sometimes up to 1 mm.

The distances between the arches is more than 10 mm, and the position of the crestal margin is more than 3 mm apical to the CEJ of the adjacent teeth **(Fig 112)**.

The indication is vertical ridge augmentation with a GBR technique and sinus elevation **(Figs 113 to 115)**.

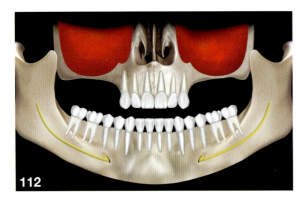
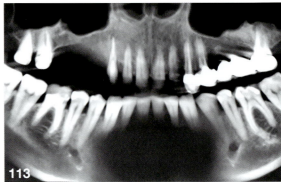

Fig 112 Class D characteristics of the posterior areas of the maxilla. The vertical dimension of the residual bone is less than 6 to 7 mm, the distance between the ridge and the CEJ of the remaining teeth is more than 3 mm, and the interarch distance is more than 10 mm. *Fig 113* CBCT of a Class D edentulous ridge. Both the severe crestal resorption and the considerable expansion of the maxillary sinus are evident.

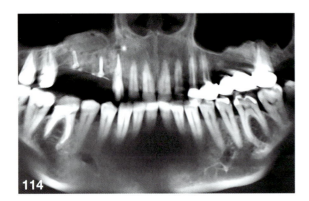
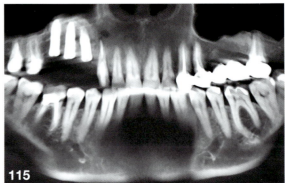

Fig 114 Vertical ridge augmentation with GBR and sinus elevation were performed simultaneously. *Fig 115* After 8 months, three hybrid iMAX implants were inserted.

Anterior areas of the maxilla and mandible

Implant rehabilitation in the anterior maxilla is probably the most complex of all rehabilitative dental procedures. Tooth loss leads to partial resorption of the alveolar bone, resulting in the frequent need for hard and/or soft tissue regenerative techniques in esthetic areas to reproduce the normal interproximal papillae and obtain an acceptable final prosthesis. A systematic review of the literature, limited to studies performed on humans, calculated a weighted average of hard tissue changes

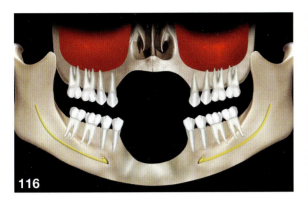
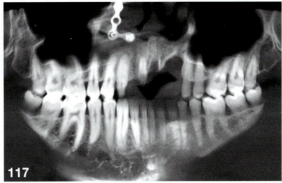

Fig 116 Severe vertical atrophy of the anterior sectors of the maxilla and mandible. The vertical dimension of the residual bone is incompatible with esthetic implant rehabilitation. *Fig 117* CBCT of an edentulous ridge with vertical atrophy in the anterosuperior sector.

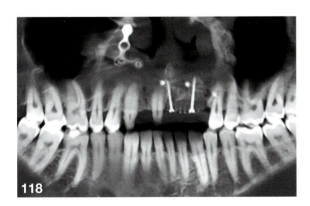
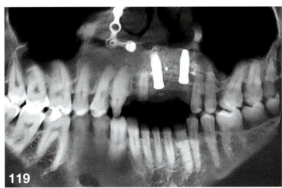

Fig 118 Vertical ridge augmentation was performed using GBR. *Fig 119* After 8 months, two hybrid iMAX implants were placed.

following tooth extraction. After 6 months, there is a dimensional reduction of 3.79 ± 0.23 mm in the horizontal dimension and 1.24 ± 0.11 mm in the vertical dimension.[16–18] This dimensional loss also results in the flattening of the interdental septa, which are responsible for supporting the papillae. In cases of massive bone resorption following trauma or periodontal disease, complex bone and soft tissue reconstruction is required, involving multiple surgeries and very prolonged treatment periods **(Figs 116 to 122)** (see chapters 17 to 19).

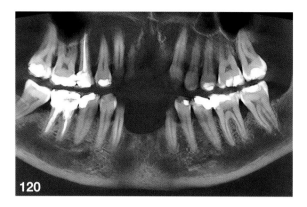

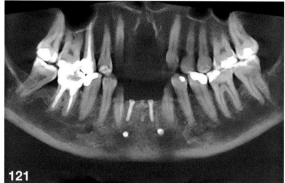

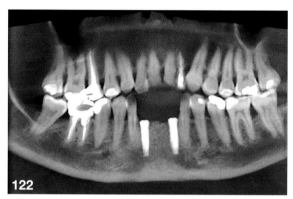

Fig 120 CBCT of an edentulous ridge with vertical bone atrophy in the anterior sector of the mandible. *Fig 121* Vertical ridge augmentation was performed using GBR. *Fig 122* After 8 months, two hybrid iMAX implants were placed.

Posterolateral mandibular areas

The inferior alveolar nerve limits the vertical dimension of bone available for implant placement in the posterolateral sectors of the mandible. Many partially edentulous patients who have worn soft tissue–supported removable prostheses for long periods have severe alveolar bone atrophy.

The indicated type of surgery, and whether it is associated with regenerative therapy, depends on the vertical dimension of the residual bone coronal to the inferior alveolar nerve.

Because a safe distance of at least 2 mm must be maintained between the apex of the implant and the nerve and the minimum implant length is 7 to 8 mm, all patients with a residual vertical dimension of bone that is less than 9 to 10 mm should be treated with regenerative techniques.

Class A

In class A posterolateral sections of the mandible, the vertical dimension of bone from the inferior alveolar nerve to the crestal margin is more than 10 mm, and the minimum thickness is at least 6 mm **(Fig 123)**.

Standard implant placement techniques are indicated, respecting the distance of 2 mm from the mandibular canal **(Figs 124 and 125)**.

Class B

In Class B posterolateral bone atrophy, bone availability between the crestal margin and the mandibular canal is 5 to 8 mm **(Fig 126)**.

It is possible to achieve implant stability in this amount of bone by performing vertical GBR and simultaneously placing implants **(Figs 127 and 128)**.

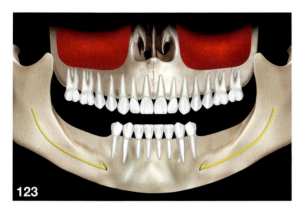

Fig 123 Class A characteristics of the posterior areas of the mandible. The distance between the residual ridge and the mandibular canal is more than 10 mm. *Fig 124* CBCT of a Class A edentulous ridge in the posterior area of the mandible. *Fig 125* Three 10-mm implants were placed according to standard protocol.

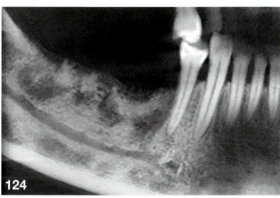

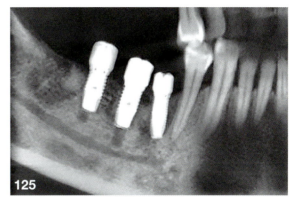

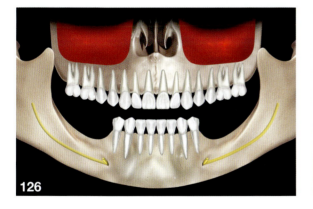

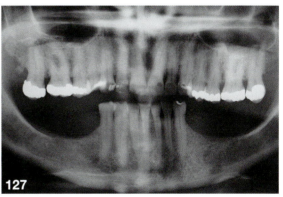

Fig 126 Class B characteristics of the posterior areas of the mandible. The distance between the residual ridge and the mandibular canal is 7 mm. *Fig 127* CBCT of a Class B edentulous ridge in a mandibular posterior area. *Fig 128* One-stage vertical ridge augmentation with GBR and immediate implant placement was performed

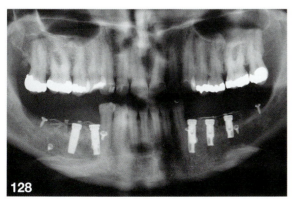

However, a two-stage technique is simpler and less risky.

Class C

Class C mandibular posterolateral bone atrophy is severe, with the mandibular canal running 2 to 4 mm from the crest **(Fig 129)**. There is no possibility of immediate implant placement, so the indication is for a two-stage procedure with vertical bone augmentation followed by implant placement after bone regeneration has taken place **(Figs 130 to 132)**.

Fig 129 Class C characteristics of the posterior areas of the mandible. The distance between the residual ridge and the mandibular canal is 2 to 3 mm. Fig 130 CBCT of a Class C edentulous ridge in the posterior area of the mandible. Fig 131 Two-stage vertical ridge augmentation was performed using GBR. Fig 132 (a and b) After 6 months, two machined implants were inserted bilaterally, and after 4 months of submerged healing, restorations were placed.

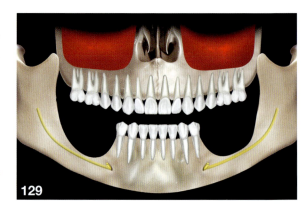

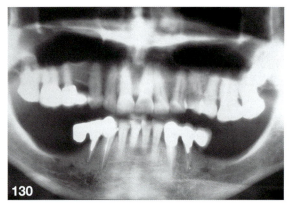

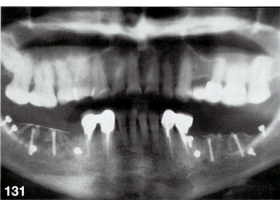

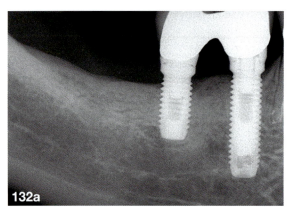

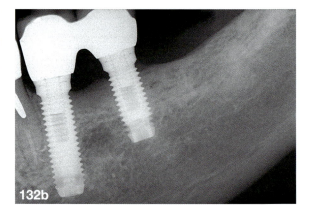

REFERENCES

1. Cawood JI, Howell RA. A classification of the edentulous jaws. Int J Oral Maxillofac Surg 1988;17:232–236.
2. Misch CE. Contemporary Implant Dentistry. Mosby, 2008.
3. Lekholm U, Zarb GA. Patient selection and preparation. In: Brånemark PI, Zarb GA, Alberktsson T, editors. Tissue-Integrated Prostheses: Osseointegration in Clinical Dentistry. Quintessence, 1985:199–209.
4. Adell R, Lekholm U, Rockler B, Brånemark PI. A 15-year study of osseointegrated implants in the treatment of the edentulous jaw. Int J Oral Surg 1981;10:387–416.
5. Brånemark PI, Hansson BO, Adell R, et al. Osseointegrated implants in the treatment of the edentulous jaw. Experience from a 10-year period. Scand J Plast Reconstr Surg Suppl 1977;16:1–132.
6. Maló P, Rangert B, Nobre M. "All-on-Four" immediate-function concept with Brånemark System implants for completely edentulous mandibles: A retrospective clinical study. Clin Implant Dent Relat Res 2003;5 (Suppl 1):2–9.
7. Esposito M, Felice P, Barausse P, Pistilli R, Grandi R, Simion M. Immediately loaded machined versus rough surface dental implants in edentulous jaws: One-year postloading results of a pilot randomised controlled trial. Eur J Oral Implantol 2015;8:387–396.
8. Sicilia A, Botticelli D. Working group 3. Computed guided implant therapy and soft- and hard-tissue aspects. The third EAO Consensus Conference 2012. Clin Oral Implants Res 2012;23(Suppl 6):157–161.
9. Vercruyssen M, Hultin M, Van Assche N, Svensson K, Naert L, Quirynen M. Guided surgery: Accuracy and efficacy. Periodontol 2000 2014;66:228–246.
10. Laleman I, Bernard L, Vercruyssen M, Jacobs R, Bornstein MM, Quirynen M. Guided implant surgery in the edentulous maxilla: A systematic review. Int J Oral Maxillofac Implants 2016;31(Suppl):S103–S117.
11. D'haese J, Ackhurst J, Wismeijer D, De Bruyn H, Tahmaseb A. Current state of the art of computer-guided implant surgery. Periodontol 2000 2017;73:121–133.
12. Becker W, Goldstein M, Becker BE, Sennerby L. Minimally invasive flap-less implant placement: Follow-up results from a multicenter study. J Periodontol 2009;80:347–352.
13. Nyström E, Nilson H, Gunne J, Lundgren S. Reconstruction of the atrophic maxilla with interpositional bone grafting/Le Fort I osteotomy and endosteal implants: An 11-16 year follow-up. Int J Oral Maxillofac Surg 2009;38:1–6.
14. Chiapasco M, Brusati R, Ronchi P. Le Fort I osteotomy with interpositional bone grafts and delayed oral implants for the rehabilitation of extremely atrophied maxillae: A 1-9-year clinical follow-up study on humans. Clin Oral Implants Res 2007;18:74–85.
15. Felice P, Pistilli R, Barausse C, Piattelli M, Buti J, Esposito M. Posterior atrophic jaws rehabilitated with prostheses supported by 6-mm-long 4-mm-wide implants or by longer implants in augmented bone. Five-year post-loading results from an within-person randomised controlled trial. Int J Oral Implantol (Berl) 2019;12:57–72.
16. Araújo MG, Lindhe J. Dimensional ridge alterations following tooth extraction. An experimental study in the dog. Clin Periodontol 2005;32:212–218.
17. Araújo MG, Silva CO, Misawa M, Sukekava F. Alveolar socket healing: what can we learn? Periodontology 2000 2015;68:122–134.
18. Chappuis V, Engel O, Shahim K, Reyes M, Katsaros C, Buser D. Soft tissue alterations in esthetic postextraction sites: A 3-dimensional analysis. J Dent Res 2015;94(9 Suppl):187S–193S.

GUIDED IMPLANT SURGERY

CHAPTER 6

Edited by Mario Beretta and Carlo Maiorana

INTRODUCTION

Guided implant surgery involves the use of 3D radiography and specific software to virtually plan implant surgery and optimize prosthetically driven implant positioning. There are two types of guided implant surgery:[1]

1. **Static guided surgery** involves the use of a physical surgical guide that reproduces the virtual position of the planned implants.
2. **Dynamic guided surgery** involves the use of a surgical navigation system that reproduces the 3D position of the drills on a monitor in real time, allowing for intraoperative modifications to the virtually planned procedure. A very complex machine is required for dynamic guided surgery. It must be equipped with infrared cameras for guiding the preparation of the implant site(s) by means of reference points mounted onto the surgical handpiece and the patient's skull. Surgery is performed without a surgical guide but through the direct simultaneous visualization of the drill, the diagnostic wax-up, and CT images of the alveolar process.[2]

This chapter examines static guided surgery, its advantages, and its clinical limitations. A clinical protocol supported by data from recent literature is also provided.[3-5] In recent years, static guided surgery has undergone considerable growth, with the development of well-defined clinical protocols that have made it possible to increase the precision and accuracy of implant placement and broaden its possible indications.

Implant surgery guided by digital platforms is one of the most important technologic acquisitions in recent years, but it cannot be done without in-depth clinical and surgical experience.

Massimo Simion

FUNDAMENTAL PRINCIPLES OF GUIDED SURGERY

Guided surgery relies upon software to create an overlay between DICOM files from CT/CBCT imaging and STL files obtained by either direct intraoral scanning or scanning of a plaster model with a laboratory scanner.[6,7] Digitally aligning these files makes it possible to plan implant treatment starting from a virtual wax-up of the definitive restoration and taking into account multiple factors, such as the volume of the bone ridges, the thickness of the soft tissues, and the esthetic and functional parameters established at the time of the initial analog or digital wax-up.

CAD/CAM processes (milling, 3D printing, or stereolithography) are then used to produce a surgical guide equipped with drill-guiding cylinders. After being stabilized inside the oral cavity with surgical pins or transcortical screws, these surgical guides allow for implant placement based on the virtually planned positions.

The great advantage of static guided surgery is that the same wax-up file used for implant planning can then be used to produce a provisional restoration that can be placed after surgery for an immediate loading procedure.

SOFTWARE FOR GUIDED SURGERY

There are numerous software packages available that are based on the principle of coupling radiographic anatomy (DICOM files from 3D imaging) with DICOM or STL files relating to the anatomy of the oral cavity.

The various software packages differ from one another in two fundamental aspects:

1. Whether the software works with only a single implant system (closed software) or can work with several implant systems thanks to different CAD libraries included in the software itself (open software).

2. The system used for aligning radiographic DICOM files with DICOM/STL files of the anatomy.[8]

COUPLING SYSTEMS IN GUIDED SURGERY

DICOM-DICOM alignment

The DICOM-DICOM protocol is referred to as the double-scan protocol and involves the use of a radiographic template (or the patient's prosthesis suitably modified with radiopaque reference points) representing the diagnostic wax-up of the future prosthetic rehabilitation. Two DICOM radiographic files are generated for this technique. The first one involves the patient wearing the radiographic template (or prosthesis with landmarks), and the second one involves only the template. The software then superimposes the radiographic reference points of the two DICOM files **(Fig 1)**. The DICOM file of the radiographic template can also be used to produce the surgical guide with CAD/CAM equipment after transforming the DICOM data into STL format.[7]

DICOM-STL alignment

DICOM-STL alignment is a more recently developed procedure based on the superimposition of DICOM data from 3D imaging with an STL file originating from an optical scan, thus requiring only one X-ray acquisition.[8] The STL file can be obtained from optical scanning of either plaster models with laboratory scanners or from direct intraoral optical scanning.

In partially edentulous patients, overlapping of the two files overlap is achieved through a process called best fit alignment, which involves matching the recognizable tooth surfaces in the DICOM file of the 3D scan and the STL file of the optical scan. In the case of an edentulous patient, a

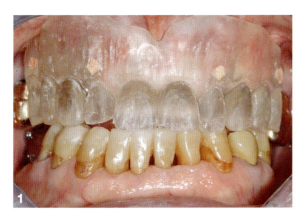 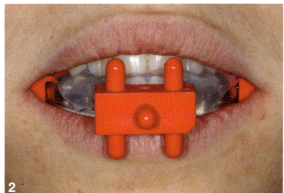

Fig 1 *Radiographic template with radiopaque landmarks for the 3D double-scan protocol.* **Fig 2** *Radiographic template with radiographic and optical marker (Evobite [3Diemme]) (red geometric object) used for a single-scan protocol. The marker enables alignment of the DICOM and STL files.*

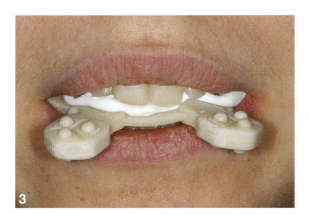 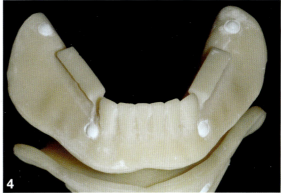

Fig 3 *Radiographic template with customized thermoplastic splint (3Diemme) equipped with radiographic markers also present in the STL library of the guided surgery software for DICOM-STL matching.* **Fig 4** *Radiographic template for edentulous patients (3Diemme) for a single-scan protocol. The thermoplastic material allows the template to be customized and used for the registration of maxillomandibular relations. The white geometric objects are made of radiopaque material recognizable in DICOM files.*

radiotransparent radiographic template representing the diagnostic wax-up of the final restoration is fitted with a radiopaque radiographic marker. This device represents a known geometric figure that the software recognizes in both the DICOM file and the STL file. Thus, matching proves to be considerably more precise than that achieved with the double-scan protocol.[9] DICOM-STL alignment also has the advantage of being able to provide a better view of the soft tissue profile and is more easily adapted to cases in which the presence of metal prosthetic restorations causes a scattering phenomenon that considerably disrupt the alignment process **(Figs 2 to 4)**.

PROTOCOL FOR GUIDED SURGERY

Guided implant surgery comprises a series of steps that must be strictly followed to reduce potential errors during the design phase, which could manifest later as dangerous inaccuracies in implant positioning.

Radiographic examination and diagnostic wax-up

In partially edentulous patients, a 3D examination can be performed without radiographic templates because the software can couple DICOM data with the STL data of the analog diagnostic wax-up to be scanned in the laboratory. A virtual wax-up can also be created using library elements (contained in the design software itself) or CAD/CAM modeling software (**Fig 5**).

For fully edentulous arches, the planning phase is based on the analysis of esthetic and functional parameters to design the diagnostic wax-up of the definitive prosthesis. This design may correspond to the patient's removable complete denture, which in this case will be used as a radiographic template.

The prosthesis itself may be used after adding radiographic markers with radiopaque material (gutta-percha), or a duplicate of the prosthesis can be made and a radiographic marker corresponding to a known geometric object can be used. If esthetic and/or functional parameters are changed, the preliminary evaluations will be the same as those carried out for full-arch rehabilitation with a traditional prosthesis (**Figs 6 to 8**).

Virtual planning

Once the 3D radiographic scans and corresponding DICOM files have been obtained, the software superimposes them with the corresponding STL or DICOM wax-up files.

This allows for prosthetically guided planning and ensures ideal 3D implant positioning.

Additionally, the volume of the bone crest and the thickness of the soft tissues are taken into consideration during virtual planning.

Virtual planning provides clinicians with the opportunities and tools to control the 3D positioning of implants and their relationships with anatomical structures, soft tissues, and the prosthetic restoration (**Figs 9 to 11**).

In sum, virtual planning enables clinicians to achieve the following:

- Establish the location of the implants
- Create a surgical guide with drill-guiding cylinders for implant site preparation
- Predefine the positions for securing the surgical guide
- Choose the type of prosthetic components (abutments) to be used

Production of the surgical guide

Surgical guides are made of light-cured resin and can be produced using guided surgery software and 3D printers. Alternatively, technicians can use laboratory and CAD software.

The various types of surgical guides are classified according to the type of hard and/or soft tissue that supports them (**Figs 12 to 14**):

- Tooth-supported guides
- Mucosa-supported guides
- Bone-supported guides
- Tooth-mucosa–supported guides

There is a consensus in the literature that tooth-mucosa–supported surgical guides are far more accurate than bone-supported ones because inaccuracies in 3D imaging or uneven bone anatomy can significantly alter the position of the surgical guide and consequently the accuracy of implant placement.[9–11]

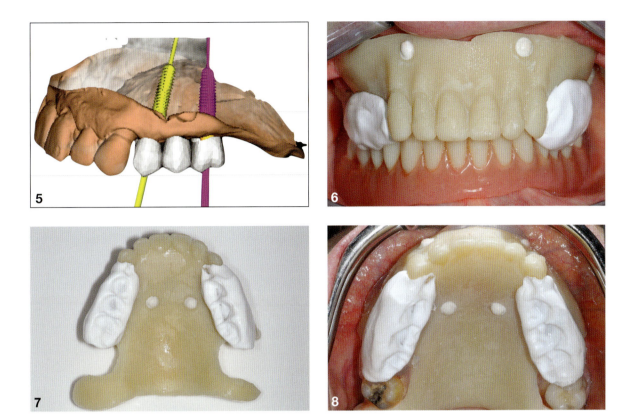

Fig 5 *Example of a virtual wax-up for guided implant placement in the sites of the maxillary left first premolar and first molar (RealGUIDE 5.0, 3Diemme).* **Fig 6** *Recording the maxillomandibular relationship in an edentulous patient. The thermoplastic radiographic template combined with the white thermoplastic material allows the vertical dimension of occlusion (VDO) to be determined.* **Fig 7** *Occlusal view of the radiographic template and the radiographic markers and thermoplastic material used to record the position of the two arches.* **Fig 8** *View of the thermoplastic radiographic template provided to the patient for the 3D radiographic examination. The thermoplastic material stabilizes the template in the correct position during radiographic scanning.*

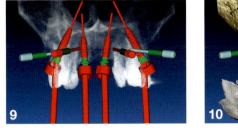
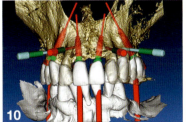
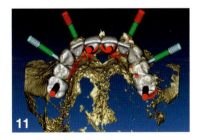

Fig 9 *Virtual planning (RealGUIDE) of All-on-4 implant rehabilitation after extraction of the remaining teeth. Bone volume, assessed via 3D imaging, and a virtual diagnostic wax-up are used to determine the correct implant positioning.* **Fig 10** *Using the 3D imaging to verify the position of implants and fixation pins to avoid interferences between the various components of the restoration.* **Fig 11** *Occlusal assessment of virtual prosthetic planning to check the emergence axis of the prosthetic screw for a screw-retained full-arch rehabilitation.*

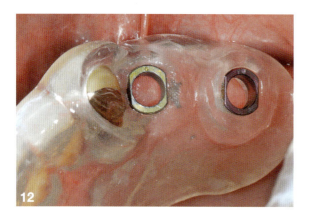
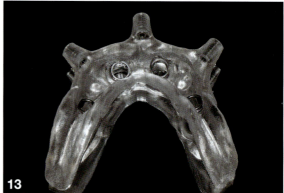

Fig 12 *Tooth-supported surgical guide for a partially edentulousness patient.* **Fig 13** *Mucosa-supported surgical guide for an edentulous mandible.*

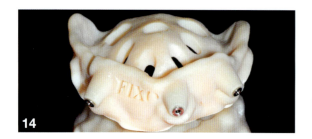
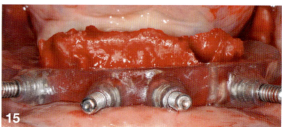

Fig 14 *Mucosa-supported surgical guide for an edentulous maxilla with mucosal support at the level of the palatine vault.* **Fig 15** *Surgical guide for performing an osteoplasty. After creating the perforations for the fixation pins with a dedicated guide, a mucoperiosteal flap can be elevated and a guide positioned by fixing it with pins in the previously prepared locations.*

Thanks to ongoing developments in guided surgery, it has recently been confirmed in the literature that surgical guides can be used to perform simultaneous resective osseous surgery in patients with irregular alveolar processes characterized by a pyramidal shape **(Fig 15)**.[12,13]

Creation of the prosthesis for immediate loading

The previously described workflow provides clinicians with all the necessary information for fabricating a provisional prosthesis that can be immediately loaded as the primary stability of the implants allows.[14–20] It is the authors' opinion that, because of the minimal distortion in implant positioning inherent in guided implant surgery caused by the resilience of the oral mucosa,[10,11,21] the placement of these prostheses should be based on bonding and intraoral stabilization onto the prosthetic abutments. This method allows for a passive screw-retained restoration characterized by a good fit of the framework on the prosthetic abutments. Examples of virtual prosthetic restoration planning are provided in **Figs 16 to 20**.

Surgical procedure

The surgical procedure is the final stage of guided implant surgery. The stable fixation of the surgical guide by means of transcortical pins is of great importance to ensure the precision and accuracy of the procedure.

Depending on the volume of bone and keratinized gingiva, different approaches are possible:

- **Flapless approach:** The flapless approach is indicated only in cases where adequate volumes of bone and keratinized tissue are present. With the use of a soft tissue punch, implants can be placed without elevating flaps and without placing sutures.

- **Flap approach:** The flap approach is indicated in cases where bone regeneration (full-thickness flaps) or soft tissue augmentation (partial-thickness flaps) is required. These needs should be taken into consideration during virtual planning to create modified surgical guides that provide access windows for flap management.

- **Postextraction approach:** The postextraction approach is indicated in cases of immediate implant placement after extracting the remaining dentition. It requires the use of two different guides. The first is a tooth-supported guide for positioning the fixation pins before tooth extraction, and the second is a mucosa-supported guide for use after the

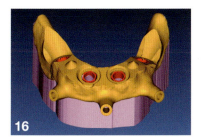 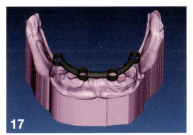 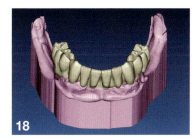

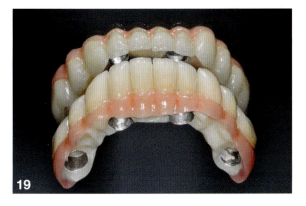 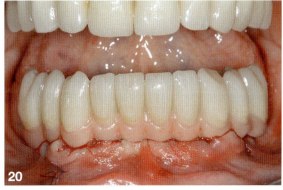

Fig 16 *All-on-4 surgical guide designed with CAD software for a mandibular restoration.* *Fig 17* *Virtual design of a reinforcement structure for an immediately loaded prosthesis.* *Fig 18* *A prosthesis for immediate loading designed via a fully digital process.* *Fig 19* *Prosthesis for immediate loading with a chrome-reinforced framework and intraoral bonding slots for temporary abutments.* *Fig 20* *Intraoral positioning of the mandibular prosthesis for immediate loading.*

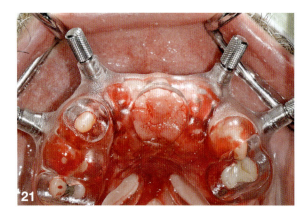 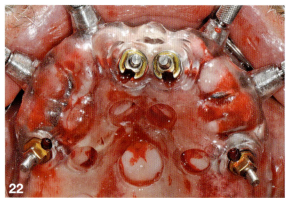

Fig 21 Tooth-supported guide for a postextraction protocol. The purpose of this device is to exploit the precision and stability offered by tooth support to create the seat of the fixation pins prior to tooth extraction. *Fig 22* Mucosa-supported guide. The guide is in contact with the portions of the maxilla that are not affected by the extractions (palate and tuber), and its position is confirmed by inserting pins into the holes made with the previous guide.

extractions, which is stabilized with fixation pins inserted in the perforations made with the first guide **(Figs 21 and 22)**.

PRECISION AND ACCURACY OF GUIDED IMPLANT SURGERY

The precision and accuracy of guided implant surgery has been the subject of numerous studies.[10,21–25] Evaluating the precision and accuracy of a guided precures involves comparing the planned virtual positions of the implants with the actual position of the implants according to postoperative 3D imaging.

Superimpositioning is performed using the bone surfaces not affected by surgery, such as the retromolar trigone, the lateral portions of the body of the mandible, the palatal vault, and the zygomatic processes.

The included studies considered three parameters:
- Position of the implant neck
- Position of the implant apex
- Angular distortion of the implant (understood as variation in the long axis of the system)

The averages of the values found were 0.56 to 1 mm for neck position, 0.64 to 1.2 mm for the apex position, and 2.42 to 3.42 degrees for the angular distortion.

In light of these data, clinicians should always maintain a minimum safe distance of approximately 2 mm from anatomical structures.

FULLY DIGITAL, MODEL-FREE PROTOCOLS FOR GUIDED SURGERY

Having ascertained the validity of guided surgery techniques with traditional methods, where digital media interact constantly with analog systems, today, guided surgery is also possible to carry out with entirely digital workflows, even in completely edentulous patients.[26–28]

As with traditional guided surgery procedures, the initial phase of fully digital guided surgery is based on a survey of the intraoral anatomy, the esthetic-functional data, and the condition of the bone to be treated.

In the traditional protocol, two initial impressions are taken to make study models, whereas in a fully digital protocol, two intraoral scans are taken with an intraoral scanner (IOS). The two scans (maxillary and mandibular) are then completed by the registration of the maxillomandibular occlusal relationship (either maximum intercuspation [MI] or centric relationship [CR]).[29,30]

It is also necessary to take intraoral and facial photographs using special markers of known size to allow CAD software to create customized virtual diagnostic wax-ups **(Fig 23)**. To create a correct prosthetic and surgical design, two preformed prostheses made of thermoplastic material with seven radiologic and optical scanning landmarks inside them are used, allowing correct measurement of the vertical dimension and accurate recording of the maxillomandibular relationship.[31,32]

The thermoplastic prostheses also have the function of maintaining the arches in the correct vertical dimension with a correct interocclusal relationship **(Fig 24)**.

After 3D scanning with thermoplastic prostheses and obtaining DICOM files, it is possible to perform alignment with the STL files from scanning of the relined prostheses and soft tissues.

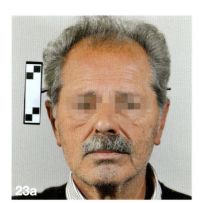 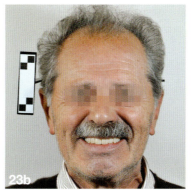 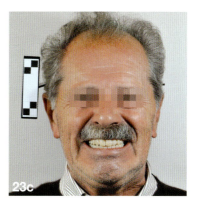

Fig 23 (a to c) *Extraoral photographs with radiographic marker used to determine the correct dimensions of the virtual CAD wax-up.*

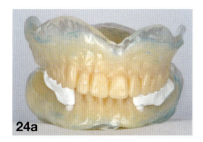 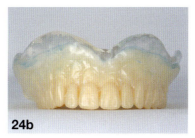 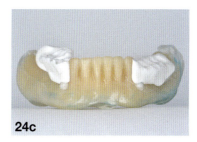

Fig 24 (a to c) *Thermoplastic prostheses relined with transparent silicone in the correct maxillomandibular ratio are used for both 3D scanning and optical scanning to achieve accurate alignment.*

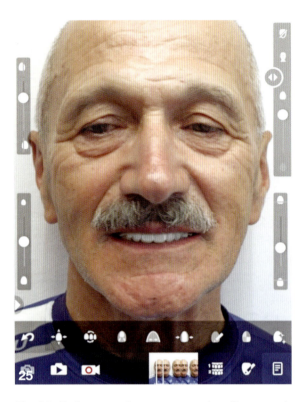

This information flow allows dental technicians to create a digital diagnostic wax-up of the two arches.

Before any kind of physical prototype is made, this wax-up is integrated into an augmented reality software (IvoSmile, Ivoclar) that allows the esthetics of the wax-up to be analyzed directly with the patient's face.

If changes are needed, the software allows corrections of the shape and position of the STL file **(Fig 25)**. Once the esthetic design has been validated, two 3D-printed prototypes are fabricated to evaluate the digital planning directly in the patient **(Fig 25)**.

Once the prototypes have been tested, the clinician can carry out implant planning using guided surgery software to produce surgical guides and ready-made prostheses for immediate loading via a fully digital and model-free workflow.

Fig 25 *Software using augmented reality to evaluate and potentially modify the virtual diagnostic wax-up file.*

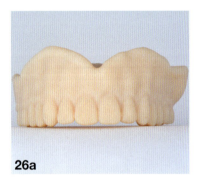
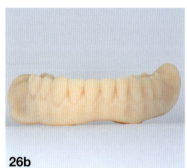
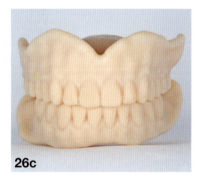

26a   26b   26c

Fig 26 *Printed prototypes for intraoral clinical evaluation of the virtual wax-up created with CAD systems and augmented reality software.*

CLINICAL CASE 1

Guided implant placement in a partially edentulous maxilla (Figs 27 to 42)

A 52-year-old, nonsmoking patient in good general health (ASA 1) presented with an edentulous site in the second quadrant. After CBCT evaluation and a virtual wax-up, the placement of two implants in the positions of teeth 24 and 26 (FDI tooth numbering system) was planned to restore the edentulous span from sites 24 to 26 with a screw-retained restoration. The presence of sufficient bone volume and keratinized mucosa allowed for placement of the two implants with guided surgery and a flapless approach. The definitive prosthetic abutments and their healing screws were positioned immediately after implant placement, ensuring transmucosal maturation. After 4 months, impressions were taken for the provisional restoration, which allowed the soft tissue morphology to be conditioned. The case was completed with a three-piece prosthetic restoration made of monolithic cubic zirconia.

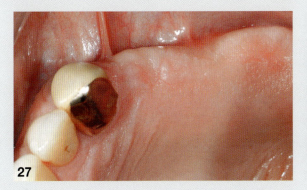
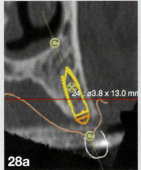
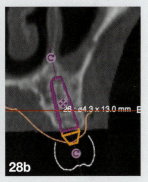

Fig 27 Edentulous span in the second quadrant in the presence of an adequate amount of keratinized tissue. **Fig 28** *(a and b)* Virtual planning for the placement of two implants in the presence of adequate residual bone ridge thickness.

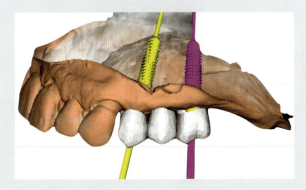
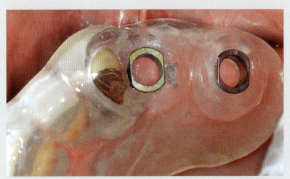

Fig 29 Virtual wax-up and prosthetically driven planning of implant positioning.

Fig 30 Tooth-supported surgical guide with cylinders for guided implant site preparation. Occlusal view.

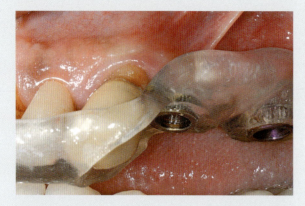

Fig 31 Tooth-supported surgical guide with cylinders for guided implant site preparation. Lateral view.

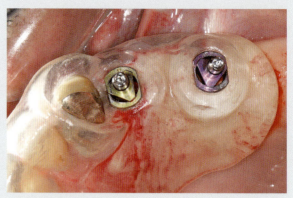

Fig 32 Placement of two implants in sites 24 and 26. Occlusal view.

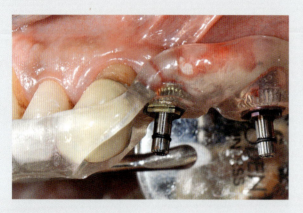

Fig 33 Placement of two implants in sites 24 and 26. Lateral view.

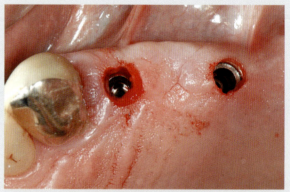

Fig 34 Intraoral view of implant placement with a flapless approach.

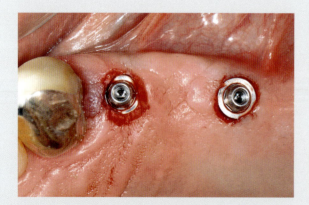

Fig 35 Placement of two definitive prosthetic abutments for a screw-retained prosthesis.

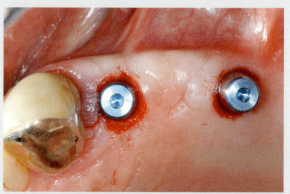

Fig 36 Placement of two healing abutments to protect the definitive abutments for transmucosal healing.

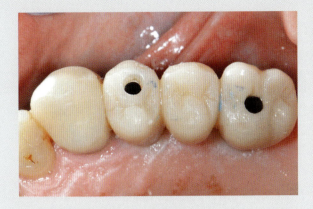

Fig 37 The screw-retained provisional restoration after 3 months of healing.

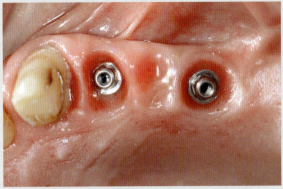

Fig 38 Occlusal view of soft tissue healing after conditioning with the provisional.

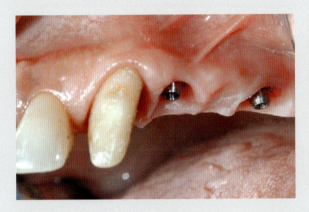

Fig 39 Soft tissue healing after conditioning with the provisional. Lateral view.

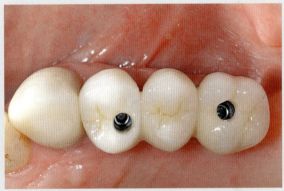

Fig 40 Screw-retained metal-ceramic final restoration. Occlusal view.

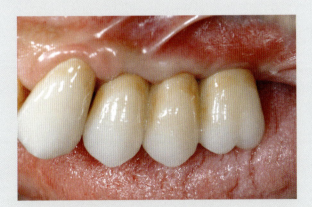

Fig 41 Permanent screw-retained metal-ceramic restoration. Lateral view.

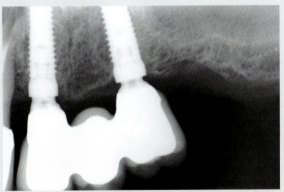

Fig 42 Radiograph showing the final restoration.

CLINICAL CASE 2

Immediate loading of maxillary and mandibular restorations after implant surgery and mandibular reduction osteoplasty performed with guided surgery (Figs 43 to 70)

A 57-year-old, nonsmoking patient in good general health (ASA 1) presented with an esthetically and functionally inadequate removable prosthesis. In the maxilla, the amount of bone and keratinized tissue were optimal, so a flapless approach was planned for the guided placement of six implants with immediate loading. In the mandible, the distal edentulous ridges were characterized by marked vertical and horizontal alveolar bone atrophy, which hindered implant placement. The patient refused a proposed treatment plan for mandibular bilateral vertical bone regeneration and a subsequent implant-supported restoration. It was therefore decided to perform remodeling of the remaining teeth and place a restoration with four implants in the intraforaminal region according to the All-on-4 method of implant placement. The horizontal atrophy of the alveolar process in the symphyseal region was treated with a reductive osteoplasty performed with a surgical guide. Four implants were then inserted with a guided approach and subsequent immediate loading. After 5 months of healing, two full-arch chrome-ceramic restorations were fabricated from intraoral scans via a fully digital method.

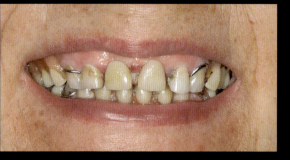

Fig 43 Preoperative situation.

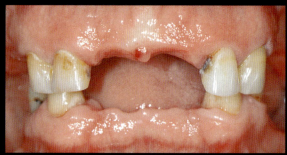

Fig 44 Intraoral view.

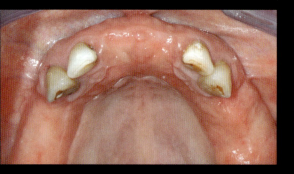

Fig 45 Adequate bone volume and keratinized mucosa in the maxilla.

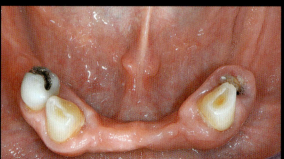

Fig 46 Horizontal bone atrophy in the symphyseal region and vertical bone atrophy in the posterior areas of the mandible.

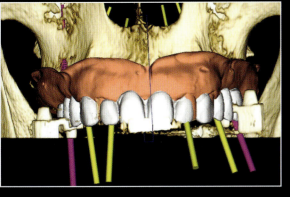

Fig 47 Planning the maxillary full-arch restoration with six immediately placed implants.

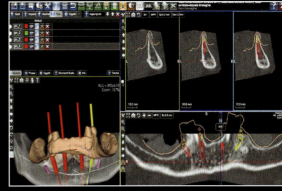

Fig 48 Planning the mandibular full-arch rehabilitation with four implants (All-on-4 method). Due to the horizontal bone atrophy, reduction osteoplasty of the alveolar process in the frontal region is planned.

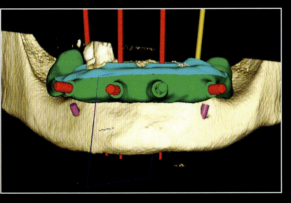

Fig 49 Design of the surgical guide for osteoplasty.

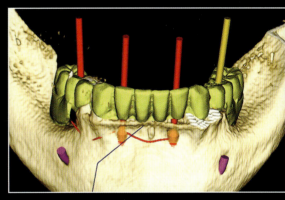

Fig 50 Virtual wax-up design of the full-arch mandibular restoration.

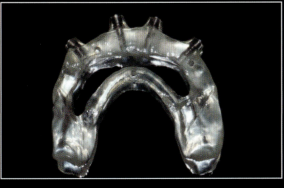

Fig 51 Surgical guide for the reductive osteoplasty.

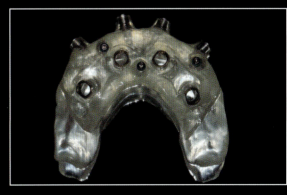

Fig 52 Second surgical guide for implant placement after the osteoplasty.

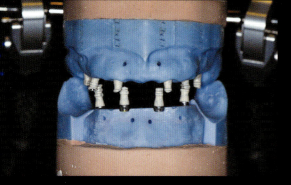

Fig 53 Printed models used to make the prostheses for immediate loading. Definitive prosthetic abutments and provisional cylinders in opaque titanium.

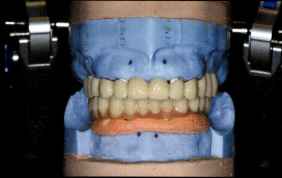

Fig 54 Prefabricated prostheses for immediate loading.

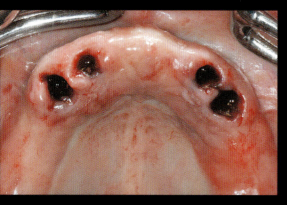

Fig 55 Extraction of the remaining maxillary teeth.

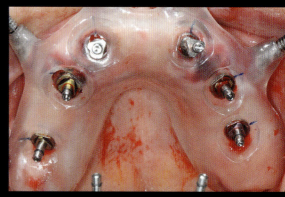

Fig 56 Six implants were placed using the flapless approach.

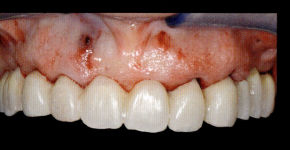

Fig 57 Immediate loading in the maxilla with a poly methyl methacrylate (PMMA) screw-retained provisional.

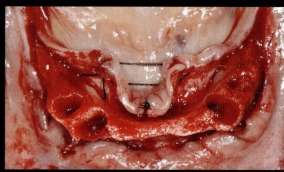

Fig 58 After preparing the sites for surgical guide fixation, the extractions and mucoperiosteal flap for the reductive osteoplasty were performed.

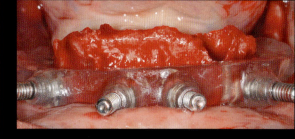

Fig 59 Surgical guide for the reduction osteo-plasty secured in the previously prepared sites.

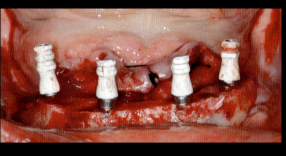

Fig 60 Alveolar ridge reduction.

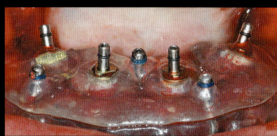

Fig 61 Second surgical guide for the insertion of four implants according to the All-on-4 method.

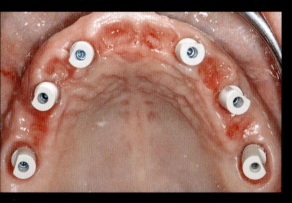

Fig 62 Placement of the definitive abutments and temporary cylinders before flap suturing.

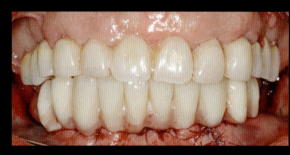

Fig 63 Immediate loading in the mandible.

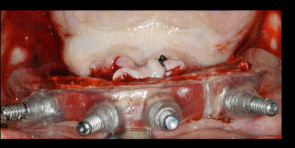

Fig 64 Soft tissue healing at 6 months with in-traoral scan bodies in place.

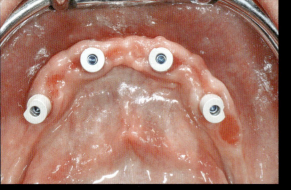

Fig 65 Soft tissue healing at 6 months and intraoral scan bodies in the mandible.

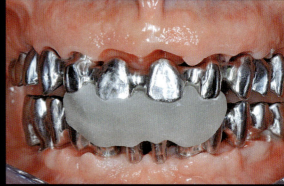

Fig 66 Try-in of the CAD/CAM-produced chrome-milled structures.

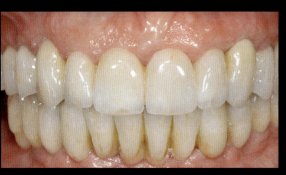

Fig 67 Frontal view of the final restorations.

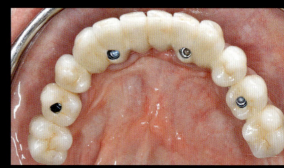

Fig 68 Occlusal view of the final mandibular restoration.

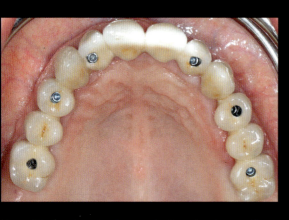

Fig 69 Occlusal view of the final maxillary restoration.

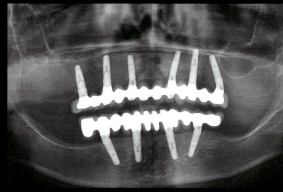

Fig 70 Radiograph showing the final prostheses.

CLINICAL CASE 3

Postextraction maxillary All-on-4 full-arch restoration with guided surgery and monophasic implants with integrated prosthetic platforms (Figs 71 to 94)

A 70-year-old, nonsmoking patient in good general health (ASA 1) presented with severe periodontal compromise and mobility of the maxillary posterior teeth, repeated episodes of abscess, and an esthetically and functionally unsatisfactory removable restoration. After causal periodontal therapy, a postextraction full-arch restoration with immediate loading was planned with digital methods. Four implants were planned according to the All-on-4 method with guided surgery and monophasic implants with an integrated prosthetic platform (Fixo, Biomec Oxy Implant). After tooth extraction, a surgical guide was used to place four implants and manage the postextraction socket with heterologous biomaterial grafting. A coronally advanced flap with a connective tissue graft was also placed at the level of the edentulous site in position 12. After 6 months of healing, a fully digital method was used to fabricate a full-arch restoration with a titanium bar and multilayer monolithic zirconia veneers.

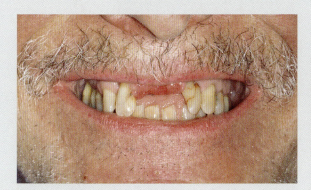

Fig 71 Preoperative view.

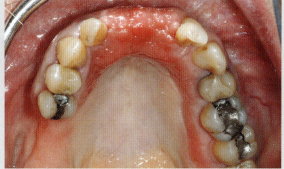

Fig 72 Intraoral view of the maxilla.

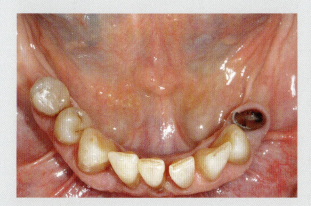

Fig 73 Intraoral view of the mandible.

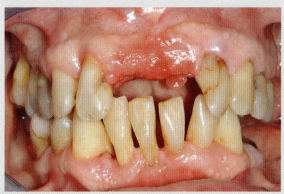

Fig 74 Intraoral view in CR.

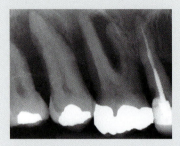
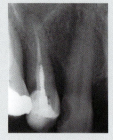
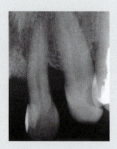
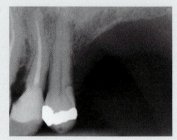

Fig 75 Preoperative radiograph demonstrating severe periodontal compromise and carious lesions of the remaining dentition.

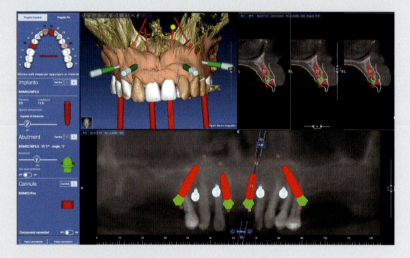

Fig 76 Virtual planning for the postextraction complete maxillary restoration via the All-on-4 method.

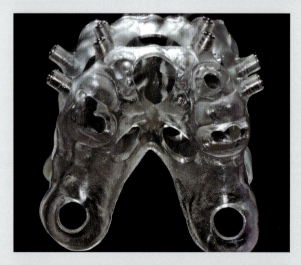

Fig 77 Tooth-supported surgical guide for positioning the fixation pins in the maxilla.

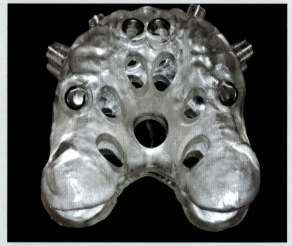

Fig 78 Mucosa-supported surgical guide for implant placement stabilized with pins inserted into the sites previously prepared with the first surgical guide.

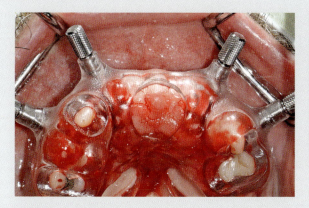

Fig 79 Intraoral view showing preparation of the fixation pin sites.

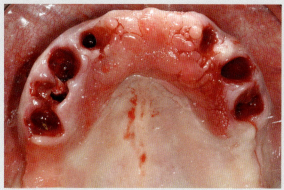

Fig 80 Extraction of the remaining teeth.

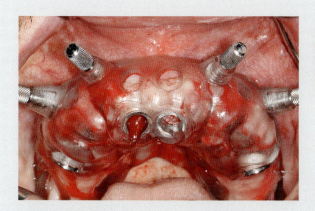

Fig 81 Stabilization of the surgical guide for implant placement.

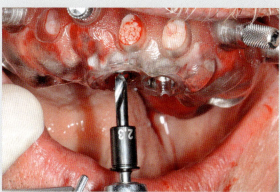

Fig 82 View of the guided preparation of implant sites.

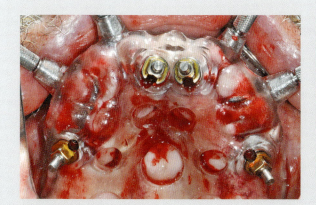

Fig 83 Placement of four one-piece implants with integrated prosthetic abutments.

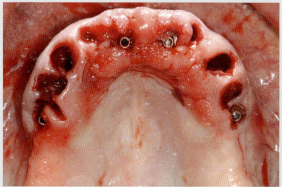

Fig 84 Intraoperative view of implant placement immediately after extraction. The prosthetic platforms of the one-piece implants with integrated abutments are visible.

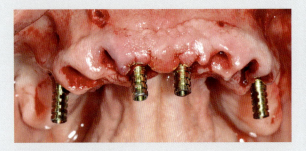

Fig 85 Provisional titanium abutments were inserted prior to immediate loading.

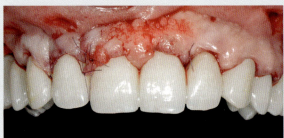

Fig 86 Immediate loading after the performance of a ridge preservation technique in the postextraction sockets and soft tissue management using connective tissue grafting and coronally repositioned flap placement in site 12.

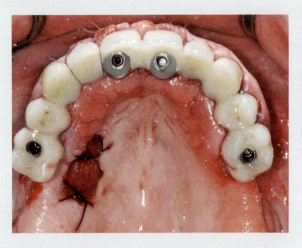

Fig 87 Occlusal view showing the donor site for the connective tissue graft.

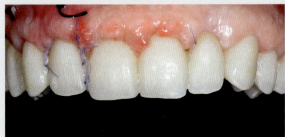

Fig 88 Healing at 10 days.

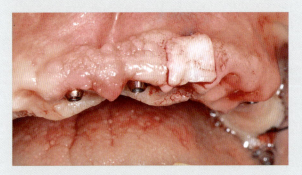

Fig 89 Connective tissue graft with the tunnel technique for the optimization of the esthetic profile of the edentulous ridge in site 22 after 3 months of healing.

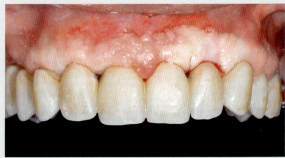

Fig 90 Provisional restoration after connective tissue grafting in site 22.

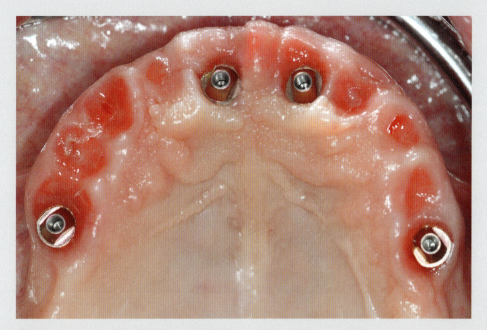

Fig 91 Occlusal view of the soft tissue healing after 6 months.

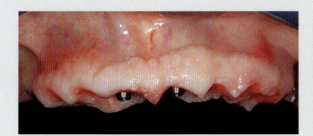

Fig 92 Frontal view of the soft tissue healing after 6 months.

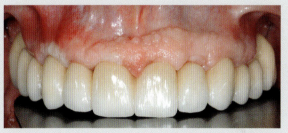

Fig 93 View of the final restoration with titanium framework and cubic monolithic zirconia veneer.

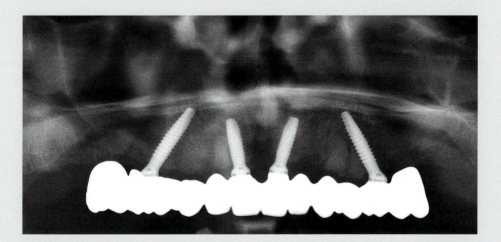

Fig 94 Radiographic follow-up.

REFERENCES

1. Hämmerle CH, Stone P, Jung RE, Kapos T, Brodala N. Consensus statements and recommended clinical procedures regarding computer-assisted implant dentistry. Int J Oral Maxillofac Implants 2009;24:126–131.

2. Ewers R, Schicho K, Undt G, et al. Basic research and 12 years of clinical experience in computer-assisted navigation technology: A review. Int J Oral Maxillofac Surg 2005;34:1–8.

3. Fortin T, Isidori M, Blanchet E, Perriat M, Bouchet H, Coudert JL. An image-guided system-drilled surgical template and trephine guide pin to make treatment of completely edentulous patients easier: A clinical report on immediate loading. Clin Implant Dent Relat Res 2004;6:111–119.

4. Pozzi A, Tallarico M, Marchetti M, Scarfò B, Esposito M. Computer-guided versus free-hand placement of immediately loaded dental implants: 1-year post-loading results of a multicentre randomised controlled trial. Eur J Oral Implantol 2014;7:229–242.

5. Fortin T, Bosson JL, Isidori M, Blanchet E. Effect of flapless surgery on pain experienced in implant placement using an image-guided system. Int J Oral Maxillofac Implants 2006;21:298–304.

6. Arisan V, Karabuda CZ, Mumcu E, Ozdemir T. Implant positioning errors in freehand and computer-aided placement methods: A single-blind clinical comparative study. Int J Oral Maxillofac Implants 2013;28:190–204.

7. Lopes A, Maló P, de Araujo Nobre M, Sanchez-Fernandez E, Gravito I. The NobelGuide® All-on-4® treatment concept for rehabilitation of edentulous jaws: A retrospective report on the 7-years clinical and 5-years radiographic outcomes. Clin Implant Dent Relat Res 2017;19:233–244.

8. Vercruyssen M, Laleman I, Jacobs R, Quirynen M. Computer-supported implant planning and guided surgery: A narrative review. Clin Oral Implants Res 2015;26(Suppl 11):69–76.

9. Arisan V, Karabuda CZ, Ozdemir T. Implant surgery using bone- and mucosa-supported stereolithographic guides in totally edentulous jaws: Surgical and postoperative outcomes of computer-aided vs. standard techniques. Clin Oral Implants Res 2010;21:980–988.

10. Beretta M, Poli PP, Maiorana C. Accuracy of computer-aided template-guided oral implant placement: A prospective clinical study. J Periodontal Implant Sci 2014;44:184–193.

11. Tahmaseb A, Wismeijer D, Coucke W, Derksen W. Computer technology applications in surgical implant dentistry: A systematic review. Int J Oral Maxillofac Implants 2014; 29(Suppl):25–42.

12. Faeghi Nejad M, Proussaefs P, Lozada J. Combining guided alveolar ridge reduction and guided implant placement for all-on-4 surgery: A clinical report. J Prosthet Dent 2016;115:662–667.

13. Beretta M, Poli PP, Tansella S, Maiorana C. Virtually guided alveolar ridge reduction combined with computer-aided implant placement for a bimaxillary implant-supported rehabilitation: A clinical report. J Prosthet Dent 2018;120:168–172.

14. Toljanic JA, Ekstrand K, Baer RA, Thor A. Immediate loading of implants in the edentulous maxilla with a fixed provisional restoration without bone augmentation: A report on 5-year outcomes data obtained from a prospective clinical trial. Int J Oral Maxillofac Implants 2016;31:1164–1170.

15. Tallarico M, Meloni SM, Canullo L, Caneva M, Polizzi G. Five-year results of a randomized controlled trial comparing patients rehabilitated with immediately loaded maxillary cross-arch fixed dental prosthesis supported by four or six implants placed using guided surgery. Clin Implant Dent Relat Res 2016;18:965–972.

16. Astrand P, Ahlqvist J, Gunne J, Nilson H. Implant treatment of patients with edentulous jaws: A 20-year follow-up. Clin Implant Dent Relat Res 2008;10:207–217.

17. Mericske-Stern R, Worni A. Optimal number of oral implants for fixed reconstructions: A review of the literature. Eur J Oral Implantol 2014;7(Suppl 2): S133–S153.

18. Maló P, de Araujo Nobre M, Lopes A, Moss SM, Molina GJ. A longitudinal study of the survival of All-on-4 implants in the mandible with up to 10 years of follow-up. J Am Dent Assoc 2011;142:310–320.

19. van Steenberghe D, Naert I, Andersson M, Brajnovic I, Van Cleynenbreugel J, Suetens P. A custom template and definitive prosthesis allowing immediate implant loading in the maxilla: A clinical report. Int J Oral Maxillofac Implants 2002;17:663–670.

20. Maló P, Rangert B, Nobre M. "All-on-Four" immediate-function concept with Brånemark System implants for completely edentulous mandibles: A retrospective clinical study. Clin Implant Dent Relat Res 2003; 5(Suppl 1):2–9.

21. Vercruyssen M, Coucke W, Naert I, Jacobs R, Teughels W, Quirynen M. Depth and lateral deviations in guided implant surgery: An RCT comparing guided surgery with mental navigation or the use of a pilot-drill template. Clin Oral Implants Res 2015;26:1315–1320.

22. Cushen SE, Turkyilmaz I. Impact of operator experience on the accuracy of implant placement with stereolithographic surgical templates: An in vitro study. J Prosthet Dent 2013;109:248–254.

23. Abduo J, Lau D. Accuracy of static computer-assisted implant placement in anterior and posterior sites by clinicians new to implant dentistry: In vitro comparison of fully guided, pilot-guided, and freehand protocols. Int J Implant Dent 2020;6:10.

24. Lin CC, Ishikawa M, Maida T, et al. Stereolithographic surgical guide with a combination of tooth and bone support: Accuracy of guided implant surgery in distal extension situation. J Clin Med 2020;9:709.

25. Cunha RM, Souza FÁ, Hadad H, Poli PP, Maiorana C, Carvalho PSP. Accuracy evaluation of computer-guided implant surgery associated with prototyped surgical guides. J Prosthet Dent 2021;125:266–272.

26. Beretta M, Poli PP, Tansella S, Aguzzi M, Meoli A, Maiorana C. Cast-free digital workflow for implant-supported rehabilitation in a completely edentulous patient: A clinical report. J Prosthet Dent 2020;125:197–203.

27. Lo Russo L, Caradonna G, Troiano G, Salamini A, Guida L, Ciavarella D. Three-dimensional differences between intraoral scans and conventional impressions of edentulous jaws: A clinical study. J Prosthet Dent 2020;123:264–268.

28. Bohner L, Gamba DD, Hanisch M, et al. Accuracy of digital technologies for the scanning of facial, skeletal, and intraoral tissues: A systematic review. J Prosthet Dent 2019;121:246–251.

29. Patzelt SB, Vonau S, Stampf S, Att W. Assessing the feasibility and accuracy of digitizing edentulous jaws. J Am Dent Assoc 2013;144:914–920.

30. Lee JH. Improved digital impressions of edentulous areas. J Prosthet Dent 2017;117:448–449.

31. Fang JH, An X, Jeong SM, Choi BH. Digital intraoral scanning technique for edentulous jaws. J Prosthet Dent 2018;119:733–735.

32. Venezia P, Torsello F, D'Amato S, Cavalcanti R. Digital cross-mounting: A new opportunity in prosthetic dentistry. Quintessence Int 2017;48:701–709.

ALVEOLAR RIDGE PRESERVATION AND IMMEDIATE IMPLANT PLACEMENT

CHAPTER 7

Edited by Luca Ferrantino, Alberto Pispero, Michele Maglione and Massimo Simion

INTRODUCTION

When a tooth is clearly compromised and cannot be maintained (for example, a tooth with a vertical root fracture), the decision to perform an extraction is simple. Similarly, in the context of a healthy mouth, it is a simple decision to maintain and treat a tooth that presents an easily solvable problem (for example, occlusal caries).

Between these two extremes, where the prognosis is easily foreseeable, there is an infinity of intermediate situations that require the careful evaluation of many factors related to the tooth, the patient, and the treatment plan, all of which must be considered when deciding whether to extract a tooth **(Table 1)**. Because these factors condition one another, they must be evaluated together.

When a tooth must be extracted, is it correct to proceed directly to extraction without thinking about what will happen next?

Of course not.

From the very beginning, implant treatment options should be considered. This chapter describes the placement of implants immediately after tooth extraction, which is a very attractive and advantageous option for patients. This chapter also delves into the consequences of tooth extraction on the surrounding tissues; the alveolus-implant interactions; and minimally invasive techniques for implant-supported prosthetic treatment, generically referred to as alveolar ridge preservation techniques.

A specific alveolar preservation technique, the socket shield, is also explored.

> *Immediate implant placement is a widely used and effective technique. However, it is not without risks. It is very reliable if the correct indications and surgical protocol are followed but totally unreliable if left to personal inventiveness and improvisation.*
>
> *Massimo Simion*

L. Ferrantino • A. Pispero • M. Maglione • M. Simion

Table 1 Factors to consider when determining the prognosis of a compromised tooth.

Tooth-related factors	Factors related to the treatment plan	Patient-related factors
Bone loss	Strategic importance of the tooth	Age
Probing depth	Occlusal stability	Health status
Mobility		Patient compliance
Furcation		Cost of therapy
Residual alveolar ridge volume		Home oral hygiene
Crown/root ratio		Smoking
Root anatomy		Subjective esthetics
Vitality		Patient desires and expectations
Caries		
Tooth position		
Objective esthetics		

ORIGINS OF IMMEDIATE IMPLANT PLACEMENT

In the first years following Brånemark's publications on osseointegration, implants were used exclusively to rehabilitate completely edentulous patients.[1]

Beginning in 1980, a growing number of clinicians began to rehabilitate partially edentulous patients with implant-supported prostheses, while adhering to Brånemark's recommendation to wait 6 to 12 months after tooth extraction to allow for complete hard and soft tissue healing before placing implants.[2]

The first documented case of immediate implant placement dates to 1976, in Germany, where Professor Wilfried Schulte of the University of Tübingen introduced the Tübingen immediate implant. This implant was a truncated conical alumina-oxide implant designed for immediate insertion into a fresh extraction socket. Because Schulte's publications were written in German, however, they remained virtually unknown outside of Germany.

The first publications in English on immediate implants date back to the late 1980s and early 1990s. At that time, another technique was also being developed that would prove to be fundamental to implantology: guided bone regeneration (GBR) using semi-permeable membranes (see chapter 14).

The combination of GBR and immediate implant placement provided encouraging results in some cases and disappointing results in others. It was probably at this stage that the hypothesis was formulated (and later disproved) that implants are responsible for the preservation of alveolar bone volume.

HEALING OF EXTRACTION SITES

By the early 2000s, knowledge of extraction site alveolus biology allowed for a more systematic approach to implant placement.[3,4] A series of studies has shown that extraction sites heal much like normal wounds. The wound-healing process is classically divided into three phases:

1. **Inflammatory phase**, which begins when the blood clot forms in the alveolus and continues for 7 to 10 days, during which the clot is stabilized by the fibrin network, new vessels form within the stabilized clot, and the clot is progressively replaced with granulation tissue.
2. **Proliferative phase**, which begins gradually and lasts several weeks, continuing with the progressive replacement of the granulation tissue and fibrin network with new vessels, mesenchymal tissue, fibrous tissue, and newly formed bone tissue (woven bone).
3. **Remodeling phase,** which continues until approximately 6 months after extraction. During this stage, the newly formed, immature bone is progressively replaced by cortical and cancellous bone.

These three phases are associated with important dimensional changes in the soft and hard tissues **(Fig 1)**.

The net result of these changes is that the total volume of the alveolar process at the extraction site tends to decrease over time. A systematic review of human studies calculated a weighted average of hard tissue changes after tooth extraction. After 6 months, there is a dimensional reduction of 3.79 ± 0.23 mm in the horizontal direction and 1.24 ± 0.11 mm in the vertical direction.[5] This reduction results from the resorption of the alveolar bundle bone, which is embryologically and functionally related to the presence of the tooth.

The bundle bone varies in thickness between 0.2 and 0.4 mm.[6] When the buccal wall of the alveolar process is thin (< 1 mm), the loss of the bundle

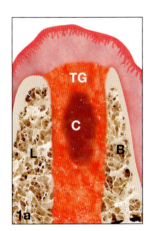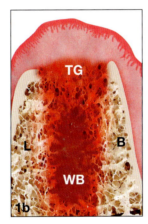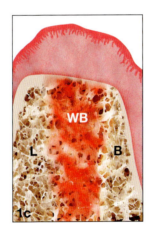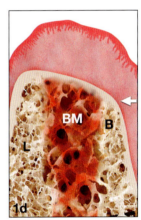

Fig 1 Four representations of animal histologic sections. From left to right, they show the healing phases of extraction sockets at 1, 2, 4, and 8 weeks. (a) At 1 week after extraction, the clot and immature granulation tissue are still evident toward the end of the inflammatory phase and the beginning of the proliferative phase. (b) The inflammatory phase is over, and immature bone is already forming at the base of the alveolus, progressively replacing the granulation tissue. (c) At 4 weeks in the animal model, the proliferative phase is already quite mature. The woven bone, which has recolonized the volume occupied by the extracted tooth, is very visible. (d) By 8 weeks, the remodeling phase is underway. The loss of bone volume due to resorption of the buccal plate is very visible (arrow). In the center of the alveolus, large bone marrow spaces covered coronally with recorticalized bone are visible.[3] L = lingual cortical; B = buccal cortical; C = clot; TG = granulation tissue; WB = woven bone; BM = bone marrow.

bone is very likely to cause a volumetric loss of the alveolar process. This is usually verifiable, especially in the anterior maxilla, where the buccal cortical thickness is very limited.

A study by Januário et al[7] showed that fewer than one in seven patients had buccal cortical bone at the maxillary central incisors thicker than 1 mm. This cortical, consisting mainly of bundle bone, resorbs in the absence of a tooth and leads to horizontal and vertical decreases of the alveolar ridge, as found in the review by Tan et al.[5]

The total volumetric contraction of the alveolar ridge becomes evident a few months after extraction, but in the first few weeks, the contraction of the hard tissues does not follow a linear pattern. A study by Chappuis et al[8] showed that simultaneously with the reduction of bone in the alveolar process, a thickening of the connective tissue is observed in the first weeks of healing, which by 8 weeks, can increase up to seven times its initial thickness, in a manner directly proportional to the bone volume that has undergone resorption.

IMPLANT AND EXTRACTION SITE INTERACTION

In consideration of the volumetric changes in the tissue that have been widely documented in the literature, what then happens when an implant is placed into an extraction socket?

From a biologic point of view, it has been shown that osseointegration is possible and predictable, even in areas where there is no initial bone-to-implant contact (BIC).[9]

On the other hand, it has become clear that the implant cannot in any way avoid or even reduce the atrophy of the alveolar process, as was hypothesized in the early 1990s. Poorly positioned implants and implants with excessive diameters can even lead to greater buccal cortical atrophy caused by compression.[4,10,11]

Implants must be appropriately sized and positioned in such a way as to leave a gap of at least 2 mm between the implant surface and the buccal plate.[12] This gap is indispensable for performing alveolar preservation procedures, which are described in the next section.

PRESERVATION OF THE ALVEOLAR RIDGE

After the extraction of a tooth, a volume of bone that could potentially have been useful for implant placement is lost. This loss is more critical if it occurs in an esthetic area, where bone volume is not only necessary to support the implant but is also essential for restoring harmony between the teeth and gingiva.[13]

Unfortunately, it is precisely in the esthetic areas (anterior maxilla) where the greatest loss of bone volume occurs after an extraction.

This is because the buccal plate of the incisors and canines is often thin (< 1 mm). The loss of bundle bone following tooth extraction results in considerable resorption, leading to a considerable volumetric reduction of the ridge. This volumetric reduction can hinder the success of implant-prosthetic rehabilitation.

Fortunately, there are methods to reduce or avoid alveolar ridge resorption and hard and soft tissue reconstruction techniques, which though predictable, inevitably increase treatment time, cost, and morbidity. This is supported by many studies in the literature,[14] among which the work published in 2006 by Nevins et al is particularly noteworthy.[15] This study showed that the use of a slow-resorbing biomaterial, such as deproteinized bovine bone mineral (DBBM), inserted into the socket immediately after extraction counteracts volumetric shrinkage.

This is particularly evident around the maxillary incisors **(Figs 2 to 5)**.

From a biologic point of view, it is important to emphasize that the preservation of the alveolar ridge with DBBM has no effect on the resorption of the buccal plate, which will follow its physiologic process regardless. Studies by Tomasi et al have shown that the use of DBBM reduces the volumetric contraction that would occur following the loss of the buccal bone plate when it is thin (< approximately 1 mm).[16,17]

This technique is effective for maintaining bone volume and is certainly indicated in posterior areas (molars and premolars), where it seems to be able to reduce the need for bone regeneration requiring maxillary sinus elevation.[18,19]

To further improve results in highly esthetic areas, it is possible to combine the heterologous bone graft with a connective graft taken from the palate to close the alveolus without modifying the mucogingival line.

It is advisable to place an epithelial-connective tissue graft of the same width as the mesiodistal diameter of the alveolus and approximately 6 mm longer than the buccopalatal dimension. The exposed central area is kept epithelialized, and the peripheral 3 mm of the long side is deepithelialized, so that they can be tunneled buccally and palatally below the mucosa to fix the graft and provide it with vascular support.

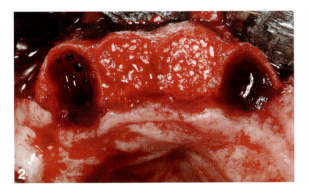 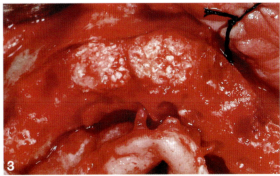

Fig 2 *The test extraction sites are the sockets of the central incisors, and the control extraction sites are the sockets of the lateral incisors.* **Fig 3** *After healing, it can be seen that the alveolar ridge has retained a good coronal thickness in the area of the central incisors, whereas at the level of the lateral incisors, the ridge has thinned due to loss of the buccal plate. (Courtesy of Int J Periodontics Restorative Dent 2006;26:19–29.)*

Fig 4 CT sections. Extraction socket filled with a biomaterial on the day of extraction (a) and 180 days later (b), with the ridge volume practically maintained. (c) Extraction socket in a control site without biomaterial. (d) After 180 days, the loss of the buccal bone plate and the resulting reduction in volume is evident. (Reprinted with permission from Int J Periodontics Restorative Dent 2006;26:19–29.)

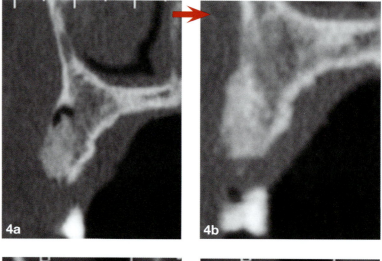

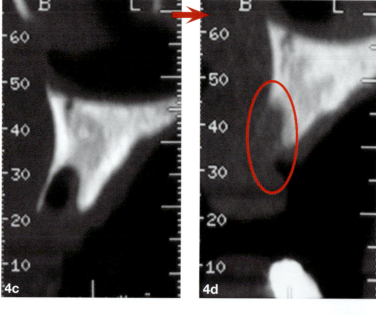

Fig 5 (a) Biopsy of an extraction site filled with DBBM at 6 months of healing. Toluidine blue staining; ×4 magnification. (b) At higher magnification, a DBBM particle surrounded by newly formed bone is visible. BO = DBBM particle; NB = newly formed bone. (Reprinted with permission from Int J Periodontics Restorative Dent 2006;26:19–29.)

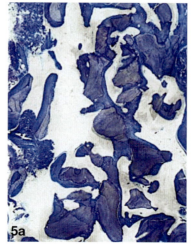

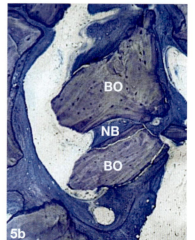

CLINICAL CASE 1

Alveolar bone preservation after maxillary central incisor extraction

A 42-year-old, nonsmoking patient in good health presented for treatment of the maxillary left central incisor, which was suffering from extensive root resorption following a traumatic accident. The CBCT examination showed almost complete involvement of the root structure up to the middle third of its length (Fig 6). Clinical examination revealed that the tooth showed a pinkish discoloration at the buccal cervical area, which was an expression of inflammatory tissue invasion within the dental tissue (Fig 7). Therefore, it was opted to extract the tooth with preservation of the alveolar bone, without immediate implant placement due to the partial loss of the buccal bone plate.

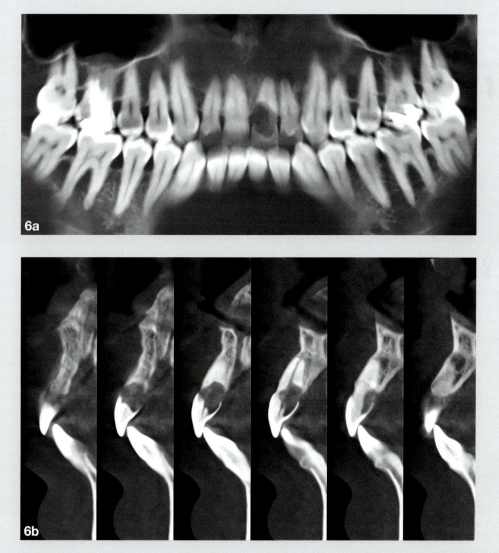

Fig 6 *(a)* Panoramic view of a CBCT showing the maxillary left central incisor with severe traumatic root resorption in the coronal third. *(b)* Cross sections show partial loss of the buccal bone plate.

The periodontal attachment was dissected with a Molt curette inserted inside the gingival sulcus (**Fig 8**), the crown was removed, and the root was sectioned longitudinally with a piezoelectric instrument (**Fig 9**). Then, the palatal portion of the root was removed (**Fig 10**), followed by removal of the buccal portion of the root by gently pushing it toward the palatal wall to completely preserve all the residual buccal bone plate (**Fig 11**). All the soft tissue present in the alveolus was removed with a long alveolar spoon (**Fig 12**).

The gingival tissue was elevated approximately 3 mm from the palatal (**Fig 13a**) and buccal (**Fig 13b**) bone plates to allow for the placement of the connective graft. A particulate deproteinized bovine bone mineral (DBBM) graft (Bio-Oss, Geistlich Biomaterials) was placed without exceeding the bone margin (**Fig 14**). An oval-shaped epithelial connective tissue graft harvested from the palate and de-epithelialized in the peripheral portions (**Fig 15**) was positioned palatally and buccally to close the alveolar defect (**Fig 16**).

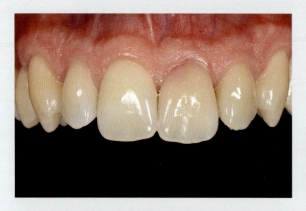

Fig 7 Clinical photo showing the reddish pigmentation of the collar of the maxillary left central incisor.

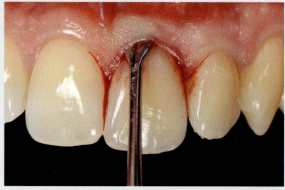

Fig 8 A Molt curette is inserted into the gingival sulcus to dissect the periodontal attachment.

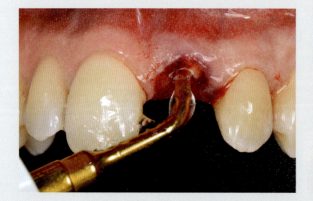

Fig 9 The root is dissected longitudinally with a piezoelectric instrument.

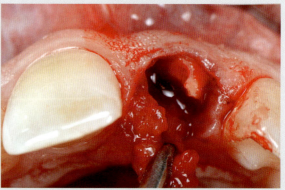

Fig 10 The palatal portion of the root is removed with tweezers, along with the inflammatory tissue.

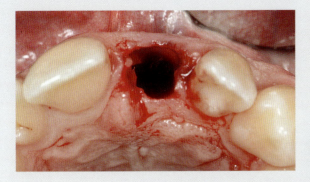

Fig 11 The buccal portion of the root was removed, showing the characteristics of the alveolus.

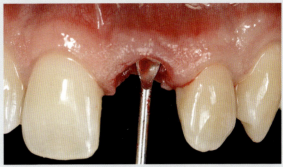

Fig 12 The alveolus is curetted with an alveolar spoon to remove all the soft tissue.

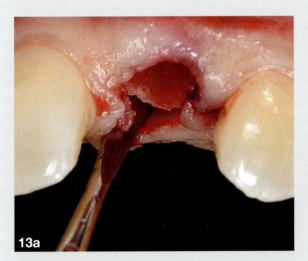

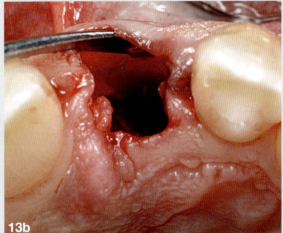

Fig 13 With a thin periosteal elevator, both the palatal mucosa (a) and buccal mucosa (b) are elevated 3 mm.

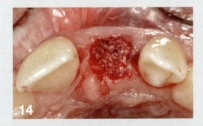

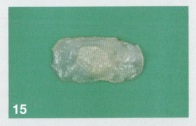

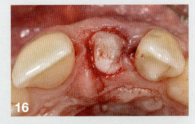

Fig 14 The socket was filled with particulate DBBM up to the level of the bone crest. **Fig 15** An epithelial-connective tissue graft was harvested from the palate and de-epithelialized in the peripheral portions, leaving an island of epithelium in the area to remain exposed to the oral cavity. **Fig 16** The graft was inserted below the buccal and palatal mucosa to cover the defect.

After applying a gel with hyaluronic acid (Hobagel Plus, Hobama), a provisional prosthesis was bonded with composite resin to the adjacent teeth, while slight pressure was exerted to keep the connective graft in place without the need for sutures **(Fig 17)**. Then 4 to 6 months were allowed to pass for healing to take place **(Fig 18)** before implant placement.

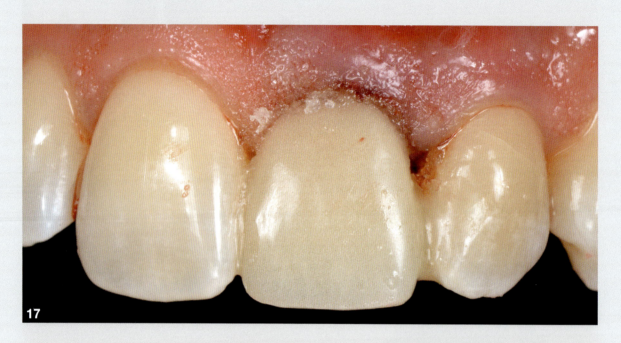

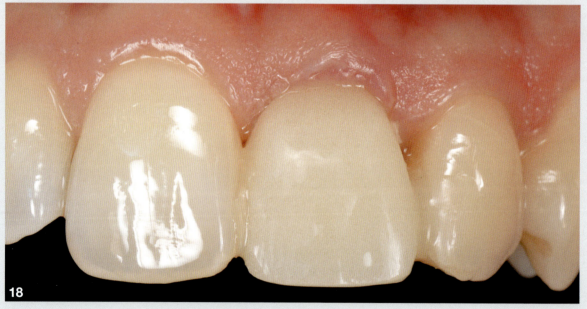

Fig 17 A hyaluronic acid gel was applied to protect the site, and a slightly compressive resin-bonded provisional prosthesis was applied to keep the graft secure. **Fig 18** Clinical photo showing the healing after 3 weeks.

RISK ASSESSMENT FOR IMMEDIATE IMPLANT PLACEMENT

The success of placing an immediate implant into a fresh extraction socket depends upon the predictability of the alveolar bone preservation technique that is used in the extraction site. The predictability of alveolar bone preservation is determined by several factors, the most important of which is the integrity and thickness of the buccal plate. Immediate implant placement is indicated only in the presence of an intact buccal cortical plate > 1 mm in thickness and when it is possible to place an implant of adequate diameter while maintaining a gap of at least 2 mm from the buccal wall.

To these requirements we must add a fundamental condition, which is necessary for any implant procedure, and that is a sufficient amount of bone for obtaining primary implant stability **(Figs 19 and 20)**. Stabilization of the implant always occurs in the 3 to 4 mm apical and palatal to the alveolus, so as not to stress its walls. For this reason, it is important that the implant design allows for effective stabilization in the few millimeters of bone apical to the alveolus. Another key factor is the absence of ongoing acute infections at the level of the tooth to be extracted, which could transfer pathogenic bacteria to the biomaterial and/or implant. Other important conditions to be assessed are the patient's subjective esthetic needs and the objective esthetics of the case, as well as patient compliance. All the factors contributing to the predictability of immediate implant placement are summarized in **Box 1**.

In the presence of all these factors, predictability is such that immediate implant placement carries no greater risk than the deferred approach, and it is advantageous for reducing the number of the surgical steps, treatment time and cost, and the invasiveness of the procedure.

When one or more of these factors is not present, the predictability of immediate implant placement decreases drastically, whereas the predictability of multistage procedures, such as deferred implant placement with or without GBR, remains relatively unaffected **(Fig 21)**.

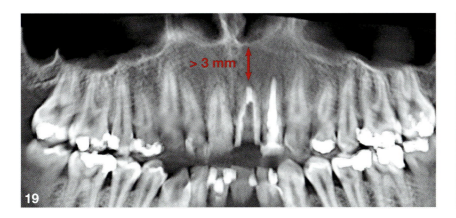
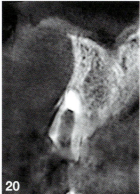

Fig 19 The presence of at least 3 mm of apical bone around the tooth to be extracted guarantees the possibility of good primary implant stability. *Fig 20* Cross-sectional view of the case presented in Fig 19.

Box 1 Favorable and unfavorable factors for performing the socket shield technique.

Absence of acute infections
Intact buccal cortical plate > 1 mm thick
Adequate implant diameter and gap > 2 mm
Sufficient bone for correct 3D implant positioning
Low esthetic risks
Patient compliance

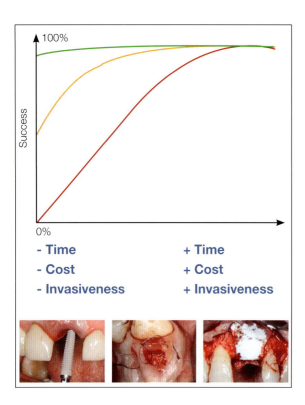

- Time   + Time
- Cost   + Cost
- Invasiveness   + Invasiveness

Fig 21 *The relationship between treatment complexity (X-axis) and treatment predictability (Y-axis). The green line represents a clinical case with a low risk profile. Because therapies of varying invasiveness, cost, and timing are shown to have similar success rates, immediate implant placement will presumably be the treatment of choice. The orange line indicates a case with a medium risk profile (ie, one or more of the factors listed in Table 2 are absent). In this case, immediate implant placement is not recommended, but with alveolar bone preservation and delayed implant placement, the case should resolve favorably. The red line represents a high-risk profile. In this type of case, an operation to restore hard and soft tissue volumes via GBR and connective grafts should be considered. Time, cost, and morbidity inevitably increase to achieve good treatment predictability for patients with high-risk profiles.*

STAGES OF IMMEDIATE IMPLANT PLACEMENT

Immediate implant placement is performed in a sequence of five steps:

1. Extraction
2. Alveolar curettage
3. Implant placement
4. Preservation of the alveolar ridge
5. Delivery of the immediate prosthesis

Extraction

Implant extraction should be performed in the least traumatic manner possible. Preserving the soft and hard tissues in their entirety is crucial for achieving a satisfactory result **(Fig 22)**. The best way is to perform an extraction is to dislodge the tooth very gently in the mesiodistal direction and potentially perform one or more odontotomies in the mesiodistal direction to gently extract the tooth

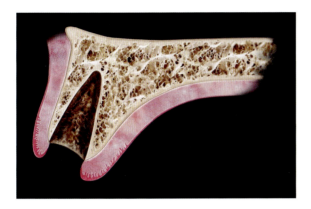

Fig 22 *Illustration of a perfectly preserved socket after tooth extraction.*

once it has been separated into several fragments. The main objective is to avoid fracturing or damaging the buccal plate.

This is the most delicate and important component of the operation. A finger can be placed during dislocation maneuvers to help the clinician perceive the application of any excessive forces on the buccal plate. Once the extraction is complete, it is important to clean the walls of the socket well to remove all granulation tissue and any remnants of infection.

Alveolar curettage

The complete removal of all granulation tissue within the alveolus is essential for achieving adequate bone regeneration and complete biomaterial integration.

Alveolar curettage is performed with alveolar spoons and sometimes takes longer than the extraction itself. The placement of a biomaterial in the presence of granulation tissue on the walls of the alveolus leads to total encapsulation of the biomaterial in the connective tissue and prevents bone neoformation.

Implant placement

Once the alveolus has been cleaned, the implant site is prepared, which as mentioned, will have to stabilize the implant in the area apical and palatal to the alveolus. In addition to these considerations, great care must be taken to obtain correct 3D implant positioning, which follows the same principles that apply to implant placement in native bone:

- **Apicocoronal position of the implant:** The implant shoulder must be assessed in relation to the future peri-implant mucosal margin, which in turn must be harmonious with the adjacent teeth. A general rule is that when using a bone-level implant, the implant shoulder should be at least 3 mm apical to the future peri-implant mucosal margin. At the same time, the implant should be completely surrounded by bone after healing, which is why immediate implants tend to be placed slightly (0.5 to 1.5 mm) subcrestal.

- **Buccopalatal position of the implant:** The implant must be in contact with the palatal plate of the alveolus, with a gap from the buccal plate of at least 2 mm. This means it is important to choose an implant diameter that is not excessive.

- **Mesiodistal position of the implant:** Immediate implants, particularly in the area of the maxillary incisors, should not be placed exactly in the center of the alveolus, but slightly distal. This makes it easier to obtain a distally shifted peri-implant mucosal zenith, which makes the prosthesis appear more natural and esthetically pleasing.

- **Angulation of the implant:** The implant must be inserted in such a way that the emergence of the screw is palatal to the incisal edge of the future crown. This allows the access hole to be masked in the case of a screw-retained prosthesis.

To achieve these results, clinicians must make careful use of the burs. The pilot drill is used to make a notch on the palatal surface of the alveolar wall **(Fig 23)**.

This avoids the risk, very frequent in this type of surgery, of the drills sliding along this wall and resulting in a too buccal implant position. The first drill is then positioned within the notch created by the pilot drill **(Fig 24)**. The drill initially has the same inclination as the pilot drill in the buccopalatal direction. Obviously, this is not the final inclination that the implant will have **(Fig 25)**.

Underpreparation and implants with aggressive apices are essential for achieving maximum primary stability (40–50 Ncm) of immediate implants. In most cases, a 2.3- to 2.8-mm drill is required for site preparation for a 3.7-mm implant. Implant insertion will also follow the same general procedure as for the preparation drills, with the implants possessing an initial buccopalatal inclination **(Fig 26)** and then gradually straightening and assuming the correct position toward the end of insertion **(Fig 27)**. In the maxilla, a manual screwdriver-type insertion tool is very useful.

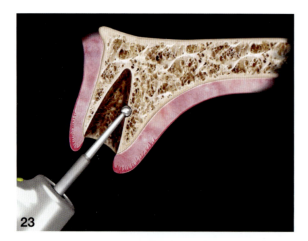
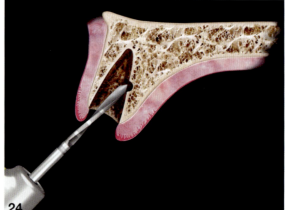

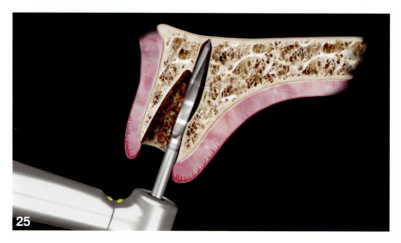

Fig 23 The pilot drill is used to make a notch in the palatal surface of the alveolar wall. Fig 24 The first drill is placed in the notch made by the pilot drill, following the same inclination. Fig 25 Gradually, as the preparation of the implant site deepens apically, the drill changes inclination, straightening and taking the angulation of the future implant.

Preservation of the alveolar ridge

Once the implant has been inserted, the gap between the buccal plate and the implant surface must be treated in the same way as an extraction site in which we want to perform alveolar ridge preservation. A slow-resorbing biomaterial is inserted in the deeper area up to the buccal bone crest, but without exceeding the level of the crest itself (**Fig 28**).

The use of the connective graft at this stage is a further aid in preserving the volume of the alveolar crest, but it is certainly not essential if the case selection and surgical procedures up to this point have been performed correctly, as demonstrated in a recent multicenter randomized clinical trial.[20]

Then, either a healing screw can be placed, as in **Fig 28**, or a prosthesis can be placed directly (**Fig 29**).

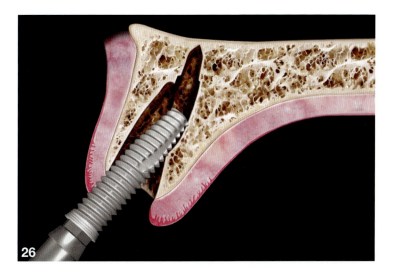

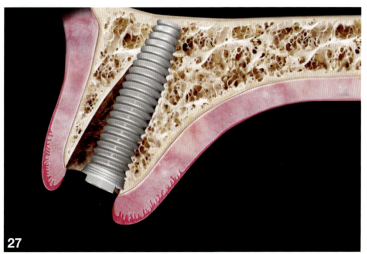

Fig 26 Insertion of the implant with an excessively buccal inclination to properly engage the implant site preparation. *Fig 27* Progressively, the inclination becomes more palatal as the implant is inserted and ends up being corrected in the last few turns.

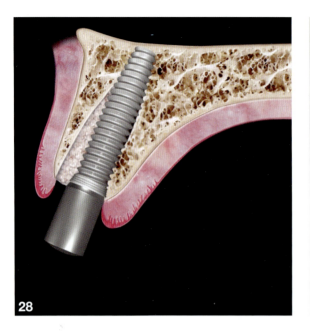
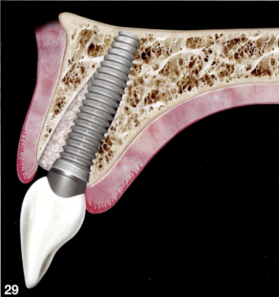

Fig 28 The implant in place and the slow-resorbing biomaterial bridging the buccal gap. *Fig 29* Completed operation with the placement of an immediate fixed prosthesis.

Delivery of the immediate prosthesis

From a patient perspective, one of the undoubted advantages of immediate implant placement is the potential to receive a fixed provisional prosthesis on the day of tooth extraction, effectively eliminating the discomfort arising from the potential (an unfortunately quite frequent) detachment of a resin-bonded provisional; from the use of removable dentures, which are always harmful to the mucosal membranes; or from being temporarily without a tooth.

Immediately restoring implants with a prosthesis also has an additional advantage: It provides support to the papillae and the free gingival margin of the newly extracted tooth, promoting stability. The material inserted in the gap between the buccal plate and the implant is also better protected by the provisional restoration **(Fig 29)**. One randomized clinical trial[21] showed that immediate implants restored with immediate prostheses achieved better esthetic results than immediate implants that were prosthetically loaded 3 months after surgery **(Fig 30)**.

The test group, in which an immediate prosthesis was placed, presented an average buccal

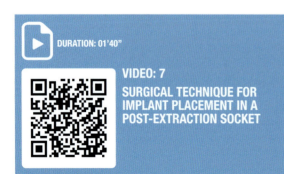

DURATION: 01'40"

VIDEO: 7

SURGICAL TECHNIQUE FOR IMPLANT PLACEMENT IN A POST-EXTRACTION SOCKET

margin recession of 0.75 mm less than the control group, which was clinically and statistically significant.

In addition to providing support to the soft tissues, the provisional crown also has the role of leaving ample space for the clot along the transmucosal path. It must therefore be characterized by a concave buccal emergence profile between the gingival margin and the implant platform **(Fig 31)**.

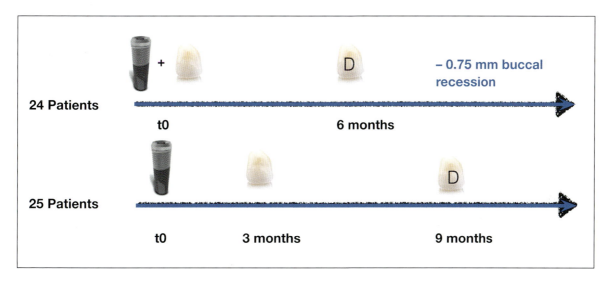

Fig 30 *Diagram of the study performed by De Rouck et al.[21] The test group, in which an immediate prosthesis was placed, presented an average of 0.75 mm less buccal margin recession than the control group, which was a statistically and clinically significant value.*

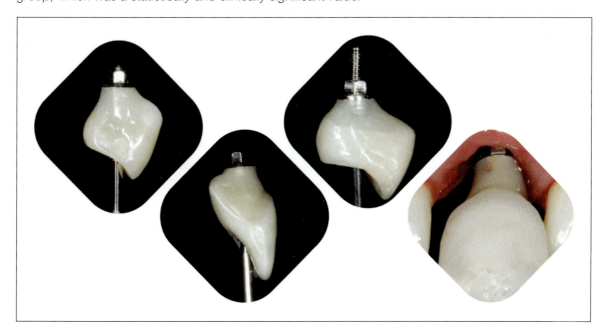

Fig 31 *Examples of transmucosal paths of provisional crowns screwed onto immediate implants.*

CLINICAL CASE 2

Alveolar bone preservation in a case of maxillary central incisor extraction and flapless implant placement

A 47-year-old, nonsmoking patient who was a carrier of thalassemia, presented for treatment of a buccal fistula at the level of the maxillary left central incisor **(Fig 32)**. CBCT imaging showed a horizontal root fracture at the level of the coronal third associated with a bony defect partially involving the buccal plate **(Fig 33)**.

The coronal portion of the tooth and the root fragment were extracted **(Figs 34 and 35)**, and the alveolus and soft tissues were curetted to remove all the granulation tissue **(Fig 36)**.

A particulate DBBM **(Fig 37)** and epithelial-connective graft were placed as previously described. The graft was secured with simple interrupted sutures (Prolene 6-0, Ethicon) to avoid compression of the provisional prosthesis in the absence of the buccal bone plate **(Fig 38)**.

After the application of Hobagel Plus, an appropriately reduced resin-bonded provisional prosthesis was placed **(Fig 39)**. Sutures were removed after 15 days **(Fig 40)**.

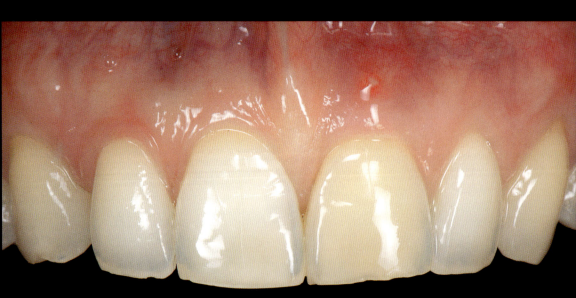

Fig 32 Clinical image of the maxillary left central incisor, where a buccal fistula is evident.

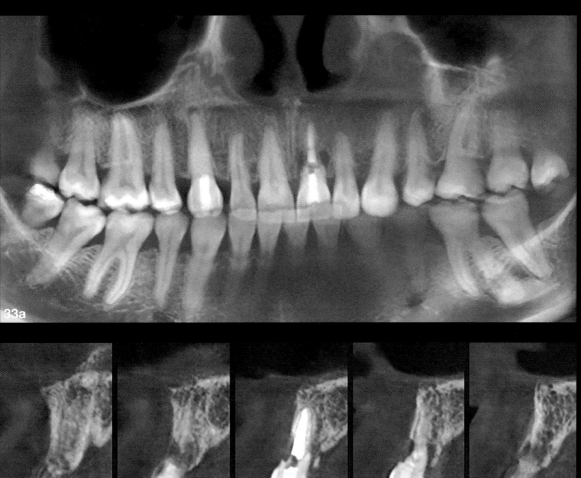

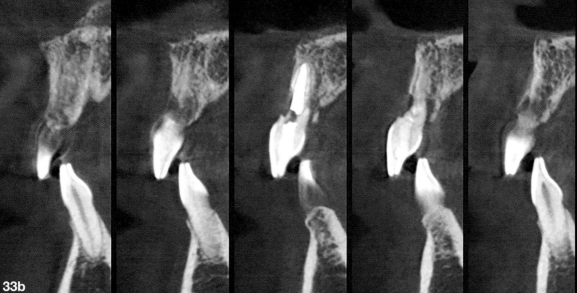

Fig 33 *(a)* CBCT showing a root fracture at the level of the coronal third of the root. *(b)* The sectional image shows the partial loss of the buccal bone plate.

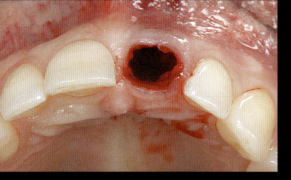

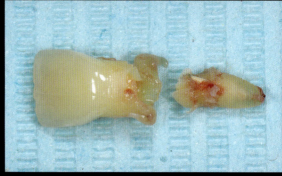

Fig 34 The tooth was extracted, and the alveolus was curetted to remove all granulation tissue.

Fig 35 Image of the extracted tooth in two sections. The extensive root resorption leading to the root fracture is evident.

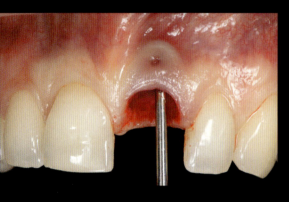

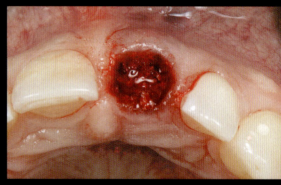

Fig 36 A Molt curette is used to evaluate the extent of buccal bone loss

Fig 37 The socket is filled with Bio-Oss collagen up to the level of the bone margin.

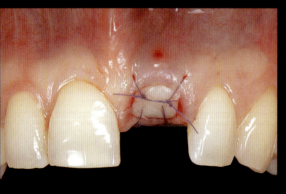

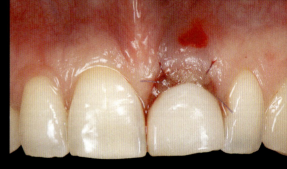

Fig 38 An oval-shaped epithelial-connective tissue graft was de-epithelialized in the portions to be inserted under the buccal and palatal mucosa and sutured with Prolene 6-0 monofilament.

Fig 39 After the application of Hobagel to protect the graft, a resin-bonded provisional prosthesis was placed.

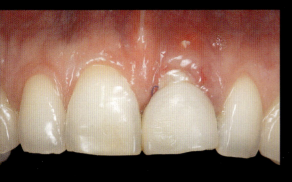
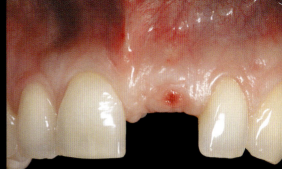

Fig 40 Healing after 15 days. Note the superficial desquamation of the graft.

Fig 41 Healing after 6 months.

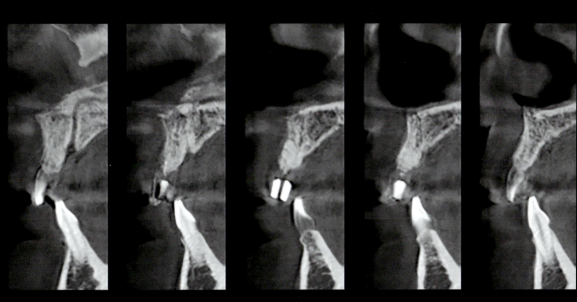

Fig 42 CBCT showing site healing after 6 months and correct positioning of a surgical guide.

After 6 months of healing **(Fig 41)**, a surgical guide was constructed based on CBCT imaging **(Fig 42)**. The implant site was prepared according to a flapless approach with the surgical guide and underpreparation of the implant site to achieve adequate primary implant stability **(Figs 43 to 45)**.

The fully machined implant was inserted 1 mm below the bone crest with a manual screwdriver instrument, and a short healing abutment of the same diameter as the implant was placed to avoid soft tissue compression **(Figs 46 to 49)**.

In the same session, a provisional was placed without occlusal contacts in centric, protrusive, or lateral movements **(Fig 50)**. After 4 months, an impression was taken **(Fig 51)**, and a zirconia abutment **(Fig 52)** was fabricated for the definitive ceramic crown **(Fig 53)**.

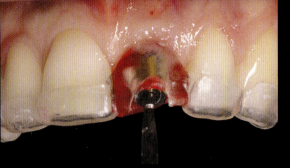

Fig 43 The implant site is prepared with the flapless technique and using a surgical guide.

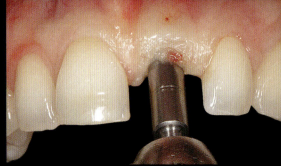

Fig 44 The mucosa is incised with a soft tissue punch mounted on a contra-angle.

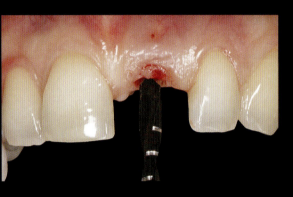

Fig 45 The final stages of implant site preparation are performed without a surgical guide.

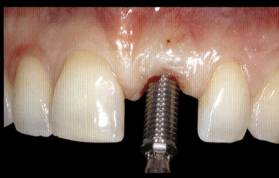

Fig 46 The fully machined implant is placed manually with a screwdriver tool for maximum control of its direction and insertion torque.

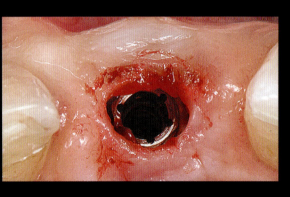

Fig 47 The implant was positioned with its head slightly below the bone crest.

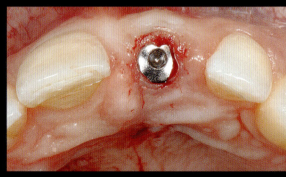

Fig 48 A healing abutment with the same diameter as the implant platform was placed to avoid soft tissue compression.

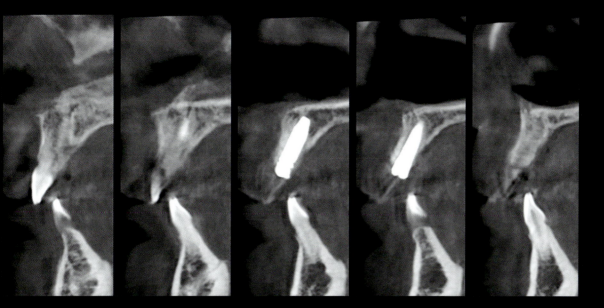

Fig 49 CBCT imagining showing correct implant positioning.

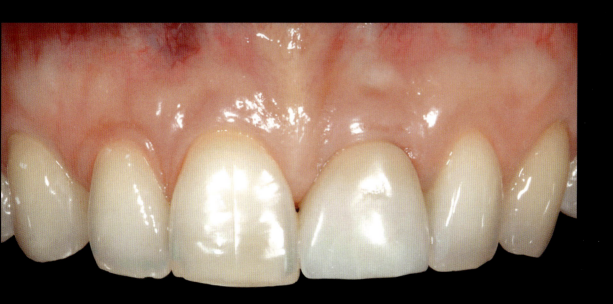

Fig 50 A provisional resin crown was placed and maintained until the emergence profile was fully mature.

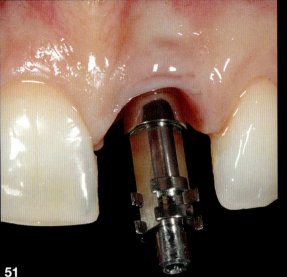
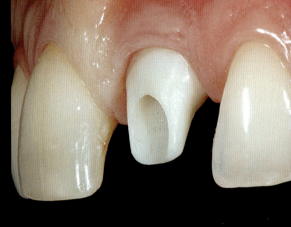

51

52

Fig 51 After 4 months, a transfer coping was placed, and an impression was taken.

Fig 52 A definitive zirconia abutment duplicating the emergence profile of the provisional crown was placed.

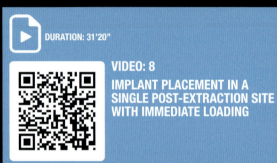

DURATION: 31'20"

VIDEO: 8
IMPLANT PLACEMENT IN A
SINGLE POST-EXTRACTION SITE
WITH IMMEDIATE LOADING

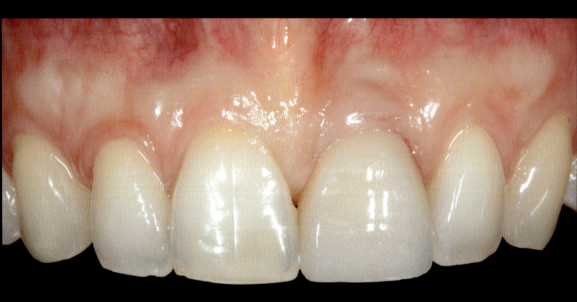

Fig 53 The final ceramic crown. The satisfactory interdental papillae and the correct shape of the gingival contour can be seen.

CLINICAL CASE 3

Immediate implant placement following maxillary premolar extraction

A 50-year-old, nonsmoking woman in good health presented with a vertical root fracture in the endodontically treated maxillary left first premolar. The fracture was evidenced by the pain response upon pressure and localized probing up to the root apex **(Fig 54)**. The periapical radiograph showed no peri-radicular bone defects **(Fig 55)**.

The tooth was extracted, the alveolus curetted, and a hybrid surface implant was placed by preparing the alveolus of the palatal root **(Fig 56)** to keep the bone defect in a buccal position **(Figs 57 and 58)**.

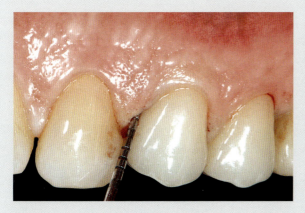

Fig 54 Maxillary left premolar showing 9 mm of localized probing as an expression of the vertical root fracture.

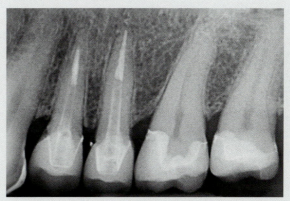

Fig. 55 The periapical radiograph shows no signs of bone loss.

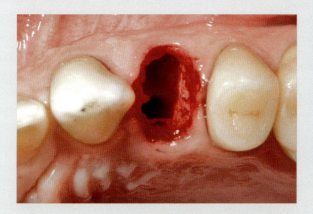

Fig 56 The tooth was extracted, and the palatal portion was prepared to receive an implant.

DURATION: 40'15"

VIDEO: 9
IMPLANT PLACEMENT IN MULTIPLE POST-EXTRACTION SITES WITH IMMEDIATE LOADING

After inserting a healing abutment of the same diameter as the implant platform, the bone defect was filled with Bio-Oss collagen up to the bone ridge margin **(Fig 59)**. The control CBCT showed the correct positioning of the implant and biomaterial **(Fig 60)**. At the same session, the healing abutment was replaced with a provisional abutment **(Fig 61)**, to which a resin crown was fitted **(Fig 62)**. The provisional crown was alleviated from all occlusal contacts in both centric and lateral excursions **(Fig 63)**.

After 4 months, the provisional was removed, a transfer coping was placed, and the tissues were rendered opaque for an impression with an intraoral scanner **(Figs 64 and 65)**. The final rehabilitation was performed with a zirconia and ceramic crown **(Figs 66 and 67)**.

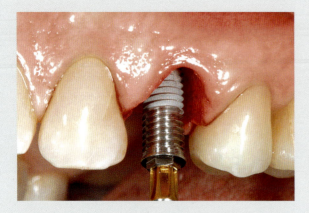

Fig 57 An iMAX (iRES) hybrid implant, 13 mm long and 3.75 mm in diameter, was inserted with a hand instrument.

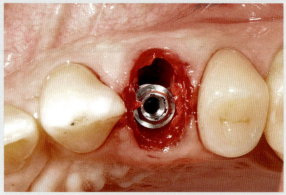

Fig 58 Occlusal view of the implant positioned slightly below the crestal margin and the residual buccal bone defect.

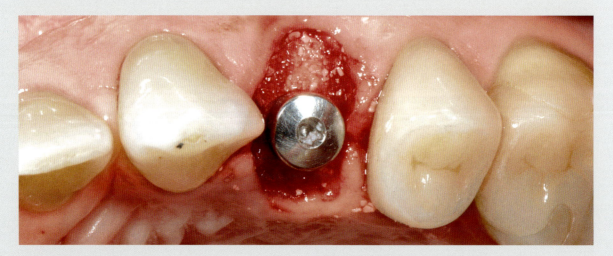

Fig 59 The healing abutment was placed, and the defect was filled with Bio-Oss collagen.

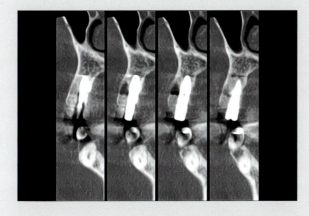

Fig 60 CBCT showing the correct implant positioning.

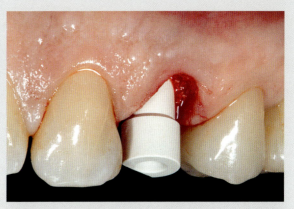

Fig 61 The healing abutment was replaced with a temporary abutment.

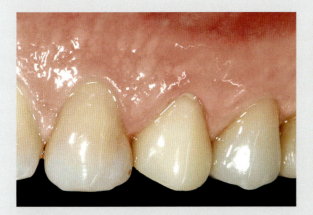

Fig 62 A provisional resin restoration was relined and adapted to the site.

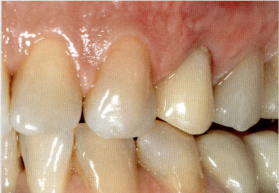

Fig 63 Checking the occlusion in a left lateral movement.

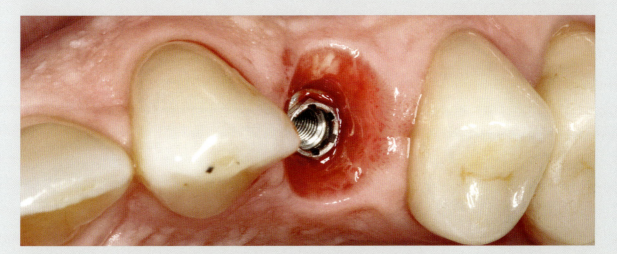

Fig 64 After 4 months of healing, the provisional prosthesis was removed. The emergence profile obtained at the level of the transmucosal portion is visible.

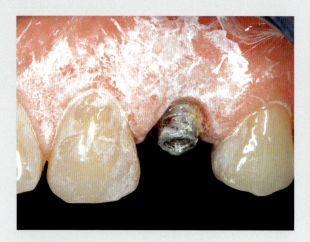

Fig 65 The transfer coping for intraoral scanning was inserted and opacified.

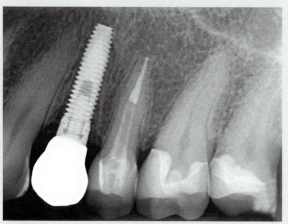

Fig 66 Control periapical radiograph. The original defect, not fully mineralized after 4 months, is still visible.

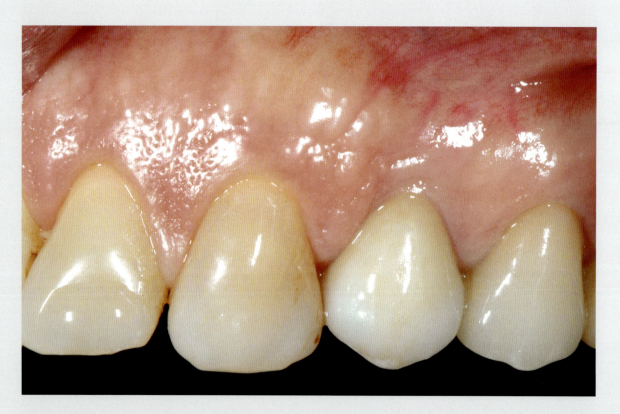

Fig 67 Definitive zirconia and ceramic crown. The interdental papillae were completely preserved.

CLINICAL CASE 4

Two adjacent immediate implants placed after extraction of the maxillary central incisors

A 50-year-old, nonsmoking man in good health presented with two severely structurally compromised maxillary central incisors. The roots appeared to be treated with excessively wide endodontic posts that compromised the integrity of the root dentin (**Fig 68**). Given the integrity of the periodontium and alveolar walls, the thickness of the gingival tissues, and the abundant amount of attached gingiva, the treatment plan involved extraction of both teeth and the immediate placement of implants and provisional restorations. The teeth were extracted gently, without damaging the buccal bone plate (**Fig 69**), and the sockets were curetted to remove any granulation tissue (**Fig 70**).

The two implants were placed after preparing the palatal bone surface, starting from the middle third of the alveolus depth, to maintain the gap between the implant and the buccal bone plate (**Fig 71**).

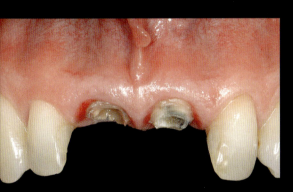

Fig 68 Structurally impaired roots of the maxillary central incisors.

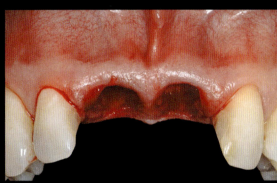

Fig 69 The roots were extracted while preserving the buccal bone plate.

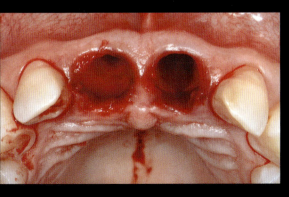

Fig 70 The sockets have been curetted and prepared to receive the implants.

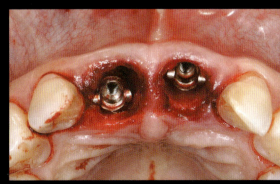

Fig 71 The implants were placed in a palatal position to maintain the entire buccal gap.

The remaining bone defects were filled with Bio-Oss DBBM. After placing the provisional restorations, appropriately reduced to the level of the buccal emergence profile, two small connective tissue grafts harvested from the palate were placed **(Fig 72)** to increase the thickness of the soft tissue. Healing after 15 days showed complete integration of the grafts, which appeared to overflow from the gingival margin **(Fig 73)**. The periapical radiograph showed the correct positioning of the implants, with the platforms 1 mm apical to the buccal bone crest **(Fig 74)**.

After 1 month of healing, the excess mucosa appeared to recede **(Fig 75)**, the provisional abutments were replaced with customized zirconia definitive abutments **(Figs 76 and 77)**, and the provisional crowns were changed **(Fig 78)**.

After 6 months of waiting for the marginal tissues to mature **(Fig 79)**, the final ceramic crowns were cemented in place **(Fig 80)**. An intraoral radiograph showed the perfect maintenance of the interproximal bone peaks after 1 year of prosthetic loading **(Fig 81)**.

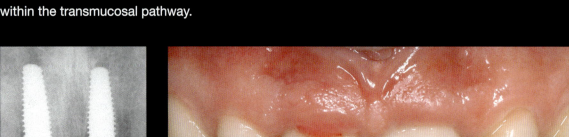

Fig 72 The defects were filled with Bio-Oss, the provisional crowns were placed, and two connective tissue grafts were inserted buccally within the transmucosal pathway.

Fig 73 Dealing after 15 days. The connective tissue grafts partially cover the buccal surface of the crowns.

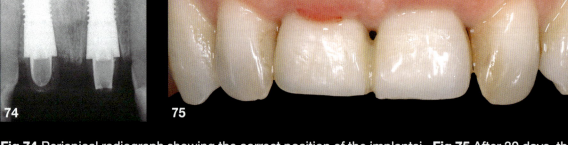

Fig 74 Periapical radiograph showing the correct position of the implantsi. **Fig 75** After 30 days, the buccal gingival margins appear to have spontaneously receded.

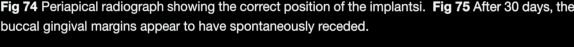

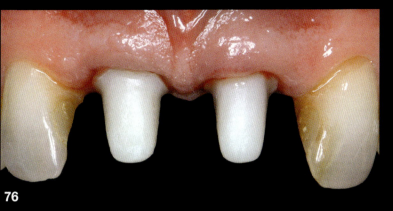

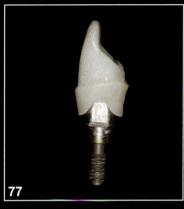

Fig 76 The final zirconia abutments were applied to the implants. **Fig 77** Customized zirconia definitive abutment.

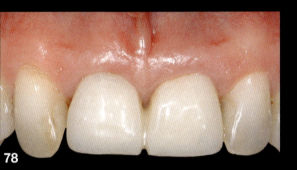

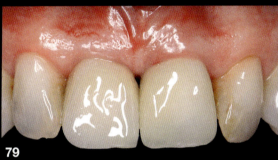

Fig 78 The provisional crowns were replaced with two new resin crowns suitable for the definitive abutments. **Fig 79** After 6 months of tissue maturation, the complete preservation of the interdental papillae and the position of the gingival margins can be seen.

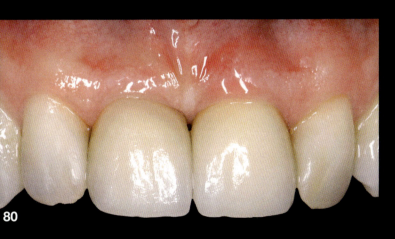

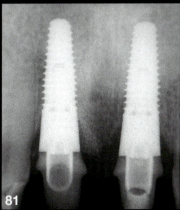

Fig 80 Definitive crowns after 1 year of function. Note the complete retention of the mesial interproximal papilla at the two central incisors. **Fig 81** Radiograph after 1 year of prosthetic loading. The interproximal bone peak is perfectly maintained.

L. Ferrantino • A. Pispero • M. Maglione • M. Simion

SOCKET SHIELD TECHNIQUE

In 2010, an article was published presenting an out-of-the-box technique for alveolar ridge preservation in which a part of the extracted tooth's root is left in place at the time of implant insertion. This is referred to as the socket shield technique, in reference to the protection offered by the root fragment to the integrity of the alveolar tissue. This section of the chapter provides a brief history of the socket shield technique, a thorough explanation of each step, and sample clinical cases, including the management of the most common complications.

Development of the socket shield technique

The creators of the socket shield technique hypothesized that retaining part of the root of the tooth to be extracted could prevent alveolar resorption.[22] The biologic principle behind this theory derived from observations that in previous studies the retention of the entire root trunk in the pontic area was shown to be a valid therapeutic alternative for maintaining alveolar volume.[23] The socket shield technique can be used to control two of the major variables that influence bone resorption after tooth extraction: buccal bone thickness and the presence of the periodontal ligament (PDL).[24]

Because good initial responses were observed in the presence of root remnants, with complete bone formation near the dentin and mucosal covering of the alveolar access, the primary hypothesis was that maintaining two-thirds of the buccal portion of the root and sectioning the crown approximately 1 mm above the bone margin would preserve the integrity of the supracrestal connective fibers and the vitality of a portion of the PDL. The latter is of paramount importance in counteracting bundle bone resorption and preserving the buccal mucosal tissues.

It was not clear, however, what the biologic response would be in the case of immediate implant placement after partial removal of the root. The first results in animal models were very encouraging, as shown by the histologic images **(Fig 82)**, and thus the technique was tested in humans. The most significant finding was the potential to maintain complete integrity of the buccal bone wall thickness and, on the palatal side of the root section, the appearance of new cementum with the induction of bone neoformation at the implant-root interface. The technique thus began to gain ground in the scientific community.

A problem immediately emerged, however: the selection of the appropriate clinical cases. The criteria for performing the socket shield technique are much stricter than for standard alveolar ridge preservation techniques with or without implant placement. The tooth in question must not be being extracted due to periodontal problems, and in fracture cases, the buccal portion of the tooth must not be involved.

The indications to perform the socket shield technique are therefore limited to teeth that are not recoverable prosthetically, teeth that have untreatable large carious lesions, and teeth with coronal-palatal fractures **(Table 2)**. It should be pointed out that the primary objective of the socket shield technique is to maintain the alveolar bone volume and that it does not increase the stability of immediately placed implants (ie, the indications and requirements for immediate implant placement and prosthetic loading remain the same). The socket shield technique can also be used as an alternative to standard alveolar ridge preservation techniques by covering the access to the alveolar cavity with an epithelial-connective graft without implant placement.

Interest in the socket shield technique, however, is predominant in cases of immediate implant placement because the clinical indications for socket shielding are often limited to situations that are

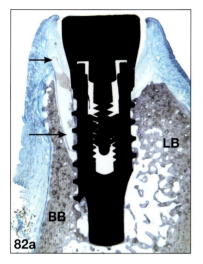
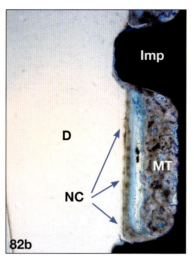

Fig 82 (a and b) *Note how the buccal and lingual bone and mucosal tissue heights are superimposable. The bundle bone is also fully preserved. On the lingual side of the root fragment, there is neoapposition of cementum, with the formation of an osteoid matrix layer. (Courtesy of Dr Markus Hüerzeler.)*

LB = lingual bone plate; BB = buccal bone plate; MT = mineralized tissue; D = dentin; NC (blue arrows) = new cementum; black arrows = dentin shield.

Table 2 Favorable and unfavorable factors for performing the socket shield technique.

Indications	Contraindications
Coronal-palatal fracture	Periodontal disease
Large, untreatable carious lesion	Vertical buccal fracture
Prosthetic failure	Acute inflammation

also favorable for immediate implant placement. In the initial version of the technique, a supracrestal portion of the root fragment was retained, which was advantageous in terms of soft tissue stability but often resulted in exposure of the coronal margin. It was therefore decided to bring the dentin tissue up to the bone profile by creating an internal chamfer to increase the distance to the implant neck.

The use of biomaterials to bridge the gap between the implant and the buccal fragment is a topic of discussion in the literature **(Fig 83)**. It is thought that the presence of the root has a membrane effect and is sufficient to allow for stabilization of the blood clot that is conducive to correct healing of the edentulous site without the need for heterologous grafts (root membrane technique) **(Fig 84)**.[24]

The literature is still insufficient and does not clearly outline each step of the technique, and there are no randomized clinical trials that could fit into a broad data analysis to define which variable influences the success or failure of the therapy. In retrospective studies with follow-ups of up to 10 years,[25] it appears that implant survival is comparable to survival with traditional techniques, that the presence of the root does not cause an inflammatory reaction that alters healing, and that complications are rare and easily managed. There is enormous potential for using this technique to achieve results comparable to those of traditional therapies with extremely limited invasiveness.

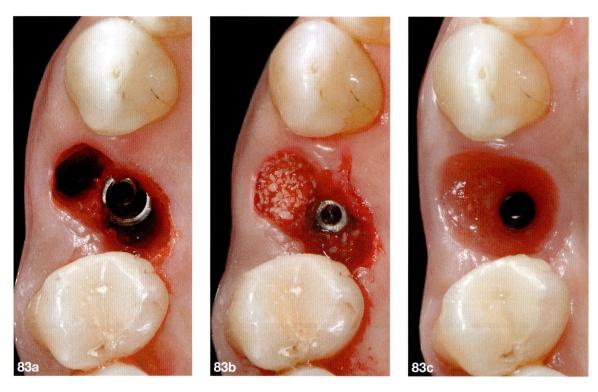

Fig 83 (a to c) *Socket shield with biomaterial insertion.*

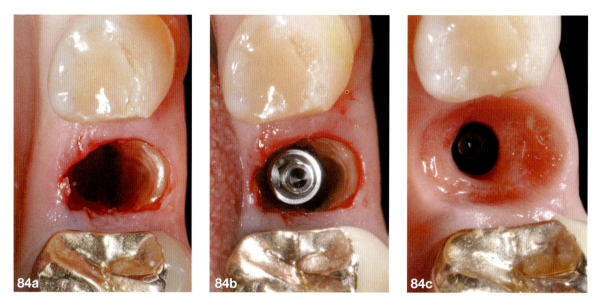

Fig 84 (a to c) *Socket shield without biomaterial insertion.*

Surgical protocol

The tooth that will be extracted must be appropriately prepared, with the buccal dentin portion left to act as the protective shield maintaining the alveolar bone volume. **Figure 85** shows the surgical procedure in an extracted tooth in which a coronal-palatal fracture has been simulated. The instruments required to perform the maneuvers described do not differ from those normally used during a dental extraction.

The first step is mesiodistal sectioning of the root, a maneuver that can be performed with a multi-blade or long diamond bur with a tip inclination such that only two-thirds of the buccal portion is included. Next, the removal of the palatal/lingual fragment of the root is performed either directly, if it is completely separated from the buccal portion, or after sectioning it into two parts to facilitate its removal.

Using a long round bur, apicocoronal movements are performed to reduce the thickness of the buccal shield to approximately 1.5 mm. A cylindric diamond bur can be used to reduce the height of the residual root down to bone level. To verify the correct execution of this maneuver, it is sufficient to perform thorough buccal bone probing until the supracrestal portion of the root has completely disappeared. Finally, a round diamond bur is used on the inner side of the coronal portion of the root to create a chamfer. This creates space for the tissue at the level of the prosthetic emergence profile.

Management of complications

The use of the socket shield technique is not without complications. The major difference between the socket shield technique and traditional treatment is the retention of a root fragment with the PDL. Properly managing this residual dental tissue is important for avoiding two of the most frequent complications: socket shield exposure within the mucosal tunnel on the tooth side and external exposure through the buccal mucosa.

Figure 86 shows a small exposure of the buccal root fragment. Exposures that are intercepted in time show no signs of inflammation, and it is possible to proceed directly to reduction of the root fragment. After anesthesia is performed, probing is carried out around the exposure area to identify the bone component, which is the reference point for the extent of reduction. A relined provisional will be used to contain the blood clot and ensure tissue maturation. After 3 weeks healing is still incomplete, but as the tissue matures, complete healing can be observed after 6 weeks.

After this simple operation, it is possible to place the definitive prosthesis. The feasibility of the treatment described, however, is restricted to cases in which apical migration of the buccal margin can be accepted as an esthetic compromise. When required, mucogingival surgery can be performed to restore the correct gingival profile.

Another complication is internal exposure of the root fragment. In this case, depending on the extent, one can proceed by reducing the fragment and using the provisional itself as a seal, or alternatively, if the exposure is superficial **(Fig 87)**, the compression of the provisional can be reduced and excellent soft tissue healing can be achieved after 1 month.

It is important to identify the exposed area as soon as possible. When the provisional crown is removed, the transmucosal path should be gently probed for areas of mucosal thinning. In these areas, yellowish discoloration of the dentin usually shines through.

The necessary time for tissue maturation should be allowed to pass after modifying the provisional so that complete healing with tissue thickening

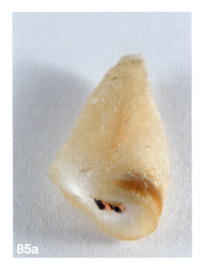
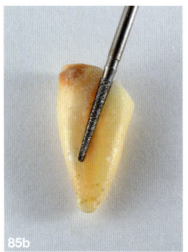
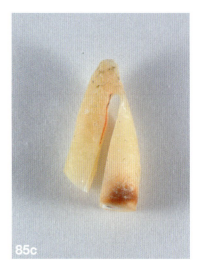

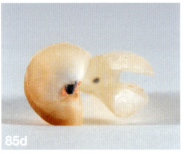
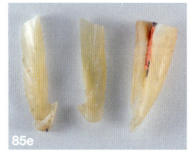
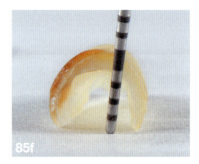

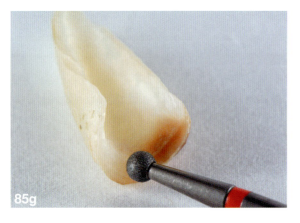

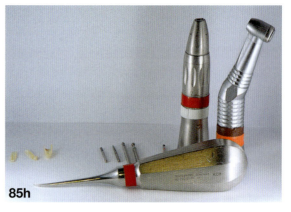

Fig 85 (a to h) *Operative sequence for creating the buccal socket shield.*

DURATION: 11'17"

VIDEO: 10
IMMEDIATE IMPLANT PLACEMENT IN A POST-EXTRACTION SITE WITH A SOCKET SHIELD

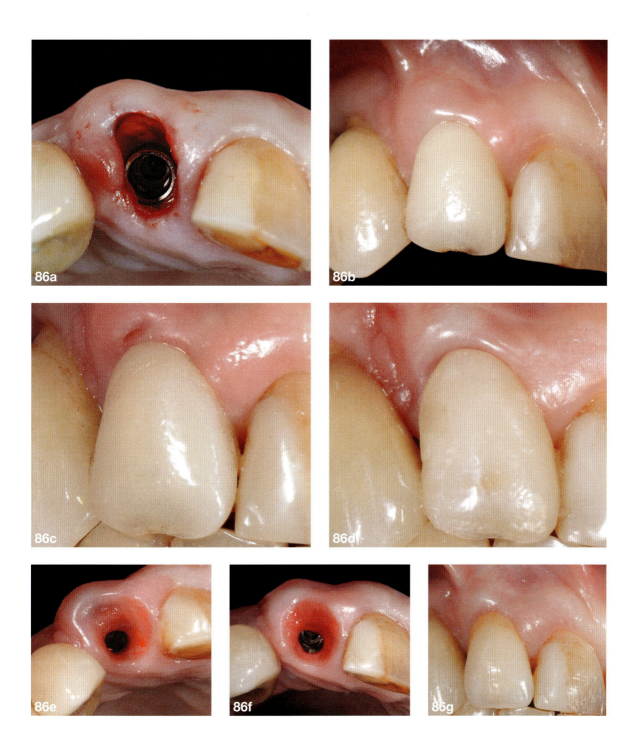

Fig 86 (a to g) *Operative sequence of socket shield exposure management on the buccal side.*

can occur. Migration of the buccal fragment during the healing phase is a very rare occurrence, especially if the technique is conducted in the manner described in this chapter. If no infection is present at the time of migration and removal of the fragment does not expose the implant, soft tissue and/or bone regeneration procedures can be performed with the vascular surface buccal to the area to be treated.[26]

Additional considerations

The socket shield technique described in this chapter has one major limitation: the selection of the clinical case. Implant rehabilitation is a therapeutic choice that is applicable only after verifying the impossibility of recovering a tooth. It is rare to find a clinical situation involving a tooth requiring extraction in which the buccal root portion is stable and free of periodontal and carious disease. Furthermore, the reduction of the supracrestal portion of the root further reduces the support of the buccal mucosal component by exposing it to minimal soft tissue recession, as previously described. This fact is negligible in the posterior sectors, but it is a variable to be carefully evaluated in esthetically relevant areas.

In all the cases described in the literature, it is emphasized that maintenance of the buccal portion of the root preserves the peri-implant volume in the least traumatic way possible, even in conditions of extremely reduced buccal plate thickness. The integrity of the PDL and the migration of cementum on the inner side of the root create conditions that protect the bundle bone from resorption. Once the long-term success of this treatment is verified, it will allow the technique to be used more and more widely.

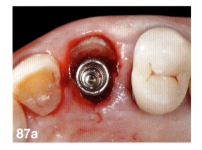 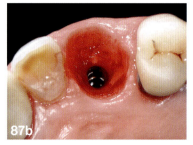 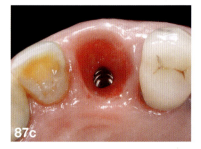

Fig 87 Internal exposure of the root dentin (a) *is visible by transparency* (b) *and completely covered by gingival tissue at the end of treatment* (c).

CLINICAL CASE 5

Immediate implant placement with the socket shield technique

An 80-year-old patient in good general health presented with a complete crown fracture of the maxillary left canine. The tooth had been previously rehabilitated with a prosthetic crown and a metal post but was not salvageable due to caries disease affecting the deep root dentin. The tooth was stable, and the buccal portion of the root appeared well preserved (**Figs 88 and 89**). There were no signs of periodontal disease in an active phase, and the CBCT images brought by the patient showed a bone thickness of less than 1 mm on the buccal side, whereas cancellous bone at the apical level was well represented (**Figs 90 and 91**).

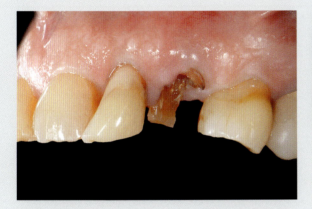

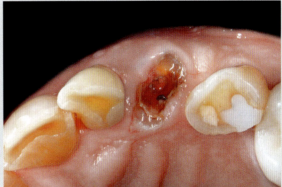

Fig 88 Lateral view of the maxillary left canine.

Fig 89 Occlusal view of the maxillary left canine.

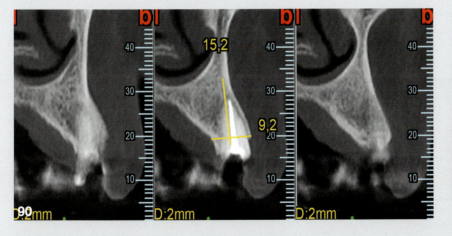

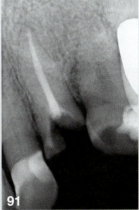

Fig 90 CT imaging shows the limited bone thickness buccal to the tooth to be treated. **Fig 91** Preoperative radiograph.

Orthodontic extrusion and clinical crown lengthening were evaluated as alternatives to implant treatment. The clinical conditions and radiographic evaluations, however, were favorable for minimally invasive implant rehabilitation, leading to the final choice of treatment with a socket shield technique. At the time of the visit, an intraoral scan was performed and the obtained STL file was aligned with the DICOM data of the CT scan for accurate planning of the implant positioning **(Fig 92)**. This is not compulsory in the case of socket shields, but it allows for precise and quicker implant placement and management of the immediate prosthetic phase.

The first surgical step involved sectioning the root to allow removal of the palatal portion. This is done, as described previously in the chapter, with a multi-blade or long diamond burs in a mesio-distal direction, trying to involve two-thirds of the buccal portion. A second perpendicular section in the palatal direction can be performed to further divide the root, facilitate removal, and prevent extractive movements from affecting the buccal shield **(Fig 93)**. The buccal margin was lowered to bone level, and the coronal chamfer was performed at the internal aspect **(Fig 94)**. At this point the implant site was prepared **(Fig 95)**.

It is important to assess the quality of the dentin, and in the case of buccal caries below the bone margin or mobility of the root remnant, it is necessary to revise the procedure and extract the last part of the root as well.

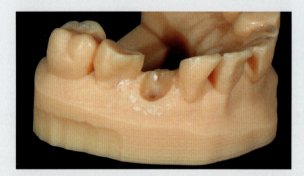

Fig 92 Stereolithographic cast with a surgical guide for the first drill used for implant site preparation.

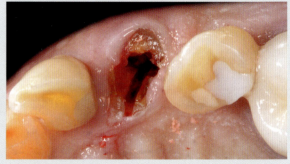

Fig 93 Mesiodistal and buccopalatal sectioning of the root.

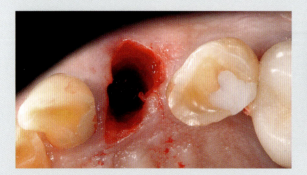

Fig 94 Preparation of the socket shield.

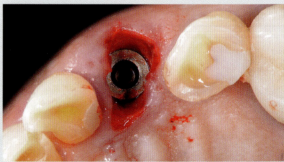

Fig 95 Implant placement.

The presence of a socket shield does not affect the position of the implant, which is placed according to standard insertion principles for fresh extraction sockets. There is no defined limit to the distance from the buccal portion, but it is important to prevent it from being mobilized during implant insertion. The apicocoronal implant placement dimension is approximately 1.5 mm below the bone margin.

Figure 95 shows the implant placed in the extraction socket of the maxillary left canine near the root fragment. **Figures 96 and 97** show other clinical cases illustrating the variability of implant placement with respect to the buccal shield.

The completion of therapy involves the placement of the provisional with the aim of not only esthetically restoring the area but also functionally stabilizing the clot (**Fig 98**).

This allows the bone and mucosal tissues to heal. When the placement of an immediate provisional is not indicated, a customized healing abutment can be fabricated to serve the same protective function for the underlying clot.

The procedure is minimally invasive, and the tissues are stable over time, though not completely unaltered. The supracrestal loss of the buccal portion of the root does not provide support for the soft tissues, and they may undergo resorption depending on their baseline buccopalatal thickness (**Fig 99**).

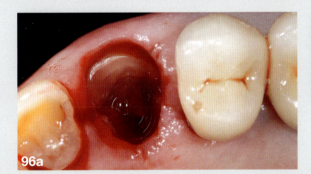 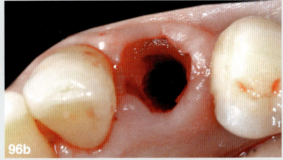

Fig 96 (a and b) Cases of socket shield preparation under different clinical conditions.

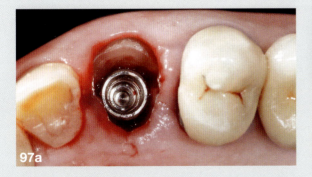 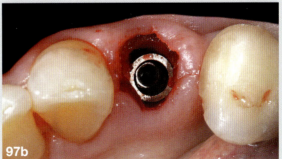

Fig 97 *(a and b)* Clinical cases of implant placement using the socket shield technique.

Upon finalization of the case, excellent tissue healing was observed after removing the provisional (**Figs 100 and 101**). From an occlusal view, the buccal profile appeared to be unchanged, but data from the digital impressions was analyzed to verify millimetric measurements.

From the chromatic variations shown in **Fig 102**, a volume reduction of more than 0.2 mm was observed around the intervention area. The final radiograph showed stability of the root fragment (**Fig 103**), and the implant emergence profile left space for the tissues. Over time, it is important to verify the stability of the results achieved (**Fig 104**).

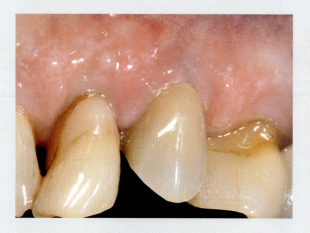

Fig 98 At 1 week, with the provisional in place.

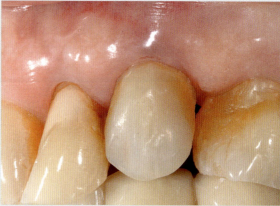

Fig 99 The tissues are stable 1 year after treatment, but limited contraction of the distal and mesial papillae is evident at the maxillary right canine and minimal apical migration of the buccal gingival parabolas is evident at the maxillary right lateral incisor and first premolar.

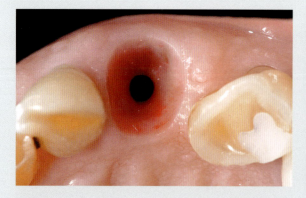

Fig 100 Occlusal view before delivery of the definitive prosthesis.

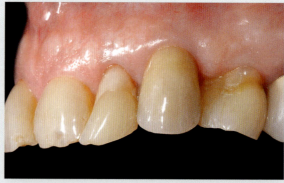

Fig 101 Lateral view after placement of the definitive prosthesis.

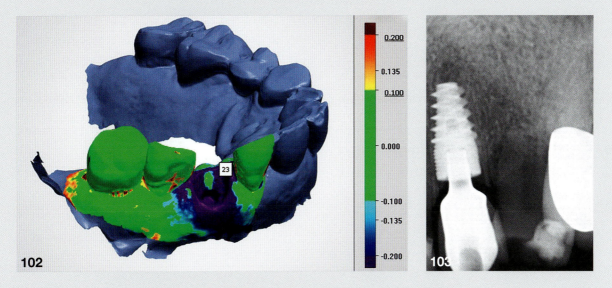

Fig 102 Superimposition of the scan images. The areas with a volume reduction of more than 0.2 mm are shown in purple. **Fig 103** Radiograph at the time of definitive prosthesis delivery.

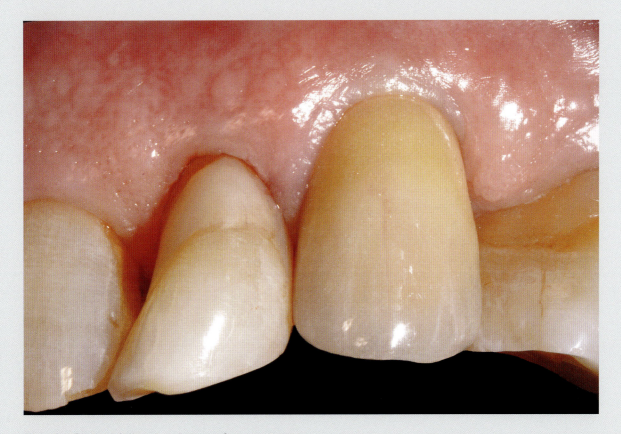

Fig 104 Clinical follow-up 1 year after treatment.

L. Ferrantino • A. Pispero • M. Maglione • M. Simion

REFERENCES

1. Brånemark PI, Hansson BO, Adell R, et al. Osseointegrated implants in the treatment of the edentulous jaw. Experience from a 10-year period. Scand J Plast Reconstr Surg Suppl 1977;16:1–132.

2. Adell R, Lekholm U, Rockler B, Brånemark PI. A 15-year study of osseointegrated implants in the treatment of the edentulous jaw. Int J Oral Surg 1981;10:387–416.

3. Araújo MG, Lindhe J. Dimensional ridge alterations following tooth extraction. An experimental study in the dog. J Clin Periodontol 2005;32:212–218.

4. Araújo MG, Wennström JL, Lindhe J. Modeling of the buccal and lingual bone walls of fresh extraction sites following implant installation. Clin Oral Implants Res 2006;17:606–614.

5. Tan WL, Wong TLT, Wong MCM, Lang NP. A systematic review of post-extractional alveolar hard and soft tissue dimensional changes in humans. Clin Oral Implants Res 2012;23(Suppl 5):1–21.

6. Araújo MG, Silva CO, Misawa M, Sukekava F. Alveolar socket healing: What can we learn? Periodontol 2000 2015;68:122–134.

7. Januário AL, Duarte WR, Barriviera M, Mesti JC, Araújo MG, Lindhe J. Dimension of the facial bone wall in the anterior maxilla: A cone-beam computed tomography study. Clin Oral Implants Res 2011;22:1168–1171.

8. Chappuis V, Engel O, Shahim K, Reyes M, Katsaros C, Buser D. Soft tissue alterations in esthetic postextraction sites: A 3-dimensional analysis. J Dent Res 2015;94(9 Suppl):187S–193S.

9. Vignoletti F, Sanz M. Immediate implants at fresh extraction sockets: From myth to reality. Periodontol 2000 2014;66:132–152.

10. Discepoli N, Vignoletti F, Laino L, De Sanctis M, Muñoz F, Sanz M. Fresh extraction socket: Spontaneous healing vs. immediate implant placement. Clin Oral Implants Res 2015;26:1250–1255.

11. Vignoletti F, Discepoli N, Müller A, De Sanctis M, Muñoz F, Sanz M. Bone modelling at fresh extraction sockets: Immediate implant placement versus spontaneous healing: An experimental study in the beagle dog. J Clin Periodontol. 2012;39:91–97.

12. Morton D, Chen ST, Martin WC, Levine RA, Buser D. Consensus statements and recommended clinical procedures regarding optimizing esthetic outcomes in implant dentistry. Int J Oral Maxillofac Implants 2014;29(Suppl):216–220.

13. Hämmerle CHF, Araújo MG, Simion M, Osteology Consensus Group 2011. Evidence-based knowledge on the biology and treatment of extraction sockets. Clin Oral Implants Res 2011;23:80–82.

14. Araújo MG, Hämmerle CHF, Simion M. Extraction sockets: Biology and treatment options. Preface. Clin Oral Implants Res 2012;23(Suppl 5):iv.

15. Nevins M, Camelo M, De Paoli S, et al. A study of the fate of the buccal wall of extraction sockets of teeth with prominent roots. Int J Periodontics Restorative Dent 2006;26:19–29.

16. Tomasi C, Sanz M, Cecchinato D, et al. Bone dimensional variations at implants placed in fresh extraction sockets: A multilevel multivariate analysis. Clin Oral Implants Res 2010;21:30–36.

17. Tomasi C, Donati M, Cecchinato D, Szathvary I, Corrà E, Lindhe J. Effect of socket grafting with deproteinized bone mineral: An RCT on dimensional alterations after 6 months. Clin Oral Implants Res 2018;29:435–442.

18. Rasperini G, Canullo L, Dellavia C, Pellegrini G, Simion M. Socket grafting in the posterior maxilla reduces the need for sinus augmentation. Int J Periodontics Restorative Dent 2010;30:265–273.

19. Lombardi T, Bernardello F, Berton F, et al. Efficacy of alveolar ridge preservation after maxillary molar extraction in reducing crestal bone resorption and sinus pneumatization: A multicenter prospective case-control study. Biomed Res Int 2018;2018:9352130.

20. Ferrantino L, Camurati A, Gambino P, et al. Aesthetic outcomes of non-functional immediately restored single post-extraction implants with and without connective tissue graft: A multicentre randomized controlled trial. Clin Oral Implants Res 2021;32:684–694.

21. De Rouck T, Collys K, Wyn I, Cosyn J. Instant provisionalization of immediate single-tooth implants is essential to optimize esthetic treatment outcome. Clin Oral Implants Res 2009;20:566–570.

22. Hürzeler MB, Zuhr O, Schupbach P, Rebele SF, Emmanouilidis N, Fickl S. The socket-shield technique: A proof-of-principle report. J Clin Periodontol 2010;37:855–862.

23. Casey DM, Lauciello FR. A review of the submerged root concept. J Prosthet Dent 1980;43:128–132.

24. Botticelli D, Berglundh T, Lindhe J. Hard-tissue alterations following immediate implant placement in extraction sites. J Clin Periodontol 2004;31:820–828.

25. Siormpas KD, Mitsias ME, Kotsakis GA, Tawil I, Pikos MA, Mangano FG. The root membrane technique: A retrospective clinical study with up to 10 years of follow-up. Implant Dent 2018;27:564–574.

26. Zuhr O, Staehler P, Huerzeler M. Complication management of a socket shield case after 6 years of function. Int J Periodontics Restorative Dent 2020;40:409–415.

IMMEDIATE
LOADING

CHAPTER 8

Edited by Massimo Simion and Michele Maglione

INTRODUCTION

According to Brånemark's original protocol, implants must remain submerged in the absence of loading for a period of 6 months in the maxilla and 3 months in the mandible to give the peri-implant bone tissue time to regenerate and mature into lamellar bone in direct contact with the implant surface.[1-3]

This two-stage approach was one of the most important conceptual differences between old implant protocols, characterized by high failure rates, and new methods for achieving osseointegration. The fundamental histologic difference is at the interface between the implant and the host tissue.

Former implantology protocols presupposed the existence of a thin layer of fibrous connective tissue that could mimic the periodontal ligament (PDL) of the natural teeth and give the implants a certain mobility, whereas osseointegrated implantology involves direct contact between the vital bone and the implant surface.

Within this context, delaying the application of loads prevents implant micromovement, which if greater than 100 to 150 μm, affects the interposition of fibrous tissue at the bone-to-implant interface.[4]

Prosthetic loading immediately after implant placement is a popular protocol with high success rates. However, it must be remembered that it violates biologic time constraints regarding bone tissue regeneration and maturation, so it should only be used after careful case selection.

Massimo Simion

Since the late 1980s, however, numerous experimental and clinical studies have shown that osseointegration can be achieved even when applying prosthetic loading immediately after implant placement, when done so under controlled conditions and with the correct indications.[5–7] The focus is therefore on keeping the implants immobile throughout the healing period rather than on maintaining the absence of loading. In other words, implant osseointegration does not necessarily require the absence of loading but the absence of micromovement at the bone-to-implant interface that would prevent normal bone healing.[8]

The advantages of a single-stage approach with immediate loading are considerable. It is a less invasive surgical technique that reduces treatment time, prevents the needs for a removable prosthesis, and results in patient satisfaction. These benefits have made the practice of immediate loading widespread and routine in daily clinical practice.

However, to avoid abuse of this technique, which increases the risk of failure, it is necessary to consider its correct indications in accordance with the biologic principles of osseointegration.

IMMEDIATE LOADING, EARLY LOADING, AND DELAYED LOADING

The concepts of immediate, early, and delayed or conventional loading are not without ambiguity in the literature. However, a practical and user-friendly classification is as follows:

- **Immediate loading** entails delivery of a prosthesis within 48 hours of surgical implant placement. It can be defined as occlusal or non-occlusal immediate loading, depending on whether occlusal contacts are present in centric relation (CR).[9] Non-occlusal loading is applicable only for partially edentulous patients, where the natural teeth can support the occlusion during the healing period.

- **Early loading** involves the delivery of a prosthesis between 2 days and 3 weeks after implant placement. The period from week 4 to month 3 is characterized by greater remodeling in the peri-implant bone, lower mechanical strength, and therefore, greater risk of implant loosening during the implant impression and prosthesis-fitting phases.

- **Delayed or conventional loading** involves prosthesis delivery after 3 to 6 months, in accordance with the traditional Brånemark protocol.

BIOLOGIC FOUNDATIONS OF LOADING

Osseointegration occurs in well-known stages that significantly condition implant stability (see chapter 3):[10]

1. In the first 2 weeks, blood clot formation occurs in the presence of residual bone particles at the bone and implant interface. Primary implant stability is ensured by implant thread engagement in the native cortical bone and compression of the residual bone particles **(Fig 1)**.

2. From week 3, osteoclastic activity begins, which leads to the demineralization of residual bone particles and native bone damaged by the trauma of surgery and also stimulates osteoblasts to begin bone regeneration **(Fig 2)**. During this period, the ability of the implant to bear loads is reduced due to the reduced bone mineralization resulting from osteoclastic activity. The bone particles are completely resorbed, but the new bone is not yet sufficiently mineralized.

3. In the following 2 to 3 months, maturation of the regenerated bone into lamellar bone occurs via the action of cutting cones **(Fig 3)**.

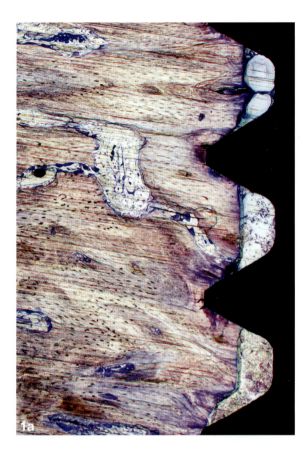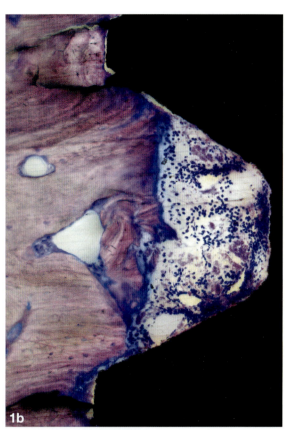

Fig 1 *Histologic image of the bone and implant interface at the time of implant placement. Note the apical threads engaged in native bone* (a) *and the blood clot and bone particles that fill the spaces between the threads* (b). *Toluidine blue/Pyronin G staining; ×10 and ×20 magnification, respectively. (Reprinted with permission from Int J Periodontics Restorative Dent 2015;35:9–17.)*

After the third month, the secondary stability of the implant is guaranteed by the presence of the new mature bone and lamellar bone.

The consequence of this healing process is the progressive reduction of implant stability from the second week until the third month, after which secondary stability generally becomes higher than initial stability **(Fig 4)**.[11] Because of the reduction in stability between the end of the second week and the end of the third month, delivery of the prosthesis during that time is discouraged. Any maneuvers of screwing/unscrewing the healing abutments and placing

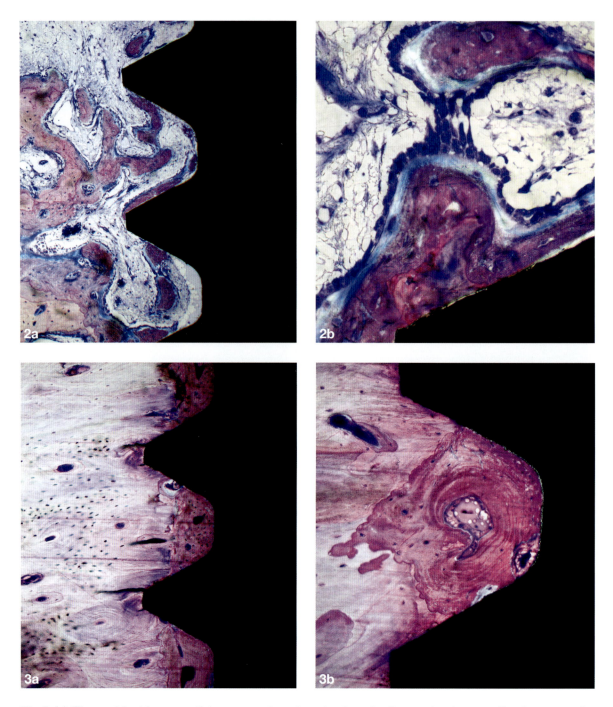

Fig 2 (a) *The residual bone particles are undergoing demineralization and act as ossification cores for bone regeneration (×10 magnification). (b) At higher magnification (×40), the orb of osteoblasts depositing osteoid tissue is evident. Toluidine blue/Pyronin G staining. (Reprinted with permission from Int J Periodontics Restorative Dent 2015;35:9–17.)* **Fig 3** (a) *At 3 months, the spaces between the implant threads are occupied by mature lamellar bone (×10 magnification). (b) At higher magnification (×20), a secondary osteon is visible in contact with the implant surface. Toluidine blue/Pyronin G staining. (Reprinted with permission from Int J Periodontics Restorative Dent 2015;35:9–17.)*

the impression copings or prosthetic abutments could lead to implant mobilization.

The importance of implant macrostructure and design are evident from the dynamics of the events that lead to osseointegration. The original Brånemark implants were completely cylindric, with a non-self-tapping apex, meaning that they could not be inserted into underprepared implant sites to increase their stability. More modern implant designs generally have a slight taper, a self-tapping apex, and double threading to allow them to be inserted into underprepared sites in bone of lower density. Underpreparation of an implant site allows for greater engagement between the implant thread and the native bone **(see Fig 1)**, and the slight taper increases lateral static forces to keep implant mobility below the 100 to 150 μm threshold. It must be emphasized, however, that excessive insertion torque (> 50 Ncm) is unnecessary and even detrimental to the peri-implant bone.[12–14]

The role of the microstructure of the implant surface is less clear. The first clinical studies and case reports on immediate loading were performed on implants with machined surfaces.[15–18] In 2003, Calandriello et al[15] published a prospective study with 2-year follow-up on a group of 26 partially edentulous patients treated with 50 machined implants supporting 30 fixed prostheses, resulting in an implant survival rate of 98%. Similar results were published by Maló et al[16] and Vanden Bogaerde et al,[17] with survival rates of 96% and 96.8%, respectively.

In the same year, Maló et al[18] presented the first retrospective study with distal inclined implants placed in edentulous patients according to the All-on-4 method: 176 machined implants placed in 44 patients showed a survival rate of 96.8%. More recently, Esposito et al[19] published a randomized controlled clinical trial comparing smooth and machined implants. They treated 50 completely edentulous patients with 300 implants, of which 137 were surface-treated and 163 machined. After 1 year of follow-up, both surfaces showed excellent and very similar results, with only two failed implants belonging to the smooth-surface group.

The results of these studies seem to indicate a rather limited influence of the roughness of the implant surface on immediate loading. Moreover, the events leading to the regeneration and maturation of bone that is sufficient to influence implant stability has a minimum duration of 3 months from surgical implant placement, regardless of the surface used.[10]

Since the year 2000, publications on immediate loading have increased exponentially **(Fig 5)**, demonstrating its clinical importance, and numerous systematic reviews of the literature limited to randomized clinical trials testify to the reliability of this method when used in an appropriate manner.[20–26]

INDICATIONS FOR IMMEDIATE LOADING

With the exclusion of general absolute contraindications for immediate loading, such as decompensated diabetes mellitus, immunodeficiencies, radiotherapy, bruxism, heavy smoking, prolonged treatment with bisphosphonates, and

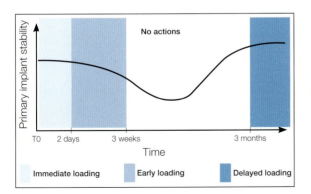

Fig 4 Prosthetic loading times.

other serious systemic diseases, the indications for immediate implant loading are rather empirical and ill-defined.

The choice to perform immediate loading is therefore left to the clinician's experience, which often leads to misuse of this protocol.

Basically, immediate loading of an implant is indicated when the load is not capable of causing micromovement greater than 150 μm at the interface between the bone and the implant itself, but because there is no way to assess or predict micromovement, the indications for immediate loading remain totally empirical.

As a general rule, immediate loading is indicated in totally edentulous patients with Class D1, D2, or D3 bone, whereas it should be avoided in patients with demineralized D4 bone in whom implants have been inserted with very low insertion torque and equally low primary stability (eg, an implant stability quotient [ISQ] < 60). Thus, immediate loading is indicated for almost all completely edentulous patients in the mandible and in most completely edentulous patients in the maxilla.

Although there is no conclusive data on the need for high insertion torques in cases of immediate loading, common sense would indicate values of more than 35 Ncm for each individual implant. Too high insertion torque values (> 50 Ncm), however, are detrimental because they cause damage to the peri-implant bone via excessive lateral static forces.[12-14] When replacing single teeth or rehabilitating limited edentulous spans, immediate delivery of the prosthesis should not be associated with true occlusal loading.[26] It is advisable to keep provisionals in subocclusion for at least 3 months (see chapters 5 to 7).

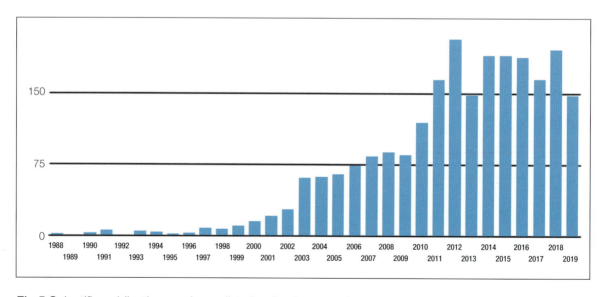

Fig 5 *Scientific publications on immediate loading by year since 1988. From the year 2000, the number of publications increased dramatically.*

CLINICAL CASE 1

Immediate loading in the maxilla in a completely edentulous patient

A 65-year-old patient presented with severe structural impairment of the maxillary teeth (**Figs 6 and 7**). Rehabilitation with a complete fixed/removable implant-supported restoration was opted for. After preparing a provisional prosthesis on the basis of the diagnostic wax-up, the teeth were extracted, and the implants were placed in the fresh extraction sites according to the flapless technique (**Figs 8 and 9**). In the same session, the impression was taken, and the provisional was relined in resin (**Fig 10**). After 6 months of adequate provisional function, the integration of the implants was verified (**Fig 11**) and the final metal-ceramic prosthesis was delivered (**Figs 12 and 13**).

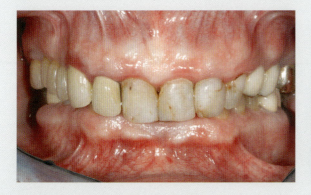

Fig 6 In the maxilla, multiple carious lesions are present in teeth that have already been extensively and inappropriately restored.

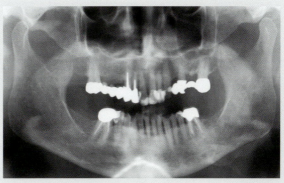

Fig 7 The structural impairment of the teeth is confirmed by the panoramic radiograph.

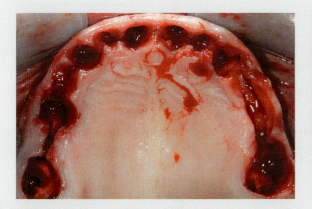

Fig 8 All teeth were extracted, and the sockets were carefully curetted.

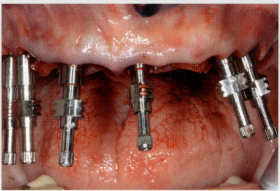

Fig 9 Six iMAX (iRES) hybrid implants were placed in the fresh extraction sites, and the bone defects were filled with deproteinized bovine bone mineral ([DBBM] Bio-Oss, Geistlich Biomaterials). Impressions were taken at the same session.

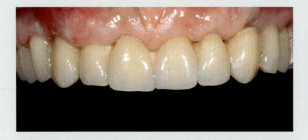

Fig 10 The provisional prosthesis was relined and applied to the temporary abutments.

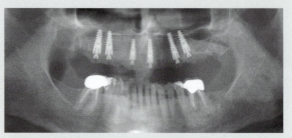

Fig 11 Control panoramic radiograph.

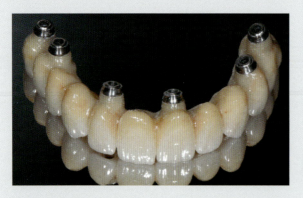

Fig 12 Final metal-ceramic prosthesis.

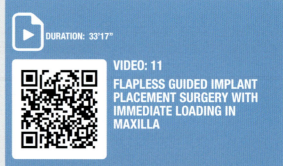

DURATION: 33'17"

VIDEO: 11

FLAPLESS GUIDED IMPLANT PLACEMENT SURGERY WITH IMMEDIATE LOADING IN MAXILLA

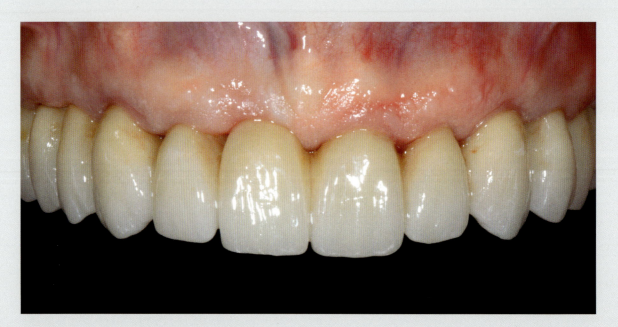

Fig 13 After 1 year of prosthetic loading.

CLINICAL CASE 2

Immediate loading in the mandible in a completely edentulous patient

A 72-year-old patient wished to receive a fixed prosthesis in the mandible. It was decided to extract the severely compromised residual teeth and place a fixed prosthesis supported on five implants (Figs 14 to 34). In the maxilla, two implants were removed, and a complete denture was placed (Fig 33).

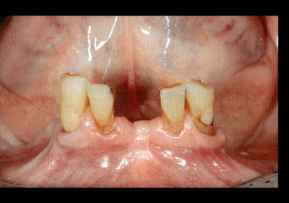

Fig 14 The mandible with four residual teeth and reduced periodontal support.

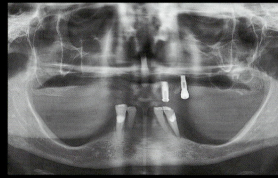

Fig 15 Panoramic radiograph showing severe bone atrophy distal to the mental foramen. The remaining teeth have severely reduced periodontal support.

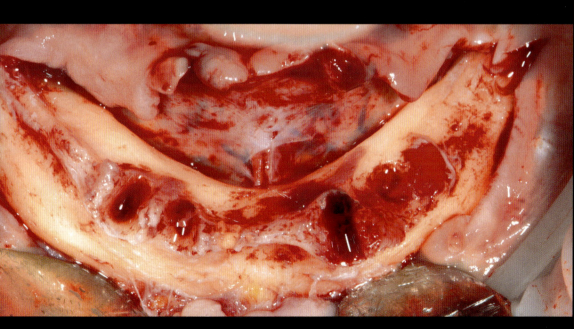

Fig 16 Tooth extraction after elevation of a full-thickness flap.

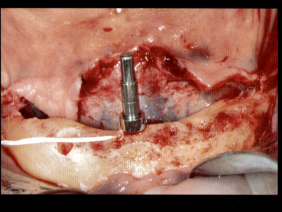

Fig 17 The sockets were curetted, and a moderate osteoplasty was performed.

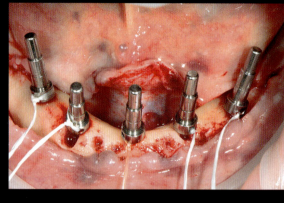

Fig 18 Implant sites were prepared, giving the distal implants an inclination of 25 degrees.

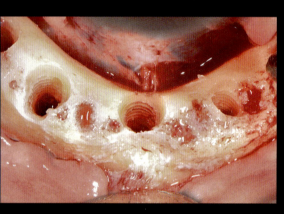

Fig 19 Countersinking and tapping were performed at all sites to avoid excessive insertion torque.

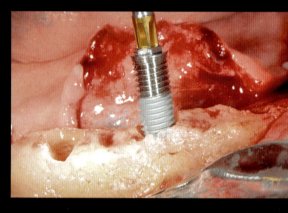

Fig 20 Five hybrid iMAX implants were placed, with insertion torques not exceeding 40 Ncm.

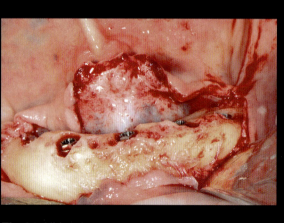

Fig 21 All implants were placed 1 mm below the bone crest.

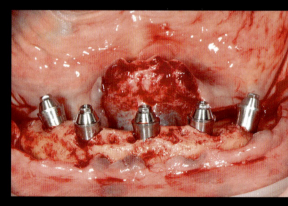

Fig 22 The multi-unit abutments (MUAs) have been positioned.

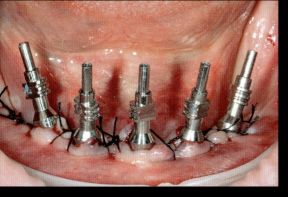

Fig 23 Impression copings were screwed onto the MUAs.

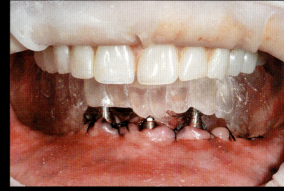

Fig 24 The occlusion and vertical dimension were recorded using a prebuilt template.

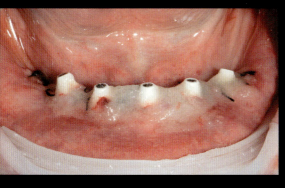

Fig 25 Healing abutments were placed on the MUAs, and a gel with hyaluronic acid (Hobagel Plus, Hobama) was applied.

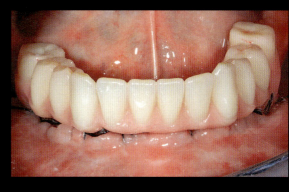

Fig 26 A reinforced resin provisional was placed on the same day.

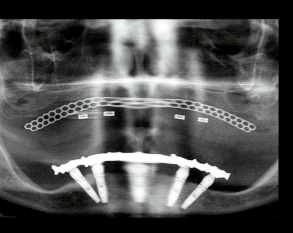

Fig 27 Control panoramic radiograph.

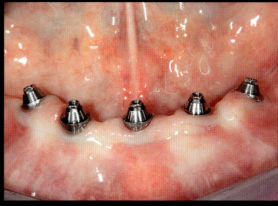

Fig 28 Tissue healing after 3 months.

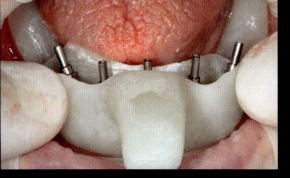

Fig 29 A new impression was taken with a personalized impression tray.

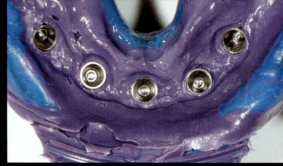

Fig 30 Polyether impression with the transfer copings in place.

Fig 31 Bar for checking the accuracy of the cast.

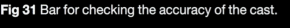

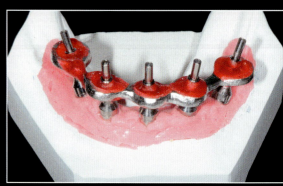

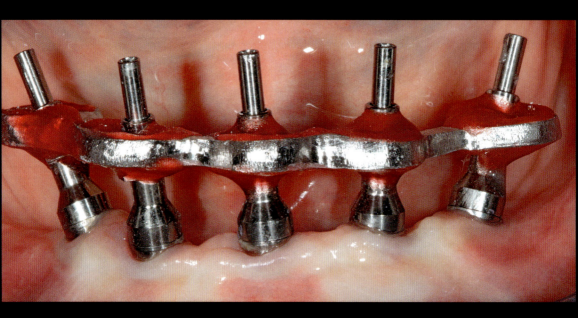

Fig 32 Verifying the accuracy of the cast in the mouth.

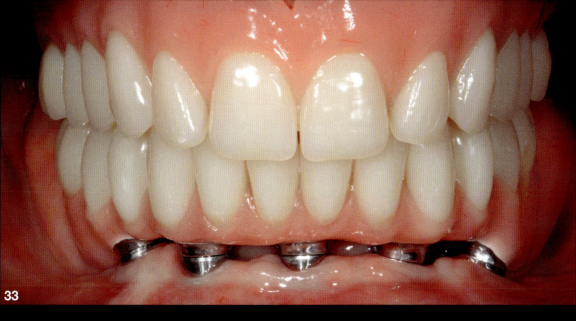

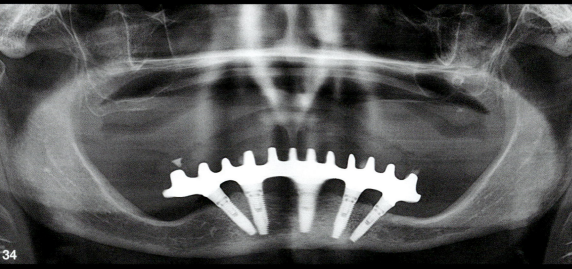

Fig 33 Metal and composite final dentures.   **Fig 34** Panoramic radiograph at the 1-year follow-up.

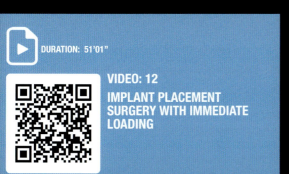

DURATION: 51'01"

VIDEO: 12
IMPLANT PLACEMENT
SURGERY WITH IMMEDIATE
LOADING

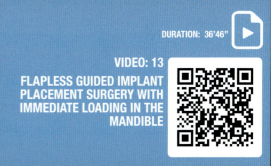

DURATION: 36'46"

VIDEO: 13
FLAPLESS GUIDED IMPLANT
PLACEMENT SURGERY WITH
IMMEDIATE LOADING IN THE
MANDIBLE

REFERENCES

1. Brånemark PI, Zarb G, Albrektsson T. Tissue-Integrated Prostheses: Osseointegration in Clinical Dentistry. Quintessence, 1985.

2. Adell R, Lekholm U, Rockler B, Brånemark PI. A 15-year study of osseointegrated implants in the treatment of the edentulous jaw. Int J Oral Surg 1981;10:387–416.

3. Brånemark PI, Adell R, Breine U, Hansson BO, Lindström J, Ohlsson A. Intra-osseous anchorage of dental prostheses. I. Experimental studies. Scand J Plast Reconstr Surg 1969;3:81–100.

4. Brunski JB. Avoid pitfalls of overloading and micromotion of intraosseous implants. Dent Implantol Update 1993;4:77–81.

5. Henry P, Rosenberg I. Single-stage surgery for rehabilitation of the edentulous mandible: Preliminary results. Pract Periodontics Aesthet Dent 1994;6: 15–22.

6. Chiapasco M, Gatti C, Rossi E, Haefliger W, Markwalder TH. Implant-retained mandibular overdentures with immediate loading. A retrospective multicenter study on 226 consecutive cases. Clin Oral Implants Res 1997;8:48–57.

7. Randow K, Ericsson I, Nilner K, Petersson A, Glantz PO. Immediate functional loading of Brånemark dental implants. An 18-month clinical follow-up study. Clin Oral Implants Res 1999;10:8–15.

8. Unthoff HK, Germain JP. The reversal of tissue differentiation around screws. Clin Orthop Relat Res 1975;123:248–252.

9. Testori T, Galli F, Del Fabbro M. Il carico immediato - La nuova era dell'implantologia orale. Acme, 2009.

10. Simion M, Benigni M, Al-Hezaimi K, Kim DM. Early bone formation adjacent to oxidized and machined implant surfaces: A histologic study. Int J Periodontics Restorative Dent 2015;35:9–17.

11. Glauser R, Sennerby L, Meredith N, et al. Resonance frequency analysis of implants subjected to immediate or early functional occlusal loading. Successful vs. failing implants. Clin Oral Implants Res 2004;15: 428–434.

12. Ferrari DS, Piattelli A, Iezzi G, Faveri M, Rodrigues JA, Shibli JA. Effect of lateral static load on immediately restored implants: Histologic and radiographic evaluation in dogs. Clin Oral Implants Res 2015;26:e51–e56.

13. Stavropoulos A, Cochran D, Obrecht M, Pippenger BE, Dard M. Effect of osteotomy preparation on osseointegration of immediately loaded, tapered dental implants. Adv Dent Res 2016;28:34–41.

14. Levin BP. The correlation between immediate implant insertion torque and Implant Stability Quotient. Int J Periodontics Restorative Dent 2016;36:833–840.

15. Calandriello R, Tomatis M, Rangert B. Immediate functional loading of Brånemark System implants with enhanced initial stability: A prospective 1- to 2-year clinical and radiographic study. Clin Implant Dent Relat Res 2003;5(Suppl 1):10–20.

16. Maló P, Friberg B, Polizzi G, Gualini F, Vighagen T, Rangert B. Immediate and early function of Brånemark System implants placed in the esthetic zone: A 1-year prospective clinical multicenter study. Clin Implant Dent Relat Res 2003;5(Suppl 1):37–46.

17. Vanden Bogaerde L, Pedretti G, Dellacasa P, Mozzati M, Rangert B. Early function of splinted implants in maxillas and posterior mandibles using Brånemark system machined-surface implants: An 18-month prospective clinical multicenter study. Clin Implant Dent Relat Res 2003;5(Suppl 1):21–28.

18. Maló P, Rangert B, Nobre M. "All-on-Four" immediate-function concept with Brånemark System implants for completely edentulous mandibles: A retrospective clinical study. Clin Implant Dent Relat Res 2003;5(Suppl 1):2–9.

19. Esposito M, Felice P, Barausse C, Pistilli R, Grandi G, Simion M. Immediately loaded machined versus rough surface dental implants in edentulous jaws: One-year postloading results of a pilot randomized controlled trial. Eur J Oral Implantol 2015;8:387–396.

20. Del Fabbro M, Bellini CM, Romeo D, Francetti L. Tilted implants for the rehabilitation of edentulous jaws: A systematic review. Clin Implant Dent Relat Res 2012;14:612–621.

21. Esposito M, Worthington HV, Thomsen P, Coulthard P. Interventions for replacing missing teeth: Different times for loading dental implants. Cochrane Database Syst Rev 2004;(3):CD003878.

22. Cochran DL, Morton D, Weber HP. Consensus statements and recommended clinical procedures regarding loading protocols for endosseous dental implants. Int J Oral Maxillofac Implants 2004;19(Suppl):109–113.

23. Esposito M, Grusovin MG, Coulthard P, Worthington HV. Different loading strategies of dental implants: A Cochrane systematic review of randomised controlled clinical trials. Eur J Oral Implantol 2008;1:259–276.

24. De Bruyn H, Raes S, Ostman PO, Cosyn J. Immediate loading in partially and completely edentulous jaws: A review of the literature with clinical guidelines. Periodontol 2000 2014;66:153–187.

25. Sanz-Sánchez I, Sanz-Martín I, Figuero E, Sanz M. Clinical efficacy of immediate implant loading protocols compared to conventional loading depending on the type of the restoration: A systematic review. Clin Oral Implants Res 2015;26:964–982.

26. Del Fabbro M, Testori T, Kekovic V, Goker F, Tumedei M, Wang HL. A systematic review of survival rates of osseointegrated implants in fully and partially edentulous patients following immediate loading. J Clin Med 2019;8:2142.

SURGICAL AND PROSTHETIC COMPLICATIONS: PREVENTION, DIAGNOSIS, AND TREATMENT

CHAPTER 9

Edited by Massimo Simion

INTRODUCTION

Exemplary surgeons are distinguished not only by achieving low complications rates in their operations but also by their ability to manage complications when they do arise and nullify or reduce their negative effects.

It is very common in clinical practice for the "management" of complications to cause more harm than the complications themselves. In most cases, implant surgery presents medium or low levels of difficulty, but complications can be very serious. Therefore, a thorough knowledge of the complications that can occur during and after implant surgery is essential before approaching this discipline. This chapter describes complication prevention and management.

COMPLICATIONS DURING THE FIRST PHASE OF SURGERY

Errors in case assessment

Many complications that occur during the first surgical phase stem from an incorrect assessment of the anatomical and dimensional characteristics of the implant site.[1] In some partially and completely edentulous patients, thick mucosa

An expert surgeon is not the one who manages to solve a few difficult cases spectacularly but the one who solves all cases with a very low percentage of complications. In the event of a complication, expert surgeons are not discouraged and know how to resolve it.

Massimo Simion

upon clinical inspection and palpation of the ridges **(Fig 1)** can mask bone atrophy that is not compatible with immediate implant placement **(Fig 2)**.

CBCT is always necessary for 3D assessment of the bone ridge and correct treatment planning.[2] In the case of atrophic ridges, regenerative techniques are indicated before or simultaneous with implant placement (see chapters 15–17). The presence of bone defects or apical undercuts at the crestal margin can cause partial exposure of the implant surface in the form of dehiscence **(Figs 3 and 4)** or fenestrations **(Fig 5)**.

These complications must be immediately treated via guided bone regeneration (GBR) (see chapter 16).

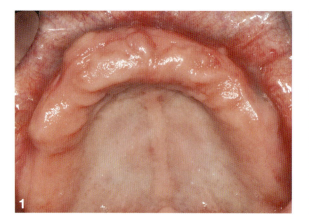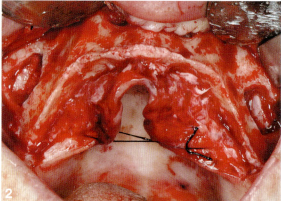

Fig 1 *A completely edentulous maxilla apparently showing considerable ridge thickness.* **Fig 2** *After elevation of the access flaps, very limited bone thickness can be observed. The misleading clinical appearance in Fig 1 was due to the unusual thickness of the soft tissue.*

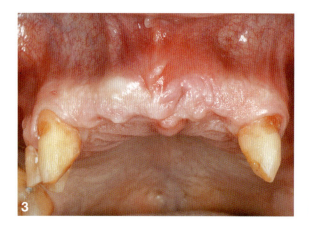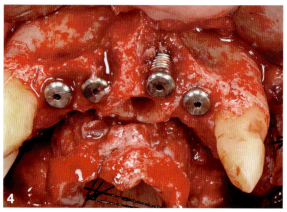

Fig 3 *Apparently regular and thick maxillary edentulous ridge.* **Fig 4** *With open flaps, two severe bone defects causing implant dehiscence are evident. Correction via GBR is necessary.*

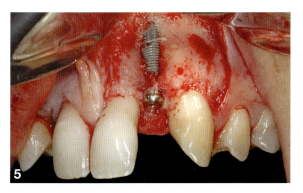 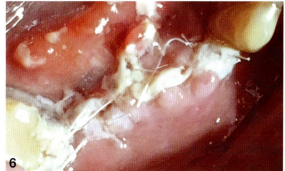

Fig 5 *Buccal undercut causing fenestration of the implant apex and requiring regenerative intervention.*
Fig 6 *Marginal flap necrosis after 15 days of healing. Whitish areas of necrosis are evident both at the margins of the flaps and in the mucosa of the oral floor. This was caused by traumatic flap elevation and excessive suture tension.*

Injury to adjacent anatomical structures

Anatomical structures can become accidentally injured during surgery, with the potential for extremely serious consequences. These injuries can include:

- Perforations in the access flap
- Damage to the roots of adjacent natural teeth
- Injuries to the inferior alveolar nerve (IAN) or lingual nerve
- Injury to the lingual artery or other vascular structures of the floor of the mouth

Access flap perforations

Access flap perforation can result from clumsy or excessively violent maneuvers during flap detachment **(Fig 6)**. Scarring from recent tooth avulsions and bony ridges with sharp buccal edges predispose a flap to perforation, which usually occurs on the buccal aspect in the maxilla and on the lingual aspect in the mandible. The laceration interrupts the vascular supply of the portion of the flap coronal to the lesion, subsequently causing necrosis during the healing phase. In the case of simple surgeries not associated with regenerative techniques, the consequences of access perforation are generally not serious, but healing of the site can be difficult and long lasting, sometimes taking up to 30 days. Treatment of perforated access flaps consists of twice-daily application of protective, healing-stimulating gels based on hyaluronic acid (eg, Hobagel Plus, Hobama) until complete healing is achieved. Attempting to suture the margins of necrotic flaps a second time is not indicated because they would not be able to withstand the tension of the sutures and further damage could be caused. The use of mobile, mucosa-supported provisional prostheses should be discouraged for the entire healing period.

Root damage to adjacent natural teeth

Incorrect angulation of the implant in a mesial or distal direction can result in involving natural teeth adjacent to the implant site with the preparation drills and subsequently the implant itself. Traumatized roots quickly undergo destructive infections that lead to the loss of both the tooth and the implant.

CLINICAL CASE 1

Injury of an adjacent tooth

A 65-year-old patient presented with painful symptoms associated with an implant in the site of the maxillary right first premolar that had been placed in a poor position 2 years before. The objective examination showed painful swelling, a probing depth of 15 mm at the first and second premolars, and in general, dental treatment of substandard level.

CBCT imaging confirmed the suspicion of injury to the periodontal tissues and root of the natural second premolar **(Fig 7)**. After the patient underwent antibiotic therapy with amoxicillin and clavulanic acid, both the compromised root and the implant were extracted. Careful curettage of the socket was performed to remove all granulation tissue, and the defect was filled with deproteinized bovine bone mineral (DBBM) and sutured with a Laurell-Gottlow suture **(Figs 8 to 11)**.

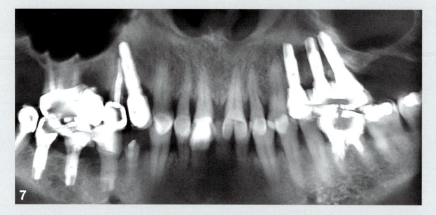 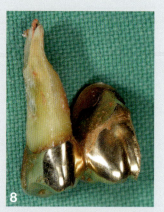

Fig 7 Malpositioned implant in the site of the maxillary right first premolar invading the periodontium and root dentin of the second premolar, which appears severely compromised. **Fig 8** The second premolar was extracted, revealing the root damage caused by the implant.

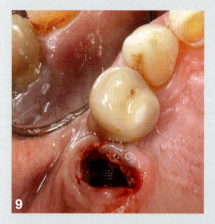 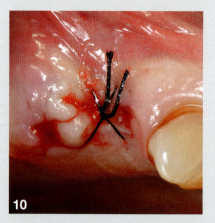 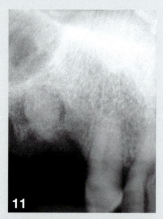

Fig 9 Through the alveolus, it is possible to observe the exposed implant surface. **Fig 10** The implant was also extracted, and the defect was treated with DBBM. **Fig 11** Postoperative periapical radiograph showing the defect filled with DBBM.

IAN injury

A complication that unfortunately occurs all too frequently in daily clinical practice is injury to the third branch of the trigeminal nerve caused by invasion of the mandibular canal during drilling or implant placement. The severity of injury depends on which of the following types it is:

- Complete severance of the nerve during drilling
- Partial nerve injury
- Partial or complete severance of the nerve at the level of the mesial loop at the mental foramen
- Compression of the nerve due to perforation of the bony roof of the mandibular canal
- Compression of the nerve due to edema or hematoma within the mandibular canal
- Straining of the incisive branch of the nerve

Complete nerve severance

Complete dissection of the IAN is caused by incorrectly assessing the position and vertical dimension of the bone crest coronal to the mandibular canal **(Fig 12)**.

A frequent error is the incorrect radiographic identification of the mandibular canal, which is sometimes confused with the radiolucent zone that runs parallel and apical to the canal itself. The complete radiographic absence of the bone canal also favors assessment errors **(Fig 13)**.

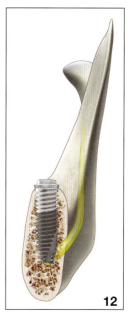

12

In these cases, it is useful to surgically visualize the mental foramen and use a preparation depth no greater than its distance from the crest, as the canal always runs 1 to 2 mm apical to it. The presence of adjacent natural teeth can provide an additional reference point if the distance from the crest to the root apices is used as the maximum preparation depth of the site. In rare cases, the mental foramen may be in an abnormal location, such as at the level of the first molar **(Fig 14)**.

Suspicion of this type of injury during operation may be provoked by a sudden feeling of collapse while drilling during the last stages of site preparation, accompanied by subsequent copious, sometimes pulsating, bleeding.

The pathognomonic symptoms include total anesthesia of the lip and skin at the chin area ipsilateral to the lesion, associated with the radiographic finding of an implant invading the mandibular canal. The symptoms are permanent and definitive unless surgically treated (see chapter 10).

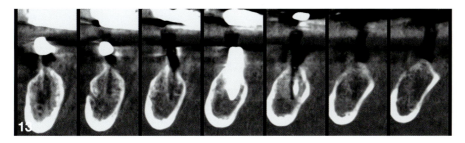

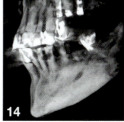

Fig 12 *Illustration of the complete invasion of the mandibular canal by an implant.* ***Fig 13*** *CBCT that does not allow for identification of the mandibular canal. The position and length of the implant are determined based on the position of the mental foramen.* ***Fig 14*** *CBCT showing an unusually located mental foramen at the level of the first molar.*

CLINICAL CASE 2

Complete severance of the IAN

A 45-year-old patient presented with complete anesthesia on the left side of the lip and chin skin after two implants had been placed in the positions of the mandibular left and right first molars 15 days earlier. The CBCT showed total invasion of the left mandibular canal at the position of the left implant **(Fig 15)**. It was decided to remove the implant immediately **(Figs 16 and 17)** and begin drug therapy, with an immediate intramuscular injection of dexamethasone (Soldesam 8 mg [EG]), then betamethasone (Bentelan, Biofutura Pharma) orally 5 mg a day for 5 days, a neuroprotectant acetyl-L-carnitine 500 mg (one pill morning and evening for 3 months), and alpha-lipoic acid/B-group vitamins (Leninerv, Grunenthal Italia) 600 mg, one pill a day for 3 months. Although the size of the affected area was reduced, symptoms were still present 1 year later.

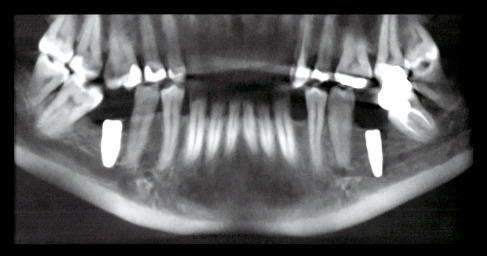

Fig 15 CBCT of a patient with anesthesia of the lower lip and left mental region, showing clear invasion of the mandibular canal by the implant in the site of the mandibular left first molar.

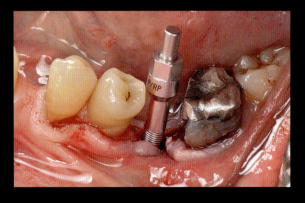

Fig 16 Removal of the implant using a reverse thread extractor.

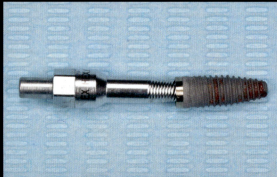

Fig 17 Extracted implant.

Partial nerve injury

Partial lesions to the IAN are essentially the same as complete severance except that the nerve is only peripherally or partially impaired **(Fig 18)**. Nothing in particularly can be felt during site preparation, but there may be profuse bleeding. Symptoms depend on the extent of the nerve lesion and may be limited to paresthesia in a small area of the lip and peri-labial skin or extend to the entire skin of the chin ipsilaterally.

After implant removal and drug therapy, symptoms may go into partial remission within a few months, but permanent symptoms usually remain.

Partial or total nerve injury at the level of the mesial loop at the mental foramen

Often, the IAN moves mesially and loops back a few millimeters distally to engage the mental foramen before exiting the mandibular canal into the alveolar mucosa. If this anatomical feature is not recognized radiographically and taken into consideration, partial or total nerve damage can occur **(Fig 19)**.

Nerve compression caused by breaking through the bony roof of the mandibular canal

An extremely thin bone septum may remain after preparing an implant site too close to the roof of the mandibular canal. Screwing an implant in can lead to the septum being forced into the canal, resulting in nerve compression. In some cases, residual bone particles produced by milling and tapping the site can be forced into the canal and contribute to compression **(Fig 20)**.

Symptoms of nerve compression may range from total anesthesia to paresthesia limited to a circumscribed area of the lip or peri-labial area.

Nerve compression due to edema or hematoma within the mandibular canal

The extreme proximity of the implant apex to the roof of the mandibular canal can cause neurologic symptoms even if there is no direct injury to the nerve. The blood clot pushed by the implant into the canal and postsurgical edema can cause a compressive effect.

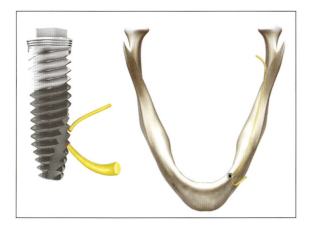

Fig 18 *Illustration of a peripheral partial lesion of the IAN.*

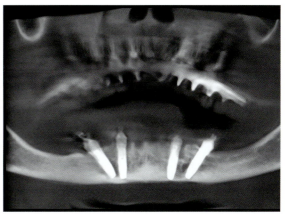

Fig 19 *Partial lesion of the IAN at the level of the loop near the mental foramen.*

Subsequently, the blood clot may become ossified and make the compression permanent **(Figs 21 and 22)**.

Symptoms usually include limited and, in the absence of ossification, transient paresthesia. After drug therapy, complete resolution may take up to several months.

Straining of the incisive branch

A very rare but possible complication is straining the incisive branch of the IAN if it is caught in and stretched by the implant during its mesial insertion near the mental foramen **(Figs 23 and 24)**. Injury of the incisive nerve does not lead to appreciable neurologic sequelae, but stretching the

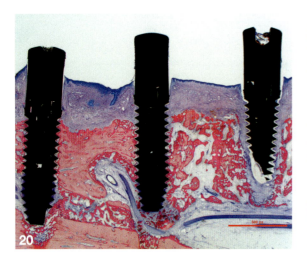

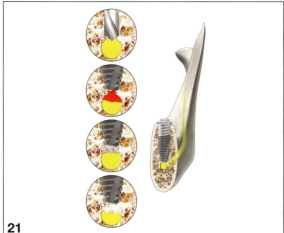

Fig 20 Histologic image of an implant that pushed the residual bone particles from the implant site into the mandibular canal, causing nerve compression. *Fig 21* Illustration of indirect compression of the IAN by edema or the blood clot pushed by the implant into the mandibular canal.

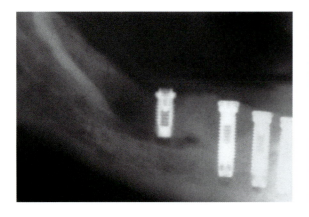

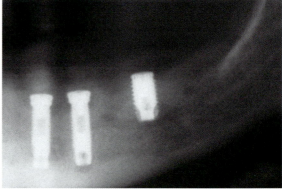

Fig 22 CBCT showing two implants in minimal relation to the IAN. The risk is of indirect nerve compression due to edema or forcing of clot and bone particles into the canal.

alveolar nerve can cause transient hypoesthesia. Neurologic symptoms, however, are minimal and limited in time.

Injury to the lingual artery or other vascular structures of the floor of the

The floor of the mouth houses a series of vessels of significant caliber that can be injured if the lingual bone is perforated during preparation of a mandibular implant site with incorrect angulation **(Fig 25)**. The consequences of injury can be very serious. Intense internal bleeding occurs in the floor of the mouth and submandibular lodge,

which compresses the upper airway and, if not recognized immediately, can lead to the death of the patient.

A predisposing anatomical factor to vascular structure injury in the floor of the mouth may be mandibular ridges that have an adequate vertical dimension for implant placement but which are extremely thin and/or have lingual undercuts. A superficial examination with panoramic or periapical radiographs alone may lead to the false impression of a wide ridge that can be easily and safely treated.

A more thorough examination with CBCT can reveal dangerous undercuts **(Figs 26 to 28)**.

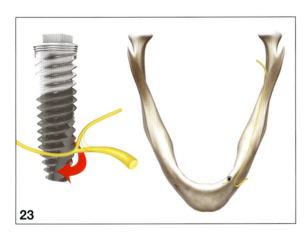

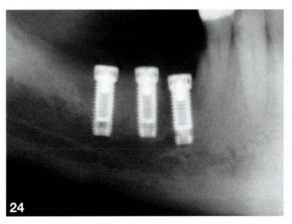

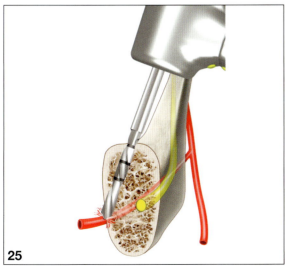

Fig 23 Illustration of stretching the incisive branch of the IAN, which is engaged by the implant threads. *Fig 24* CBCT showing an implant with the apex engaged in the incisive branch of the IAN.

Fig 25 Illlustration of lingual artery injury due to incorrect angulation of the implant site preparation.

Another predisposing factor for vascular lesions is the presence of terminal perforating branches of the anastomosis between the sublingual and submental artery **(Fig 29)**. They are located in the mandibular symphysis, close to the midline, and can be severed by preparing an implant site with an overly lingual angle. The interruption of these vessels at the endosseous level generally does not cause hemorrhagic consequences because the subsequent insertion of the implant completely occludes the injured vessel, but an injury at the point of penetration of the arteriole into the bone canal can cause dangerous hemorrhaging within the soft tissues of the floor of the mouth.

The prevention of such complications hinges on careful analysis of the mandibular morphology at the level of the implant sites, with CBCT used to identify any undercuts or lingual perforating branches not detectable via 2D radiographic examination.[1]

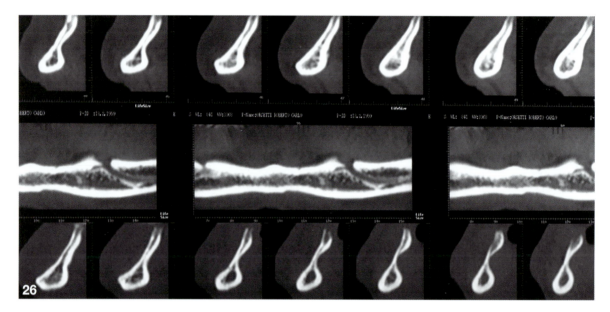

Fig 26 *CBCT showing an optimal vertical dimension of the body of the mandible but a significant undercut in the middle third. Horizontal bone augmentation using GBR techniques will be required prior to implant placement.*

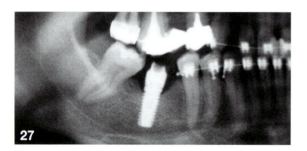
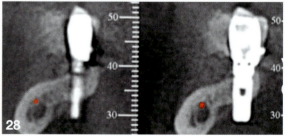

Fig 27 *CBCT in panoramic view showing an implant apparently positioned correctly within the alveolar crest.* **Fig 28** *Cross-sectional images of the same CBCT show a pronounced lingual undercut and the apical third of the implant dangerously protruding into the floor of the mouth.*

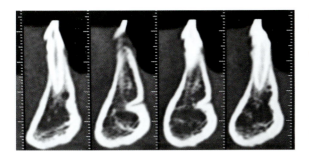

Fig 29 *CBCT showing a perforating branch of the anastomosis between the sublingual and submental artery at the level of the mental symphysis.*

During surgery, it is important to perform an extensive full-thickness elevation of the lingual flap for direct visualization of the mandibular lingual wall and undercuts. A wide reflection in the apical direction also allows the soft tissue to be displaced and protected by means of a periosteal (Prichard) elevator.

Insufficient primary implant stability

Good implant osseointegration requires sufficient primary implant stability (ie, an insertion torque between 30 and 50 Ncm or an ISQ value > 60). An implant that has even minimal mobility or that can be rotated freehand after insertion into the bone has little chance of integration.

Insufficient primary stability can be caused by extremely poor bone quality at the recipient site, inadequate site preparation, or an unsuitable implant design.

It is advisable to remove the implant, deepen the preparation if possible, and insert a longer implant with a larger diameter.

If primary implant stability is limited (insertion torque < 30 Ncm), it is advisable to submerge the implant and wait 6 months without loading (see chapter 4).

COMPLICATIONS BETWEEN THE FIRST AND THE SECOND PHASES OF SURGERY

Complications that can occur during the healing period between the first and second surgical phases include the following:

- Suture granuloma
- Wound dehiscence
- Early exposure and infection of the cover screw
- Apical fistula
- Early implant failure

Edema, bruising, and pain

To a certain extent, modest edema and ecchymosis confined to the surgical area is a normal occurrence after implant surgery.

Severe ecchymosis, however, is rare and usually caused by predisposing factors, for example, in patients with loose subcutaneous tissue and vascular fragility or in patients being treated with antiplatelets or anticoagulants **(Fig 30)** (see chapter 11). In general, edema and ecchymosis occur on the third day of the postoperative period. Certain types of surgery, such as regenerative techniques requiring periosteal releasing incisions at the base of the flaps, may also predispose patients to increased ecchymosis. In these cases, bleeding may continue after suturing and cause blood to spread to the surrounding tissues. Prevention and treatment consist of administering a single dose of dexamethasone (Soldesam 4–8 mg) intramuscularly at the end of surgery along with nonsteroidal anti-inflammatory drugs (NSAIDs; eg, ketoprofen or paracetamol) orally over the next 3 to 4 days, as well as the application of ice packs in the hours following surgery. Pain is typically modest and can be easily controlled with common anti-inflammatory drugs and/or painkillers.

Suture granuloma

Suture granuloma can occur if excessively tight sutures are placed, especially in the alveolar mucosa. The thread strangles the tissue and tends to become embedded, leading to secondary bacterial infection **(Fig 31)**. This is a minor complication that resolves spontaneously after suture removal.

Wound dehiscence

Wound dehiscence is caused by partial necrosis of the flaps during the healing period **(see Fig 6)**. Its etiopathogenesis can be traced back to intraoperative trauma to the flaps from the periosteum elevator or retractors, or to flap perforation. Vascular damage leads to necrosis of the portion of the flap coronal to the injury and subsequent loss of the sutures.

Another reason for partial flap necrosis is excessive tension of the sutures leading to strangulation of the coronal portion of the flaps, which is particularly dangerous in the case of regenerative techniques with horizontal or vertical augmentation of alveolar ridges.

Therapy consists of disinfecting the site with 0.2% chlorhexidine rinses twice a day and applying antiseptic gels based on hyaluronic acid (eg, Hobagel Plus).

Resuturing the margins of necrotic flaps is not indicated. The healing time is generally very long and can last up to 1 month.

Early exposure and infection of cover screws

In two-stage surgical techniques, partial exposure of the implant cover screw may occur through perforated mucosa **(Fig 32)**. This is caused by compression from mucosa-supported removable prostheses and/or an overly exposed position of the implant head above the crest.

The mucosal pocket created by the perforation allows for rapid colonization of the cover screw by pathogenic bacteria. If early action is not taken to remove the cover screws, disinfect the implant, and place healing abutments **(Fig 33)**, the infection can spread apically and cause small peri-implant bone defects 2 to 3 mm deep.

A similar complication is the direct infection of the cover screw without exposure.

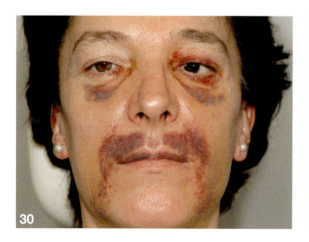
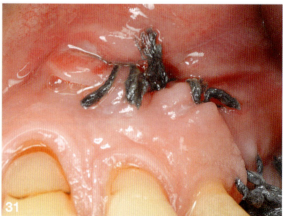

Fig 30 Massive localized hematoma on the eyelids and upper lip in a 52-year-old patient 1 week after implant placement in the maxilla. *Fig 31* Suture granuloma caused by excessive knot tension in the alveolar mucosa.

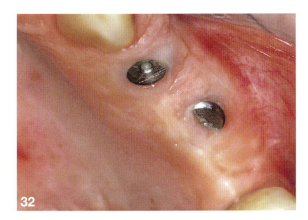
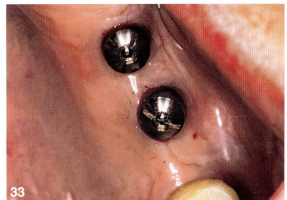
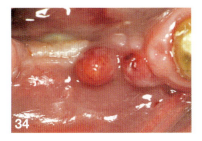
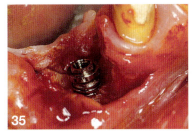
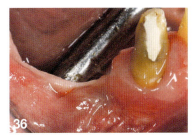

Fig 32 Partial exposure of the cover screws of two implants in the sites of the maxillary right first and second premolars caused by their excessively coronal position and protrusion above the bone crest. *Fig 33* The cover screws were removed, the implants disinfected with chlorhexidine, and the healing abutments screwed in. *Fig 34* Fistula at the level of an implant's cover screw. *Fig 35* A small flap was elevated so that the inflammatory tissue and cover screw could be removed. The implant surface was disinfected with hydrogen peroxide and tetracycline, and a new sterile screw was placed and the flap sutured. *Fig 36* After 1 month of healing, the tissues appear completely healed.

This usually occurs when it is not completely screwed into the implant and manifests as a small swelling of the mucosa and a fistula at the head of the implant **(Fig 34)**.

It too causes marginal bone loss of several millimeters.

Therapy consists of immediately reopening the site by elevating a small flap. After ensuring that the implant is stable, the infected tissue and the cover screw are removed, and both the exposed implant surface and the inside of the implant are disinfected with hydrogen peroxide and an antibiotic solution.

A new sterile cover screw is then screwed in, and a Laurell-Gottlow suture and additional simple sutures are placed **(Figs 35 and 36)**.

Alternatively, a healing abutment can be screwed in, with the implant left in a transmucosal position. If the implant surface is smooth, these maneuvers generally lead to healing without further complications in the long-term.

Apical fistula

A rather rare complication is the development of a fistulous infection at the level of the implant apex

(Fig 37), associated with a radiographic image of an apical bone lesion (**Fig 38**).

The etiopathogenesis of this complication is difficult to identify, but in most cases, it can be traced back to excessive heating of the apical bone during drilling or to excessive compression of the most apical portion of the implant site. The resulting massive necrosis of the periapical bone is a predisposing factor for bacterial infection. The persistence of residual apical granulomas from previous extractions has also been considered a cause of peri-implant granulomas.[3] Therapy consists of opening a flap via a horizontal incision in the alveolar mucosa, removing the inflammatory tissue with titanium curettes, and decontaminating the implant surface with hydrogen peroxide and antibiotic solution (**Fig 39**). In many cases, when the presence of apical implant threads makes effective decontamination impossible, it is necessary to perform a true implant apicoectomy (**Figs 40 to 42**).

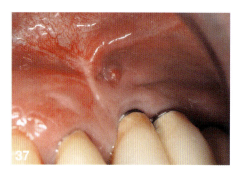 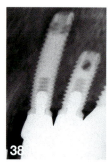 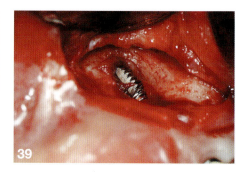

Fig 37 *Fistula at the apex of the implant in the site of the maxillary left second premolar.* **Fig 38** *Periapical radiograph showing the presence of a periapical granuloma* **Fig 39** *After flap elevation, the periapical bone defect can be seen.*

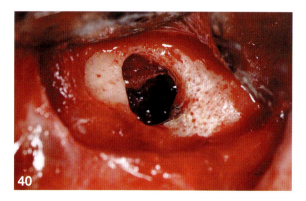 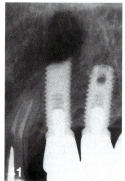 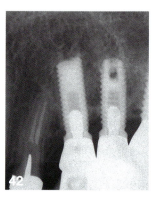

Fig 40 *The apex of the implant was cut and removed under profuse irrigation with saline, and the defect was curetted and disinfected with hydrogen peroxide and tetracycline.* **Fig 41** *Postoperative periapical radiograph showing the apicoectomy of the implant.* **Fig 42** *Periapical radiograph showing total bone healing after 6 months.*

Early implant failure

An implant that is not osseointegrated presents histologically with a layer of fibrous connective tissue interposed along the entire interface between the bone and the implant surface **(Fig 43)**. The connective tissue may be thick, allowing for clinically discernible implant mobility, or extremely thin, making early recognition of implant failure more difficult.

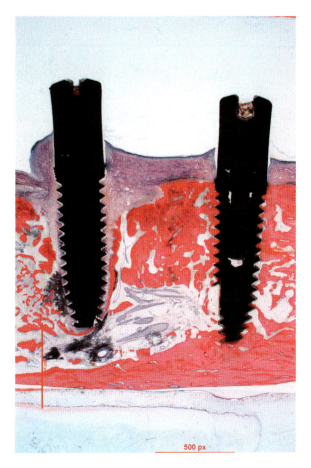

500 px

Fig 43 Histologic image of a nonintegrated implant. An interposed layer of scar connective tissue at the implant and bone interface is evident.

Bone resorption after prosthetic loading, which inevitably occurs if the implant is not integrated,[4,5] causes increased mobility and pain symptoms, making diagnosis easier. For this reason, even in the first studies of Brånemark's patients,[6–9] the evaluation of implant success is postponed until 1 year after the application of prosthetic loading. Implant failure, which can be observed at the time of the second surgical phase or during the first loading times, can be attributed to several unfavorable factors that may occur separately or in association with each other, including poor quality of the recipient bone and insufficient primary implant stability or excessive insertion torque greater than 50 to 60 Ncm. Excessive heating of the bone (> 47°C) during implant site preparation and early infection of peri-implant tissues are also common causes of the failure of an implant to osseointegrate.[10]

Recognizing a lack of osseointegration is not always easy and is based on diagnostic findings that are sometimes certain and sometimes unclear. Sure signs of failure include implant mobility in the lateral or rotational direction and the presence of evident radiolucency upon radiographic examination.

Uncertain signs, which can lead only to the suspicion of failure, are a dull sound upon percussion with a metal instrument, ISQ values between 50 and 60, and slight pain caused by screwing/ unscrewing the prosthetic abutments. In these cases, a safe diagnosis can only be made by attempting forced manual unscrewing of the implant under local anesthesia, with torques not exceeding 15 Ncm. An implant that is not osseointegrated must be removed immediately, along with all connective or inflammatory tissue on the bone walls with an alveolar spoon. After about 2 months, a new implant can be inserted.

PROSTHETIC COMPLICATIONS
(Edited by Stefano Pieroni)

When discussing prosthetic complications in implantology, the first distinction to be made concerns the level of the prosthetic structure where the complication occurs. Prosthetic complications can be classified as follows:

- Deep complications, which occur at the deep aspect of the transmucosal pathway
- Intermediate complications, which occur at the marginal level of the transmucosal pathway
- Superficial complications, which involve only the supragingival esthetic materials

All three types of prosthetic complications can have biomechanical and biologic implications.[11] Mechanical complications involve events that lead to alteration(s) in the prosthetic components. Biologic complications entail impairment to the health of peri-implant tissues. As a rule, the deeper the complication is, the more serious the mechanical or biologic damage can be.

Deep complications

Deep prosthetic complications concern the connection between the implant and the prosthesis. Prosthetic structures are secured onto the implant with a screw, tightening either the connection between the implant and abutment (in the case of a cemented prosthesis) or between the implant and crown (in the case of a screw-retained prosthesis).

Loss of preload

Loss of preload of a screw is the most common prosthetic complication. It involves loosening of the screw tightening an abutment to an implant and is generally related to the continuous stress on the framework by masticatory loads. In the case of external hexagon connections, particularly, there is little opposition to lateral loads due to the limited height of the hexagon. Consequently, the loads are concentrated on the abutment screw.

A further consideration is related to the type of restoration. Restorations for single teeth can present this type of complication much more easily than restorations for multiple teeth. In a single-tooth restoration, masticatory forces can potentially develop infinite lever arms, whereas in multiple-tooth restorations, the connection of all the elements contributes to the absorption of masticatory loads.[12]

Clinically, loss of screw preload is indicated by mobility of the crown. Often, patients will alert clinicians of mobility of the prosthetic crown that is not associated with any discomfort. If the angle of rotation is greater than the normal tolerances of the antirotational components, axial movement of the crown may also be observed because the loosening of the screw is such that the axial excursion of the prosthesis is greater than the height of the antirotational component.

Loss of preload in a screw-retained prostheses is easily remedied. Removing the filling and the materials used to close the screw access hole make it possible to proceed with mechanical tightening of the abutment screw. Clinicians should also always remove the framework to check the integrity of the internal parts and replace the screw if it has suffered any deformation. Before screwing the components together again, the deep structures and the inside of the implant must be disinfected with 0.2% chlorhexidine.

In cemented prostheses, the procedure is more complex. The first approach is always to try to remove the crown with special pliers or a sliding hammer crown remover. If this fails, an extreme solution before cutting open the crown may be to drill an occlusal hole to access the underlying screw and screw the abutment back in. This effectively transforms a cemented crown into a screw-retained structure.

Loss of screw preload is not a serious complication, and resolution is generally simple, but the complications that can occur if this problem is neglected can be serious. Loss of preload tends to evolve negatively, and it can result in fracture of the screw and loss of the crown. From a biologic point of view, micromovement causes continuous trauma at the level of the peri-implant soft tissue and results in a simultaneous accumulation of potentially pathogenic bacteria. The combination of bacterial infiltrate and untreated mechanical trauma can trigger the onset of peri-implantitis. Fortunately, however, the introduction of dynamometric ratchets for torque-controlled screw tightening has drastically decreased the incidence of loss of preload.[13–15]

Screw fracture and abutment fracture

If a screw fracture occurs **(Fig 44)**, the main challenge is to remove the fragment of the screw that is still inside the implant. The difficulty lies in the fact that the remaining fragment does not have a screwdriver slot.

If the fragment has some mobility, ultrasonic tips can be used counterclockwise to create vibrations to slowly unscrew the fragment. If the screw is still tightly screwed in, it is necessary to create a horizontal notch on the coronal part of the screw with a thin diamond bur and use a thin screwdriver mounted on a contra-angle handpiece. Alternatively, smooth cylindric cutter kits with cutting blades at the apex can be used counterclockwise.

Abutment fracture **(Figs 45 and 46)** is treated by removing the abutment and replacing both it and the crown.

If a fractured screw or abutment cannot be removed, it may be necessary to extract the implant. This is the case with broken screws that have incongruously engaged the internal threading of the implant, irreparably damaging it and fusing within it.

Misfit of the prosthesis

Prosthetic misfits can be classified as major or minor. Minor misfits may be related to inaccuracies and procedural flaws within the workflow between the practice and the laboratory. These can result in imperfect seating of the abutment due to stresses in the overlying structures in the case of multiple elements.

Major misfits are related to more gross clinical errors that are easily avoidable, though unfortunately, not very rare.

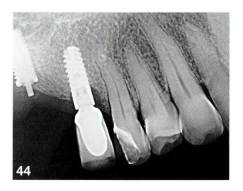 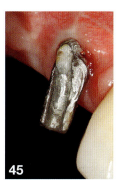 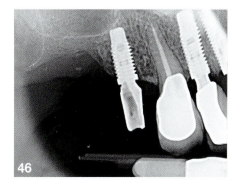

Fig 44 Fracture of the screw. **Fig 45** Case of abutment fracture. **Fig 46** Radiographic appearance of the abutment fracture.

Misfits at the level of the implant-abutment connection are more easily identified in multi-unit screw-retained prostheses because they are caused by tensions in the structure due to imperfect passivation **(Fig 47)**. In this case, it is possible to clinically perceive a progressive increase in tension while screwing the prosthesis in. The earlier this resistance to screwing occurs, the greater the degree of inaccuracy is. Frequently, these inaccuracies are observable radiographically **(Figs 48 and 49)**.

Major prosthetic misfits are generally related to macroscopic inaccuracies and have very obvious clinical and radiographic signs **(Fig 50)**. The failure of cemented structures to fit onto the abutments immediately suggests a major procedural flaw, and the clinician is obliged to repeat all procedures, starting from the impression taking. In these cases, it is common to observe excessive occlusal precontact (even greater than 1 mm), a total absence of contact points, or the impossibility of tightening one or more screws.

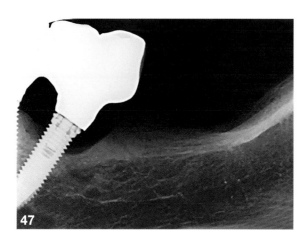
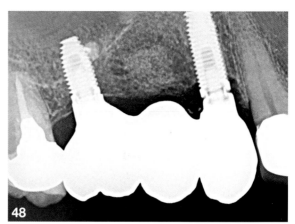

Fig 47 *Minor prosthetic misfit related to inadequate passivity of the structure. One can observe the peri-implant defect likely triggered by this inaccuracy.* **Fig 48** *Evidence of an inaccurate prosthesis created using digital technology.*

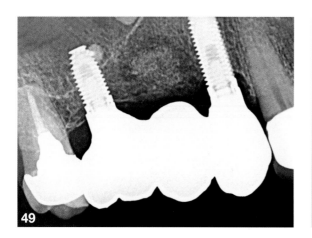
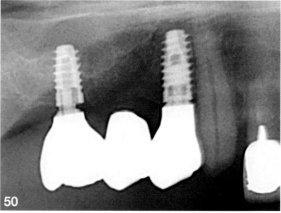

Fig 49 *Resolving the problem by taking a new impression.* **Fig 50** *In this case, it was easy to identify the inaccuracy of the restorations due to the impossibility of screwing in the distal element.*

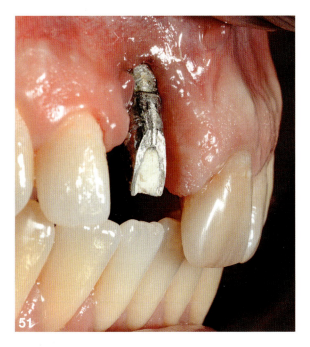

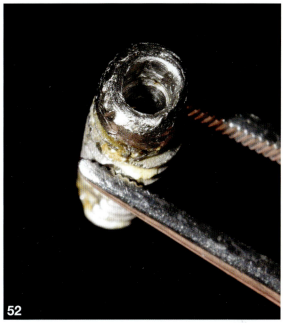

Fig 51 *Clinical image of a severe esthetic defect on the maxillary right central incisor. There is rotational abutment mobility due to the damage of the implant connection caused by use of an inappropriate abutment.* **Fig 52** *Macrophotograph showing the severe impairment of the implant connection structure.*

Deterioration of the Implant connection

Deterioration of the implant connection is a rare but extremely serious complication involving damage at the implant level.

The use of nonoriginal abutments can lead to micromovement that, under excessive forces, can strip the internal implant thread **(Figs 51 and 52)**. Most implants are made of Grade 4 titanium, which is purer and more biocompatible but softer than TiAl6V4 (Grade 5 titanium), from which the prosthetic components are made.

Under conditions of excessive tolerance between the antirotational components, micromovement results in friction that inevitably damages the implant. The most common cause of damage to the implant connection is the development of excessive insertion torque (> 50 Ncm) during surgical maneuvers.

The only remedy is implant removal.

Excessive overcontouring of prosthetic profiles

Invasion of the biologic spaces with excessive prosthetic contours can lead to soft tissue injury **(Figs 53 to 56)**. This is a complication of more biologic nature, although closely related to prosthetic complications.

Intermediate complications

Intermediate-level complications occur in the paramarginal portion of the transmucosal pathway, which is generally accessible to probing.

Crown and abutment misfit

In cemented prostheses, there is potential for a misfit between the prosthetic crown and the abutment at the level of the marginal closure. Minor misfits are difficult to notice, but major misfits present with obvious clinical indications **(Figs 57 to 61)**.

The deeper the closure line is positioned, the greater the negative role of a microgap between the crown and the abutment is on peri-implant bioenvironment.

In patients with multiple missing teeth, even slight inconsistencies in implant position between the mouth and cast may lead to imperfect passivation and, consequently, the presence of microgaps in the mouth that would not be apparent on the cast. With this in mind, the testing of structures to verify their correct fit by means of a fit checker and intraoral radiographs is important.

Cement residue

The risk of leaving apically displaced cement residue at the crown margins is why screw-retained rather than cemented structures tend to be preferred whenever possible. There is ample evidence in the literature that cement residue is a frequent cause of peri-implantitis.[16]

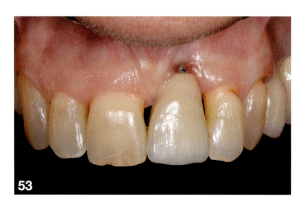
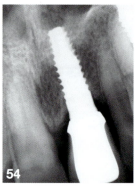
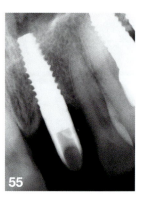

Fig 53 *The excessive bulk of the prosthetic abutment at the level of the transmucosal path caused gingival inflammation and soft tissue recession.* **Fig 54** *Periapical radiograph showing the compression zone.* **Fig 55** *Thinning the deep part of the abutment and using a new provisional with a paramarginal finishing line resolved the inflammation.*

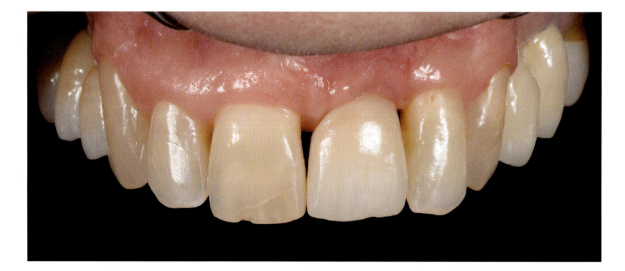

Fig 56 *Crown replacement after connective tissue grafting associated with a coronally advanced flap.*

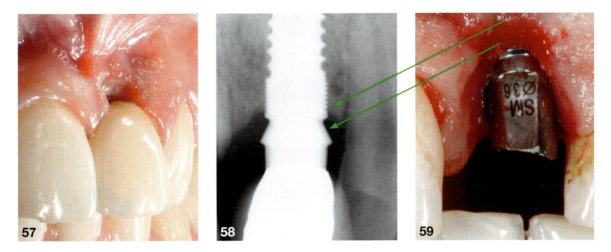

Fig 57 Severe prosthetic misfit resulting in esthetic damage to the peri-implant soft tissue. The photo shows mucositis with the presence of exudate. *Fig 58* Periapical radiograph showing the crown margin 1.5 mm coronal to the abutment shoulder. *Fig 59* The level of the closure margin in relation to the abutment shoulder. This situation made hygienic maintenance impossible in this area, and the anatomy was too irregular to be tolerated by the peri-implant soft tissue.

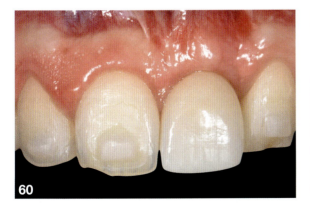

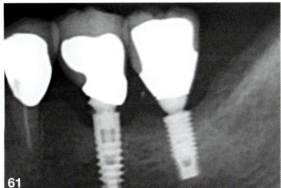

Fig 60 Removing the abutment shoulder, conditioning the tissues with a new provisional, and placing a final ceramic restoration with adequate margins led to the resolution of the inflammatory process. *Fig 61* Major prosthetic misfit on a crown placed 7 years earlier on the mandibular left first molar. The severe misfit resulted in marginal bone loss.

For this reason, it is very important to pay attention to the placement of the finish line. If it is too apical, cement removal is extremely difficult. Periapical radiographs are only able to highlight the interproximal areas, whereas the radiopacity of the abutments hides buccal and palatal residues. It is important to make a distinction between cements and the flowable composites that are used to reline temporaries: cement is generally arranged as irregular granules, whereas flowable composite shows a homogeneous surface (Fig 62).

Superficial complications

Superficial prosthetic complications include the fracture or partial or total detachment of prosthetic crowns. Either individual portions or the entire volume of restorative material can detach from the underlying structure (Figs 63 to 65). Generally, detachments occur in areas bearing the greatest stress (occlusal guidance) and in the areas at the implant access holes where the restorative material is thinnest. These complications are unlikely to have a biologic impact because the damage occurs outside the transmucosal portion of the restoration. The patient, however, will perceive them as being more traumatic.

Completely edentulous patients rehabilitated with implants have a greater tendency to develop this type of complication due to decreased proprioceptive sensitivity.

Other prosthetic complications

Additional prosthetic complications involve the complete fracture of the provisional or definitive prosthesis.

A fracture that occurs early on jeopardizes the osseointegration process for immediately loaded implants (Figs 66 to 69). In other cases, the integrity of the implant connection may be at risk due to the significant lever arm that develops because of the fracture.

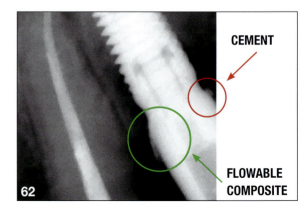

Fig 62 *Provisional element recontoured with flowable composite. A periapical radiograph was taken due to marginal tissue inflammation. Cement residues are evident in the distal portion of the abutment, which have caused a bone defect.*

CEMENT

FLOWABLE COMPOSITE

62

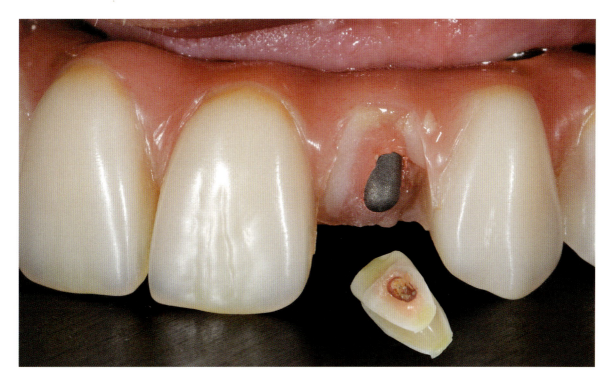

Fig 63 *Tooth detached from a full-arch implant-supported prosthesis.*

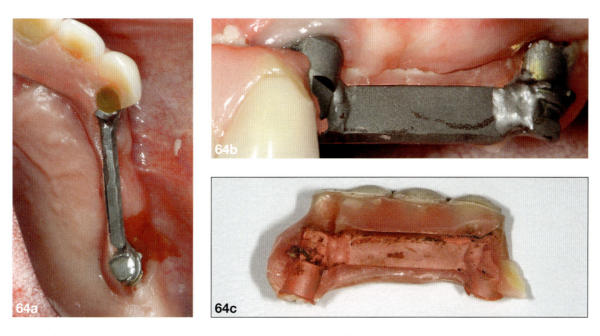

Fig 64 (a to c) *Detachment of the entire restorative material from the underlying structure.*

Fig 65 *Detachment of resin from bonding links caused by slight distortion of the transmucosal portion of the resin.* Fig 66 *Early fracture of the poly methyl methacrylate (PMMA) provisional in a situation with immediately loaded implants.* Fig 67 *The lever arm caused the implant in the site of the maxillary left second premolar to fail.* Fig 68 *The implant was removed, and the site was curetted to remove all granulation tissue.* Fig 69 *After 2 months, a new implant was inserted.*

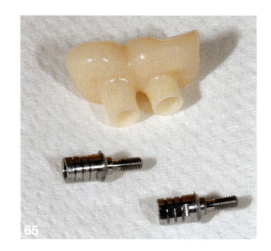

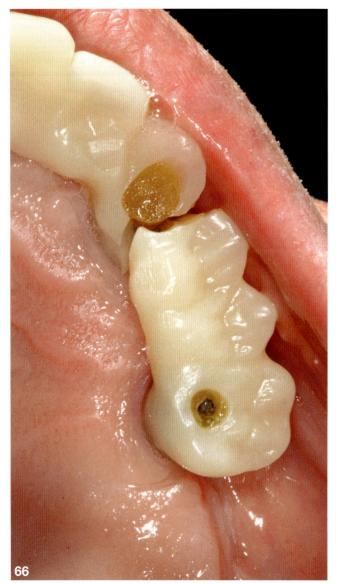

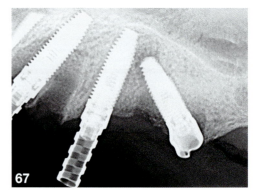

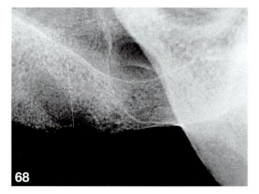

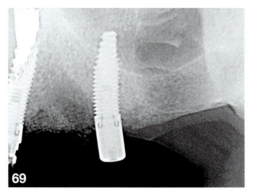

REFERENCES

1. Pistilli R, Felice P. Anatomy and Surgery of the Oral Cavity: Mandible and Oral Floor. Pescara, 2018.

2. Bornstein MM, Scarfe WC, Vaughn VM, Jacobs R. Cone beam computed tomography in implant dentistry: A systematic review focusing on guidelines, indications, and radiation dose risks. Int J Oral Maxillofac Implants 2014;29(Suppl):55–77.

3. Feller L, Jadwat Y, Chandran R, Lager I, Altini M, Lemmer J. Radiolucent inflammatory implant periapical lesions: A review of the literature. Implant Dent 2014;23:745–752.

4. Pilliar RM, Lee JM, Maniatopoulos C. Observations on the effect of movement on bone ingrowth into porous-surfaced implants. Clin Orthop Relat Res 1986;(208):108–113.

5. Søballe K, Hansen ES, B-Rasmussen H, Jørgensen PH, Bünger C. Tissue ingrowth into titanium and hydroxyapatite-coated implants during stable and unstable mechanical conditions. J Orthop Res 1992;10:285–299.

6. Adell R, Lekholm U, Rockler B, Brånemark PI. A 15-year study of osseointegrated implants in the treatment of the edentulous jaw. Int J Oral Surg 1981;10:387–416.

7. Brånemark PI, Zarb G, Albrektsson T. Tissue-Integrated Prostheses: Osseintegration in Clinical Dentistry. Quintessence, 1985.

8. Albrektsson T, Sennerby L. State of the art in oral implants. J Clin Periodontol 1991;18:474–481.

9. Albrektsson T, Zarb G, Worthington P, Eriksson AR. The long-term efficacy of currently used dental implants: A review and proposed criteria of success. Int J Oral Maxillofac Implants 1986;1:11–25.

10. Eriksson AR. Heat-induced bone tissue injury. An in vivo investigation of heat tolerance of bone tissue and temperature rise in the drilling of cortical bone [thesis]. University of Gothenburg, 1984.

11. Berglundh T. A systematic review of the incidence of biological and technical complications in implant dentistry reported in prospective longitudinal studies of at least 5 years. J Clin Periodontol 2002;29(Suppl 3):197–212.

12. Kim SS, Yeo IS, Lee SJ, et al. Clinical Use of alumina-toughened zirconia abutments for implant-supported restoration: Prospective cohort study of survival analysis. Clin Oral Implants Res 2013;24:517–522.

13. Jemt T, Pettersson P. A 3-year follow-up study on single implant treatment. J Dent 1993;21:203–208.

14. Cho SC, Small PN, Elian N, Tarnow D. Screw loosening for standard and wide diameter implants in partially edentulous cases: 3-to-7 year longitudinal data. Implant Dent 2004;13:245–250.

15. Jemt T. Single implants in the anterior maxilla after 15 years of follow-up: Comparison with central implants in the edentulous maxilla. Int J Prosthodont 2008;21:400–408.

16. Staubli N, Walter C, Schmidt JC, Weiger R, Zitzman NU. Excess cement and the risk of peri-implant disease - systematic review. Clin Oral Implants Res 2017;28:1278–1290.

MANAGEMENT OF INFERIOR ALVEOLAR NERVE INJURIES

CHAPTER 10

Edited by Federico Biglioli and Fabiana Allevi

INTRODUCTION

The inferior alveolar nerve (IAN) is a sensory branch of the third trigeminal branch (V3, mandibular nerve). It runs for most of its course within the mandibular canal, which it enters medial to the mandibular branch and exits anteriorly, on the buccal side, through the mental foramen immediately after dividing into the incisive and mental branches. The incisive branch continues its course intraosseously up to the symphyseal area, and the mental branch exits the bony canal and continues into the soft tissues of the symphysis region.

The anatomical position of the IAN is highly relevant to oral surgery. IAN injuries have increased over the years in proportion to the increase in the practice of oral surgery, implantology, and periodontal surgery.

Fortunately, the intraosseous course of the nerve favors reparative processes, with the bone canal acting as a guide for the regeneration process of the nerve fibers.

However, with regard to lesions of the extraosseous portion of the nerve (eg, at the mental nerve), spontaneous repair mechanisms are almost impossible.

Injury to the inferior alveolar nerve is one of the most serious complications that can occur during implant placement, and surgeons must exercise the utmost care to avoid it. In the event of nerve injury, patients must be referred to nerve regeneration experts who can provide them with the best treatment.

Massimo Simion

In the absence of the mandibular canal walls, regenerating axons are not directed toward the distal nerve stump. The partial nerve recovery that is generally witnessed in these cases is due to the occupation of the denervated region by nerve fibers from adjacent sensitive regions.

Knowledge of nerve self-repair mechanisms is essential for avoiding unnecessary delays to diagnosis and treatment. If the nerve has the capacity to spontaneously resume its function, recovery will begin within 2 to 3 months after the infliction of the injury and continue until a high degree of function is restored after 6 to 8 months. This is also the timeframe within which to decide whether to undertake treatment. If there has been very little or no nerve recovery within this timeframe, it can be deduced that a mechanical impediment to nerve regeneration has occurred, and only a microsurgical restoration of nerve continuity will lead to recovery. The management of a painful lesion of the IAN is different. In the case of neuralgia, urgent intervention is required to avoid chronic symptoms that will have strong negative effects on the patient's quality of life.[1,2]

CLASSIFICATION OF NERVE INJURIES

Nerve injuries are classified, as proposed by Seddon in 1943, as neurapraxia, axonotmesis, or neurotmesis. Neuropraxia (nerve ischemia/edema) generally has a good prognosis, with complete spontaneous recovery within 4 to 8 weeks. Axonotmesis (nerve stretching/compression) has a fairly good prognosis, with partial spontaneous recovery within 3 to 6 months. Neurotmesis (nerve sectioning) has a very poor prognosis, with no possibility of spontaneous recovery.[3] As mentioned previously, however, the location of the IAN within a bony canal makes the prognosis in case of nerve sectioning better than that of other nerve structures located in soft tissue, such as the lingual nerve.[1,2]

ETIOPATHOGENESIS OF IAN INJURY

Many factors may contribute to temporary or permanent injuries to the IAN and its terminal incisive and mental branches.

Various aspects of oral surgery, including the type of surgical technique being performed and the instrumentation being used, can jeopardize the integrity of the IAN.

By far, the most frequent cause of IAN injury is iatrogenic.[1,2,4]

Surgical removal of impacted or partially impacted mandibular third molars is the most common situation in which damage to the IAN occurs, with an estimated incidence of between 0.4% and 25%, according to the literature. The estimate for permanent injuries ranges between 1 out of 100 and 1 out of 2,500 cases.

To reduce the risk of injury in select cases, such as in the presence of root ankylosis, the apices of third molars can be left in place if they are in close proximity to the mandibular canal and the IAN.

In this situation, however, there is a risk of infection and/or mobilization of the remaining root pieces, which, although unlikely, must always be considered.[5–13]

Other possible causes of injury include root canal therapy with an overflow of endodontic material into the bone canal, which results not only in compression of the canal's content but also in chemical damage to the nerve structures it contains;[14–16] implant surgery (in up to 8% of IAN injury cases, the cause is related to the placement of dental implants in the region posterior to the mental foramen[17–21]); peri-implant surgery; and the performance of regional nerve blocks at the entry of the IAN into the mandibular canal and/or its exit from the mental foramen[22,23] (with an estimated incidence of between 1 out of 30 and 1 out of 300 cases being due to direct needle trauma, chemical toxicity, or internal or epineural hematoma with compartment syndrome).

Orthognathic surgery,[24,25] trauma, the removal of bony neoformations of the mandible (in the literature, 3.2%–8% of reported IAN injuries occur during enucleation of cystic lesions[26]), and oncologic surgery are other potential causes of injury.

Etiology of specific types of nerve injuries

Nerve injuries are distinguished as being compression injuries, stretch injuries, partial nerve section injuries, or complete nerve section injuries.

Compression injuries occur when the nerve trunk is compressed, for example, by instruments like retractors and protective clevises. This type of injury is usually characterized by an excellent prognosis, with complete spontaneous functional recovery in a period of weeks to a few months.

Stretch injuries occur when the nerve is stretched along its major axis. Its etiology is similar to that of compression injuries, for example, the inappropriate use of retractors and protective spreaders. The prognosis for this type of injury is also good, but if the stretching has resulted in some nerve fibers being severed, recovery may be incomplete.

A partial nerve section involves partial interruption of the nerve fibers and is generally caused by the use of sharp instruments (eg, scalpel blades, periosteal elevators) or electric instruments (eg, bipolar forceps, electroscalpels). The prognosis is variable, depending on the percentage of interrupted fibers, and spontaneous recovery is never complete and may take up to 12 months.

In instances of complete nerve severance, macroscopic severance of the nerve structure involving all the nerve fibers is evident. This type of damage occurs in situations similar to those that generate partial nerve sections. Once dissected, nerve stumps naturally tend to retract, resulting in a highly unfavorable prognosis in the case of extraosseous injury (ie, in the part of the nerve proximal to its entry into the mandibular canal or distal to its exit from the mental foramen). This unfavorable prognosis is due to the distance between the stumps, which makes nerve regeneration impossible. When nerve severance takes place within the canal, the prognosis becomes more favorable, with the canal acting as a natural guide for the regeneration of nerve fibers from the proximal stump to the distal one. In the case of intraosseous nerve severance, the prognosis becomes comparable to that of a partial section lesion. Recovery can begin within 2 to 3 months and take up to 24 months. Spontaneous recovery is possible, although rarely complete. Recovery must occur quickly to prevent the formation of a postoperative scar giving rise to a second injury, in this case, for tearing of the epineural sheath. Sometimes, the healing process results in the formation of scar tissue that joins the nerve fibers in the regeneration process. This can result in the formation of a traumatic (ie, amputation) neuroma at the site of the injury, which results in spontaneous or pressure-induced pain in 50% of patients **(Fig 1)**. If these symptoms are present, microsurgical intervention should be performed as quickly as possible to reduce the risk of chronic pain symptoms.[1,2,27]

CLINICAL SYMPTOMS AND DIAGNOSIS OF IAN INJURIES

The diagnosis of lesion of the IAN and/or its terminal branches is based on the collection of a careful anamnesis and the evaluation of the symptoms reported by the patient. It is essential to establish not only whether an IAN injury has occurred, but also what type of lesion it is, which affects both the chances of spontaneous recovery and the indications and timing for surgery.

Therefore, the symptomatology and its changes from the time of injury, as well as the time that has elapsed since the injury, must be considered during diagnosis.

Careful planning of oral surgery, whether it is for the extraction of impacted third molars or implant placement (particularly in the posterior mandible),

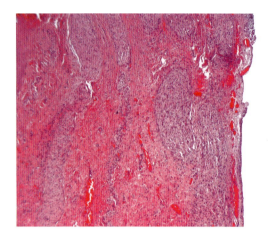

Fig 1 *Microscopic image of a traumatic/amputation neuroma.*

undoubtedly makes it possible to reduce the incidence of nerve lesions.[28] Preoperative imaging, including panoramic radiographs, CT scans, and CBCT, can provide clinicians with accurate information on the anatomy of the regions involved in the surgical procedure for proper planning of all the intraoperative steps, including incision, flap elevation, protection of the soft tissue, and the selection of appropriate instrumentation.

The clinical manifestation of a lesion of the IAN and/or its peripheral branches is very variable and may involve symptoms such as hypoesthesia of the ipsilateral lower lip (82.6% of cases), painful anesthesia (8.7% of cases), and other forms of altered sensation, including paresthesia (8.7% of cases).[1,2,27] The assessment of the symptomatologic pattern is crucial because the need for treatment and the time within which it must be delivered vary greatly depending on the presence or absence of neuralgia.

Patients who present with pain must be treated as quickly as possible to avoid the onset of chronic pain that would seriously affect their quality of life. Better results are also obtained when early intervention is performed. In patients who present with a total or partial deficit of sensibility without pain,

however, particularly if nerve injury is not certain, it is better to wait and give the nerve a chance to spontaneously recover before deciding to intervene surgically. In these cases, symptoms tend to slowly resolve spontaneously and the patient learns to live with the deficit in sensation, which does not cause significant functional impediments. As time passes, the symptomatology associated with IAN injuries generally changes. In the case of a mild injury, anesthesia will become hypoesthesia within a few weeks and disappear within a few months. In the case of a more severe injury, marked hypoesthesia will still be present 2 to 3 months after the original onset of symptoms, even though the area affected by the sensory deficit tends to be reduced in size due to the partial migration of other nerve endings from adjacent areas. If the deficit of sensation is still complete by 6 to 8 months, it is likely that spontaneous regeneration cannot take place due to a mechanical impediment, such as blockage of the canal by a foreign body (eg, implant, residual root, bone spicule). Immediate intervention must be favored when the canal is occupied by a foreign body obstructing nerve regeneration. The foreign body, usually a dental implant, must be removed.[1,2,27]

Besides the clinical evaluation, including simple puncture **(Fig 2)** and rubbing **(Fig 3)** tests to delimit the area of hypoesthesia, it is necessary to objectify what the patient reports.

Undoubtedly, the most effective method for this is an electrophysiologic test, which is an exteroceptive suppression test/trigeminal sensitivity test to evaluate the masseter inhibitory reflex (MIR) with an exteroceptive stimulus **(Fig 4)**. This diagnostic investigation analyzes a suppression reflex of the masticatory musculature with an electrical stimulus at the level of the perioral and oral trigeminal innervation.

The MIR has the trigeminal sensitive and motor endings as afferent and efferent branches and is integrated at the brain stem level, causing two periods of short (SP1) and long latency (SP2) suppression. Stimulation of the area affected by the sensory deficit is very precise thanks to the use of small needle electrodes, with only the tip being electrically active and the needle body insulated with Teflon.

The patient is instructed to communicate the intensity of perception of the stimulus in both the affected and the healthy side, signaling the tactile threshold (ie, the perception of low-intensity electrical stimulation) and distinguishing it from the pain threshold. The intensity of the stimulus is expressed in milliamperes (mA) as a control parameter both pre- and postoperatively. By means of electrical stimulation, increasing the intensity of the electrical stimulus by 6 to 9 times the intensity corresponding to the pain threshold, the suppression reflex of the masseter muscle activity recorded with surface electrodes is then investigated by evaluating its two components, SP1 and SP2, with an electromyograph (EMG) device (Neuro-MEP-Micro, Neurosoft).[29–32]

In anticipation of microsurgical reconstruction of the IAN, preoperative imaging is also fundamental and should always be correlated with the clinical evaluation.

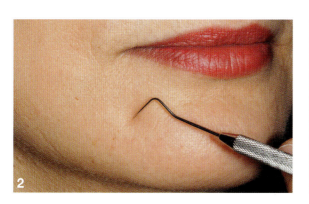

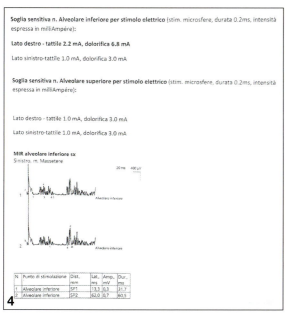

Soglia sensitiva n. Alveolare inferiore per stimolo elettrico (stim. microsfere, durata 0.2ms, intensità espressa in milliAmpére):

Lato destro - tattile 2.2 mA, dolorifica 6.8 mA

Lato sinistro-tattile 1.0 mA, dolorifica 3.0 mA

Soglia sensitiva n. Alveolare superiore per stimolo elettrico (stim. microsfere, durata 0.2ms, intensità espressa in milliAmpére):

Lato destro - tattile 1.0 mA, dolorifica 3.0 mA

Lato sinistro-tattile 1.0 mA, dolorifica 3.0 mA

MIR alveolare inferiore sx
Sinistro. m. Massetere

N	Punto di stimolazione	Dist., mm	Lat., ms	Amp., mV	Dur., ms
1	Alveolare inferiore	SP1	13,3	0,3	31,7
2	Alveolare inferiore	SP2	62,0	0,7	60,5

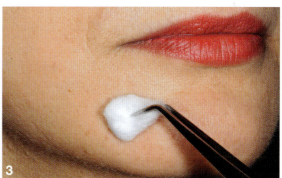

Fig 2 Clinical puncture test to assess skin sensitivity. **Fig 3** Clinical rubbing test to assess skin sensitivity. **Fig 4** Trigeminal sensitivity test.

CBCT imaging can highlight the presence of any foreign bodies (eg, root remnants, implant apices, bone fragments, endodontic material), but unfortunately, it cannot offer information about the integrity of the nerve or the presence of a traumatic neuroma. The use of MRI with nerve tractography, on the other hand, is currently being developed and can be used to confirm the presence of a lesion, without quantifying it[33–36] **(Fig 5).**

TREATMENT OF IAN INJURIES

The timing of treatment depends on the symptomatology that is reported. An immediate intervention should be undertaken in the presence of neuralgia.[27] On the other hand, delayed interventions are indicated in the case of painless sensory deficits, during which any changes in the reported symptoms should be evaluated at follow-ups.

Microsurgical intervention should be considered only if the loss of sensation remains at a high degree 8 months after the event causing injury and if the patient has difficulty tolerating the situation. In the case of a modest residual deficit in sensation at 8 months after the traumatic event, which is a sign that the nerve regeneration process has taken place within the mandibular canal, surgery would at best lead to a modest improvement in sensitivity and is generally not recommended. If,

there has been no sign of spontaneous recovery by 8 months, regeneration has probably not taken place, and it is therefore permissible to discuss the possibility of reconstructing the likely injured nerve with microsurgery.

When more than 24 months have passed since the time of injury, surgical success rates drop slightly, although positive data have been documented in the literature, particularly for late lingual nerve corrections.[32,37,38]

Surgical treatment is not the only option for managing IAN injuries. Medical therapy can also be carried out **(Box 1)**. Medical/pharmacologic therapy with supplements and neuroprotective drugs is undertaken in the period immediately following the injury to promote nerve regeneration. Pain relief therapy can also be provided, possibly with the aid of antiepileptic drugs in the case of pain that is unresponsive to surgical therapy.[39]

Surgical protocol

Surgical therapy[1,2,27] consists of removing any foreign bodies from the bony canal. In most cases, these foreign bodies are dental implants that need to be unscrewed by a few turns to free the canal as quickly as possible. If too much time has passed since the placement of the dental implants, however, and they have become osseointegrated, it is not prudent to remove them with burs because of the risk of further damaging the part of the IAN in contact with the implant.

It is therefore more appropriate to proceed with a surgical procedure under general anesthesia to access the mandibular canal.

Then the IAN can be moved to maintain its integrity, and the part of the implant protruding into the canal is milled.

This intervention is referred to as nerve decompression and can be performed alone if the nerve macroscopically appears intact or be paired with microsurgical reconstruction of the damaged/

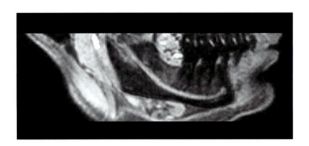

Fig 5 *Sagittal MRI section with tractography of the IAN.*

Box 1 Therapy with supplements and neuroprotective drugs.

Prednisone 50 mg daily on a full stomach for 5 days
Ranitidine 150 mg in the evening before going to bed for 10 days
Leninerv (Grunenthal Italia) 600 mg daily for 3 months (alpha lipoic acid/vitamin B group); *Alternative:* Tiobec (Laborest) 800 mg fast-slow
Nicetile (Alfasigma) 500 mg morning and evening for 3 months (carnitine)
Nicetile cp. 500 mgr mattina e sera per 3 mesi (carnitina)

sectioned nerve tract, which can be carried out by either of the following means:

- Direct suturing of the nerve stumps.
- Insertion of an autologous nerve graft, cryopreserved nerve, decellularized nerve, autologous vein graft, or alloplastic tube (most frequently collagen).

Microsurgery must be performed under general anesthesia because the patient must remain perfectly still throughout the entire procedure. The mucosa of the vestibular fornix on the side of the lesion is infiltrated with local anesthetic and vasoconstrictor to reduce intraoperative bleeding.

Next, a mucosal incision is made in the vestibular fornix, and the mandibular bone is exposed. Care should be taken to identify and preserve the mental nerve as it exits the canal through the mental foramen. With piezoelectric instrumentation, which allows for greater cutting precision and better preservation of the soft tissue, an access osteotomy must be performed on the buccal side of the mandible at the area affected by the nerve lesion. Before removing the bony plate, a guide must be made with titanium plates and screws to facilitate its repositioning at the end of surgery.

This type of osteotomy may not always be sufficient to reach the damaged portion of the nerve. Sometimes, in injuries inflicted during the extraction of included third molars, the lesion is very posterior, and to reach the site and have freedom of movement during the reconstructive microsurgical phase, it is better to perform a sagittal osteotomy, as is done for orthognathic surgery.

Once the transosseous access has been made, the nerve is identified, and its appearance is evaluated under the microscope. It may appear severed, thinned, or simply have an irregular profile. The damaged section of the nerve is then removed, and immediate reconstruction is undertaken. Even if the nerve appears to be completely severed, the proximal and distal nerve stumps that generally appear macroscopically remodeled are removed until macroscopically healthy nerve tissue is reached. The damaged nerve piece is then sent to pathologic anatomy specialists for definitive histopathologic examination **(see Fig 1)**.

Microsurgical reconstruction takes different forms depending on the damaged nerve section. If the mental nerve is affected, it is possible to consider freeing the nerve stumps, which can slide within the soft tissue, and direct neurorrhaphy of the proximal and distal stump can be performed. Because other portions of the IAN lie inside a bony canal, however, the nerve tissue there is not very flexible. In the case of a lesion in an intraosseous section of the IAN, it is not possible to carry out a direct neurorrhaphy of the nerve stumps due to the lack of tissue. In these cases, it is necessary to bridge the gap between the proximal and distal stumps with an interpositional graft. The best functional results are obtained with an autologous nerve graft. Usually, the sural nerve or the great auricular nerve is used.

Neurorrhaphy consists of an epineural suture and is performed under the operating microscope with inert suture thread, usually polypropylene 10-0 suture[27] **(Figs 6 to 10).**

Harvesting an autologous nerve graft inevitably involves side effects at the donor site (eg, sensory deficits and skin scarring).

Several alternatives have therefore been proposed, including the use of collagen tubules[40,41] and reconstruction with cryopreserved[42] and decellularized[43] homologous nerve grafts. These techniques are still being developed, however.

At the end of the microsurgical reconstruction, the bone plate is repositioned and stabilized with titanium microplates and screws **(Fig 11)**, and the mucosal access is sutured with resorbable suture material **(Fig 12).**

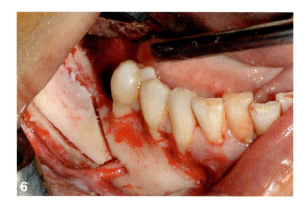
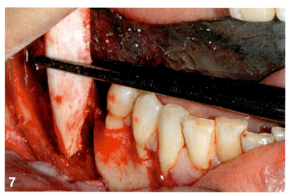

Fig 6 *An osteotomy on the buccal right side of the mandible to allow access to the mandibular canal and the injured IAN.* **Fig 7** *Removal of the buccal bone plate to access the mandibular canal.*

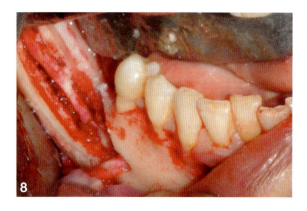
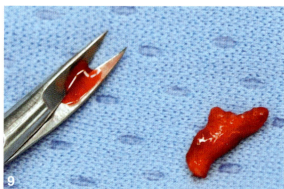

Fig 8 *Damaged portion of the right IAN.* **Fig 9** *Damaged portion of the IAN removed and sent to anatomical pathology specialists for definitive histopathologic examination.*

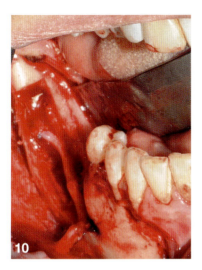 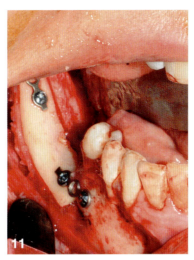 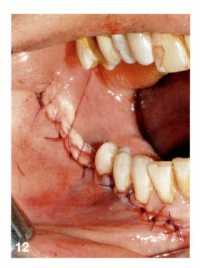

Fig 10 *Reconstruction of the injured IAN with a sural nerve interpositional graft.* **Fig 11** *Repositioning of the buccal osteotomy access plate and stabilization with microplates and titanium screws.* **Fig 12** *Suturing of the mucosal surgical access with resorbable monofilament thread.*

REFERENCES

1. Biglioli F. Diagnosis and therapy of nerve lesions of the oral cavity. Modern Dentist 2010;4:39–59.
2. Biglioli F, Allevi F, Lozza A. Diagnosis, treatment and follow-up of trigeminal lesions of the oral cavity. Dental Cadmos 2014;82:31–47.
3. Seddon HJ. Three types of nerve injury. Brain 1943;66:237–288.
4. Hillerup S. Iatrogenic injury to the inferior alveolar nerve: Etiology, signs and symptoms, and observations on recovery. Int J Oral Maxillofac Surg 2008;37: 704–709.
5. Gülicher D, Gerlach KL. Sensory impairment of the lingual and inferior alveolar nerves following removal of impacted mandibular third molars. Int J Oral Maxillofac Surg 2001;30:306–312.
6. Gülicher D, Gerlach KL. Incidence, risk factors and follow-up of sensation disorders after surgical wisdom tooth removal. Study of 1,106 cases. Mund Kiefer Gesichtschir 2000;4:99–104.
7. Robert RC, Bacchetti P, Pogrel MA. Frequency of trigeminal nerve injuries following third molar removal. J Oral Maxillofac Surg 2005;63:732–735.
8. Alling CC 3rd. Dysesthesia of the lingual and inferior alveolar nerves following third molar surgery. J Oral Maxillofac Surg 1986;44:454–457.
9. Goldberg MH, Nemarich AN, Marco WP 2nd. Complications after mandibular third molar surgery: A statistical analysis of 500 consecutive procedures in private practice. J Am Dent Assoc 1985;111:277–279.
10. Kipp DP, Goldstein BH, Weiss WW Jr. Dysesthesia after mandibular third molar surgery: A retrospective study and analysis of 1,377 surgical procedures. J Am Dent Assoc 1980;100:185–192.

11. Queral-Godoy F, Valmaseda-castellon E, Berini-Aytes L, Gay-Escoda C. Incidence and evolution of inferior alveolar nerve lesions following lower third molar extraction. Oral Surg Oral Med Oral Pathol Oral Radiol Endod 2005;99:259–264.

12. Valmaseda-Castellon E, Berini-Aytes L, Gay-Escoda C. Inferior alveolar nerve damage after lower third molar surgical extraction: A prospective study of 1117 surgical extractions. Oral Surg Oral Med Oral Pathol Oral Radiol Endod 2001;92:377–383.

13. Jerjes W, Swinson B, Moles DR, et al. Permanent sensory nerve impairment following third molar surgery: A prospective study. Oral Surg Oral Med Oral Pathol Oral Radiol Endod 2006;102:e1–e7.

14. LaBanc JP, Epker BN. Serious inferior alveolar nerve dysesthesia after endodontic procedure: Report of three cases. J Am Dent Assoc 1984;108:605–607.

15. Biglioli F, Kutanovaite O, Autelitano L, et al. Surgical treatment of painful inferior alveolar nerve injuries following endodontic treatment: A consecutive case series of seven patients. Oral Maxillofac Surg 2017;21:461–466.

16. Lorenzini G, Viviano M, Di Vece L, Parrini S, Autelitano L, Biglioli F. Surgical treatment of bifid mental nerve damaged by root canal therapy. A case report. Minerva Stomatol 2008;57:369–373, 373–376.

17. Gregg JM. Neuropathic complications of mandibular implant surgery: Review and case presentations. Ann R Australas Coll Dent Surg 2000;15:176–180.

18. Kraut RA, Chahal O. Management of patients with trigeminal nerve injuries after mandibular implant placement. J Am Dent Assoc 2002;133:1351–1354.

19. Bartling R, Freeman K, Kraut RA. The incidence of altered sensation of the mental nerve after mandibular implant placement. J Oral Maxillofac Surg 1999; 57:1408-1412.

20. Dao TT, Mellor A. Sensory disturbances associated with implant surgery. Int J Prosthodont 1998;11:462–469.

21. Ellies LG, Hawker PB. The prevalence of altered sensation associated with implant surgery. Int J Oral Maxillofac Implants 1993;8:674–679.

22. Pogrel MA, Thamby S. Permanent nerve involvement resulting from inferior alveolar nerve blocks. J Am Dent Assoc 2000;131:901–907.

23. Hillerup S, Jensen R. Nerve injury caused by mandibular block analgesia. Int J Oral Maxillofac Surg 2006;35:437–443.

24. Gianni AB, D'Orto O, Biglioli F, Bozzetti A, Brusati R. Neurosensory alterations of the inferior alveolar and mental nerve after genioplasty alone or associated with sagittal osteotomy of the mandibular ramus. J Craniomaxillofac Surg 2002;30:295–303.

25. Ylikontiola L, Kinnunen J, Oikarinen K. Factors affecting neurosensory disturbance after mandibular bilateral sagittal split osteotomy. J Oral Maxillofac Surg 2000;58:1234–1239.

26. Sumer M, Baş B, Yildiz L. Inferior alveolar nerve paresthesia caused by a dentigerous cyst associated with three teeth. Med Oral Pathol Oral Cir Bucal 2007;1;12:E388–E390.

27. Biglioli F, Allevi F, Lozza A. Surgical treatment of painful lesions of the inferior alveolar nerve. J Craniomaxillofac Surg 2015;43:1541–1545.

28. Tantanapornkul W, Okouchi K, Fujiwara Y, et al. A comparative study of cone-beam computed tomography and conventional panoramic radiography in assessing the topographic relationship between the mandibular canal and impacted third molars. Oral Surg Oral Med Oral Pathol Oral Radiol Endod 2007;103:253–259.

29. Cruccu G, Inghilleri M, Fraioli B, Guidetti B, Manfredi M. Neurophysiologic assessment of trigeminal function after surgery for trigeminal neuralgia. Neurology 1987;37:631–638.

30. Renton T, Thexton A, McGurk M. New method for the objective evaluation of injury to the lingual nerve after operation on third molars. Br J Oral Maxillofac Surg 2005;43:238–245.

31. Biasiotta A, Cascone P, Cecchi R, et al. Iatrogenic damage to the mandibular nerve as assessed by the masseter inhibitory reflex. J Headache Pain 2011;12:485–488.

32. Biglioli F, Lozza A, Colletti G, Allevi F. Objective assessment of lingual nerve microsurgical reconstruction. J Craniofac Surg 2018;29:e740–e744.

33. Assaf AT, Zrnc TA, Remus CC, et al. Evaluation of four different optimized magnetic-resonance-imaging sequences for visualization of dental and maxillomandibular structures at 3 T. J Craniomaxillofac Surg 2014;42:1356–1363.

34. Cassetta M, Pranno N, Pompa V, Barchetti F, Pompa G. High resolution 3-T MR imaging in the evaluation of the trigeminal nerve course. Eur Rev Med Pharmacol Sci 2014;18:257–264.

35. Kotaki S, Sakamoto J, Kretapirom K, Supak N, Sumi Y, Kurabayashi T. Diffusion tensor imaging of the inferior alveolar nerve using 3T MRI: A study for quantitative evaluation and fiber tracking. Dentomaxillofac Radiol. 2016;45:20160200.

36. Manoliu A, Ho M, Piccirelli M, et al. Simultaneous multislice readout-segmented echo planar imaging for accelerated diffusion tensor imaging of the mandibular nerve: A feasibility study. J Magn Reson Imaging 2017;46:663–677.

37. Biglioli F, Allevi F, Colletti G, Lozza A. Cross-tongue procedure: A new treatment for long-standing numbness of the tongue. Br J Oral Maxillofac Surg 2015;53:880–882.

38. Cabib C, Biglioli F, Valls-Solé J, et al. Traumatic lingual nerve injury assessed by sensory threshold and masseter inhibitory reflex. J Neurol 2013;260(Suppl 1):S230.

39. Backonja MM. Use of anticonvulsants for treatment of neuropathic pain. Neurology 2002;59:S14–S17.

40. Meyer RA, Bagheri SC. A bioabsorbable collagen nerve cuff (NeuraGen) for repair of lingual and inferior alveolar nerve injuries: A case series. J Oral Maxillofac Surg 2009;67:2550–2551.

41. Farole A, Jamal BT. A bioabsorbable collagen nerve cuff (NeuraGen) for repair of lingual and inferior alveolar nerve injuries: A case series. J Oral Maxillofac Surg 2008;66:2058–2062.

42. Wolford LM, Rodrigues DB. Autogenous grafts/allografts/conduits for bridging peripheral trigeminal nerve gaps. Atlas Oral Maxillofac Surg Clin North Am 2011;19:91–107.

43. Squintani G, Bonetti B, Paolin A, et al. Nerve regeneration cryopreserved allografts from cadaveric donors: A novel approach for peripheral nerve reconstruction. J Neurosurg 2013;119:907–913.

PATIENTS UNDERGOING ANTIPLATELET AND ANTICOAGULANT THERAPY

CHAPTER 11

Edited by Riccardo Nocini and Daniele De Santis

INTRODUCTION

Practicing modern oral surgery requires constant and exhaustive evaluation and study of the protocols that are most effective for managing patients undergoing anticoagulant and antiplatelet therapies. The main goal must always be to achieve consolidated hemostasis.

HEMOSTASIS

Hemostasis is a physiologic process involving a finely regulated dynamic balance between procoagulant and anticoagulant factors, the aim of which is to preserve blood flow, limit blood loss, and allow for the repair of vascular lesions.

The repair of vascular lesions is achieved by the creation of a clot (a fibrin-reinforced platelet plug) to restore the continuum of the vessel wall. The mechanisms controlling hemostasis are coordinated by the following biologic components **(Box 1)**:

- platelets
- the vascular wall (endothelial cells and smooth muscle cells)
- procoagulant and anticoagulant plasma and tissue proteins
- the fibrinolytic system

Hemostasis can be altered by states of disease or drugs, leading to the risk of massive bleeding or thrombosis.

Implant placement in patients who have been treated with drugs that interfere with coagulation is always a source of serious risk and concern. It is essential to have a perfect understanding of the biologic mechanisms underlying hemostasis and to adapt safe protocols to each patient.

Massimo Simion

Box 1 Phases of hemostasis.

Seconds	**Surgical trauma** → Loss of vascular wall integrity.
	Vascular phase → Vascular damage induces the local activation of the endothelium, which immediately releases molecules responsible for vasoconstriction. This phenomenon is indispensable for reducing bleeding, which is permanently blocked by the following phases.
	Primary hemostasis → Formation of the platelet plug at the level of the vessel lesion within seconds from the trauma. Primary hemostasis is the result of complex interactions between platelets, the endothelium, and sub-endothelial tissue. It occurs in three consecutive stages: 1. Platelet adhesion. 2. Platelet activation. 3. Platelet aggregation.
Minutes	**Clinical finding.** A disorder or drug that alters primary hemostasis requires attention from the clinician within the first few minutes following surgical incision. Maneuvers that involve breaking the platelet plug (eg, the use of continuous suction) should be avoided.
Ours	**Secondary hemostasis** → Coagulation cascade, a set of proteolytic enzymatic reactions carried out by coagulation factors. Within a few minutes from the trauma, secondary hemostasis leads to the production of a fibrin network that harnesses the platelets of the platelet plug, thus forming the clot.
	Clinical finding. A disorder or drug that alters secondary hemostasis does not lead to early bleeding but does cause a risk of late bleeding. Schedule interventions in the morning and early in the week, and monitor patients until late afternoon.

PRIMARY HEMOSTASIS[1]

Platelets

Platelets, also known as thrombocytes, are small, anucleate, discoid cell fragments derived from megakaryocytes. There are between 150,000 and 400,000 platelets per mm^3 in the blood, and their life cycle lasts 5 to 9 days. They have numerous glycoprotein (GP) receptor complexes on the plasma membrane, which are essential for hemostasis.

Within the cytoplasm, a high number of alpha and dense granules can be found, containing substances necessary for the hemostatic process, such as calcium ions (Ca^{2+}), von Willebrand factor (vWF), serotonin (5-HT), and adenosine diphosphate (ADP). Surgery is not recommended if a patient's platelet count is < 50,000/mm^3 due to the increased risk of hemorrhage. Surgery should not be performed in patients with platelet counts < 30,000/mm^3.

Platelet adhesion

Surgical trauma results in the exposure of the subendothelial tissue, which is rich in collagen fibers.

Circulating platelets adhere to the subendothelial collagen by means of vWF, which is released by endotheliocytes and activated platelets following trauma.

Platelet activation

Platelet activation is enabled by the interaction between platelet receptors and ligands, represented by collagen, ADP, and thrombin, which is produced during the coagulation cascade. This activation causes a change in the morphology of platelets, which emit cytoplasmic extensions (ie, pseudopodia). It also triggers the secretion of alpha and dense granule contents, including calcium ions, into the surrounding environment (degranulation phenomenon).

Platelet aggregation

The aggregation of activated platelets is enabled by thromboxane A2 (TXA2), a product of the cyclo-oxygenase 1 (COX-1) enzyme pathway. Thromboxane A2 is a potent platelet activator and vasoconstrictor, similar to 5-HT and ADP. In this phase, platelets are joined to each other by fibrinogen, which acts as a bridge.

SECONDARY HEMOSTASIS[2]

The coagulation cascade consists of a succession of proteolytic enzymatic reactions producing fibrin monomers, which spontaneously polymerize to form a fibrin network that stabilizes the platelet plug. This is how the clot is formed. Coagulation factors are present in plasma in an inactive state (ie, as zymogens/proenzymes). The initial stimulus, represented by the pathologic or traumatic damage, leads to the activation of a first coagulation factor, which takes on serine protease activity and activates the next factor according to a cascade mechanism, resulting in the activation of prothrombin into thrombin.

Thrombin is then responsible for the hydrolysis of fibrinogen into fibrin monomers. The classical coagulation cascade was proposed in 1964[1] and consists of two pathways converging on factor X:

- the intrinsic pathway, in which all coagulation factors are present and activated within the blood
- the extrinsic pathway, which is triggered by proteins of tissue origin (subendothelial) and is carried out by factors present in the blood

For the various stages of the coagulation cascade to occur, the presence of calcium ions is necessary. These ions bind to the phospholipids of activated platelets and act as cofactors for the enzymatic reactions. Coagulation factors are produced by hepatocytes within the liver. Hepatocytes also carry out a post-transcriptional modification of factors II (prothrombin), VII, IX, and X and proteins C and S— γ-carboxylation of vitamin K–dependent glutamic acid residues. This modification enables these factors to bind to calcium ions and thus participate in the coagulation cascade **(Fig 1)**.

Hepatic problems, including HBV-HCV–dependent liver cirrhosis and alcoholism, can cause bleeding disorders due to the decreased production of coagulation factors.

Intrinsic pathway[3,4]

The intrinsic pathway is triggered and terminated entirely by factors present within the plasma and is measured by the activated partial thromboplastin time[5] (aPTT). It begins when, due to the loss of integrity of the endothelium alone (endothelial discontinuity), exposure of the basement membrane occurs. This exposure results in the activation of factor XII (FXII) to active FXII (FXIIa). Causes relevant within a dental context may include blood stasis from orthostatism or immobility in bedridden patients.

Extrinsic pathway

The extrinsic pathway is measured with the prothrombin time (PT), from which the international normalized ratio (INR) is derived.[5] It is activated when trauma disrupts the continuity of the entire vessel wall, thus exposing tissue factor (TF), with which plasma factors come into contact. It ends with the formation of the tenase complex, consisting of TF and FVIIa.

Common pathway

The tenase complexes produced at the end of the intrinsic and extrinsic pathways are responsible for the activation of FX to FXa. FXa combines with FVa to form the prothrombin complex, which is responsible for the activation of prothrombin into thrombin. The latter hydrolyses fibrinogen, thus forming fibrin monomers. In addition, thrombin is co-responsible for the activation of factors XIII (necessary for stabilizing the fibrin network), V, VII, VIII, and XI.

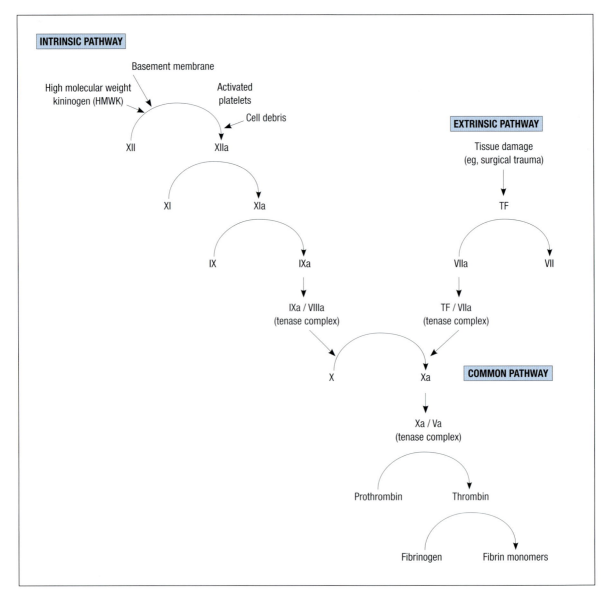

INTRINSIC PATHWAY

Basement membrane

High molecular weight
kininogen (HMWK)

Activated
platelets

Cell debris

XII → XIIa

EXTRINSIC PATHWAY

Tissue damage
(eg, surgical trauma)

XI → XIa

TF

IX → IXa

VIIa   VII

IXa / VIIIa
(tenase complex)

TF / VIIa
(tenase complex)

X   Xa   **COMMON PATHWAY**

Xa / Va
(tenase complex)

Prothrombin   Thrombin

Fibrinogen   Fibrin monomers

Fig 1

NEW CONCEPT OF COAGULATION (CELL-BASED MODEL)[6]

The model of the coagulation process described in the previous section provides a very good interpretation of in vitro tests, but it is not as indicative with regard to the process that occurs *in vivo*. Therefore, instead of talking about a cascade model of coagulation, a cell-based model is now proposed. In this model, the process of

hemostasis is completed in three steps: initiation, amplification, and propagation.

Initiation

Blood coagulation begins with the exposure of circulating blood to cells expressing TF, usually fibroblasts and smooth muscle cells surrounding the endothelium. At this point, FVII binds to TF and is activated. The FVIIa/TF complex activates FX and FIX. This activation of FIX by the FVII/TF complex acts as a bridge between the classic extrinsic and intrinsic pathways. FXa activates and binds to FVa, forming the prothrombin complex, which is responsible for the initial formation of thrombin **(Fig 2)**.[7]

Amplification

Because the amount of thrombin generated in the previous stage is not sufficient to create a fibrin network to stabilize the clot, a series of positive loops are activated in the amplification stage. The thrombin generated in the initiation stage is responsible for several events: it activates both platelets, leading to their degranulation, and FV and FVIII. The circulating vWF/FVIII complex is cleaved by thrombin, which determines the release of FVIII. Finally, thrombin also activates FXI **(Fig 3)**.[7]

Propagation

The propagation phase is characterized by the formation of tenase (FIXa/FVIIIa) and prothrombin (FXa/FVa) complexes on the surface of platelets, with the final effect of producing a high amount of thrombin. Therefore, this phase can be regarded as a direct continuation of the previous

amplification phase. The IXa/VIIIa tenase complex formed on the surface of platelets is responsible for FX activation.

FXa also binds to the surface of thrombocytes, on which it forms a complex with the cofactor FVa. The prothrombin complex FXa/FVa cleaves the inhibitory domain of prothrombin, leading to its activation to thrombin.

The large amount of thrombin that is produced hydrolyses fibrinogen into fibrin. In addition, thrombin activates FXIII, which is responsible for stabilizing the fibrin network **(Fig 4)**.[7]

ANTIPLATELET DRUGS

Antiplatelet agents are drugs that hinder thrombus formation by inactivating platelet aggregation during primary hemostasis. Secondary hemostasis, on the other hand, is not affected by the action of these drugs.

There are three categories of antiplatelet drugs:
1. ADP receptor antagonists (P2Y12)
2. COX-1 inhibitors
3. GP FIIa/FIIIb receptor antagonists

Once hemostasis is ensured at the end of surgery, there is no risk of major late bleeding in patients undergoing antiplatelet drug therapy.

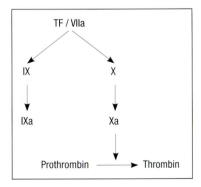

Fig 2

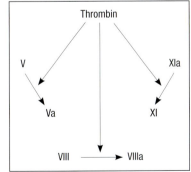

Fig 3

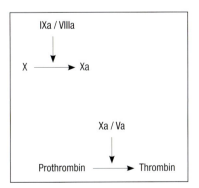

Fig 4

ANTICOAGULANT DRUGS

Anticoagulant drugs are molecules that take direct or indirect action against one or more of the factors involved in secondary hemostasis. Their purpose is to reduce blood coagulability in patients with an increased thrombotic risk. Therefore, these drugs do not impede any stage of primary hemostasis. Instead, the platelet plug is formed as usual at the level of vascular damage but is not reinforced by the fibrin network **(Fig 5)**. A patient taking anticoagulant medication has a low risk of intraoperative bleeding but will be at increased risk of postoperative hemorrhage.

Therefore, these patients should be monitored for several hours following surgery.

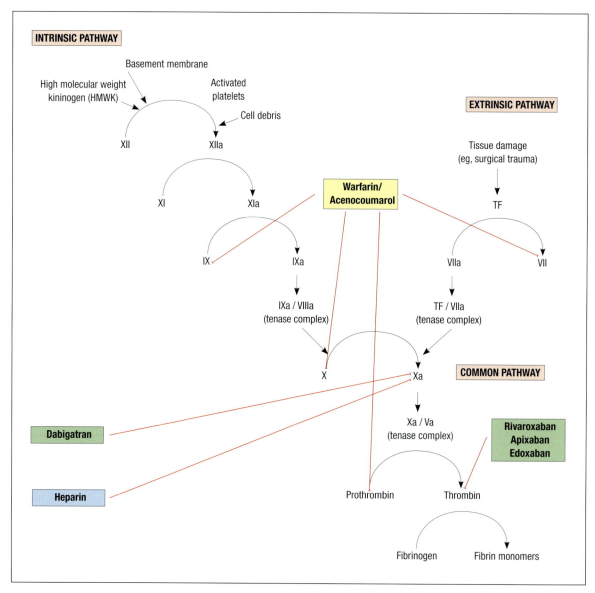

Fig 5

PHARMACOLOGY

Antiplatelet drugs (Table 1)

COX-1 inhibitors

The main representative of COX-1 inhibitors is aspirin (acetylsalicylic acid [ASA]), which irreversibly inhibits COX-1 by acetylation of the enzyme. Consequently, the effect of a dose of ASA is maintained until the platelets are removed. The action of this drug affects prostaglandin metabolism, inhibiting the intracellular production of thromboxane A2. This results in a prolonged bleeding time.

ADP (P2Y12 receptor) antagonists

Ticlopidine, clopidogrel, and prasugrel belong to this group of antagonists for ADP receptors. These drugs bind to the ADP receptor, blocking it irreversibly.
Consequently, the antiplatelet effect is maintained throughout the platelet life cycle.

GP FIIb/FIIIa receptor antagonists

Antagonists for GP FIIb/FIIIa receptor include abciximab, eptifibatide, and tirofiban, which are administered parenterally.
They exert an antiplatelet action by inhibiting the GP FIIb/FIIIa receptor, which is responsible for binding activated platelets to fibrinogen (acting as a bridge between one thrombocyte and another to allow platelet aggregation).[8] The antiplatelet effect of abciximab lasts for a long time (weeks), whereas that of the drugs eptifibatide and tirofiban lasts only a few hours.[8]
Antiplatelet therapy is administered in various cerebrovascular ischemic conditions, particularly for the primary and secondary prevention of venous thrombosis and pulmonary embolism. Dual antiplatelet therapy (DAPT) is indicated as secondary prevention of acute coronary syndrome.

Heparins

Heparins can be divided into two classes based on their molecular weight (Table 2):
1. **Unfractionated heparin (UFH)** sodium and calcium, which are only used in special situations and only in hospitals. These molecules have a high molecular weight. Sodium UFH has a more prolonged effect because it accumulates in the adipose tissue.
2. **Low molecular weight heparins (LMWHs)**, which are the most common. They include enoxaparin, nadroparin, dalteparin, parnaparin, reviparin and bemiparin. In addition, there is a pentasaccharide, fondaparinux.

Heparin acts as a cofactor of antithrombin (AT), to which it binds to increase its anticoagulant effect by 1,000 to 2,000 times.
The coagulation factors that are mainly inhibited are thrombin (FIIa) and FXa **(Fig 6)**.
Because the inhibitory effect is mediated by TA, heparins are defined as indirect inhibitors of factors IIa and Xa. UFH exerts a potent anticoagulant activity against thrombin and FXa, whereas LMWH inhibits FXa only.
Both high and low molecular weight heparins are administered parenterally. LMWHs are injected subcutaneously.

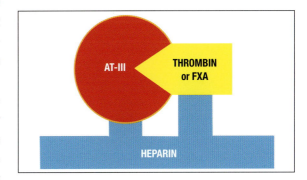

Fig 6

Table 1 Antiplatelet drugs.

Class	Active ingredient	Brands	Half-life*	Protocol
COX-1 inhibitors	ASA	Aspirin (eg, Bayer), Cardio Aspirin (Apohealth), Cardirene (Sanofi)	20–30 min	
ADP receptor antagonists	Ticlopidine	Antigreg (Piam), Ticlid (Sanofi)	30–50 h	
	Clopidogrel	Plavix (Bristol-Myers Squibb–Sanofi)	6–8 h	No discontinuation of drugs before surgery
	Prasugrel	Effiant (Daiichi Sankyo–Eli Lilly)	7 h	
GP FIIb/ FIIIa receptor antagonists	Abciximab	ReoPro (Janssen)	< 10 min	
	Eptifibatide	Integrillin (Millennium Pharmaceuticals)	2–3 h	
	Tirofiban	Aggrastat (Medicure)	2–3 h	

*The times listed in the table relate to the plasma half-life and not to the duration of the antiplatelet effect. The duration of the antiplatelet effect of ASA is 7–10 days.

Table 2 Heparins.

Class	Active ingredient	Brands	Half-life
Unfractionated heparin (UFH)	UFH calcium	Calciparina (Italfarmaco)	1–2 h
	UFH sodium	Eparina Sodica Athena (Pharma Italia)	1–2 h
Fractionated heparin	Fondaparinux	Arixtra (Mylan)	17–21 h
	Enoxaparin	Clexane (Sanofi)	4.5 h
	Nadroparin	Fraxiparine (Aspen), Seledie (Italfarmaco)	3.5 h
	Dalteparin	Fragmin (Pfizer)	4 h
	Parnaparina	Fluxum	6 h
	Reviparina	Clivarina	3 h
	Bemiparina	Ivor	4–5 h

The long half-life of LMWHs (3–6 hours on average, even up to 12 hours) allows for fewer daily doses (1–2/day), whereas UFHs, which have a shorter half-life (1–2 hours), generally require three administrations per day.

Heparins are indicated for acute coronary syndrome, atrial fibrillation, cardiopulmonary bypass in cardiac surgery, hemofiltration, at prophylactic doses in patients with a low thrombo-embolic risk, and (of considerable relevance in dentistry) in patients treated with vitamin K antagonist (VKA) therapy who have to discontinue anticoagulant medication to undergo surgical procedures (bridging therapy).

Vitamin K antagonists

VKA drugs, also known as old oral anticoagulants, include the coumarin anticoagulants warfarin and acenocoumarol, which share the same mechanism of action but have different half-lives **(Table 3)**. They act indirectly by inhibiting the hepatic production of vitamin K–dependent coagulation factors: factors II (prothrombin), VII, IX, and X and proteins C and S.

The remarkable success of VKA drugs stems from their oral method of delivery. Moreover, in contrast to the new oral anticoagulants, they possess a high bioavailability after oral administration, close to 100%. A disadvantage of warfarin is its unpredictable pharmacokinetics, which is responsible for the considerable variation in the doses administered from one patient to another. Therapy with this drug requires continuous monitoring via the INR:[9]

$$\text{INR} = \left(\frac{\text{Patient PT}}{\text{Reference PT}} \right)^{\text{ISI}} = (\text{PT ratio})^{\text{ISI}}$$

Another disadvantage of warfarin lies in its numerous food and drug interactions. Treatment with VKA drugs is indicated in cases of deep vein thrombosis (DVT), pulmonary embolism (PE), and to prevent the recurrence of atrial fibrillation and stroke in patients with nonvalvular atrial fibrillation (NVAF), patients with previous acute myocardial infarction, and patients with vasculopathies or cardiac valve prostheses. These drugs are also used as prophylaxis for venous thromboembolism (VTE) in patients at high thromboembolic risk.

New oral anticoagulants

New oral anticoagulants (NOAs) are drugs that have recently been discovered and introduced to the market. They carry the advantage of oral delivery. To date, the NOAs authorized by the Italian Medicines Agency for clinical use are dabigatran, rivaroxaban, apixaban, and edoxaban **(Table 4)**.[10] Compared to old oral anticoagulants (VKAs), NOAs have more predictable anticoagulant effects. Another salient difference lies in the mechanism of action.

Table 3 VKAs.

Class	Active ingredient	Brands	Half-life	Average time of drug discontinuation before surgery*
Cumarolics	Warfarin	Coumadin (Bristol-Meyers Squibb	32 h (L) 42 h (R)	5 days before surgery; resume 2 days after surgery
	Acenocoumarol	Sintrom (Juvisé Pharmaceuticals)	12–24 h	5 days before surgery; resume 2 days after surgery

*The indicated timelines are relevant to interventions that carry a high risk of hemorrhage.

Table 4 Anticoagulants: active ingredients and their pharmacokinetics.

	Warfarin	Dabigatran[11]	Rivaroxaban[11]	Apixaban[11]	Edoxaban[11]
Mechanism of action	Inhibits synthesis of vitamin K-dependent factors (II, VII, IX, X)	Direct thrombin (FIIa) antagonist	Direct FXa antagonist	Direct FXa antagonist	Direct FXa antagonist
Bioavailability	100%	6–7%	80% (variable with food intake)	50%	58–62%
Onset of effects	36–72 h	0.5–2 h	2–4 h	1–3 h	1–2 h
Half-life	32 h (L) 42 h (R)	12–17 h	5–9 g (young patients); 11–13 g (senior patients)	8–15 h	9–11 h
Renal clearance	0%	80%	70%	25%	33%
No. of doses/day	1	2	1	2	1

NOAs directly inhibit coagulation factors IIa (thrombin) or FXa, which is why they are also called direct oral anticoagulants (DOACs). Furthermore, whereas the dose of a VKA is determined on an individual basis (by checking the INR), NOAs have standard dose prescriptions, except for in patients with severe liver or kidney disease. For this reason, NOAs do not require monitoring with the INR.[12,13]

NOAs have been successfully used for the prevention and treatment of VTE in patients following elective hip and knee arthroplasty, for the treatment of acute coronary syndrome, and to prevent stroke and systemic embolism in patients with NVAF. NOAs are not indicated in cases of valvuloplasty **(Table 5)**.[14]

OPERATIVE PROTOCOLS

Before delving into operative protocols, it is important to distinguish our use of the terms hemorrhage and bleeding. Hemorrhage is the traumatic or iatrogenic interruption of a large-caliber vessel. Repairing the vessel requires the intervention of a maxillofacial surgeon or, in severe cases, a vascular surgeon. Bleeding, on the other hand, represents the outflow of blood from gingival capillary vessels or small endosteal vessels. Bleeding can be managed with the protocols described in this section. Oral anticoagulant therapy (OAT) in candidates for oral surgery presents dentists with a challenge that requires continuous dialogue with the specialists who manage and monitor the patient's coagulative status.[15] Health care providers must cooperate to define the hemorrhagic risk arising from the oral surgical procedure and the thromboembolic risk arising from any reduction or temporary suspension of anticoagulant therapy. The first risk should be communicated by the oral surgeon and the second should be determined by the patient's treating physician in relation to the patient's underlying pathology.

Dental procedures are classified with a bleeding risk scale **(Table 6)**.[16] Many classifications of the bleeding risk associated with various dental procedures are proposed in the literature. The classification presented here is based on classifications proposed by the Scottish Dental Clinical Effectiveness Programme (2017),[17] the American College of Chest Physicians (2012)[18] and the Federation of Centers for the Diagnosis of Thrombosis and Surveillance of Antithrombotic Therapies (2016).[19]

SURGERY IN PATIENTS ON ANTIPLATELET THERAPY

Antiplatelet drugs can be administered as single antiplatelet therapy (SAPT) or DAPT to increase the antithrombotic effect. Use of these drugs increases

Table 5 NOAs.

Active ingredient	Brands	Half-life	Average time for drug discontinuation before surgery*
Dabigatran	Pradaxa (Boehringer Ingelheim)	12–17 h	24–48 h
Rivaroxaban	Xarelto (Janssen)	5–9 h (young patients) 11–13 h (senior patients)	24–48 h
Apixaban	Eliquis (Bristol-Myers Squibb)	8–15 h	24–48 h
Edoxaban	Lixiana (Daiichi Sankyo), Savasya (Daiichi Sankyo)	9–11 h	24–48 h

*The indicated timelines are relevant to interventions that carry a high risk of hemorrhage. In the case of impaired renal function and for low-risk interventions, other precautions are required.

Table 6 Classification of oral procedures according to the risk of hemorrhage.

Unpredictable risk	Low risk	High risk
Local infiltration or intraligamentary anesthesia	Simple extractions (1–3 teeth with a small wound)	Complex extractions (> 3 teeth and an associated extensive wound)
Regional nerve block	Incision and drainage of intraoral abscesses	Procedures involving flap elevation
Basic periodontal examination	Complete (six-point) periodontal examination	Surgical extractions
Supragingival removal of plaque, calculus, or stains	Scaling and root planing	Periodontal surgery
Supragingival direct and indirect restorations	Subgingival direct and indirect restorations	Preprosthetic surgery
Orthodontic endodontics		Crown lengthening
Implants and other prosthetic procedures		Implant surgery
Nonsurgical orthodontics		Gingivioplasty/gingivectomy
		Biopsy

the risk of intraoperative bleeding. The guidelines of the major international associations of cardiovascular experts agree that preoperative discontinuation of antiplatelet drugs carries a thromboembolic risk that is significantly higher than the limited hemorrhagic risk of performing surgery without suspending use of the drug.

Therefore, the continuation of SAPT and DAPT is recommended whether performing dental surgeries with a low or high risk of bleeding. Hemorrhage can be prevented and managed intraoperatively with resorbable fibrin or collagen sponges, hemostatic sutures, tranexamic acid, etc.[20]

SURGERY IN PATIENTS ON VKA THERAPY

When performing surgery with a low risk of hemorrhage in patients with an INR < 3, the patient's VKA therapy should be continued in combination with local pro-hemostatic agents. When performing surgery with low hemorrhagic risk in patients with INR > 3, the surgical intervention should be postponed, and if the patient's underlying pathology does not require keeping the INR value > 3, the patient's attending physician should be asked to reduce the INR value to between 2.5 and 3.

If the patient's underlying pathology require an INR > 3, the attending physician must be asked to discontinue the VKA drug and replaced it with heparin (ie, bridging therapy). When performing oral surgery with high hemorrhagic risk, the patient's doctor should be asked to discontinue the VKA drug and implement bridging therapy.

The patient's INR must be measured either the morning of surgery or the day before. The decision to replace the VKA drug with heparin must made by the treating physician with regard for the patient's thromboembolic risk. If the thromboembolic risk is low, bridging therapy is not necessary.

SURGERY IN PATIENTS UNDERGOING NOA THERAPY

When performing a surgical intervention with a low risk of hemorrhage in patients undergoing NOA therapy, suspension of the drug is not required in patients with normal renal function. If possible, it is preferable to perform the operation after the peak effect of the NOA (ie, 12 or 24 hours after the last intake of the drug and shortly before the next intake.[21] When performing surgery with a high risk of hemorrhage, suspension of the drug for at least 48 hours is recommended, consistent with the patient's renal function. Unlike in patients receiving VKA therapy, bridging therapy is not required when the NOA is discontinued.[21]

CLINICAL CASE 1

Performing surgery with a high risk of hemorrhage in a patient on oral antiplatelet therapy with clopidogrel

An 81-year-old man presented with a history of stroke, hypertensive heart disease, and familial hypertriglyceridemia and required the extraction of all maxillary teeth in an outpatient setting. The patient was taking clopidogrel, bisoprolol, and atorvastatin. According to international guidelines for antiplatelet therapy, drug discontinuation was not required before surgery but a consultation with the patient's attending physician was. In this case, the patient's physician decided to discontinue clopidogrel and replace it with Clexane (Sanofi), an LMWH, to promote better management of bleeding risk due to its shorter half-life.

On the morning of surgery, however, the patient did not discontinue Clexane. Because the dental procedure could not be postponed due to the patient's motor difficulties, the profuse intraoperative bleeding was managed by topical injections of tranexamic acid, which is an antifibrinolytic agent that opposes the lysis of the fibrin network, thus favoring clot stabilization **(Fig 7)**.

At the end of the operation, the patient was instructed to use ice packs (every 30 minutes for 12–18 hours) and follow a soft, cold diet. He was recommended to sleep with his head elevated and not to use rinses that could dislodge the clot. In the case of late bleeding, the patient was instructed to perform compressive hemostasis for 15 minutes with gauze soaked in tranexamic acid. The patient was placed on a 1-week follow-up program and examined the day after surgery.

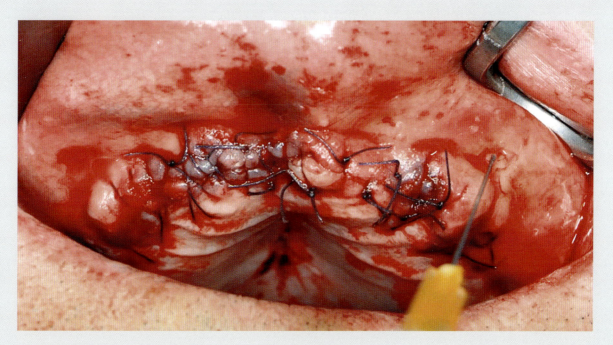

Fig 7 Bleeding did not stop with suturing and compression with moist gauze alone, so topical injections of tranexamic acid (Ugurol, Rottapharm) were used (5 ml).

CLINICAL CASE 2

Management of a postoperative complication in a patient undergoing antiplatelet and NOA therapy

A 73-year-old woman with a history of venous thrombosis and atrial fibrillation presented with postoperative bleeding secondary to extraction of the mandibular right lateral incisor. The patient was taking ASA (Cardio Aspirin, Apohealth) and apixaban (Eliquis, Bristol-Meyers Squibb). SAPT with Cardio Aspirin does not require discontinuation of the drug, but proper postoperative management protocols must be followed. Likewise, anticoagulant therapy with apixaban did not need to be discontinued because the operation performed (single tooth extraction) is classified as presenting a low risk of hemorrhage.

In this case, the patient had continued both antiplatelet therapy with Cardio Aspirin and anticoagulant therapy with Eliquis before undergoing surgery. Coadministration of apixaban and ASA, however, increases the risk of hemorrhage, so a more cautious protocol would have required temporary discontinuation of the NOA drug (apixaban). Furthermore, the patient had not been given postoperative instructions. In fact, at the anamnestic investigation, the patient reported continuous rinsing, which caused the clot to break up and bleeding to occur.

We managed the patient with compressive hemostasis by means of gauze soaked in tranexamic acid, which is an antifibrinolytic agent useful for preventing lysis of the fibrin network and increased stabilization of the platelet plug. In addition, in agreement with the treating physician, apixaban was suspended for 12 hours (the patient was instructed to skip the evening dose and resume administration normally the following day). We provided the appropriate postoperative recommendations to the patient and followed up with her the following day **(Fig 8)**.

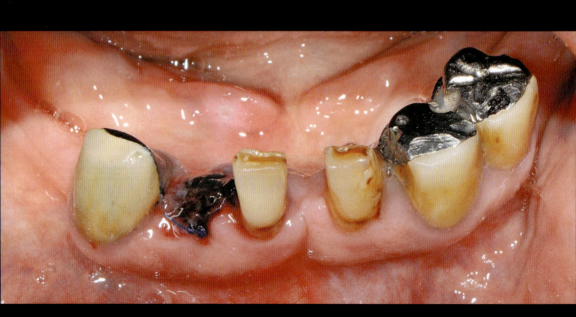

Fig 8 Confirmation of the achievement of good hemostasis.

CLINICAL CASE 3

Performing surgery with a high risk of hemorrhage in a patient undergoing oral anticoagulant therapy with VKA

A 75-year-old woman with a history of atrial fibrillation and familial hypercholesterolemia presented with the need for multiple biopsies of the left oral mucosa for suspected oral Lichen Planus **(Fig 9)**. According to the classification proposed in this chapter, this operation is characterized by a high risk of hemorrhage. The patient was taking warfarin (Coumadin, Bristol-Meyers Squibb) and rosuvastatin. The patient's attending physician was contacted, and the necessary intervention and the relative hemorrhagic risk were described. The physician gave clearance to proceed with surgery, which was performed after discontinuing Coumadin and replacing it with an LMWH (bridging therapy).

On the day scheduled for biopsy, the patient's INR was 2.1, so surgery was performed. Intraoperative measures can be taken to reduce bleeding in these situations, including using local anesthesia with vasoconstrictor if possible, Spongostan (Ethicon), Tabotamp (Ethicon), electrocautery or photocoagulation (with laser), and hemostatic sutures, as well as performing flap closure for healing by primary intention.

Postoperative management includes preferably performing surgical procedures in the morning and discharging the patient 2 to 3 hours after surgery. Ice packs (every 30 minutes for 12–18 hours) are recommended, along with a soft and cold diet for 4 to 5 days and careful oral hygiene. A 7-day follow-up is recommended.

In this patient, heparin was resumed 1 day after surgery, and Coumadin was reintroduced on the second day postoperatively, in the absence of hemorrhagic complications **(Fig 10)**.

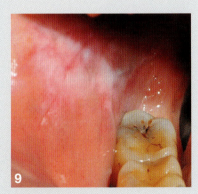

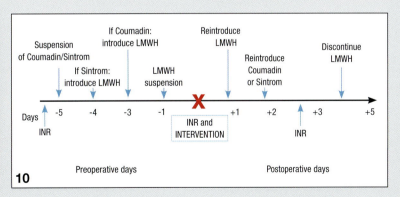

Fig 9 Intraoral image of the lesion of suspected Lichen Planus, for which a biopsy examination was planned. **Fig 10** Diagram of the bridging therapy to be implemented for the proper management of the surgery.

CLINICAL CASE 4

Management of a postoperative complication in a patient undergoing VKA therapy

A 75-year-old man with a history of coronary atherosclerosis, atrial fibrillation, myocardiopathy, hypertension, and type 2 diabetes mellitus presented with hematomas in the face following multiple tooth extractions in the first and second quadrants. The patients was taking Coumadin, spironolactone, furosemide, bisoprolol, and metformin.

In this case, appropriate patient management protocols had been followed. Coumadin had been discontinued and replaced with an LMWH. Nevertheless, there were postoperative submucosal **(Fig 11)** and perioral hematomas extending to the suborbital level and chin **(Fig 12)**. These were due to the vitamin K hydroquinone deficiency caused by warfarin administration and the slow recovery of vitamin K–dependent coagulative factors due to partial liver failure.

Postoperatively, Coumadin should be discontinued for an additional 2 days, during which the patient should continue heparin therapy.

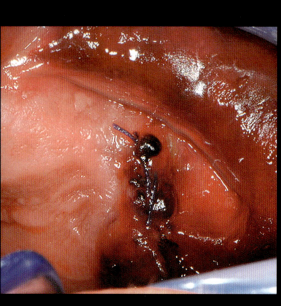

Fig 11 Intraoral clinical appearance of submucosal hematoma.

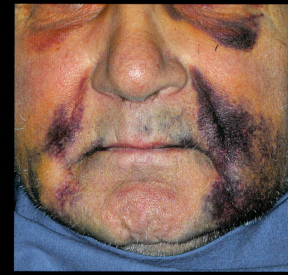

Fig 12 Extraoral clinical appearance of multiple perioral hematomas.

CLINICAL CASE 5

Management of a postoperative complication in a patient undergoing NOA therapy

A 67-year-old man with a history of mastocytosis, thrombophlebitis, hiatal hernia, and thyroidectomy presented with diffuse deep hematomas at the neck level following the surgical extraction of the mandibular right second and third molars and the insertion of an implant in the site of the second molar. The patient was taking dabigatran (Pradaxa, Boehringer Ingelheim), euthyrox, and omeprazole. Due to overly aggressive intervention and the limited withdrawal of the NOA drug (only 12 hours), diffuse skin hematomas at the base of the neck **(Fig 13)** and hemorrhagic suffusion at the floor of the mouth **(Fig 14)** occurred, with the danger of upper airway blockage.

As a precautionary measure only, the patient was admitted for 1 day in the hospital's department of dentistry and maxillofacial surgery, where tranexamic acid was administered intravenously and the suspension of dabigatran was extended until discharge the following day.

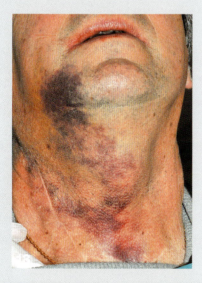
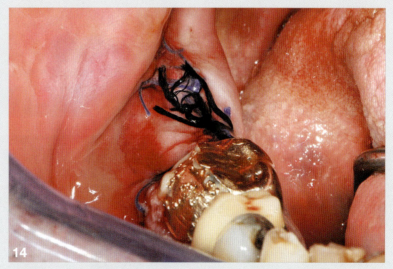

Fig 13 Widespread distribution of deep hematomas secondary to extraction of the mandibular right second and third molars and simultaneous implant placement. **Fig 14** Intraoperative image of the treated area.

CLINICAL CASE 6

Surgery with a high risk of hemorrhage in a patient undergoing oral anticoagulant therapy with a NOA

A 56-year-old man with a history of venous thromboembolism following knee arthroplasty requested an implant-supported prosthesis for the maxillary central incisors. He was taking Pradaxa.

It was planned to place two implants in the sites of the maxillary central incisors, a surgery classified as having a high risk of hemorrhage **(see Table 6)**, so the patient's doctor was contacted and received a description of the operation and the associated bleeding risk. It was considered appropriate to suspend the administration of dabigatran 48 hours before surgery.

To reduce the invasiveness of the incision and the associated bleeding, it was decided to perform computer-guided implant placement. Therefore, the implant position was determined with the multilayer CT scan, which was also used for the fabrication of the surgical guide. During surgery, the surgical guide was positioned **(Fig 15)**, and a small incision was made **(Fig 16)**. Postoperatively, the patient was instructed to use ice packs (every 30 minutes for 12–18 hours), maintain a soft and cold diet, avoid the use of NSAIDs (especially aspirin) for pain control and instead use paracetamol, sleep with the head elevated, and avoid rinses while maintaining adequate oral hygiene.

The patient resumed the usual dose of dabigatran the day following surgery and was placed on a follow-up program until complete healing of the surgical wound (this lasts at least until the sutures are removed). No bleeding complications were reported.

Clinical tip: when implant placement is required in patients undergoing oral anticoagulant therapy, the use of computer-guided surgery is suggested to avoid the need for large mucogingival incisions, periosteal dislocation and osteoplasty, thus reducing bleeding.

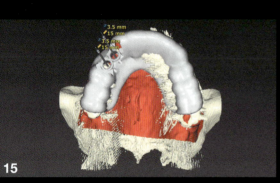
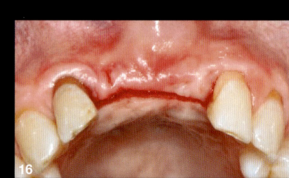

Fig 15 Screenshot of static guided surgical planning to optimize implant placement and reduce the risk of hemorrhage. **Fig 16** Clinical image of the conservative flap incision.

CLINICAL CASE 7
Pre- and postoperative management of a patient undergoing NOA therapy

A 90-year-old woman with a history of ischemic stroke, atrial fibrillation, chronic renal failure, and chronic obstructive pulmonary disease presented with bleeding following the extraction the maxillary left second molar **(Fig 17)**. She was taking Pradaxa, metoprolol, furosemide, and esomeprazole. The extraction of a single tooth is classified as having a low risk of hemorrhage **(see Table 6)**, but the oral surgeon did not take into account the patient's history of chronic renal insufficiency, which results in a lower clearance of the NOA drug and, consequently, a greater anticoagulant effect and a greater risk of postoperative bleeding. In the case of renal insufficiency, it is necessary to extend the period of withdrawal from the NOA drug **(Table 7)**.

Figure 11-18 shows an inefficient clot (ie, an unstable platelet plug reinforced by the fibrin network). Patient management involved removal of the inefficient platelet plug and the placement of Spongostan soaked in tranexamic acid. Compressive hemostatic sutures were then placed. The patient's attending physician was contacted, to whom the patient's oral condition was reported. In light of the patient's compromised renal function and comorbidities, the doctor suggested a 48-hour suspension of dabigatran. The patient was recommended ice packs and a cold, liquid diet for 4 to 5 days. Oral rinses were prohibited for the first 2 to 3 days. The patient was followed up with until the wound was completely healed.

Table 7 Guidelines for the last intake of NOAs before elective surgery.

CrCl* (mL/Min)	Dabigatran		Apixaban, edoxaban, rivaroxaban	
	Low risk of hemorrhage	High risk of hemorrhage	Low risk of hemorrhage	High risk of hemorrhage
≥ 80	≥ 24h	≥ 48h	≥ 24h	≥ 48h
50-80	≥ 36h	≥ 72h	≥ 24h	≥ 48h
30-50	≥ 48h	≥ 96h	≥ 24h	≥ 48h
15-30	Not indicated	Not indicated	≥ 36h	≥ 48

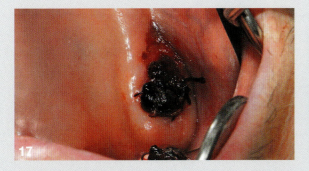
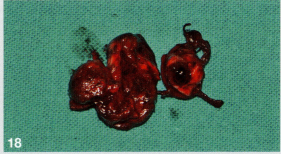

Fig 17 Ineffective clot in the site of the extracted maxillary second molar. **Fig 18** Removal of the ineffective clot to allow proper wound management and the consolidation of hemostasis.

CLINICAL CASE 8

Panagement of a postoperative complication in a patient undergoing NOA therapy

A 65-year-old man with a history of acute coronary syndrome and hypertension presented for uncovering of implants in the sites of the mandibular left second premolar and first and second molars and the placement of healing screws. He was taking Pradaxa and spironolactone.

In agreement with the attending physician, the morning dose of dabigatran was foregone to reduce the plasma concentration of the drug, and the drug was reintroduced normally on the evening of the operation.

Despite the suspension of dabigatran, copious bleeding did not occur because primary hemostasis allows for the formation of the platelet plug.

The following day the patient returned to the dental clinic reporting bleeding from the surgical wound **(Fig 19)**. This bleeding was due to the failure of the fibrin network to stabilize the platelet plug due to slower clearance of the drug (which varies from patient to patient), resulting in an inefficient clot **(Fig 20)**. It was decided to remove the inefficient clot and add a few hemostatic sutures **(Fig 21)**. Compressive hemostasis was performed with gauze soaked in tranexamic acid (10 to 15 minutes). The patient was kept under observation for 1 hour and was discharged as no bleeding was observed. Postoperative instructions were then reinforced to the patient.

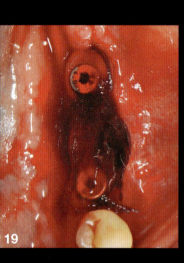 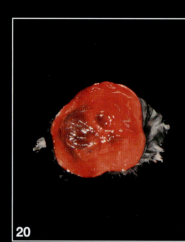 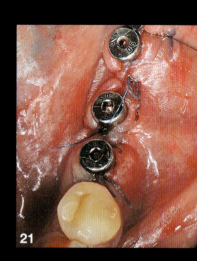

Fig 19 Inefficient clotting found the day after uncovering the implant. **Fig 20** Removal of the inefficient clot. **Fig 21** Successful hemostasis at the 1-hour follow-up after removal of the ineffective clot and appropriate surgical wound management.

REFERENCES

1. Palta S, Palta A, Saroa R. Overview of the coagulation system. Indian J Anaesth 2014;58:515–523.

2. Saba HI, Saba SR. Vascular endothelium, influence on hemostasis: Past and present. In: Saba HI, Roberts HR (eds). Hemostasis and Thrombosis: Practical Guidelines in Clinical Management. John Wiley & Sons, 2014.

3. Cooley BC. The dirty side of the intrinsic pathway of coagulation. Thromb Res 2016;145:159–160.

4. Gailani D, Renné T. Intrinsic pathway of coagulation and arterial thrombosis. Arterioscler Thromb Vasc Biol 2007;27:2507–2513.

5. Bonar RA, Lippi G, Favaloro EJ. Overview of hemostasis and thrombosis and contribution of laboratory testing to diagnosis and management of hemostasis and thrombosis disorders. Methods Mol Biol 2017;1646: 3–27.

6. Vine AK. Recent advances in haemostasis and thrombosis. Retina 200-;29;1–7.

7. Monroe AD, Hoffman M. Theories of blood coagulation: Basic concepts and recent updates. In: Saba HI, Saba SR (eds). Hemostasis and Thrombosis: Practical Guidelines in Clinical Management. John Wiley & Sons, 2014.

8. Cacciapuoti F. Antiplatelet drugs. Trends Med 2015;15:11–16.

9. Palareti G. Guidelines for monitoring anticoagulant therapy. Riv Med Lab JLM 2001;2:S.1.

10. Harder S, Graff J. Novel oral anticoagulants: Clinical pharmacology, indications and practical considerations. Eur J Clin Pharmacol 2013;69:1617–1633.

11. Ferri N, Corsini A. New oral anticoagulants: Clinical pharmacology considerations. G Ital Cardiol 2015;16(11 Suppl 1):3S–16S.

12. Becattini C, Vedovati M. C, Agnelli G. Old and new oral anticoagulants for venous thromboembolism and atrial fibrillation: A review of the literature. Thromb Res 2012;129:392–400.

13. Galanis T, Thomson L, Palladino M, Merli GJ. New oral anticoagulants. J Thromb Thrombolysis 2011;31: 310–320.

14. Agnelli G, Becattini C, Franco L. New oral anticoagulants for the treatment of venous thromboembolism. Best Pract Res Clin Haematol 2013;26:151–161.

15. Ageno W, Büller HR, Falanga A, et al. J. Managing reversal of direct oral anticoagulants in emergency situations. Anticoagulation Education Task Force White Paper. Thromb Haemost 2016;116:1003–1010.

16. Finazzi G, Palareti G, Filippi A, Zaninelli A. Guide to oral anticoagulant therapy for general practitioners. FCSA-SIMG 2000.

17. Dézsi CA, Dézsi BB, Dézsi AD. Management of dental patients receiving antiplatelet therapy or chronic oral anticoagulation: A review of the latest evidence. Eur J Gen Pract 2017;23:196–201.

18. Douketis JD, Spyropoulos AC, Spencer FA, et al. Perioperative management of antithrombotic therapy: Antithrombotic Therapy and Prevention of Thrombosis, 9th ed: American College of Chest Physicians Evidence-Based Clinical Practice Guidelines. Chest 2012;141(Suppl):e326S–e350S.

19. Parretti D, Grilli P, Bastiani F, Manotti C, Poli D, Testa S. SIMG-FCSA consensus document on correct anticoagulation procedures. J Ital Soc Gen Med 2018;25:35–47.

20. Li L, Zhang W, Yang Y, Zhao L, Zhou X, Zhang J. Dental management of patient with dual antiplatelet therapy: A meta-analysis. Clin Oral Investig 2019;23: 1615–1623.

21. Johnston S. An evidence summary of the management of patients taking direct oral anticoagulants (DOACs) undergoing dental surgery. Int J Oral Maxillofac Surg 2016;45:618–630.

BISPHOSPHONATES AND IMPLANTOLOGY

CHAPTER 12

Edited by Daniele de Santis and Pier Francesco Nocini

INTRODUCTION

The relationship between dental implants and the administration of bisphosphonates is controversial and deserves in-depth attention. Bisphosphonate therapy exposes patients to the risk of complications that, according to the most recent guidelines on the subject, are connected not so much to the surgical act of implant insertion but rather to the potential for peri-implant inflammation in the long-term.[1] The aim of this chapter, therefore, is to provide oral surgeons with a general overview of the management of patients who are or will be taking bisphosphonates and who require or have already undergone implant placement. Bisphosphonates are a group of drugs widely used in the treatment of diseases involving the skeletal system. The diseases that bisphosphonates are used to treat include the following **(Table 1)**:

- oncologic and hematologic diseases that are responsible for adverse skeletal events
- metabolic bone diseases, which alter bone turnover and lead to bone fragility

Bisphosphonates are also increasingly used for the prevention of osteoporosis in conditions of postmenopausal osteopenia or iatrogenic osteopenia from drugs (eg, chronic cortisone therapy).

Bisphosphonate therapy has become far more widespread in recent years. Clinicians involved in oral and implant surgery must be aware of the risks presented by bisphosphonate therapy and use the correct protocols to avoid serious complications.

Massimo Simion

Bisphosphonate prescription is widespread, and a high percentage of women in the menopausal period take these drugs.

Therefore, there is a high probability that oral surgeons will treat patients who are taking or have taken bisphosphonates.[2]

CLINICAL USE OF BISPHOSPHONATES

Bisphosphonates were synthesized in 1897 by Bayer and Hoffman and immediately proved useful in inhibiting bone resorption. They consist of two phosphoric chains linked to a central ring consisting of a carbon atom that is in turn linked to an R1 and an R2 chain **(Fig 1)**.[3]

Based on the presence of an amine group in the R2 chain, there are two pharmacologic classes of bisphosphonates:

- aminobisphosphonates: zoledronate, pamidronate, alendronate, risedronate, ibandronate, and neridronate

- non-aminobisphosphonates: clodronate, tiludronate, and etidronate

Bisphosphonates increase bone density by inhibiting the function of osteoclasts **(Fig 2)**. When bone is activated by trauma or inflammation, the hydroxyapatite dissolves, resulting in the release of the bisphosphonates bound to it. Released bisphosphonates then bind to osteoclasts, blocking their action. Aminobisphosphonates have a higher affinity for hydroxyapatite and a 10 to 1,000 times greater potency than bisphosphonates that do not contain amine groups **(Fig 3)**.

In the case of peri-implantitis, a rapid spread of bacteria into the deeper peri-implant tissues occurs. The resulting inflammatory process causes the dissolution of hydroxyapatite and the release of bisphosphonates that have accumulated in the bone tissue. This process results in peri-implant bone necrosis, which if left untreated, can progress to become diffuse in the jaw bones.[4]

Table 1 Indications for bisphosphonate therapy.

Oncologic and hematologic pathologies	Benign metabolic bone diseases
Malignant hypercalcemia	Osteoporosis
Bone metastases of solid tumors (from breast, kidney, or prostate cancer)	Osteitis deformans (Paget's disease)
Multiple myeloma	

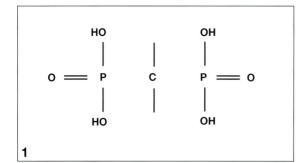

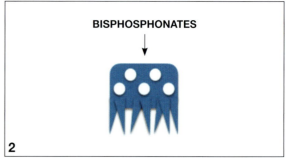

Fig 1 Molecular structure of a bisphosphonate. Unlike in a pyrophosphate, the central atom has been replaced by a carbon atom. *Fig 2* Anti-osteoclastic effect via the suppression of proinflammatory cytokines and receptor activator of nuclear factor kappa beta ligand (RANKL).

This pharmacodynamic mechanism explains why suspending the administration of bisphosphonates in patients undergoing long-term treatment is controversial.

Even after relatively few administrations, a high concentration of bisphosphonates remains accumulated within the jaw bones, which can be released and thus inhibit osteoclastic activity secondary to any event that causes dissolution of the hydroxyapatite.

The pharmacokinetics of bisphosphonates are affected by the method of administration (oral, intravenous, or intramuscular; **Table 2**), the duration of therapy (often prolonged over years), and the various doses that may be prescribed. Intravenous administration is associated with greater effects, explaining why intravenously administered aminobisphosphonates are associated with a greater risk of osteonecrosis complications than those administered orally. In fact, less than 1% of the dose of orally administered bisphosphonates is absorbed. The administration of 150 mg of ibandronate orally once a month is equivalent to a dose of 3 mg intravenously every 3 months.[2]

MEDICATION-RELATED OSTEONECROSIS OF THE JAW

Bisphosphonate-related osteonecrosis of the jaw (BRONJ) was first defined in 2007 by the American Association of Oral and Maxillofacial Surgeons (AAOMS) as the presence of exposed necrotic bone in the oral cavity for more than 8 weeks in patients receiving bisphosphonate therapy and who had never undergone radiotherapy of the head and neck region. To allow for early diagnosis, this definition was modified in 2012 to describe a drug-related adverse reaction characterized by the progressive destruction and necrosis of the mandibular and/or maxillary bone of subjects exposed to treatment with aminobisphosphonates in the absence of previous radiation treatment.

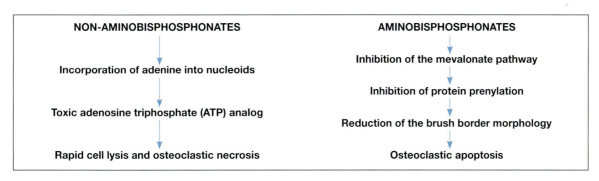

Fig 3 *Pharmacodynamics of aminobisphosphonates and non-aminobisphosphonates.*

Table 2 Methods of delivery of bisphosphonates.[3,5]

Drug (active ingredient)	Brands	Method of delivery
Alendronate	Fosamax (Merck)	Oral
Risedronate	Actonel (Proctor and Gamble)	Oral
Ibandronate	Bonviva (Roche)	Oral/intravenous
Neridronate	Nerixia(Abiogen Pharma)	Intravenous/intramuscular
Zoledronate*	Zometa (Novartis), Aclasta (Novartis)	Intravenous

*Zoledronate is nephrotoxic, so in case of renal insufficiency, it is replaced with ibandronate.[6]

Recently, several cases of osteonecrosis of the jaw bones have been described in cancer patients being treated with biologically targeted anti-angiogenic anticancer drugs (eg, bevacizumab, sunitinib, and sorafenib, whether in combination with bisphosphonates or not) and also with anti-resorptive drugs consisting of monoclonal antibody alternatives to bisphosphonates (eg, denosumab [Prolia and Xgeva from Amgen]) that bind to receptor activator of nuclear factor kappa beta ligand (RANKL) but have a lower affinity for hydroxyapatite than bisphosphonates, thus resulting in a lower accumulation effect in the bone. For this reason, the term MRONJ (medication-related osteonecrosis of the jaw) is now preferred over BRONJ.

One of the peculiarities of bisphosphonate-related osteonecrosis is its almost exclusive limitation to the jaw bones, particularly at the level of the posterior mandible. This is due to the high rate of bone turnover in the maxillary alveolar processes; the terminal vascularization of the mandible; the presence of a thin mucoperiosteal lining to protect the underlying bone tissue, which is easily subject to trauma; the peculiar microflora/biofilm of the oral cavity; and the characteristic dentoalveolar interface.

Numerous studies have made it possible to correlate the occurrence of osteonecrosis of the jaws with the administration of intravenous bisphosphonates in patients with neoplastic pathology, as well as to identify risk factors for this pathology. Studies have shown that the risk of MRONJ is 1% within the first 3 years of therapy, 6% within 4 years, and 11% beyond 4 years (see Table 6). Moreover, cases of osteonecrosis are always linked to the use of aminobisphosphonates. No cases have ever been linked with the use of non-aminobisphosphonates.[2] The estimated ratio of osteonecrosis of the jaws with intravenous bisphosphonates is between 1 and 10 out of 100 cases, whereas that number is 1 out of every 100,000 cases of orally administered bisphosphonates.

BRONJ: BIPHOSPHONATE RELATED OSTEONECROSIS OF THE JAW

Bisphosphonate-related osteonecrosis of the jaw (BRONJ) was first defined in 2007 by the American Association of Oral and Maxillofacial Surgeons (AAOMS) as the presence of exposed necrotic bone in the oral cavity for more than 8 weeks in patients receiving bisphosphonate therapy and

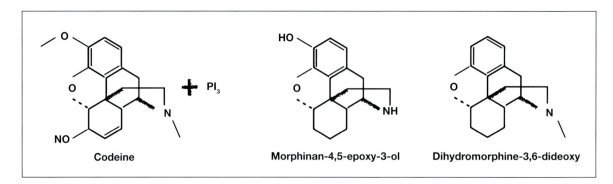

Fig 4 *Phosphorus is used in the synthesis of Krokodil as a catalyst in the reaction to create morphine from codeine. The intravenous use of phosphorus results in osteonecrosis of the jaws that is difficult to treat.*[6]

who had never undergone radiotherapy of the head and neck region. To allow for early diagnosis, this definition was modified in 2012 to describe a drug-related adverse reaction characterized by the progressive destruction and necrosis of the mandibular and/or maxillary bone of subjects exposed to treatment with aminobisphosphonates in the absence of previous radiation treatment.

Recently, several cases of osteonecrosis of the jaw bones have been described in cancer patients being treated with biologically targeted anti-angiogenic anticancer drugs (eg, bevacizumab, sunitinib, and sorafenib, whether in combination with bisphosphonates or not) and also with anti-resorptive drugs consisting of monoclonal antibody alternatives to bisphosphonates (eg, denosumab [Prolia and Xgeva from Amgen]) that bind to receptor activator of nuclear factor kappa beta ligand (RANKL) but have a lower affinity for hydroxyapatite than bisphosphonates, thus resulting in a lower accumulation effect in the bone. For this reason, the term MRONJ (medication-related osteonecrosis of the jaw) is now preferred over BRONJ.

One of the peculiarities of bisphosphonate-related osteonecrosis is its almost exclusive limitation to the jaw bones, particularly at the level of the posterior mandible. This is due to the high rate of bone turnover in the maxillary alveolar processes; the terminal vascularization of the mandible; the presence of a thin mucoperiosteal lining to protect the underlying bone tissue, which is easily subject to trauma; the peculiar microflora/biofilm of the oral cavity; and the characteristic dentoalveolar interface. Numerous studies have made it possible to correlate the occurrence of osteonecrosis of the jaws with the administration of intravenous bisphosphonates in patients with neoplastic pathology, as well as to identify risk factors for this pathology. Studies have shown that the risk of MRONJ is 1% within the first 3 years of therapy, 6% within 4 years, and 11% beyond 4 years **(see Table 6)**. Moreover, cases of osteonecrosis

are always linked to the use of aminobisphosphonates. No cases have ever been linked with the use of non-aminobisphosphonates.[2] The estimated ratio of osteonecrosis of the jaws with intravenous bisphosphonates is between 1 and 10 out of 100 cases, whereas that number is 1 out of every 100,000 cases of orally administered bisphosphonates.

Clinical criteria for the diagnosis of MRONJ

Pain is one of the most frequent symptoms associated with MRONJ. It may present as odontalgia; severe bone pain, either well delimited in the site or irradiated to the masticatory and cervical muscles; sinus pain; or trigeminal-type pain. Pain is considered as a factor to define the transition to a more advanced disease state in the presence of exposed bone in the oral cavity. The color of the bone affected by osteonecrosis should also be assessed and has a major impact on treatment. Necrotic, gray-blue bone needs to be removed. Conversely, red, bleeding bone tissue should not be removed because it is considered healthy.

A patient can be diagnosed with MRONJ if all the following criteria are met[8] **(Table 3) (Figs 5 to 11)**:

1. Current or previous treatment with antiresorptive or anti-angiogenic drugs
2. Exposed bone or bone that can be probed through an intraoral or extraoral fistula in the maxillofacial region and that persists for at least 8 weeks
3. No history of radiation therapy or metastases to the jaw bones

Radiologic criteria for the diagnosis of MRONJ

No radiologic sign is pathognomonic for MRONJ, so radiography must always be correlated with the anamnestic and clinical investigations. In fact, radiology is used to assist in diagnosis of the disease only when the clinical picture is doubtful (ie, characterized by the presence of only minor clinical signs). The major clinical sign of MRONJ (exposed or probably necrotic bone) is sufficient for its diagnosis in the presence of a positive pharmacologic history of treatment with aminobisphosphonates and without previous radiotherapy of the jaws. The most commonly used radiologic tools are periapical radiographs, panoramic radiographs, and CT without contrast medium. Periapical and panoramic radiographs are performed first. CT is required only at a later stage to confirm the diagnosis or for treatment planning. The radiologic criteria for the diagnosis of MRONJ are divided into early and late signs (**Table 4**) (**Figs 12 to 15**).

Table 3 Clinical criteria for the diagnosis of MRONJ.

Major clinical signs and symptoms	Minor clinical signs and symptoms
Exposure of necrotic bone tissue in the oral cavity	Halitosis
	Odontogenic abscess
	Mandibular asymmetry
	Pain of tooth or bone origin
	Mucosal fistula
	Extraoral fistula
	Failure of the alveolar mucosa to heal after tooth extraction
	Rapid onset of tooth mobility
	Preternatural mobility of the jaw, with or without preserved occlusion
	Paresthesia/dysesthesia of the lips (Vincent's symptom)
	Leaking of fluids from the nose
	Purulent discharge
	Spontaneous sequestration of bone fragments
	Trismus
	Soft tissue swelling

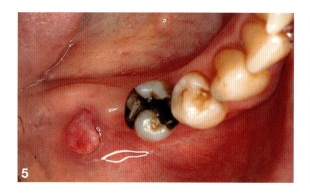
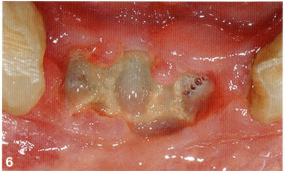

Fig 5 Mucosal fistula. **Fig 6** Purulent discharge.

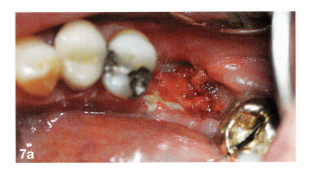
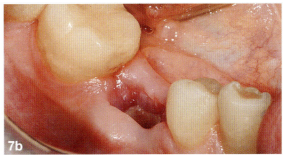

Fig 7 (a) *Delayed mucosal healing in an extraction site.* (b) *Failure of alveolar mucosa to heal after 8 weeks.*

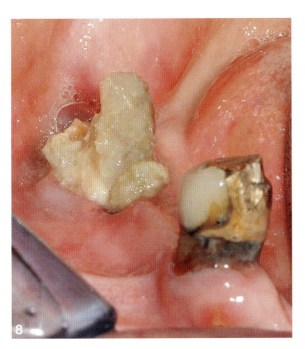
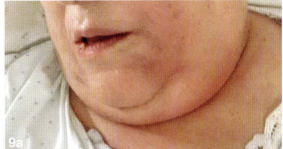
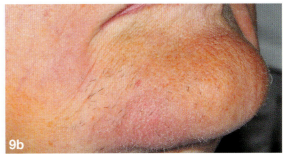

Fig 8 *Spontaneous sequestration of bone fragments.* **Fig 9** (a) *Abscess in the floor of the oral cavity.* (b) *Paresthesia/dysesthesia of the lip and soft tissue swelling.*

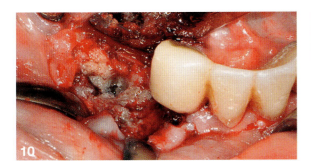
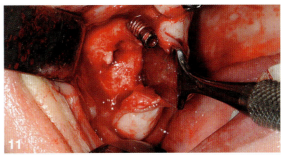

Fig 10 *Bluish-gray bone.* **Fig 11** *Healthy bone that is bleeding after curettage with piezosurgery.*

Stages of MRONJ

There have been numerous attempts in the literature to classify the stages of MRONJ, which would be useful not only to delineate the clinical picture of the patient but also to help clinicians plan the correct treatment for osteonecrosis. Here, the classification proposed by the Italian Society of Maxillofacial Surgery (SICMF) and the Italian Society of Oral Pathology and Medicine (SIMPO) are provided. In this classification, MRONJ is classified into three stages of increasing severity: focal, diffuse, and complicated MRONJ, in relation to the clinical and radiologic signs and the extent of the process in the maxillary/mandibular bone **(Table 5)**.

DENTAL TREATMENT IN MRONJ PATIENTS

When bisphosphonates are deposited in bone tissue for many years, they interfere with its metabolism. Therefore, it is necessary that patients about to start bisphosphonate therapy are in an optimal state of oral health. Prevention remains the most significant approach to protecting the oral health of these individuals. The type of bisphosphonate that will be used, the indication for aminobisphosphonate therapy (eg, oncologic pathology or metabolic bone pathology), and the timing of the dental procedure (before, during, or after the patient begins taking bisphosphonates) must be considered. **The main objective is to achieve and maintain an adequate state of oral hygiene and periodontal health.**

Management of patients before bisphosphonate therapy begins

The problem with placing implants in patients who will take (or are taking) bisphosphonates lies in the long-term potential for the development of peri-implant inflammation and the easy spread of germs in the bone tissue around the implant. This has the potential to induce MRONJ. For this reason, rigorous quarterly follow-ups with thorough professional oral hygiene care should be performed around all implants. Furthermore, implant rehabilitation is contraindicated in cancer patients, even before bisphosphonate administration,

Table 4 Radiologic criteria for the diagnosis of MRONJ

	Early	Late
Panoramic radiograph	Thickening of alveolar crest and lamina dura	Oroantral, oronasal, mucocutaneous fistula
	Persistence of the extraction alveolus	Pathologic fracture
	Bony sequestrum	Osteolysis extended to the maxillary sinus
	Widening of the periodontal ligament (PDL)	Mandibular canal thickening
TC	Cortical erosion	Diffuse atherosclerosis
	Thickening of the alveolar crest and lamina dura	Osteosclerosis of the zygoma and/or hard palate
	Trabecular thickening	Periosteal reaction
	Focal medullary osteosclerosis	Sinusitus
	Bony sequestrum	
	Widening of the PDL space	

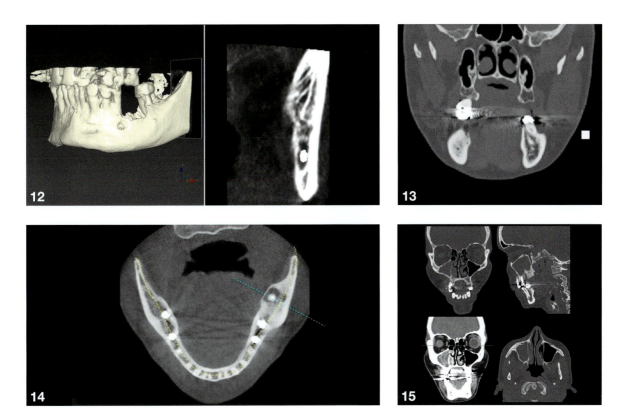

Fig 12 Persistence of extraction alveolus. *Fig 13* Bony sequestrum visible on the right with augmented density. *Fig 14* Diffuse osteosclerosis. *Fig 15* Sinusitis.

Table 5 SICMF/SIMPO stages of MRONJ.

Stage 1	Stage 2	Stage 3
Focal MRONJ requires the presence of at least one minor clinical sign of MRONJ with CT evidence of bone thickening limited to the dentoalveolar process, with or without other radiologic signs	Diffuse MRONJ requires the presence of at least one minor clinical sign with CT evidence of bone thickening extended to the basal process, with or without late radiologic signs	Complicated MRONJ requires the presence of one or more of the following signs
Minor clinical signs and symptoms: halitosis, odontogenic abscess, mandibular asymmetry, pain of dental or bone origin, bone exposure, mucosal fistula, failure of the alveolar mucosa to heal following tooth extraction, rapid onset of tooth mobility, paresthesia/dysesthesia of the lips, purulent discharge, spontaneous sequestration of bony fragments, lockjaw, swelling	Minor clinical signs and symptoms as for stage 1	Minor clinical signs: Extraoral fistula, nasal fluid discharge, preternatural mobility of the mandible with or without preserved occlusion
CT signs: Trabecular thickening, focal medullary osteosclerosis with or without thickening of the alveolar crest and lamina dura, persistence of the extraction alveolus, widening of the periodontal space a. Asymptomatic b. Symptomatic (presence of pain and/or suppuration)	CT signs: Diffuse osteosclerosis with or without oroantral/oronasal fistula, thickening of the alveolar canal, periosteal reaction, seizure, sinusitis a. Asymptomatic b. Symptomatic (presence of pain and/or suppuration)	CT signs: Mucocutaneous fistula, pathologic fractures, osteolysis extended to the maxillary sinus, osteosclerosis of the zygoma and/or hard palate

precisely because of the increased risk of MRONJ in the long-term.

For patients who have to start therapy with antiresorptive agents, ie, bisphosphonates or denosumab and/or antiangiogenics, it is important to implement primary prevention measures. Patient oral health should be assessed via a clinical and radiologic examination before the drug is started.

1. If the patient's oral health is optimal, they can safely start bisphosphonate therapy with a follow-up clinical examination every 4 months, during which the dental, periodontal, and mucosal conditions must be assessed, possibly with radiographic evaluation (periapical or panoramic radiographs). It is important to remember to always evaluate the adequacy of any removable prostheses and to make modifications where necessary. In the case of implants, always use screw-retained prostheses and avoid overdentures.

2. If the patient's oral health is suboptimal, all procedures to restore the oral cavity to a healthy state must be performed, including professional oral hygiene, topical fluoride treatment, supportive periodontal therapies, conservative, endodontics, and dentoalveolar or periodontal surgery.

It is very important to motivate patients to perform appropriate home oral hygiene and attend regular check-ups and to educate them about the clinical signs and symptoms of MRONJ (eg, pain and swelling). Patients should be well informed about the possible failure of implants in the long-term and the risk of MRONJ.

Ultimately, in both cancer patients and patients with metabolic bone diseases, any procedure aimed at maintaining or restoring oral health, whether invasive or not, is indicated prior to the use of bisphosphonates.

Bisphosphonate administration should be postponed until the surgical site is completely healed.

In patients with metabolic bone disease, implant-supported prosthetic rehabilitation can be carried out with informed consent from the patient regarding the potential for the development of peri-implant osteonecrosis in the long-term.

Patient management during and after bisphosphonate therapy

For patients already on bisphosphonate therapy, measures must be implemented to preserve or achieve good oral health. Supportive and conservative periodontal therapy and endodontic treatment are indicated.

Invasive procedures, such as tooth extractions, are also indicated if such interventions are aimed at eliminating an infectious state that could potentially cause MRONJ.

In the case of surgical intervention in patients taking bisphosphonates, it is important to perform a surgical protocol that allows for the use of a mucoperiosteal flap, involves minimal bone manipulation, includes interalveolar irrigation with antibacterial solution (eg, rifampicin sodium or ceftazidime pentahydrate 1 g/3 ml for local use), and entails wound closure with double-layered sutures that will promote healing by primary intention. Prosthetic and orthodontic treatments are possible, whereas elective invasive procedures such as implant placement and bone surgery are contraindicated (Table 6).

Practical advice

If implants will be placed in a patient who has been taking bisphosphonates/antiresorptives orally for less than 3 years, it is advisable to use computer-guided protocols for both the prosthetic design and for surgical guide fabrication. It is also possible to use real-time surgical navigation systems. Guided surgery makes it possible to eliminate or minimize periosteal elevation and reduce the time that bone is exposed in the oral environment.

Table 6 Bisphosphonates and implantology.

	Risk of MRONJ	Operative protocol	Follow-up	Suspension of therapy
Orally administered bisphosphonates	Low within the first 3 years	Antibiotic prophylaxis	Every 3 months with hyperbaric oxygen therapy (screwed-retained prostheses are preferable to facilitate disassembly)	Evaluate the suspension or modification of the current therapy with an internist or general practitioner
	Medium from year 4 of therapy	Regenerative techniques		
	High if associated with corticosteroids, methotrexate, anti-angiogenic agents, or immunosuppressants	Verify the absence of osteonecrosis with CT		
Intravenously administered bisphosphonates	High	Implant placement contraindicated		

Insight
CTX and the risk of MRONJ

Taking intravenous bisphosphonates is an important and irreplaceable therapy. As described earlier, these drugs inhibit the function of osteoclasts and thus reduce bone resorption.

The extent of bone resorption, and indirectly the extent of osteoclastic activity, correlates with a hematochemical marker known as C-terminal telopeptide of type I collagen (CTX). The greater the bone resorption there is, the higher the serum levels of this marker are.

Because bisphosphonates reduce osteoclastic activity, CTX levels decrease in association with the administration of these drugs. Recently, CTX serum levels have been used in oral and maxillofacial surgery to assess the action of bisphosphonates indirectly and to predict the risk of developing osteonecrosis of the jaws after oral surgery[8,9] **(Table 7)**. Thus, an increase in serum CTX titers would indicate only a reactivation of bone metabolism but could not be used to assess the risk associated with previous therapy. However, it must be remembered that there is a fair degree of skepticism about the use of the CTX test as a risk assessment parameter for MRONJ.[10] Caution must be exercised when using this test because though it certainly indicates a possible resumption of bone metabolism, this does not exclude the unfavorable effect of accumulation of doses of the drug.

PERFORMING EXTRACTIONS FOR IMPLANT PLACEMENT IN PATIENTS TAKING BISPHOSPHONATES/ANTIRESORPTIVES

When performing extractions for implant placement in patients undergoing bisphosphonate/antiresorptive therapy, it is advisable to postpone implant placement by at least 2 to 3 months. This approach is recommended for various reasons:

Table 7 CTX levels and the risk of developing osteonecrosis.

CTX	Risk of developing osteonecrosis of the jaw
< 100 pg/ml	High
100-150 pg/ml	Moderate
> 150 pg/ml	Minimal

1. Complete mucosal healing can be achieved.
2. Guided implant placement is facilitated.
3. There is no need to use biomaterials.
4. By 8 weeks after extraction, the absence of latent osteonecrosis can be confirmed in a healed socket.

Surgery in patients taking bisphosphonates disrupts the integrity of the mucosa, leading to the spread of bacteria from the oral environment to the bone tissue.[11]

This can lead to local infection and potentially osteonecrosis.

To avoid this complication, numerous pharmacologic and operative protocols have been proposed that oral surgeons must follow when performing tooth extraction in patients taking oral or intravenous bisphosphonates.

It should be emphasized that all protocols in the literature lack conclusive scientific evidence; the authors recommend the following protocol:

1. Prophylaxis with 0.12% chlorhexidine rinses to be performed three times per day, starting 7 days before extraction; antibiotic therapy (amoxicillin and clavulanic acid together with metronidazole) to be administered the day before surgery and continued for at least 6 days after surgery.[1]

2. Intraoperatively, it is best to use locoregional anesthesia without a vasoconstrictor and to perform a partial-thickness flap and gently extract the tooth. This should be accompanied with possible smoothing of the inter-radicular bone peaks or interdental bone septa when they are prominent or sharp. Cleansing the extraction socket with sterile saline is very important. Finally, suturing should be performed to allow healing by primary intention,[1] thus minimizing the risk of wound dehiscence. This entails closing the flap without tension and using releasing incisions and periosteal scoring. Suturing must be accurate, with overlapping and double layers.

3. For postoperative management, antibiotic therapy should be combined with topical therapy with 0.12% chlorhexidine rinses three times a day for 15 days. Topical treatment with hyaluronic acid three times daily for 15 days is recommended to promote wound healing. Sutures should be removed between 7 and 10 days after surgery. The patient should then return for follow-up at 3, 6, and 12 months.[1]

CLINICAL CASE 1

Tooth extraction in a patient with a history of taking oral bisphosphonates

A 60-year-old woman with a history of osteoporosis underwent extraction of the mandibular left second premolar. The patient had undergone therapy with orally administered alendronate (Fosamax, Merck), which had been discontinued 1 year before extraction.

Preoperative management: Preoperatively, the patient was prescribed antibiotic therapy (amoxicillin and clavulanic acid 1 g every 8 hours combined with metronidazole 250 mg every 12 hours) to be started the day before surgery, along with rinses with 0.12% chlorhexidine to be performed three times a day starting 7 days before extraction.

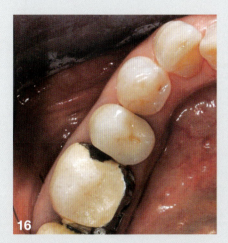
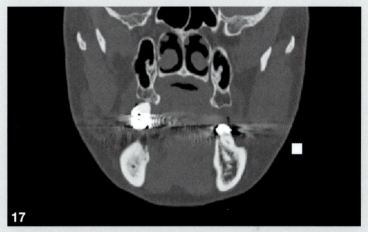

Fig 16 Planning extraction of the mandibular left second premolar. **Fig 17** 3D cross-section of the area to be treated.

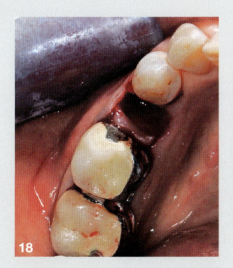
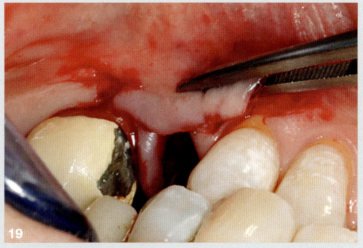

Fig 18 The extraction socket. **Fig 19** Management of the surgical flap.

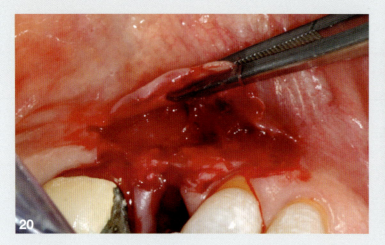
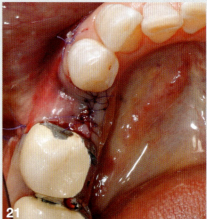

Fig 20 Management of the partial-thickness flap to allow for wound closure via primary intention healing. **Fig 21** Complete closure of the defect to promote healing by primary intention.

Intraoperative management: After administration of locoregional anesthesia without vasoconstrictor, a partial-thickness sliding flap was performed for the extraction of the mandibular left second premolar and sutured to allow for healing by primary intention **(Figs 16 to 21)**.

Postoperative management: Antibiotic therapy (amoxicillin and clavulanic acid 1 g every 8 hours combined with metronidazole 250 mg every 12 hours) was prescribed for 6 days. After 14 days, the sutures were removed, and the patient attended follow-ups until the surgical wound was completely healed.

In recent years, new cases of bisphosphonate-related osteonecrosis are appearing in patients who started therapy after undergoing implant placement. For patients who already have implants and start therapy with bisphosphonates, it is necessary to perform an individualized follow-up and, if possible, to exchange removable prostheses for fixed screw-retained ones. In these patients, it is recommended to perform a periapical radiograph once a year to intercept any peri-implantitis or early-stage MRONJ. Finally, the patient should be instructed to recognize early signs of MRONJ (eg, pain, swelling) and to promptly alert the dentist. If MRONJ is suspected, treatment should be implemented as soon as possible. The pathophysiologic effects will begin with peri-implantitis that is associated with focal MRONJ; if not adequately treated, the focal MRONJ will become diffuse, extending to the basal bone of the jaws.[9]

CLINICAL CASE 2

Treatment of a patient who started therapy with intravenous Zometa after implant placement

A 71-year-old man with a history of prostate adenocarcinoma with bone metastases presented with pain in the fourth quadrant, and the radiographic examination revealed osteonecrosis and peri-implantitis at the implant in the site of the mandibular right first premolar **(Figs 22 and 23)**. The patient had been taking intravenous zoledronic acid (Zometa, Novartis) for 4 years (starting after implant placement).

Preoperative management: The patient was prescribed antibiotic therapy (amoxicillin and clavulanic acid 1 g every 8 hours combined with metronidazole 250 mg every 12 hours) to be started the day before surgery, along with rinses with 0.12% chlorhexidine to be performed three times a day starting 7 days before surgery.

Intraoperative management: After administration of locoregional anesthesia without vasoconstrictor, the implant in the site of the mandibular right first premolar was removed **(Fig 24)**, and bone curettage was performed until healthy, bleeding bone was reached (all necrotic bone with the typical gray-blue appearance was removed) **(Fig 25)**. Finally, the mucoperiosteal flap was sutured to allow for healing by primary intention **(Fig 26)**.

Postoperative management: Antibiotic therapy (amoxicillin and clavulanic acid 1 g every 8 hours combined with metronidazole 250 mg every 12 hours) was prescribed for 10 days. The sutures were removed at 14 days, and the patient was placed on a nonsurgical follow-up schedule to treat dehiscence via chlorhexidine rinses. In fact, this was a case of diffuse MRONJ, so treatment was limited to the management of painful symptoms and associated infections while relying on medical therapy with chlorhexidine for progressive healing via secondary intention **(Figs 27 and 28)**.

Some authors are finding positive results with the use of hydrogen peroxide and ozone therapy.[12,13]

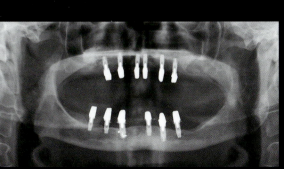

Fig 22 Panoramic radiograph upon report of pain in the fourth quadrant.

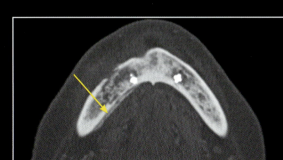

Fig 23 A careful 3D radiologic examination showed osteonecrosis and peri-implantitis at the implant in the site of the mandibular right first premolar.

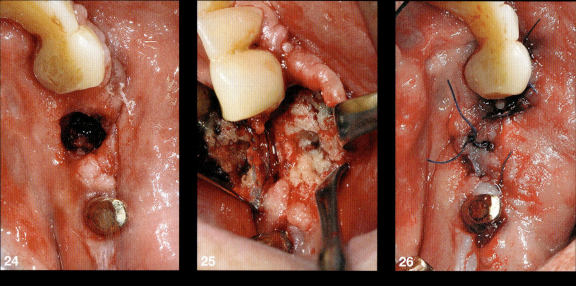

Fig 24 Delayed healing after tooth extraction.   **Fig 25** Exposure of the necrotic bone. **Fig 26** Correct flap management with closure to promote healing by primary intention.

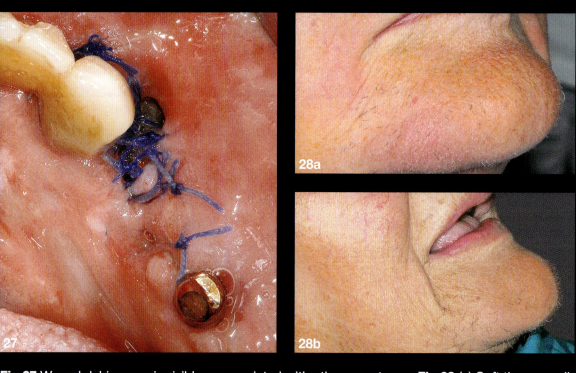

Fig 27 Wound dehiscence is visible unassociated with other symptoms.   **Fig 28** (a) Soft tissue swelling, pain on palpation, and paresthesia were present before surgery. (b) After surgery, swelling and spontaneous or provoked pain disappeared, and there was an absence of paresthesia.

CLINICAL CASE 3

Treatment of a patient who started therapy with intravenous Zometa 2 years after implant placement

A 60-year-old woman with a history of breast cancer and osteoporosis presented with peri-implantitis and implant-related bone sequestration. She had been taking zoledronic acid (Zometa) for 10 years (starting 2 years after implant placement).

Preoperative management: The patient was prescribed antibiotic therapy (amoxicillin and clavulanic acid 1 g every 8 hours combined with metronidazole 250 mg every 12 hours) to be started the day before surgery, along with rinses with 0.12% chlorhexidine to be performed three times per day starting 7 days before surgery.

Intraoperative management: After the administration of locoregional anesthesia without a vasoconstrictor, the implant and bone sequestration were removed **(Fig 29)**, and scrupulous bone curettage with piezosurgery was carried out until healthy bleeding bone was achieved **(Fig 30)**. Finally, the surgical flap was closed and sutured to allow for healing via primary intention.

Postoperative management: Antibiotic therapy (amoxicillin and clavulanic acid 1 g every 8 hours combined with metronidazole 250 mg, every 12 hours) was prescribed for 10 days. After 14 days, the sutures were removed, and the patient attended follow-ups until the surgical wound was completely healed.

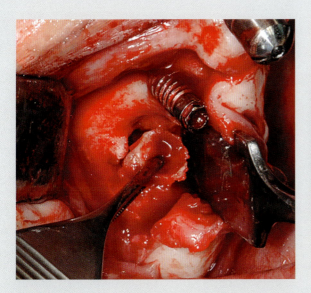

Fig 29 After the administration of locoregional anesthesia without vasoconstrictor, the implant and bone sequestrum were removed.

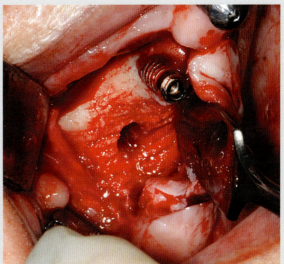

Fig 30 Scrupulous bone curettage with piezo-surgery was performed until healthy, bleeding bone was reached. Finally, the surgical flap was closed and sutured to allow for healing by primary intention.

TREATMENT OF MRONJ

There are currently two possible approaches to the treatment of MRONJ—medical and surgical. The medical approach is based on the use of drugs to control infection and pain, and its main aim is stabilization and prevention of disease progression. This approach entails very limited use of surgery, which is reserved for only refractory and advanced forms of MRONJ.[14]

The surgical approach, on the other hand, uses surgery in combination with medical therapies from the earliest stages of the disease, with the aim of halting disease progression as early as possible. Medical therapy involves:

- Antiseptic therapy with chlorhexidine, with transitional use limited to flare-ups.
- Antibiotic therapy with penicillin and metronidazole in case of suppuration or pain, even in the absence of clinical evidence. In the event of allergy, ciprofloxacin (500 mg twice per day) is recommended. There is currently no consensus regarding the best type of antibiotic or the dose and/or duration that it should be used. Clinicians must consider the stage of the disease and the route of administration of the bisphosphonate therapy.[15]
- Pain relief therapy.
- Biostimulation with ozone therapy or hyperbaric oxygen therapy. Ozone therapy has an important antimicrobial action, stimulates the circulatory system, modulates immune cells, and reduces pain, whereas hyperbaric oxygen therapy increases dissolved oxygen in the plasma and stimulates tissue neoangiogenesis.

NEW APPROACH TO THE TREATMENT OF FOCAL MRONJ

A new approach to the surgical treatment of MRONJ involves taking mesenchymal cells from healthy gums using a Rigenera machine (Esacrom) and injecting them into the osteonecrosis site using a Mucogain membrane (Nobel Biocare). This treatment represents a new frontier in the treatment of focal MRONJ, and clinical studies on this technique are still ongoing, though showing promising results. Using this technique also reduced pain and results in better healing, thanks to mesenchymal cells grafted into the site of osteonecrosis.

MANAGEMENT OF THE THERAPEUTIC WINDOW (DRUG HOLIDAY)

The suspension of bisphosphonate therapy, a "drug holiday," is used here to refer to the temporary and preventive withdrawal of bisphosphonates, denosumab, and sometimes anti-angiogenic drugs in patients at risk of developing MRONJ before needed dental treatment begins (eg, tooth extraction or alveolar surgery).

Discontinuation of drug therapy may induce various risk-benefit balances depending on the type of drug that is taken.

In patients on bisphosphonate therapy, temporary drug discontinuation may be useful starting from the week before surgical treatment.

Bisphosphonate intake can be resumed once healing is established (at least 4–6 weeks after surgery). In patients on denosumab therapy, (eg, Prolia, Xgeva), it is possible to manipulate the pharmacokinetics to create a window within which to manage noncritical dental/periodontal conditions that require invasive treatment.

This "delayed dosing window" lasts approximately 2 months, ideally starting 5 months after the last dose of denosumab and ending at the beginning of month 8. If the surgical dental procedure is considered urgent and cannot be postponed, bisphosphonates should be discontinued 1 week before surgery and resumed 4 to 6 weeks after wound healing.[16]

CLINICAL CASE 4

Medical therapy of MRONJ in a patient who started intravenous bisphosphonate therapy 2 years after implant placement

A 68-year-old man with a history of multiple myeloma presented at a routine check-up without any symptoms apart from some discomfort around the implants that had not been present before starting treatment with intravenous Zometa for 7 months. Upon clinical examination, there were no signs of gingival inflammation, but considerable peri-implant bone resorption was discovered with probing **(Figs 31 and 32)**. Radiographic investigation with a periapical and panoramic radiograph and CT revealed areas of radiolucency around the implants in the first quadrant **(Figs 33 and 34)**. Given the suspicion of focal MRONJ but the absence of symptoms, a conservative approach was adopted, with hyperbaric oxygen therapy (repeated every 3 months) and local application of chlorhexidine gel together with the application of a chemical desiccant in gel capable of disintegrating the bacterial biofilm **(Fig 35)**.

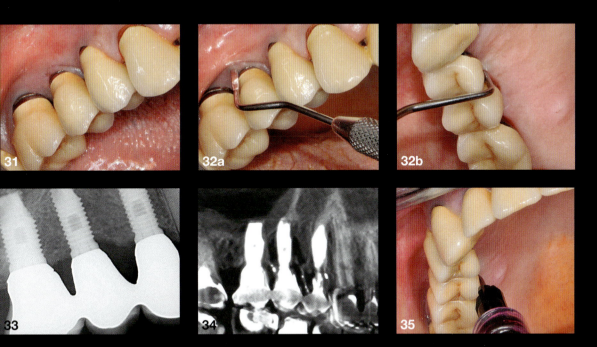

Fig 31 Clinical appearance, apparently without signs of mucositis or gingivitis. **Fig 32** (a and b) Probing was associated with considerable peri-implant bone resorption, evident on both the buccal and palatal aspects. **Fig 33** Radiograph of the corresponding area. **Fig 34** 3D image showing the bone lesion associated with the peri-implant area. **Fig 35** The suspicion of focal MRONJ without associated symptoms called for a conservative approach with hyperbaric oxygen therapy (to be repeated every 3 months) and the local application of chlorhexidine gel in conjunction with applications of a chemical desiccant in gel capable of attacking and disrupting the bacterial biofilm.

CLINICAL CASE 5

Rigenera technique in a patient taking intravenous Zometa

The use of a newly developed collagen matrix (Mucogain) enriched with autologous fibroblasts promoted gingival tissue regeneration even in a subject with low, drug-induced cell turnover.

An 83-year-old man with a history of multiple myeloma underwent tooth extraction. He was taking intravenous Zometa.

The patient underwent extraction of the mandibular left first molar, with a surgical flap for healing via primary intention. After 2 months, the patient returned due to lack of healing of the extraction socket, bone sequestration, and pain **(Figs 36 to 38)**. It was decided to intervene with a Rigenera technique with a Mucogain membrane.

Preoperative management: The patient was prescribed antibiotic therapy (amoxicillin with clavulanic acid 1 g every 8 hours combined with metronidazole 250 mg every 12 hours) to be started the day before surgery, along with rinses with 0.12% chlorhexidine to be performed three times per day starting 7 days before surgery.

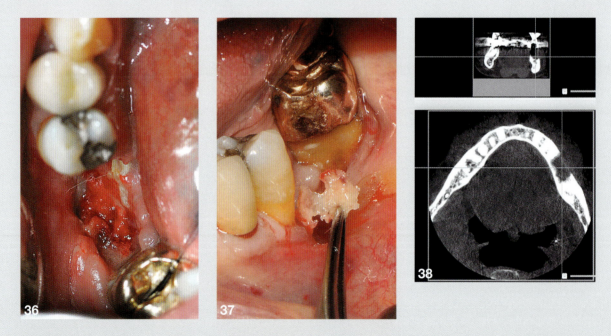

Fig 36 Intraoral clinical appearance of the extraction site 2 months after surgery was performed correctly with appropriate closure of the alveolus for healing by primary intention. **Fig 37** Removal of the bone sequestrum that was associated with intense symptoms. **Fig 38** With close 3D radiographic examination, the extent of the affected area can be appreciated.

Intraoperative management: After the administration of locoregional anesthesia without vasoconstrictor, a full-thickness surgical flap was performed to allow for thorough curettage of the alveolus and rinsing with hydrogen peroxide and physiologic saline solution. At the surgical flap, a mucosal harvest was carried out to obtain mesenchymal cells using the Rigenera device **(Fig 39)**. These cells were then injected along with physiologic saline onto the Mucogain membrane, on which small incisions were made to promote stabilization of the cells inside. The membrane was then placed at the extraction socket. Finally, the surgical flap was sutured to allow for healing by primary intention **(Fig 40)**. As in the previous clinical cases, the sutures were placed without tension in overlapping double layers.

Postoperative management: Antibiotic therapy (amoxicillin with clavulanic acid 1 g every 8 hours combined with metronidazole 250 mg every 12 hours) was prescribed for 10 days. After 14 days, the sutures were removed, and the patient attended follow-ups until the surgical wound was completely healed. **Figure 41** shows complete healing 1 year after surgery.

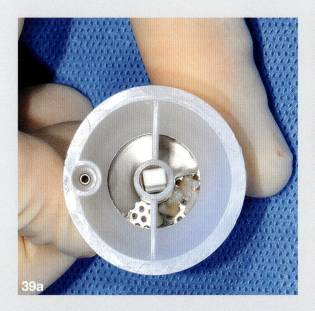 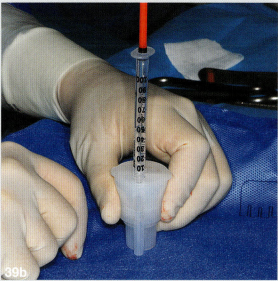

Fig 39 *(a and b)* With the Rigenera device, autologous mesenchymal cells can be harvested and reinjected into the recipient site after appropriate surgical management.

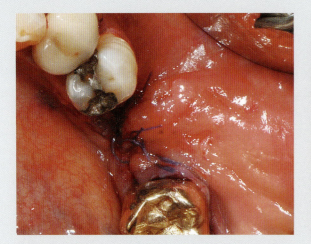

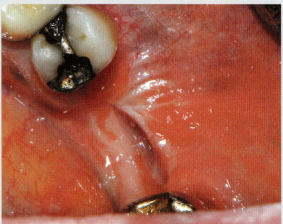

Fig 40 These mesenchymal cells are injected along with physiologic saline into the Mucogain membrane. The membrane is then placed at the extraction socket. Finally, the surgical flap is sutured to allow for healing by primary intention.

Fig 41 Complete healing observed 1 year after surgery.

REFERENCES

1. Di Fede O, Panzarella V, Mauceri R, et al. The dental management of patients at risk of medication-related osteonecrosis of the jaw: New paradigm of primary prevention. Biomed Res Int 2018;2018:2684924.

2. Saia G, Blandamura S, Bettini G, et al. Occurrence of bisphosphonate-related osteonecrosis of the jaw after surgical tooth extraction. J Oral Maxillofac Surg 2010;68:797–804.

3. Ebetino FH, Hogan A-ML, Sun S, et al. The relationship between the chemistry and biological activity of bisphosphonates. Bone 2011;49:20–33.

4. Drake MT, Clarke BL, Khosla S. Bisphosphonates: Mechanism of action and role in clinical practice. Mayo Clin Proc 2008;83:1032–1045.

5. Marx RE. Drug-Induced Osteonecrosis of the Jaws. Quintessence, 2009.

6. Hughes JP, Baron R, Buckland DH, et al. Phosphorus necrosis of the jaw: A present-day study. Br J Ind Med 1962;19:83–99.

7. Marx RE. Uncovering the cause of "phossy jaw" circa 1858 to 1906: Oral and maxillofacial surgery closed case files. J Oral Maxillofac Surg 2008;66:2356–2363.

8. Ruggiero SL, Dodson TB, Fantasia J, et al. American Association of Oral and Maxillofacial Surgeons position paper on medication-related osteonecrosis of the jaw–2014 update. J Oral Maxillofac Surg 2014;72: 1938–1956.

9. Rosen HN, Moses AC, Garber J, et al. Serum CTX: A new marker of bone resorption that shows treatment effect more often than other markers because of low coefficient of variability and large changes with bisphosphonate therapy. Calcif Tissue Int 2000;66:100–103.

10. Enciso R, Keaton J, Saleh N, Ahmadieh A, Clark GT, Sedghizadeh PP. Assessing the utility of serum c-telopeptide cross-link of type 1 collagen as a predictor of bisphosphonate-related osteonecrosis of the jaw: A systematic review and meta-analysis. J Am Dent Assoc 2016;147:551e11–560.e11.

11. Schmitt CM, Buchbender M, Lutz R, Neukam FW. Oral implant survival in patients with bisphosphonate (bp)/antiresorptive and radiation therapy and their impact on osteonecrosis of the jaws. A systematic review. Eur J Oral Implantol 2018;11(Suppl 1):S93–S111.

12. De Santis D, Gelpi F, Luciano U, et al. New trends in adjunctive treatment and diagnosis in medication-related osteonecrosis of the jaw: A 10-year review. J Biol Regul Homeost Agents 2020;34(Suppl 2):37–48.

13. Nocini R, De Santis D, Luciano U, et al. The rule of hydrogen peroxide long term rinse during a particular alveolar bone healing after ONJ injuries in a patient with periodontal disease: A 4-year radiological follow up report of a mental nerve emergence migration. J Biol Regul Homeost Agents 2020;34(6 Suppl 2):69–76.

14. Abu-Id MH, Warnke PH, Gottschalk J, et al. "Bis-phossy jaws" – high and low risk factors for bisphosphonate-induced osteonecrosis of the jaw. J Craniomaxillofac Surg 2008;36:95–103.

15. Bermúdez-Bejarano EB, Serrera-Figallo MÁ, Guitiérrez-Corrales A, et al. Prophylaxis and antibiotic therapy in management protocols of patients treated with oral and intravenous bisphosphonates. J Clin Exp Dent 2017;9:e141–e149.

16. Campisi G, Mauceri R, Bertoldo F, et al. Medication-related osteonecrosis of jaws (MRONJ) prevention and diagnosis: Italian consensus update 2020. Int J Environ Res Public Health 2020;17:5998.

DIAGNOSIS AND TREATMENT OF PERI-IMPLANTITIS

CHAPTER 13

Edited by Massimo Simion, Eleonora Idotta, and Alessandra Sironi

INTRODUCTION

There are three clearly definable periods in the history of dental implants and osseointegration: the developmental era, the classic (golden) era, and the era of bioactive implant surfaces.

The developmental period ran from 1965, when Professor P-I Brånemark began preclinical studies on osseointegrated implants, to the beginning of the 1980s, when implants were made available to clinicians all over the world. Next, Brånemark-style surgical protocols and implants, characterized by a two-stage surgical procedure to place threaded, cylindric implants with almost smooth, machined surfaces, were used to treat millions of patients worldwide with overwhelmingly favorable success rates[1,2] **(Fig 1)**. Since the beginning of 2000, however, a number of researchers, supported by implant companies, have tried to increase the already high success rates and to reduce the waiting time for implant loading. To this end, modified implants with rougher or even porous surfaces have been produced by means of air-borne particle abrasion, acid etching, plasma spray, and anodizing techniques (see chapter 3) **(Fig 2)**. These new surfaces have been received enthusiastically by clinicians and researchers worldwide, so much so that the traditional machined surfaces fell into disuse and were taken off the market.

For the first 4 to 5 years, the new surfaces were used successfully and received general acceptance, but by year 5, purulent inflammation of the peri-implant soft tissue associated with progressive marginal bone loss began to be observed around some of the new implants, a condition that became referred to as peri-implantitis **(Fig 3)**. In the following years, the incidence of peri-implantitis increased exponentially, to the extent that some clinicians warned of a wave of peri-implantitis cases that would hit clinicians in the near future.[3]

Peri-implantitis has been the scourge of modern implant dentistry since the adoption of bioactive implant surfaces in the year 2000. Very often, this pathology, which leads inexorably to implant loss and the development of serious residual bone defects, is misunderstood or shamefully ignored.

Massimo Simion

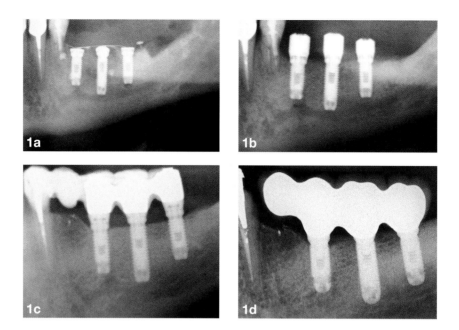

Fig 1 *Radiographic series showing implant placement in a vertically regenerated bone ridge with smooth-surface implants. The follow-up at 16 years showed the maintenance of crestal bone levels. (a) In 1997, implant placement was performed with concomitant vertical bone regeneration using a nonresorbable Gore-Tex membrane reinforced with titanium and autologous bone. (b) In 1998, reopening and placement of the healing abutments was performed. (c) The 2005 8-year follow-up. (d) The 2013 16-year follow-up.*

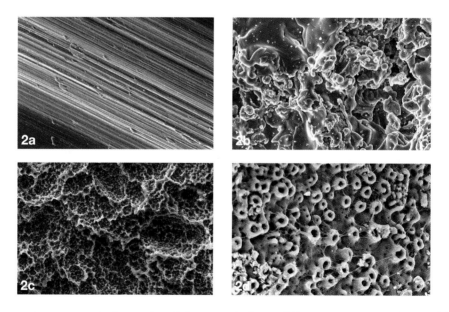

Fig 2 *Electron microscope photographs of the morphology of the most commonly used implant surfaces. (a) Smooth, machined surface. (b) TPS (titanium plasma–sprayed) surface. (c) Air-borne particle–abrased and etched surface. (d) Anodized surface. ×5,000 magnification. (Courtesy of Dr Clara Cassinelli, Nobel Bio Ricerche.)*

DEFINING PERI-IMPLANT CONDITIONS

According to the consensus meeting of Estepona in 2012, peri-implantitis is as an infection of the peri-implant tissues associated with suppuration and progressive marginal bone loss[4,5] **(Fig 4)**. More recently, in the consensus of the Seventh European Workshop on Periodontology,[6] the requirement of suppuration was eliminated because, peri-implantitis being a cyclic disease, suppuration may be more or less evident merely depending on the phase of increased or decreased disease activity. A key aspect that is considered in all definitions of peri-implantitis is progressive marginal bone resorption. To develop an unambiguous definition of peri-implantitis so that standardized

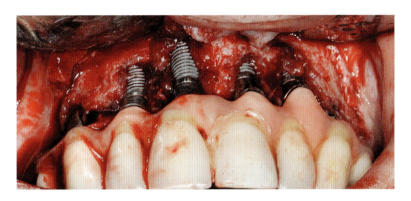

Fig 3 *Intraoral view of peri-implantitis after elevation of the maxillary mucoperiosteal flap. Peri-implant bone resorption and the presence of granulation tissue within the bone defects can be observed.*

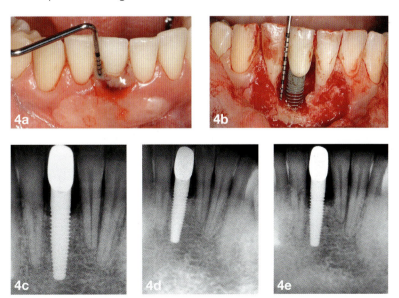

Fig 4 *Patient with peri-implantitis at the implant in the site of the mandibular right central incisor. (a) Probing depth of 10 mm and purulent discharge. (b) With the flap reflected, the severe bone defect involving the adjacent natural teeth can be seen. Periapical radiographs show the progression of the disease at the time of prosthetic loading* (c) *and after 3* (d) *and 4 years* (e). *Rapid and early bone resorption is evident.*

research protocols and diagnoses can be caried out, the scientific community formulated the following classification of the different peri-implant health and disease states:[7]

1. Peri-implant health
2. Peri-implant mucositis
3. Peri-implantitis
4. Peri-implant hard and soft tissue deficits

PERI-IMPLANT HEALTH

Peri-implant health is a purely clinical condition, and every implant will show a modest degree of inflammation on a histologic level **(Fig 5)**. An implant is defined as "clinically healthy" when there are no clinical signs of inflammation.

The symptom of bleeding on probing, which is pathognomonic of inflammation around a natural tooth, is not as indicative around implants due to the anatomical and histologic differences between implants and natural teeth.

Peri-implant health is also possible around implants with either normal or reduced bone support. Loss of initial bone support may be due to adaptive or traumatic factors secondary to surgery and not necessarily related to peri-implantitis **(Fig 6)**.

Peri-implant probing depth is another diagnostic parameter that is difficult to interpret because it is not possible to define a maximum probing depth compatible with peri-implant health. The depth of the sulcus around an implant cannot be directly related to a state of health or inflammation but rather must be considered in light of the implant's positioning in relation to the bone crest and the thickness of the mucosa at the time of its insertion. In other words, for probing depth to have diagnostic significance, it must be recorded at the time of the final prosthetic rehabilitation and monitored over time. In the absence of inflammatory signs such as hyperemia, swelling, bleeding on probing, or purulent exudate, an implant with a probing depth of 7 mm is not compromised.

Despite the difficulty in interpreting peri-implant probing depths, peri-implant probing is integral to a complete intraoral examination.

It can be used to detect bleeding, the presence of pus, tissue resistance, probing depth, and pain, which are all useful factors for diagnosing peri-implantitis.

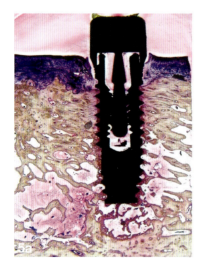 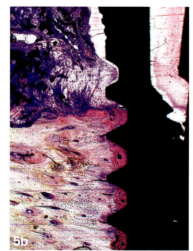 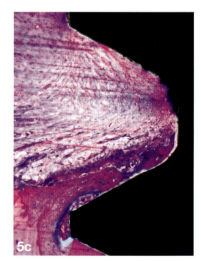

Fig 5 *Histologic appearance of a clinically healthy implant. ×5 magnification* (a)*, ×20 magnification* (b)*, ×40 magnification* (c)*. Toluidine blue/Pyronine G staining.*

The diagnosis of peri-implant health requires the absence of the following clinical signs:

- Clinical signs of inflammation
- Bleeding and/or suppuration with gentle probing
- Increases in probing depth compared to previous examinations
- Radiographic signs of bone loss after initial remodeling
- Peri-implant mucositis

PERI-IMPLANT MUCOSITIS

Mucositis is defined as inflammation of the peri-implant mucosa that is not associated with crestal bone loss. It is caused by the accumulation of bacterial plaque and is a reversible process if the etiologic factor is eliminated **(Fig 7)**. The peri-implant mucosa manifests rather intense signs of inflammation, such as bleeding on gentle probing, redness, and swelling, and the superficial characteristics of the tissue are also altered. Decreased mucosal resistance to probing may result in a slight increase in probing depth. Mucositis has no radiographic signs, and it is not accompanied by any crestal bone loss. A human biopsy study of peri-implant mucosal tissue affected by mucositis (induced by undisturbed plaque accumulation for 21 days) allowed observation of the presence of an inflammatory infiltrate dominated by B and T lymphocytes and rich in vascular structures and plasma cells.[8] This inflammatory infiltrate is present lateral to the sulcus epithelium and occupies approximately 0.14 mm.

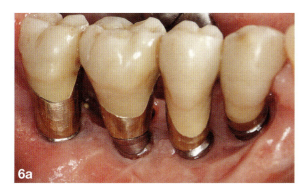
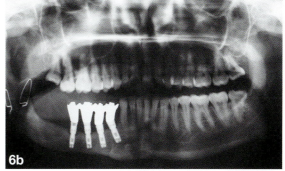
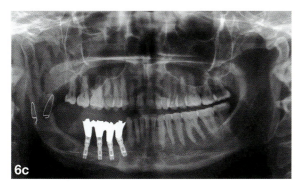
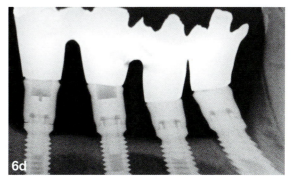

Fig 6 (a) *Healthy peri-implant tissue with reduced bone support due to adaptive remodeling of a hemi-mandibular reconstruction using a free bone graft taken from the hip.* (b) *Panoramic radiograph after 1 year.* (c) *Panoramic radiograph after 23 years.* (d) *Periapical radiograph after 27 years. Horizontal bone remodeling in the absence of inflammation is evident.*

It is separated from the underlying bone tissue by a layer of healthy connective tissue. Several authors have pointed out that this infiltrate does not extend apically with respect to the junctional epithelium (ie, it does not invade the supracrestal connective tissue).[9] The removal of the bacterial biofilm and the resumption of home oral hygiene procedures results in the resolution of mucositis, with the tissues returning to normal.

However, the healing time may exceed 3 weeks.[10] Just as gingivitis precedes periodontitis, mucositis precedes peri-implantitis. However, not all cases of mucositis will evolve into peri-implantitis.

The diagnosis of peri-implant mucositis requires the following clinical signs:

- Reddening and swelling of the mucosa and bleeding after gentle probing with or without increased probing depth compared to previous examinations
- No bone loss beyond normal crestal bone level changes resulting from initial remodeling

Peri-implantitis

Peri-implantitis is a pathologic condition associated with bacterial plaque affecting the tissues

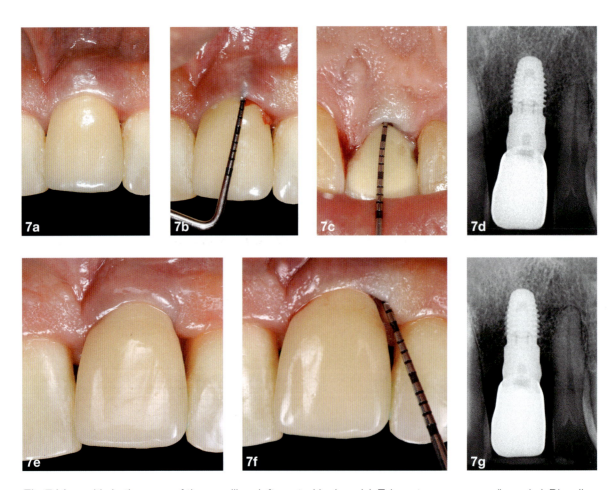

Fig 7 *Mucositis in the area of the maxillary left central incisor.* (a) *Edematous mucosa.* (b and c) *Bleeding on probing.* (d) *A periapical radiograph showing no detectable bone defect.* (e and f) *Healing of the lesion after causal therapy. Clinically healthy mucosa with an evident reduction of the bleeding index upon probing.* (g) *Periapical radiograph.*

around dental implants. It is characterized by inflammation of the mucosa and progressive bone resorption **(Figs 8 and 9)**, which are the two fundamental aspects to consider when making a diagnosis. Diagnosing peri-implantitis on the basis of clinical or radiographic signs in which only bone resorption or deep probing depths are evident is erroneous if there are no signs of inflammation paired with tissue loss and if probing depths are not compared with previously measured values. Adaptive changes in crestal bone levels may occur unrelated to peri-implantitis.

Resorption may occur due to excessive surgical trauma caused by the clinician or by implant insertion, or as a result of aging. Implants that have been in place for 20 years may frequently show radiographic signs of exposed threads.

It is important to emphasize that a substantial initial loss of peri-implant hard tissue not associated with inflammation may remain years without progressing and not affect the long-term success of the rehabilitation.

The onset of peri-implantitis can occur very early. Many implants show signs of progressive bone resorption after only a few years.

Derks et al[11] evaluated radiographs of 596 patients and identified 105 implants with peri-implantitis spread across 62 patients.

The study, which had a 9-year follow-up, showed that 52% of the implants already showed the first signs of bone loss at 2 years. At 3 years, the percentage rose to 66%.

Peri-implantitis has an acute, very aggressive and non-linear course.

The bone loss is progressive, but the speed at which it occurs is not constant and does not follow the same course in all patients.

PREDISPOSING FACTORS FOR THE DEVELOPMENT OF PERI-IMPLANTITIS

All factors recognized in the literature as predisposing a patient to the development of peri-implantitis either directly or indirectly favor the formation of bacterial biofilm or reduce the immune response. Predisposing factors include the following:[12]

• Patient susceptibility to periodontal pathology and the presence of periodontally affected teeth.

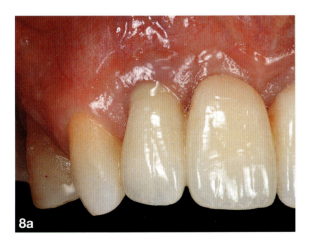
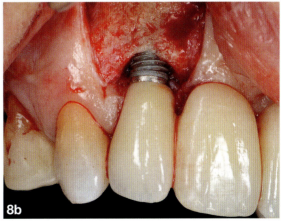

Fig 8 (a) *Purulent exudate in the site of a maxillary lateral incisor in a 35-year-old patient treated with a rough-surface implant with anodic oxidation 4 years earlier.* (b) *A full-thickness flap was elevated, and the inflammatory tissue removed, revealing the peri-implant bone defect.*

- Surface characteristics of dental implants. Pathology is more frequent and more acute around implants with completely rough, especially porous, surfaces because they are more susceptible to bacterial adhesion.

- Diabetes mellitus and smoking. These conditions reduce the effectiveness of the immune response and promote the formation of periodontal-pathogenic plaque.

- Absence of keratinized mucosa. Numerous studies[13–18] suggest that the absence or reduced presence of keratinized mucosa adversely affects the ability to perform proper home oral hygiene and thus favors plaque accumulation.

- Iatrogenic damage.[19] The presence of a buccal dehiscence[20] at the time of implant insertion causes early exposure of the rough implant surface in the sulcus and is associated with an increased risk of developing pathology. This applies to regenerative procedures in general.[21,22] Residual cement in the peri-implant sulcus is also a risk factor because it prevents effective hygiene maintenance of the peri-implant sulcus and encourages plaque build-up. Finally, implant placement in areas that are difficult to clean and ill-fitting prostheses also prevent thorough cleaning.

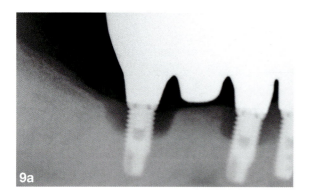
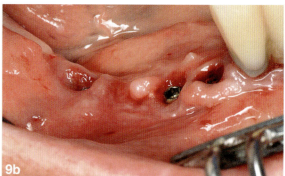
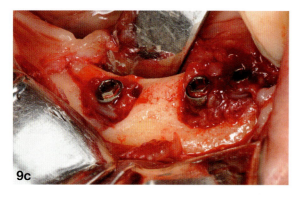
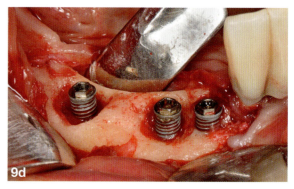

Fig 9 (a) *Periapical radiograph showing saucer-shaped bone defects in the sites from the mandibular right canine to the right first molar.* (b) *The peri-implant mucosa is edematous and hyperemic.* (c) *With the flap reflected, the severe bone defects and the massive inflammatory reaction are evident.* (d) *The defects were cleared of inflammatory tissue, and the implants were decontaminated with curettes, hydrogen peroxide, and antibiotics.*

CLINICAL CASE 1

Peri-implantitis in regenerated bone

This clinical case documents progressive osteolysis in sites previously subjected to vertical bone regeneration. In 7 years, three of five implants with porous surfaces treated with anodic oxidation were lost. The other two implants, in the sites of the mandibular left second premolar and the mandibular right first premolar were also affected by peri-implantitis **(Figs 10 to 17)**.

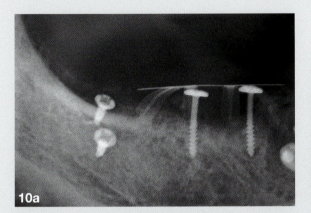 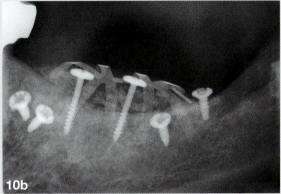

Fig 10 Periapical radiographs of mandibular posterior sectors after guided bone regeneration (GBR) using Gore-Tex polytetrafluoroethylene (PTFE) membranes. Right *(a)* and left *(b)* sides.

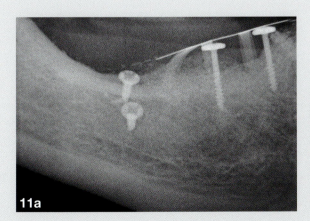 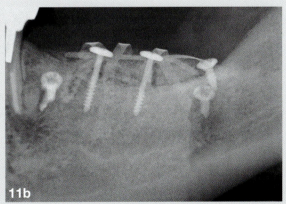

Fig 11 *(a and b)* Radiographs 6 months after guided bone regeneration. The satisfactory mineralization of the regenerated bone is evident.

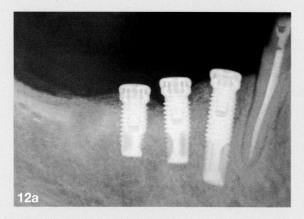
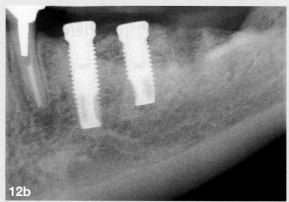

Fig 12 *(a and b)* Periapical radiographs 12 months after the insertion of porous-surface implants treated with anodic oxidation.

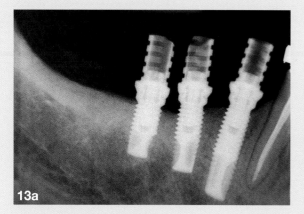
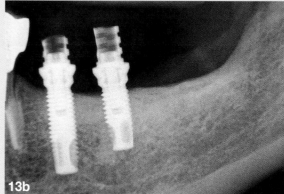

Fig 13 *(a and b)* Periapical radiographs taken at the delivery of the provisional. Slight crestal bone remodeling can be observed, which resulted in the exposure of some implant threads.

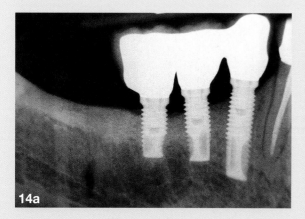
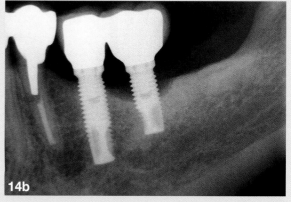

Fig 14 *(a and b)* Radiographs at 18 months. Initial angular bone resorption can be observed at the implant in the site of the mandibular left first molar.

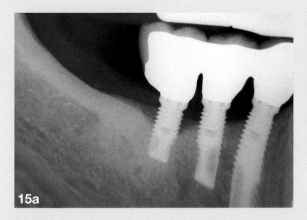
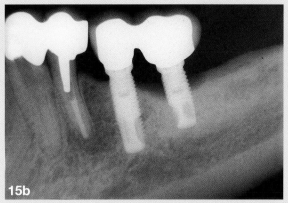

Fig 15 *(a and b)* Radiographs at 2 years that also show the early involvement of the implant in the site of the mandibular right first molar.

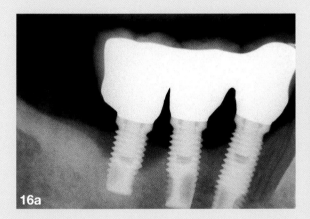
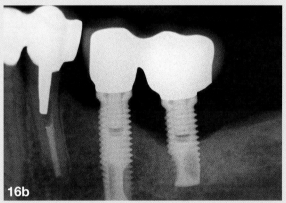

Fig 16 *(a and b)* Radiographs at 4 years showing the clear progression of bone loss extending to the adjacent implant sites.

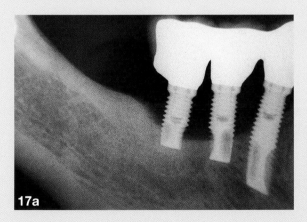
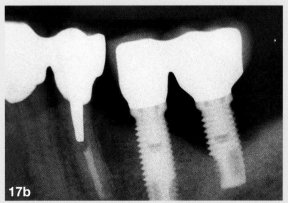

Fig 17 *(a and b)* Radiographs at 7 years showing the complete impairment of the implants in the positions of the mandibular left first molar and right second premolar and first molar. The implants in the sites of the mandibular left second premolar and the right first premolar are also affected by the pathology.

EPIDEMIOLOGY OF PERI-IMPLANTITIS

Epidemiology involves the study of the distribution and frequency of health-relevant events in the population and the identification of their triggers or risk factors. In particular, epidemiologic analysis assesses the incidence and prevalence of a health event. Incidence is defined as the number of new cases of a specific pathology over a certain period of time in a given population.

Prevalence, on the other hand, is defined as the ratio of the number of health events detected in a population at a defined time (or over a short period of time) to the number of individuals in the population at the same time.

A reliable assessment of the prevalence of peri-implantitis is impossible because the values are strongly influenced by a large number of variables, such as the size and quality of the sample that is analyzed (eg, the level of patient compliance and quality of oral hygiene), the duration of follow-up, the expertise of the clinician, and above all, the type of implant and its surface. For this reason, it is not surprising that prevalence and incidence values vary considerably across reports.

In a recent systematic review[23] assessing peri-implantitis prevalence, incidence, and risk factors, a search for studies on peri-implantitis published between January 1980 and March 2016 was performed on 9 databases, and ultimately 56 papers were selected for analysis. Smoking, diabetes mellitus, lack of antibiotic prophylaxis, and a history of periodontitis were identified as risk factors for peri-implantitis, with a medium to medium-high level of supporting evidence.

The importance of the role of implant surfaces is also emerging, both in daily clinical experience and in clinical studies. A study by Astrand et al[2] on 21 patients treated with 123 machined implants and followed for 20 years showed an implant survival rate of 99.2% and an extremely low prevalence of peri-implantitis (2.5%).[2] Similar results were obtained in a study by Simion et al[24] on implants placed in the posterior maxillary region with a success rate of 93.5% and the complete absence of peri-implantitis with a follow-up of 12 years.

In another recent long-term retrospective study, Simion et al[25] showed implant success and survival rates of 92.7% and 97.7%, respectively, and a prevalence of peri-implantitis of only 1.8% in 105

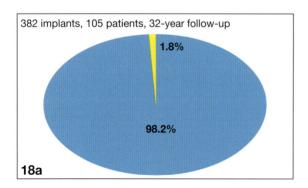

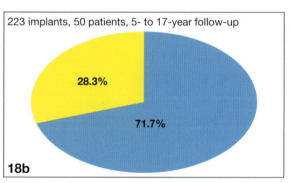

Fig 18 *Prevalence of peri-implantitis in a retrospective study conducted on smooth-surface (a) and anodized-surface (b) implants. The prevalence of peri-implantitis was 28.3% for anodized implants and only 1.8% for machined implants. These results suggest that surface roughness plays a role in the pathogenesis of peri-implantitis. (Reprinted with permission from Int J Periodontics Restorative Dent 2018;38:489–493 and 2019;39:799–807.)*

patients treated with 382 machined implants with a follow-up of up to 32 years **(Fig 18a)**. Completely different results were obtained in a similar study by Ferrantino et al[26] (with the same authors) on implants with anodically oxidized surfaces: 223 implants in 59 patients were re-evaluated after a period ranging between 5 and 17 years, showing implant survival rates of 91.9%, success rates of 66.3%, and a prevalence of peri-implantitis of 28.3% (with peri-implantitis present in 44% of patients) **(Fig 18b)**.

In a randomized clinical trial with a 5-year follow-up, Raes et al[27] compared 42 machined implants with 42 rough-oxidized implants in 15 patients with a previous history of severe periodontitis. In their conclusions, the authors highlighted a clear difference in results in that more loss of supportive bone was associated with the moderately rough implants than the machined ones. On a microbiologic level, the rough-surface implants also showed more pathogenic microorganisms. A systematic literature review by Esposito et al[28] showed a 20% higher risk of developing peri-implantitis for rough implants compared to smooth implants after a 3-year period.

ETIOLOGY OF PERI-IMPLANTITIS

During the Sixth European Workshop on Periodontology in 2008, it was postulated that peri-implantitis is an infectious disease caused by bacterial plaque.[29] The composition of the periodontal microbiota is similar to that found in peri-implant pockets,[30–32] and there is no evidence that the greater aggressiveness of peri-implant pathology compared to periodontitis is related to the composition of the plaque. In addition, colonization of implant surfaces follows the same pattern as that observed in natural teeth[33,34] **(Fig 19)**.

The microorganisms present in peri-implant pockets are also found suspended in saliva. The bacteria adhere by means of specific receptors (adhesins) to a substrate of a few microns that covers all oral surfaces. This layer is formed by adsorption by the surfaces of salivary lipids and glycoproteins and is known as the acquired salivary pellicle. Adhesion of the first bacteria, predominantly cocci mediated by adhesins, is rather labile and occurs within hours of exposure to any surface in the oral cavity. This adhesion is strengthened by an extracellular matrix rich in polysaccharides and nucleic acids produced by the microorganisms, which begin to manifest bacterial-bacterial interactions.

If bacterial accumulation is not prevented by cleansing processes, small communities of cells begin to form. Through their metabolism and co-adhesion and the microenvironment they establish, along with genuine intercellular chemical communication, these cells create a microecosystem that is predisposed to accommodate more and more species.

Within 24 hours, an organized multilayer biofilm is formed, in which several hundred bacterial species coexist. This number is destined to grow exponentially over time.

The biofilm is therefore a sessile community of cells that are irreversibly attached to a substrate or to each other. This community is immersed in an extracellular matrix produced by the bacteria themselves. The first populations to arise in the periodontal and peri-implant grooves are predominantly gram-positive, aerobic, and nonmotile, often belonging to the streptococci family.[35] This type of microflora is the predominant one in marginal inflammatory states (eg, gingivitis/mucositis). As the biofilm matures, thanks in part to the production of the extracellular matrix, the levels of oxygen in the deeper layers are lowered enough to allow for the survival and proliferation of anaerobic species, such as motile spindle cell species (eg, *bacteroides, actinomycetes*, etc) and *spirochetes*. In the oral plaque, the microorganisms organize in symbiotic relationships and form corncob-like structures.[36]

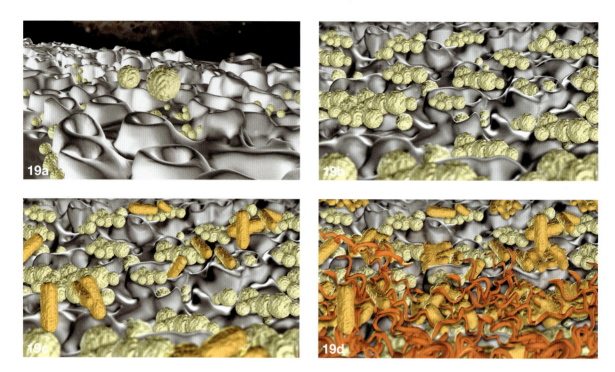

Fig 19 *Stages of bacterial colonization on implant surfaces exposed to the oral cavity. (a) In the first few hours, mainly aerobic gram-positive cocci adhere to the implant surface. (b) In the following hours, the number of bacteria increases, along with their adhesive capacity. (c) Subsequently, rods adhere to the first layer of cocci, forming a more complex ecosystem. (d) Within 24 hours, an organized multi-layered biofilm forms, in which several hundred bacterial species, including spirochetes and spindle forms, co-exist. The number of bacteria increases exponentially over time.*

There are 19 bacterial species associated directly with periodontal and peri-implant pathology, among them *Porphyromonas gingivalis* and *Tannerella forsytia*.[37] The so-called red complex (*Porphyromonas gingivalis, Tannerella forsythia*, and *Treponema denticola*), considered pathogenic for periodontitis, is also present in peri-implant pockets, in the plaque of which *Actinobacillus actinomycetemcomitans* or *Aggregatibacter actinomycetemcomitans* (the bacterium by which the characteristic corncob shape is formed) is also detected.

In partially edentulous patients with implant-supported prostheses, the bacteria present on implant surfaces are the same as those found on neighboring teeth, mucous membranes, and the tongue.[38,39]

If periodontal-pathogenic bacterial species are already present in the oral cavity, they are more likely to colonize other surfaces as well. Compared to other patients, patients with a history of periodontitis tend to have a higher prevalence of putative periodontal pathogens after 6 months of exposure of implant surfaces in the oral cavity.[40]

It does not appear that the composition of the biofilm is influenced by the roughness of the implant surfaces, but it is evident that rougher surfaces can offer more protected niches to the bacteria residing in the oral cavity and thus increase their quantity.[41]

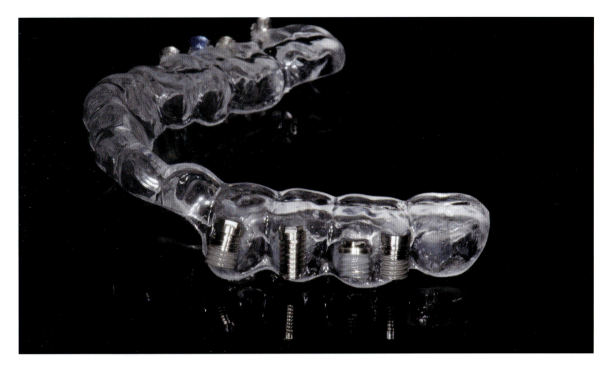

Fig 20 Fragments of four implants with different surfaces glued onto an acetate retainer.

In an experimental pilot study on biofilm formation on different implant surfaces, removable acetate retainers were placed in the mandibles of four volunteers. Eight implant fragments with four different surfaces (machined, double acid-etched [DAE], hybrid [coronal 3 mm machined and apical 3 mm DAE], and roughened with anodic oxidation) had been randomly bonded to the retainers **(Fig 20)**. After 48 hours without cleansing, the fragments were analyzed morphologically via scanning electron microscopy (SEM), and the following features were revealed:

- **Machined surface** (Sa: 0.40 µm; Sdr: 25%): The surface had a uniform acquired film with rare bacterial aggregates consisting exclusively of cocci **(Fig 21)**.
- **DAE surface** (Sa: 0.45 µm; Sdr: 80%): The samples showed an irregular biofilm that was very thick in some areas. In these areas, cracks due to dehydration were colonized by polymorphous bacterial aggregates consisting of cocci and rods **(Fig 22)**.
- **Hybrid surface** (similar characteristics to the previous two implants in relation to the two different surfaces): the immediate quantitative and qualitative change of bacterial flora was evident between the two surfaces **(Fig 23)**.
- **Oxidized surface** (Sa: 1.1 µm; Sdr: 50%; porous): The samples showed a thick bacterial biofilm distributed over a large part of the surface so that the morphologic characteristics of the surface were no longer visible **(Figs 24a and 24b)**. In areas of lower bacterial aggregation, coccoid and rod forms were recognizable **(Fig 24c).**

The study showed that rough surfaces can accelerate biofilm formation in the first hours of exposure to the oral cavity and influence bacterial adhesion, especially with regard to quantity of bacteria.

Fig 21 (a) *Seminal analysis of an implant fragment with a machined surface. Scattered aggregates of bacteria are visible in large areas of the still uncolonized implant surface at ×5,000 magnification. (b) At higher magnification (×10,000) only cocci are visible.*

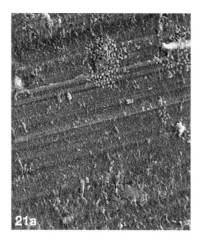
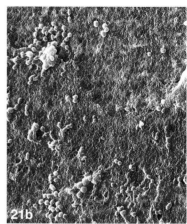

Fig 22 (a) *Very thick, irregular biofilm with cracks due to dehydration (×5,000 magnification). (b) Magnification of a crack showing polymorphic aggregates of bacteria consisting mainly of cocci and rods (×10,000 magnification).*

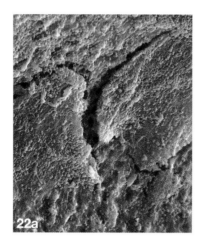
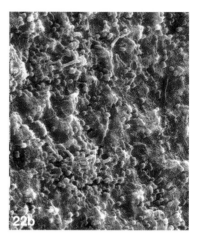

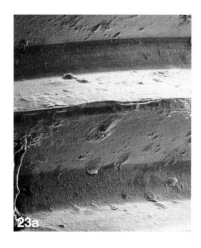
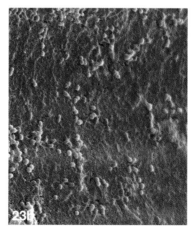
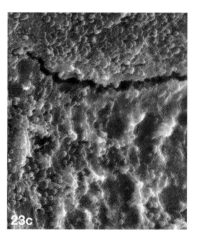

Fig 23 (a) *SEM image of a hybrid implant at the boundary between the machined section and the DAE section (×500 magnification). (b) Higher magnification of the machined surface (×10,000 magnification). (c) Higher magnification of the DAE surface (×10,000 magnification).*

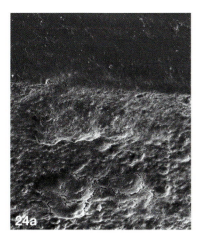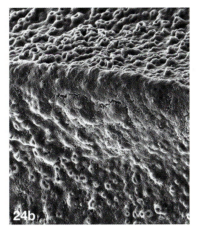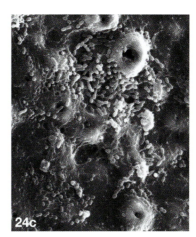

Fig 24 (a) *SEM image of an implant treated with anodic oxidation at the boundary between the smooth collar and the treated surface (×500 magnification).* (b) *The morphologic features of the surface are hardly recognizable due to the thick bacterial biofilm (×1,000 magnification).* (c) *At higher magnification, an area of less bacterial aggregation allows coccoid and rod-like forms to be identified (×10,000 magnification).*

It is therefore not the quality of the plaque that changes between periodontitis and peri-implantitis but rather the conditions that favor the early formation and growth and thus the quantity of a periodontal-pathogenic plaque with a consequent host immune response.

This explains why peri-implantitis can occur early and progress more rapidly on rough-surface implants than in natural teeth and smooth-surface implants.[42,43]

There is no marked qualitative microbiologic difference between mucositis and severe peri-implantitis. In fact, pathogenic bacteria are present in the grooves affected by both of these diseases, which could mean that the disease gradually evolves from a more superficial to a more profound condition if the pathogenic insult persists in predisposed individuals.[44]

In a 2006 study, it was noted that by 1 week after the insertion of a transmucosal implant or the reopening of a submerged implant, it was possible to find red complex bacteria in the peri-implant sulcus, though in very small quantities compared to all the species present in the plate. For pathology to develop, therefore, the mere presence of bacteria does not seem to be sufficient. Rather the development of pathology depends upon the consolidated persistence of the bacteria in terms of time and above all quantity. In the study cited, it was found that the periodontal-pathogenic species present in the peri-implant furrows after 3 months represented 50% of the species present in the biofilm.[45]

Therefore, peri-implantitis is not a monobacterial infection. Pathology sets in or recurs when the following conditions are met:

- Host is predisposed to develop peri-implantitis
- Biofilm has time to organize itself to accommodate an adequate amount of gram-negative anaerobic bacteria and induce an abnormal inflammatory response

A study on an implant extracted due to peri-implantitis provides a very precise morphologic picture of the bacterial population found on contaminated implant surfaces[46] **(Fig 25)**.

Five zones of interest were identified in this study:
1. Smooth titanium prosthetic abutment
2. Exposed supramucosal implant surface
3. Submucosal implant surface
4. Apical implant surface at the biofilm margin
5. Osseointegrated bone-implant interface

On the surface of the smooth prosthetic abutment, islands of bacterial plaque alternated with cleaner areas, in which the texture of the titanium was easily distinguishable **(Fig 26a)**. At higher magnification, spherical and rod-like shapes were visible as the expression of a relatively young plaque **(Fig 26b)**. Immediately below the abutment-implant interface, where the surface became rough and porous, the picture was completely different.

A thick aggregate of polymorphic bacteria coated the implant surface, penetrating into the porosity caused by anodic oxidation and masking the surface characteristics **(Fig 27a)**. Despite being a supramucosal zone, the main forms were of the rod-shaped and filamentous type **(Fig 27b)**.

More apically, at the level of the peri-implant pocket, a thick and complex bacterial biofilm was

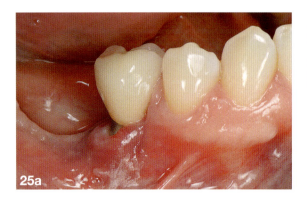
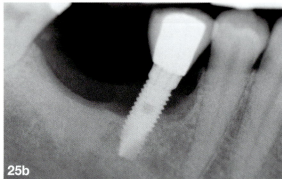

Fig 25 (a) *An implant in site of the mandibular right second premolar with an oxidized surface affected by peri-implantitis. Signs of mucosal inflammation, such as edema, hyperemia, bleeding, and suppuration, are evident. (b) Periapical radiograph showing the characteristic saucer-shaped angular bone defect involving two-thirds of the implant surface.*

Fig 26 (a) *SEM image of an implant extracted due to peri-implantitis. On the smooth titanium abutment there are islands of bacterial plaque alternating with large, essentially clean areas (×20 magnification). (b) At higher magnification (×500), bacterial deposits are visible, with the expression of relatively young plaque.*

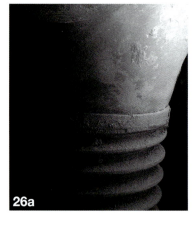
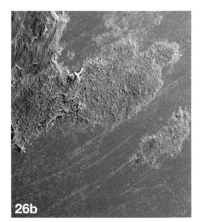

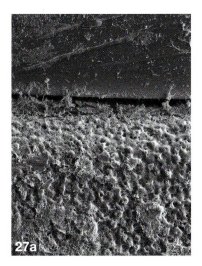
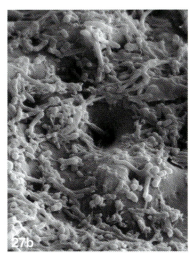

Fig 27 (a) *Abutment-implant interface. Whereas the smooth abutment appeared almost clean, a thick aggregate of polymorphic bacteria can be seen on the oxidized implant surface (×5,000 magnification). (b) At higher magnification (×20,000), rod and filamentous forms can be seen penetrating the porosity caused by the anodic oxidation and masking the surface characteristics.*

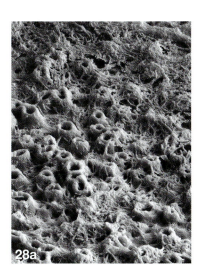
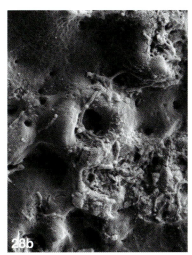

Fig 28 (a) *At the level of the peri-implant pocket, a thick and complex bacterial biofilm consisting predominantly of spindle-rod–like forms can be seen (×10,000 magnification). They deeply infiltrate the surface porosities (b) (×20,000 magnification).*

evident, consisting mainly of spindle-rod–like forms **(Fig 28a)** that deeply infiltrated the surface porosities **(Fig 28b)**. At the lower limit of the mucous pocket, a dense infiltrate of leukocytes was observed immediately below the advancing front of the bacterial biofilm **(Fig 29)**.

Deeper and apical to the inflammatory infiltrate was the osseointegrated zone, in which the mineralized bone matrix was visible in intimate contact with the implant surface **(Fig 30a)**. Bacteria and inflammatory cells were absent **(Fig 30b)**.

PATHOGENESIS OF PERI-IMPLANTITIS

The formation of biofilm on implant surfaces provokes a local immune response that, in addition to playing a defensive role, is paradoxically also highly destructive toward the peri-implant tissues. This is the biologic price the body pays to prevent the spread of plaque bacteria into the blood stream. The mucosal seal around implants is less effective and the blood supply is much reduced compared to that around a natural tooth, so

Fig 29 (a) *Dense infiltrate of inflammatory cells immediately below the advancing front of the bacterial biofilm (×10,000 magnification).* (b) *Higher magnification (×20,000).*

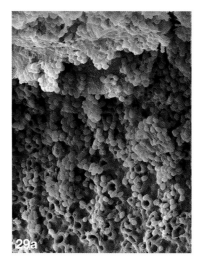
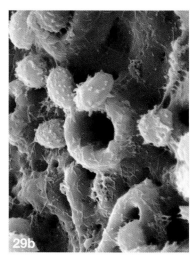

Fig 30 (a) *Osseointegrated area apical to the inflammatory infiltrate. The mineralized bone matrix is in intimate contact with the implant surface (×5,000 magnification).* (b) *Neither bacteria nor inflammatory cells were present (×10,000 magnification).*

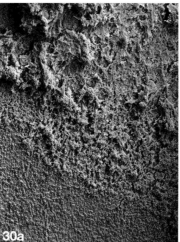
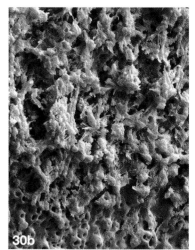

bacterial aggression is dealt with less effectively. Pathogenic plaque flora induces periodontal/peri-implant damage on three levels:

1. Directly by releasing metabolic products, enzymes, and bacterial endotoxins
2. Indirectly by triggering an innate/nonspecific immune response
3. Indirectly by triggering an acquired/specific immune response

Innate (ie, natural) immunity is the body's armor against any kind of physical, chemical, or biologic insult. It involves cellular and biochemical mechanisms that exist in the body prior to exposure to the pathogenic damage, which are ready to react immediately.

There are three main components of innate immunity:

1. Physical and chemical barriers, such as epithelia and the antimicrobial substances produced by epithelial surfaces. The mucous membranes, in addition to continuously desquamating, are coated with a layer of immunoglobulin A (IgA), an antiseptic varnish that hinders bacterial adhesion.

2. Phagocytes (neutrophil granulocytes and macrophages) and natural killer cells (NK lymphocytes).
3. The release of mediators of inflammation, such as vasoactive factors like histamine, serotonin, kinins, prostaglandins, and leukotrienes and factors of the complement system.

The presence of bacteria and their derivatives stimulates the epithelial cells of the sulcus lining to produce proinflammatory cytokines and other chemical mediators that have vasoactive and chemotactic actions against phagocytes. The polymorphonuclear neutrophil granulocytes are the first leukocytes to intervene, after which macrophages also rush in. Macrophages, known as tissue scavengers because they phagocytose microorganisms and waste present in the tissues, have a marked motility that allows them to migrate even outside the furrow by crossing the epithelial barrier.

Macrophages also evoke the second level of defense—specific immunity. These cells digest intruders, reprocess their substances, and present certain bacterial fragments in the form of antigens on their membrane, giving the alarm to the other immune cells, the lymphocytes. This activity, called antigen presentation, makes macrophages fall into the APC (antigen-presenting cell) family. This form of defense is known as acquired or specific immunity because it is elaborated on the basis of the present/infecting pathogens. Cells are trained to destroy a precise target after the initiation of innate immunity. Acquired/specific immunity is characterized by specificity and memory (ie, the ability to "remember" a specific pathogen by responding to repeated exposures over time, thus resulting in responses of greater intensity and precocity).

The main players in specific immunity are the lymphocytes and their secretion products, such as antibodies. Antigen presentation activity occurs between APC cells and T lymphocytes, which in turn activate B lymphocytes. Once activated, B lymphocytes turn into plasma cells and start producing antibodies.

Antibodies are specific for various types of antigens and adhere to the bacterial membranes with a marking, which is known as opsonization. Because receptors for antibodies are present on neutrophils and macrophages, the labelled bacteria are recognized and neutralized via phagocytosis or the production of toxic substances.

Many structural components of the peri-implant connective tissue are reabsorbed during the active phase of inflammation to make physical space for the inflammatory infiltrate, but the continuous release of collagenase and lytic enzymes by immune cells becomes the main cause of periodontal tissue damage. For example, when macrophages are overstimulated, their membranes fail to close externally before coming into contact with lysosomal enzymes, which are then released into the extracellular environment. This regurgitation phenomenon leads to a massive release of lytic enzymes into the tissues.

Plaque harbors hundreds of bacterial species and induces a huge activation of lymphocytes in the host, which are therefore the cells most present in the inflammatory infiltrate of both periodontitis and peri-implantitis. Due to inflammation, the junctional epithelium migrates apically, and the bone tissue resorbs to make room for the inflammatory cells. In the peri-implant connective tissue, a granulation tissue rich in blood vessels and plasma cells, which produce antibodies, is formed. If timely action is not taken, the process progresses in an apical direction to the apex of the implant.

In peri-implant tissues the immune response is even more extreme than in periodontal tissues, and it deeply affects the supracrestal connective tissue. There is a strong presence of macrophages and neutrophils, a sign that innate and acquired immunity processes occur in conjunction with one another.[47–49]

The clinical finding of pus, a very frequent occurrence in the diseased peri-implant, is a clear sign of acute inflammation and also a sign of the intensity with which tissues react to insults. Pyocytes, which are leukocytes with severe degenerative and necrotic changes, represent the vast majority of the cellular elements that make up the purulent collections.

HISTOPATHOLOGY OF PERI-IMPLANTITIS

Animal studies have described the morphologic characteristics of peri-implantitis and shown important differences between rough and smooth implant surfaces. Berglundh et al[50] induced peri-implantitis in five dogs. A total of 3 months after extraction of the mandibular premolars, they placed 15 implants with a smooth surface and 15 implants of an identical shape but with a surface roughened by airborne particle abrasion and etching. After 3 months of healing, they placed ligatures in the peri-implant sulcus to promote bacterial plaque accumulation and induce experimental peri-implantitis. When the loss of bone support reached 40%, they removed the ligatures and kept the animals under observation without treatment for a further 6 months. Radiographic and histologic findings showed a spontaneous arrest of the progression of peri-implantitis around the smooth implants but an average progression of 1.12 mm of bone resorption and a larger inflammatory infiltrate around the rough implants.

In another animal experiment,[51] peri-implantitis induced in machined implants and in implants roughened with anodic oxidation were compared to periodontitis induced in natural teeth. Teeth were extracted from only one side of the jaw of six dogs, and after a healing period of 3 months, four implants with the two different surfaces were placed. After a further 3 months, ligatures were placed in the peri-implant sulcus and the gingival sulcus of the contralateral premolars. After 9 weeks, the ligatures were removed to observe the spontaneous progression of peri-implantitis and periodontitis.

After 6.5 months, periapical radiographs and biopsies were used for histologic examination. At the time the ligatures were removed, the natural teeth had lost an average of 1.74 mm of attachment, the machined implants had lost 2.69 mm, and the oxidized implants had lost 3.14 mm. At the biopsy after 6.5 months of observation without treatment, the natural teeth and machined implants showed a spontaneous cessation of bone loss, whereas the oxidized implants had lost an additional 1.34 mm of attachment.

These observations demonstrate, albeit with an experimental pathology induction technique, that natural teeth and machined implants are less susceptible to the development and progression of periodontitis and peri-implantitis than anodically oxidized implants.

This study also revealed another substantial difference between periodontitis and peri-implantitis. In natural teeth, the bacterial biofilm was separated from the gingival connective tissue by an intact sulcular epithelium. Furthermore, between the inflammatory infiltrate and the bone margin, there was a capsule of healthy, noninflamed connective tissue. Around the implants, however, there was a larger inflammatory infiltrate (3.5 mm² versus 1.5 mm²) and an ulcerated sulcular epithelium. Thus, peri-implant lesions lack an epithelial barrier and have the characteristics of an open wound, leaving them less able to defend themselves against bacterial insult **(Fig 31)**.

It is now evident that as long as a rough implant surfaces remain confined inferior to the bone crest, and are thus not colonizable by bacteria, only small, 1.5-mm angular defects are usually formed **(Fig 32)**.

However, the peri-implant alveolar ridge may undergo postsurgical resorption phenomena for innumerable reasons, including traumatic surgery, excessive pressure of the implant on the walls of the recipient site caused by a very high insertion torque (> 50 Ncm), the pressure of a provisional mucosa-supported prosthesis, the use of regenerative techniques involving a certain amount of bone remodeling **(Fig 33a)**, and the presence of very thin bone or even small areas of implant dehiscence **(Fig 33b)**.

In all these cases, in the presence of an exposed rough surface, there is a strong local predisposing factor for plaque accumulation and thus peri-implantitis **(Figs 34 and 35)**.

In conclusion, a dental implant constitutes an intermediary between the heavily bacteria-contaminated environment of the oral cavity and the deep structures of the peri-implant mucosa-bone complex. It is not surprising, therefore, that even around a clinically healthy implant, there is a certain number of inflammatory cells constantly engaged in mitigating the migration of toxins and bacteria along the surface of the implant into the interior.

A clinically healthy implant is in a state of equilibrium between the bacterial load on the crown and the host's defense systems. If at some point the bacterial load becomes excessive, for example if a rough or porous implant surface becomes exposed above the bone crest and is colonized or if the patient's compliance worsens, the balance breaks down in favor of peri-implant pathology. If, on the other hand, the bacterial load is kept low, thanks to a smoother, nonporous implant surface and proper oral hygiene, the balance is maintained. Conversely, if the immune defenses are lowered due to reasons such as diabetes mellitus, smoking, or other systemic diseases, the balance shifts toward pathology even with the same bacterial load **(Fig 36)**.

For this reason, there is currently a tendency to use more and more hybrid implants with a rough surface in the apical half and a machined, smoother surface in the more coronal half of the implant that is closer to the marginal tissues.

DIAGNOSIS OF PERI-IMPLANTITIS

Peri-implant probing is the first and indispensable procedure for diagnosing peri-implant disease. The clinical signs of peri-implantitis are those of an inflammatory process in the peri-implant soft and hard tissues: bleeding on probing and/or suppuration, edema and reddening of the mucosa, and increased probing depth and/or recession of the marginal tissues.

During probing, there will be no resistance from the tissues, and the bone surface will be easily reached. Patients rarely experience spontaneous pain in the peri-implant tissues, but probing and brushing are often uncomfortable. Radiographic signs of pathology can be used to confirm clinical findings and document crestal bone loss over time.

The intraoral examination cannot be entirely replaced by the peri-implant radiographic finding. However with peri-implantitis, the bone defect is usually circumferential and has a characteristic saucer-like appearance **(Fig 37)**. Depending on the thickness of the ridge, the defect may be complete (with four walls) or incomplete (with two or three walls) **(Fig 38)**.

In contrast, adaptive bone resorption generally has a more linear, horizontal, and supraosseous pattern. Radiographically, inflamed bone appears with blurred and poorly radiopaque margins, whereas healthy bone tissue is more radiopaque and has sharp, well-defined margins. If left untreated, peri-implantitis takes a nonlinear but progressive and significantly faster course than periodontitis, and it always results in implant loss.

Destruction of the supporting tissues progresses without obvious signs of mobility because osseointegration is maintained in the most apical portion of the implant.

A mobile implant indicates the complete loss of osseointegration and total implant failure.

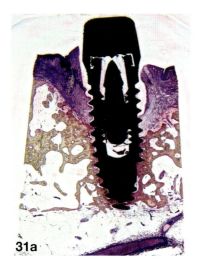 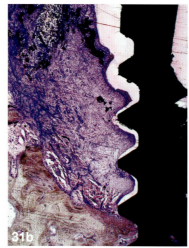 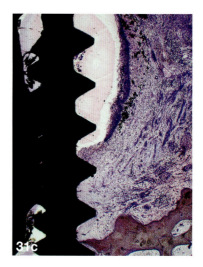

Fig 31 (a) *Histologic preparation showing an implant affected by peri-implantitis. Toluidine blue/Pyronine G staining; ×2 magnification.* (b) *At higher magnification (×4), the absence of an epithelial barrier and the penetration of the inflammatory infiltrate to the bone is evident. Toluidine blue/Pyronin G staining.* (c) *Howship lacunae are present at the level of the ridge, a sign of bone resorption. Toluidine blue/pyronine G staining; ×4 magnification.*

The diagnosis of peri-implantitis requires the presence of the following clinical signs:

- bleeding and/or suppuration with gentle probing
- greater probing depth than in the previous examination
- radiographic bone loss beyond crestal bone level changes resulting from initial bone remodeling

TREATMENT OF PERI-IMPLANTITIS

In most scientific publications, the treatment strategy for peri-implantitis is left to the experience of the author. The literature offers no definitive method to eradicate this pathology, and the treatment of peri-implantitis therefore does not follow evidence-based guidelines and is not predictable. Prevention remains the best means to control it. Paradoxically, the long-term successes encountered with Brånemark-style osseointegrated implants have led to the perception of implant therapy as an ad vitam treatment, inevitably leading both clinicians and patients to neglect the importance of preventing infectious complications by using appropriate implant surfaces and reducing all risk factors and applying prevention protocols along with periodic follow-ups and appropriate home oral hygiene maintenance.

Nonsurgical therapy

Nonsurgical therapy of peri-implantitis has three main objectives:

1. Breakdown and removal of the bacterial biofilm present on the implant
2. Removal of granulation tissue present in inflamed mucosal membranes
3. Maintenance of oral hygiene that is compatible with a state of health

It has been claimed that nonsurgical therapy is essentially ineffective in the treatment of peri-implantitis but that it improves the health of soft

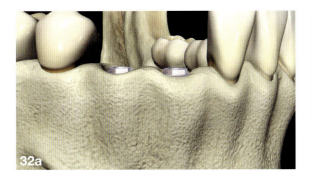 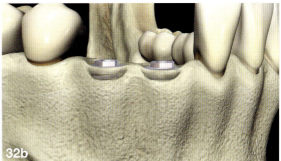

Fig 32 *Formation of the physiologic angular defect common to all implants with few exceptions. (a) The position was just below the bone crest at the time of insertion. (b) Angular reabsorption of 1.5 mm after application of the prosthetic load.*

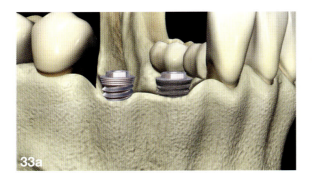 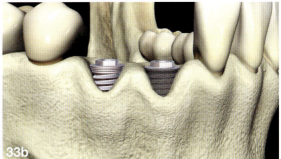

Fig 33 *(a) Abnormal adaptive remodeling of the bone ridge caused by traumatic surgery, excessive torque, provisional prosthesis pressure, grafting, or regenerative techniques. (b) Implant dehiscence due to reduced crestal bone thickness.*

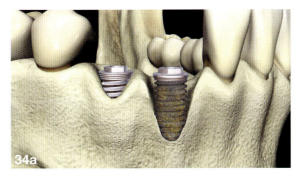 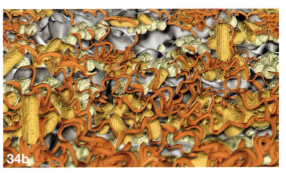

Fig 34 *(a) Evolution of the dehiscence-type defect with peri-implantitis in an implant with a totally rough/ porous surface. (b) Biofilm formation on the rough/porous surface.*

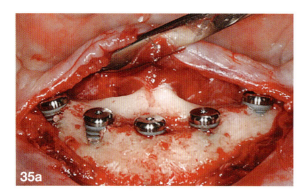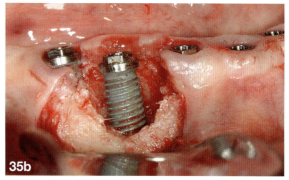

Fig 35 *Implants placed in a thin mandibular ridge.* (a) *Part of the rough surface is exposed above the bone ridge.* (b) *Bone defect caused by peri-implantitis after 4 years of function.*

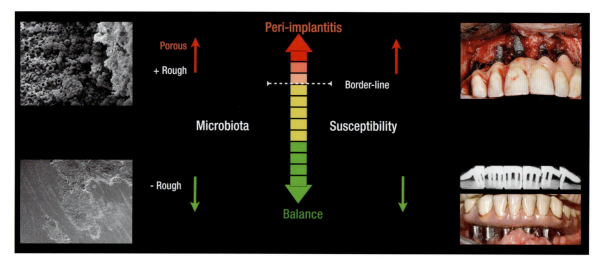

Fig 36 *A clinically healthy implant is in a state of equilibrium between bacterial load and host defense systems. In the presence of an exposed rough implant surface, the bacterial load may increase, and the balance will be broken in favor of pathology. In the presence of a smooth surface, the bacterial load is kept low, and the balance is maintained. If immune defenses are lowered due to diabetes mellitus, smoking, or other systemic diseases, the balance shifts in favor of pathology.*

tissue.[52] It was therefore recommended only as a therapy for mucositis and as preparation for surgical treatment. Clinical experience gained in recent years, however, has led to a critical review of this statement and a reassessment of the nonsurgical approach. The decontamination and instrumentation of a threaded implant with a rough surface, without first elevating a flap and without removing the threads, is very complex. Here, we describe a procedure with promising results, discuss its rationale, and finally, present some cases that support it.

The protocol described here is not only for nonsurgical therapy but is also essential to achieve high success rates with surgical therapy and regenerative techniques.

The technique is based mainly on the use of local mechanical nonsurgical treatment, the application of local antiseptics and irrigants, the administration of systemic antibiotic therapy, and a strict supportive program. If subjects with peri-implantitis also present with symptoms of periodontitis, they must be given periodontal therapy at the same time. Periodontitis sites act as a reservoir of pathogenic bacteria, with colonization of the most aggressive species occurring as early as the first week after exposure of an implant surface to the oral environment.[45] Candidates for this treatment must achieve a full-mouth plaque score of less than 25%.

The procedure begins with a careful study of the site and the implant to be treated.

The type of surface and morphology of the implant is important for making the best use of manual and mechanical tools.

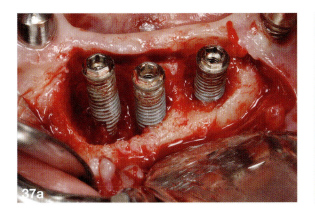
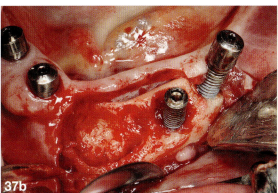
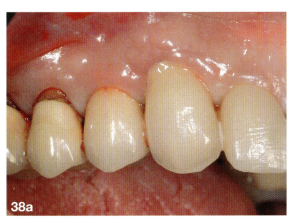
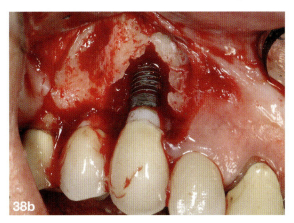

Fig 37 (a) *Porous-surface mandibular implants affected by peri-implantitis. Large, saucer-shaped defects involve most of the implant surface.* (b) *The implants are removed for regeneration of the bone in the defect areas and replaced with hybrid implants.* **Fig 38** (a) *Purulent discharge at the level of the sulcus of the implant in the position of the maxillary right canine.* (b) *After elevation of an access flap, a three-walled defect is visible.*

Additionally, clinicians must know whether heterologous grafting materials were used during extraction and implant placement. These slow-resorbing materials may be secondarily involved in the peri-implant infectious process and amplify the destructive effects of infection.

Finally, it is necessary to assess the depth, width, morphology, and accessibility of the defect because the procedure is effective only if the entire surface of the implant can be decontaminated.

Nonsurgical therapy involves the following steps **(Table 1)**:

1. Determination of defect characteristics
2. Dissolution of bacterial biofilm
3. Decontamination of the implant
4. Local antibiotic and antiseptic therapy
5. Posttreatment maintenance protocol
6. Long-term maintenance protocol

A consequence of this protocol is contraction of the marginal soft tissues, so caution must be exercised in areas of significant esthetic value. In such areas, surgical therapy combined with regenerative techniques is probably indicated.

Determination of defect characteristics

Under local anesthesia, a PCP-15 periodontal probe is used to assess the depth, morphology, and characteristics of the bone defect **(Fig 39a)**. Further analysis is carried out by determining the number of threads involved in the defect using a mini titanium curette tip and comparing the result with what was previously identified in the periapical radiograph **(Fig 39b)**.

Breakdown of bacterial biofilm

An air-polishing procedure is performed with glycine/erythrol powders to remove the superficial bacterial biofilm. This is followed by subgingival debridement with an ultrasonic handpiece with an NSK P21L periodontal metal tip to break up the bacterial biofilm and create an anatomical space between the implant and the soft tissue to allow better access to the base of the pocket.

The granulation tissue is then carefully and gently removed with mini titanium Gracey curettes (11/12 or 13/14), the working parts of which are oriented toward the soft tissue with respect for its anatomy and the avoidance of excessive recession **(Fig 40a)**. The inflammatory tissue has a different

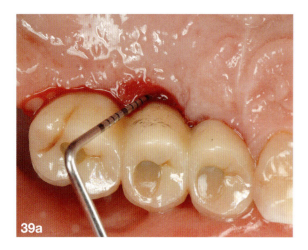
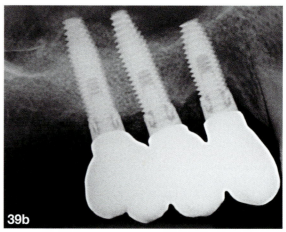

Fig 39 (a) *Probing down to the bone crest with a PCP 15-mm probe.* (b) *Comparison of data obtained with the periapical radiograph.*

consistency from the noninfiltrated tissue, and its removal can be performed without the use of a scalpel, as the curette blade easily finds the cleavage plane offered by the healthy mucosal tissue. At this stage, it is usually possible to remove any small sequestrations of heterologous bone previously detected with radiography.

The complete removal of the granulation tissue leads to an immediate reduction in bleeding and increased visibility of the bone defect and implant surface **(Fig 40b)**. The NSK P21L ultrasonic tip is then used to perform a final wash and completely remove any granulation tissue still present inside the pocket.

Implant decontamination

The mini 11/12 or 13/14 curettes should be inserted into the pocket parallel to the implant surface and then angled so that only the first third of the blade is working, just as in traditional periodontal root planing.

The most important aspect of this part of the procedure is the meticulous decontamination of the implant surface, which begins with apicocoronal movements aimed at removing the bacterial agglomerates present on the apex of the implant threads **(Fig 41)**. It continues with horizontal (mesiodistal and distomesial) movements that follow the course of the recess between each thread and the next. This smoothing must be performed for each individual thread exposed within the peri-implant defect and requires good tactile sensitivity, especially because the threads are often located several millimeters below the mucosal margin **(Fig 42)**. This slow and meticulous movement makes it possible to remove biofilm and any fragments of necrotic bone tissue adhered to the implant threads and to smooth the surface.

Valuable aids for this procedure are titanium brushes mounted on a micromotor used at low speed (between 200 and 1,000 rpm) and with irrigation. This can reduce the roughness of the implant surface **(Figs 43a and 43b)**. Several studies have shown that titanium curettes and brushes are able to reduce the roughness of the implant by burnishing its surface and making it less retentive to plaque, without causing any structural changes to the implant design.[53] Because the brushes are made of titanium, the surface chemistry is also not altered, and contaminants are not released.

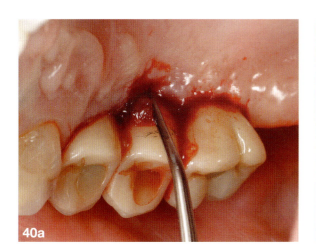
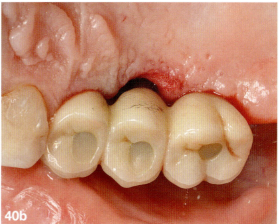

Fig 40 (a) *Curettage of the mucosal wall of the pocket with mini Gracey curettes.* (b) *After removing the granulation tissue, the defect and implant surface are more visible.*

Brush-type inserts have filaments that are too thin to abrade the titanium surface but can be useful in deep, narrow peri-implant defects **(Fig 43c)**. It is advisable to perform frequent irrigation with 10% hydrogen peroxide during polishing to disinfect the pocket and remove debris and titanium shavings produced by mechanical polishing. The final stage of decontamination involves once again applying air polish with erythritol or glycine above and below the mucosa, for 5 seconds at each site, to perfect the removal of hard and soft deposits from the implant surface without altering it.

Local posttreatment antibiotic and antiseptic therapy

At the end of treatment, an antiseptic hyaluronic acid–based gel (Hobagel Plus, Hobama) is applied to the site to create a protective film and promote soft tissue healing.

Gel applications are repeated twice a day for 20 days at the end of home oral hygiene practices. Patients must be carefully instructed on how to perform correct hygiene from the day of surgery. Various aids are prescribed: an electric toothbrush, a single tuft toothbrush, antiseptic toothpaste

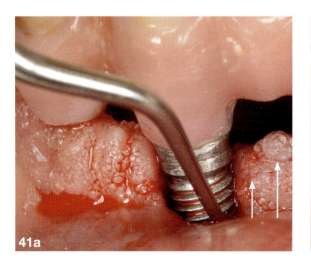
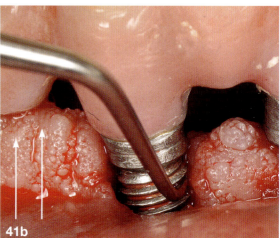

Fig 41 (a and b) *Apicocoronal movements with the mini 13/14 Gracey curette for the removal of the biofilm present on the apex of the threads.*

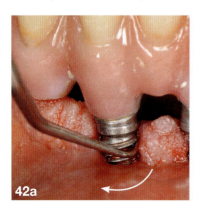
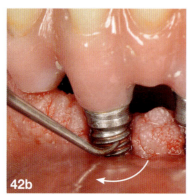
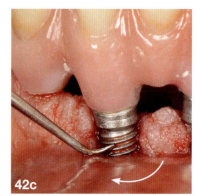

Fig 42 *Horizontal (mesiodistal and distomesial) movements that follow the course of the notch between one thread and the next, from the deepest to the most superficial areas, over the entire exposed implant surface.*

(Hobagel, Hobama), and interdental brushes. Interdental brushes are chosen according to the size of the interdental/interimplant spaces.

They work by friction, so they should be the most voluminous possible without damaging the soft tissue. The use of interdental brushes helps to reposition the interdental papillae by reducing the transmucosal path. We recommend the application of 1% chlorhexidine gel with the interdental brush twice a day for 2 weeks.

The procedures described in this section remove and disrupt the biofilm present on the implant surface, but they also cause a fair amount of bacteremia and the dispersion of pathogenic bacteria onto neighboring oral tissues and into the salivary fluid. Therefore, systemic antibiotic therapy is indicated to lower the bacterial load.

Broad-spectrum antibiotics are a valuable aid in periodontal and peri-implant therapy.

The protocol includes the prescription of amoxicillin and clavulanic acid (1 g every 12 hours for 7 days) and metronidazole (250 mg every 8 hours for 7 days).

Amoxicillin/clavulanic acid is a broad-spectrum antibiotic and, combined with metronidazole, is particularly effective against gram-negative anaerobic bacteria.

In 1992, Mombelli and Lang[54] indicated its use and emphasized its efficacy. Their study proposed a pharmacologic treatment similar to that mentioned here, involving the taking and culturing of subgingival plaque samples at the treated sites after 10 days and 1, 2, 3, 4, 6, 9, and 12 months. The combination of mechanical, systemic antibiotic, and home antiseptic therapy for 10 days resulted in a substantial reduction of pathogenic bacteria.

As time passed, the presence of anaerobic gram-negative bacteria increased progressively, reaching a peak of relapse after 3 months. Based on this information, the need arose to undertake a particularly intensive postsurgical support therapy

in the first 4 months and a long-term maintenance therapy with appointments every 3 months in the following years. Preventing the natural formation of pathogenic plaque is essential to prevent pathology from recurring.

Posttreatment maintenance protocol

The posttreatment maintenance protocol involves a 30-minute session every month for the first 4 months. Zitzmann et al[8] demonstrated that mucositis in humans can be experimentally induced by undisturbed plaque accumulation for 21 consecutive days.

This observation demonstrates the need to maintain close monitoring in the period immediately after treatment.

Initial monthly recalls make it possible to intercept any deficiencies in home oral hygiene and to motivate the patient to prevent the bacterial biofilm from having time to organize itself.

In these short sessions, a plaque test is performed: If plaque is present, it is removed gently with air polishing with erythritol or glycine, without inserting any submucosal instruments. This procedure, in addition to improved home hygiene, is intended to promote healing of the deeper areas of the defect.

Long-term maintenance protocol

At the end of the 4-month period, the site is reevaluated and assigned a full-mouth plaque score. A periodontal examination, periapical radiograph, and a comprehensive oral hygiene session are also carried out.

During this period, patients should attend several appointments to refine their home hygiene practices. They are then placed on a customized maintenance protocol with bimonthly or quarterly supportive therapy recalls.

This timing is determined by the knowledge that it takes about 3 months of plaque accumulation for a recurrence of the disease.

Table 1 Protocol for nonsurgical peri-implantitis therapy after anesthesia and bone probing.

Active treatment	Air polishing
Postoperative protocols	Ultrasound ablation
Posttreatment maintenance	Soft tissue curettage
Re-evaluation	Irrigation with hydrogen peroxide
Long-term maintenance	Implant decontamination with curettes
	Implant decontamination with brushes
	Application of Hobagel Plus
	Antibiotic therapy (amoxicillin/clavulanic acid 1 g every 12 h for 7 days)
	Topical application of 1% chlorhexidine gel once per day for 2 weeks
	Topical applications of Hobagel Plus
	Monthly follow-ups with hygiene procedures for 4 months
	Calculus removal and clinical and radiographic evaluations
	Follow-ups every 2 to 3 months with calculus removal

Results of nonsurgical therapy

Nonsurgical treatment has considerable advantages. A nonsurgical operation is simpler and less invasive than surgery with access flaps, and management of the pathology by the hygienist significantly reduces treatment costs. Between 2005 and 2015, the treatment of peri-implantitis consisted of treatment inspired by that used to manage periodontitis. After an initial preparation and causal therapy phase, surgical treatment was performed with access flaps, potentially associated with either resective or regenerative surgery. Thereafter, the patient entered a normal maintenance protocol with follow-ups every 3 to 4 months. This method of treatment had very low

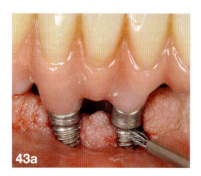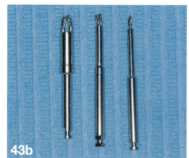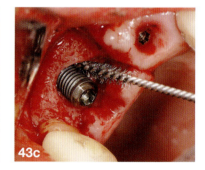

Fig 43 (a) *Finishing the surface of an implant with a titanium brush mounted on a slow-speed micromotor with abundant irrigation.* (b) *Types of brushes.* (c) *Use of a titanium brush in an angular defect.*

success rates (between 30% and 40%) because it did not include the phase of active therapy during the first 4 months after surgery, which is essential to avoid the rapid recolonization of the implant surface by pathogenic bacteria. Under the new protocol, the indications for surgical therapy are drastically reduced, and success rates have increased. In many patients, true bone regeneration with partial or total filling of the defects or stabilization of the defects with more regular margins and reappearance of the lamina dura has been observed **(Fig 44a)**.

The success, stabilization, and failure rates of 34 consecutively treated patients with a follow-up of 1 to 4 years were calculated, and it was found that 27 patients (79.4%) showed both remission of inflammatory symptoms and the filling of bone defects. In three patients (8.8%), remission of clinical symptoms was observed, but the defects were still present radiographically, although they showed signs of stabilization. In another 3 patients, pathology was still present.

Similar figures were obtained when considering each individual implant in the same group of 34 patients **(Fig 44b)**. Of 45 implants affected by peri-implantitis and treated with nonsurgical therapy, 36 (80%) showed partial or total radiographic filling of the bone defect, 3 (6.6%) showed signs of stabilization (ie, more regular margins and the reappearance of the lamina dura), and 6 implants (13.3%) showed persistence of the inflammatory pathology.

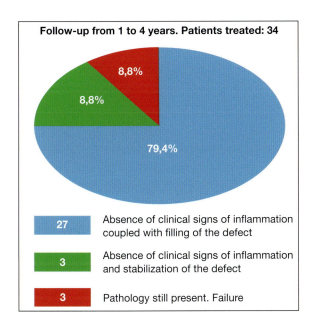

Fig 44a Success, stabilization, and failure rates in the 34 patients treated, with follow-ups between 1 and 4 years. Twenty six patients (79.4%) showed remission of symptoms and radiographic filling of the defects. Three patients (8.8%) showed stabilization of the defect, and five patients (8.8%) showed persistence of the pathology.

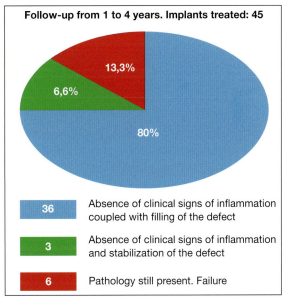

Fig 44b Success, stabilization, and failure rates of 45 implants treated for peri-implantitis, with follow-ups between 1 and 4 years in the same 34 patients as in a. A high percentage of implants (80%) showed radiographic filling of the defect, 6.6% showed stabilization of the defect, and 13.3% showed persistence of the pathology.

CLINICAL CASE 2

Nonsurgical therapy to treat peri-implantitis in a distal implant used for complete mandibular rehabilitation

A patient with a completely edentulous mandible with a fixed/removable prosthesis supported by four implants presented with localized peri-implantitis at the distal left implant after 6 years of function **(Figs 46 to 48)**. Slight marginal bone resorption had been observed around an implant, which had an anodized porous surface, with a periapical radiograph after 3 years of prosthetic loading **(Fig 45)**, and by the sixth year, a classic crater-shaped defect involving five threads was visible. The bone adjacent to the defect appeared radiolucent due to demineralization **(Fig 46)**. The patient underwent nonsurgical therapy as described in this chapter, resulting in the complete remission of symptoms and disappearance of the defect **(Fig 47)**.

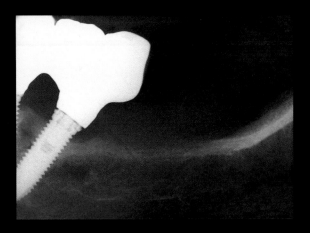

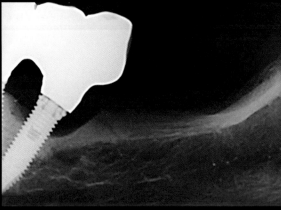

Fig 45 Periapical radiograph of the implant in the site of the mandibular left first premolar after 3 years of prosthetic loading. A small marginal defect is visible.

Fig 46 Periapical radiograph after 6 years of loading. A typical peri-implantitis defect extending up to the sixth thread is present.

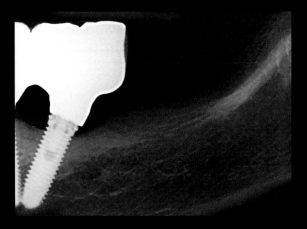

Fig 47 Radiograph 4 years after nonsurgical therapy showing almost complete bone regeneration and flattening of the defect.

CLINICAL CASE 3

Nonsurgical therapy to treat peri-implantitis in intermediate implants used for a complete mandibular rehabilitation

A completely edentulous patient who had received anodized implants for a complete fixed restoration 2 years earlier presented with peri-implantitis at the level of the two intermediate implants **(Fig 48a)**. After 4 years of ineffective conventional nonsurgical therapy, the loss of bone support progressed to the tenth implant thread **(Fig 48b)**. Nonsurgical treatment with the protocol described in this chapter resulted in filling of the intraosseous component and flattening of the defect **(Fig 48c)**.

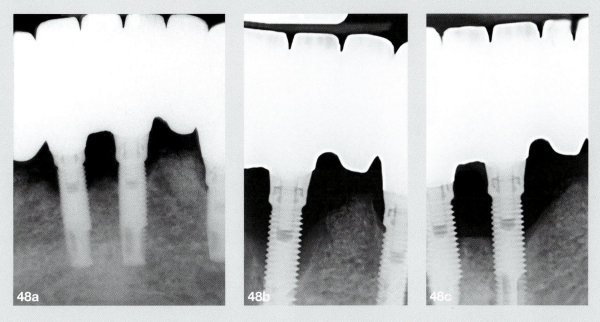

Fig 48 *(a)* Periapical radiograph showing peri-implantitis at the level of the intermediate implants of a full-arch implant prosthesis after 2 years of function. *(b)* After another 4 years of ineffective nonsurgical therapy, the defects reached the tenth implant thread. *(c)* A radiograph taken after 4 years of therapy with the new nonsurgical protocol revealed filling of the intraosseous component of the defects and bone remineralization.

Nonsurgical therapy for a single implant at the level of the mandibular left first molar

A patient was treated with an implant with a wide platform and an anodized surface in the site of the mandibular left first molar **(Fig 49a)**. After prosthetic rehabilitation, physiologic adaptive bone remodeling occurred with resorption up to the first thread **(Fig 49b)**. After 4 years, the implant underwent severe peri-implantitis that developed a crater-shaped defect extending up to the sixth thread **(Fig 49c)**. Nonsurgical treatment, performed according to the protocol described in this chapter, led to complete bone regeneration in the defect and reformation of the lamina dura after 1 year **(Fig 49d)**.

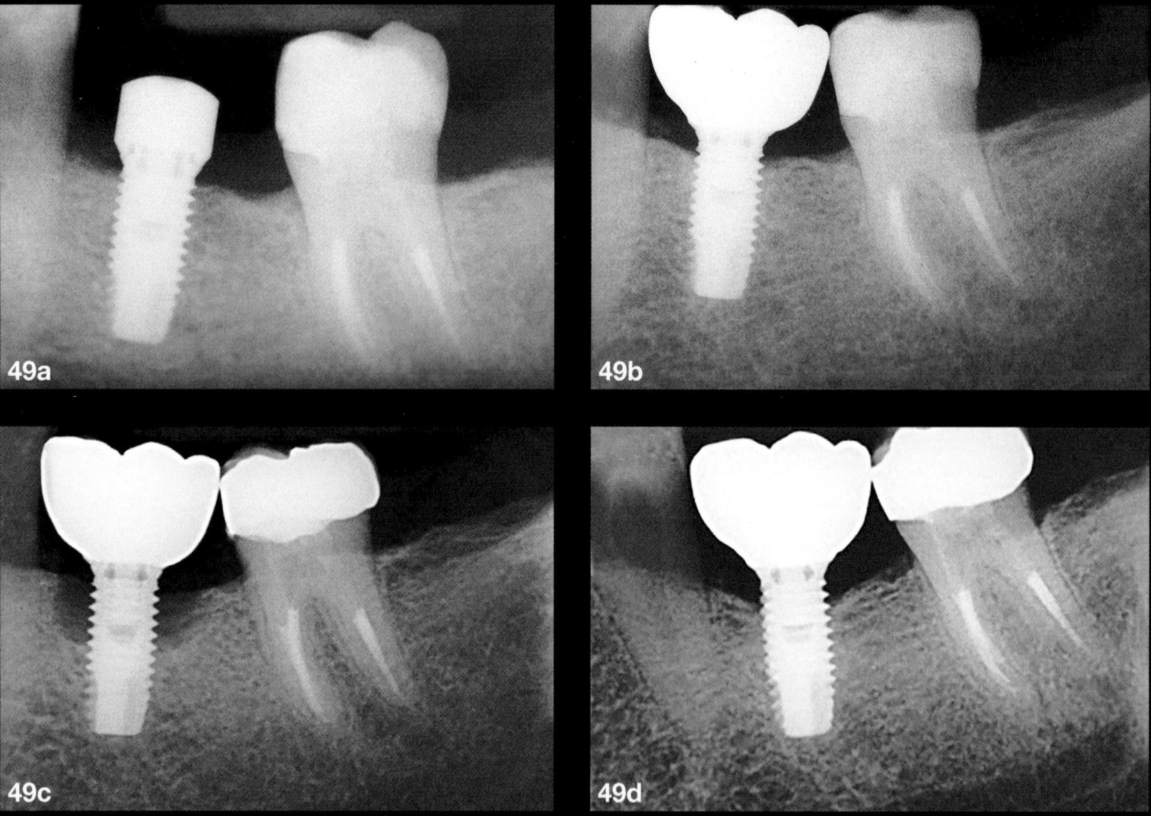

Fig 49 *(a)* Periapical radiograph after the insertion of an implant with a wide platform in the site of the mandibular left first molar. *(b)* After prosthetic loading, physiologic bone remodeling led to exposure of the first thread. *(c)* At the 4-year follow-up, a crater-shaped defect typical of peri-implantitis was found extending to the sixth thread. *(d)* Complete bone regeneration within the defect and the appearance of the lamina dura were evident 1 year after nonsurgical therapy.

Surgical therapy

Surgical peri-implant therapy is aimed at decontaminating the open implant surface and removing the implant or the structures that favor plaque accumulation (eg, surface roughness, exposed threads, and excessively deep bone defects). In some cases, partial or complete bone regeneration within the defect is intended so that a rough implant surface can be submerged as deeply as possible, far from the peri-implant sulcus area that is potentially colonized by bacteria. Surgical therapy is reserved for patients in whom nonsurgical therapy alone has been unsuccessful, and it should therefore be performed only after a complete course of nonsurigcal treatment that includes all the steps described in the previous section, with a period of supportive therapy of at least 8 months. Unfortunately, surgical therapy is often considered a solution in itself, and the subsequent maintenance phases are therefore neglected. A surgical act that is not followed by adequate supportive therapy, however, cannot be effective. The postsurgical and long-term maintenance treatment protocols are the same as for nonsurgical therapy. Surgical therapy involves the following steps:

1. Determination of the defect characteristics
2. Design and elevation of the mucosal flap
3. Thread removal and decontamination of the implant surface
4. Possible regenerative technique and suturing
5. Local postsurgical antibiotic and antiseptic therapies
6. Postsurgical maintenance protocol
7. Long-term maintenance protocol

Determination of the defect characteristics, local postsurgical antibiotic and antiseptic therapy, postsurgical maintenance, and long-term maintenance are performed identical to the corresponding steps in nonsurgical therapy. The other steps are described in the following sections.

Design and elevation of the mucosal flap

Surgery should be undertaken only after removal of the crowns and prosthetic abutments to gain better access to the site.

A full-thickness flap should extend to an adjacent element in edentulous spans surrounded by natural teeth to provide ample visibility of the bone defect. In completely edentulous patients, the incision should be extended a few millimeters beyond the defect, and vertical releasing incisions can be made.

Ideally, the incision should be paramarginal and directed over the bone crest at the margins of the defect to isolate any granulation tissue. The granulation tissue should be meticulously removed with ultrasonic instruments and titanium curettes. It is important to perform frequent rinses with 10% hydrogen peroxide.

Thread removal and decontamination of the implant surface

Once all the granulation tissue has been removed, the thread is removed with fine-grain diamond burs mounted on a handpiece. This step is time-consuming and delicate. Clinicians must avoid overheating the implant and weakening its structure by removing too much material, for which a microscope or ×4 magnification and abundant irrigation with physiologic saline solution are used. Healing screws are recommended to protect the implant head from drills and hand instruments. From time to time, the titanium dust produced by the drilling should be removed with ultrasonic instruments, and abundant irrigation should be performed with hydrogen peroxide. Finishing is performed with a smooth, multiblade bur and titanium brushes.

There is no consensus in the literature on the most effective methods for intraoperative disinfection of the implant surface. The authors use 10% hydrogen peroxide irrigation combined with the application of tetracyclines.

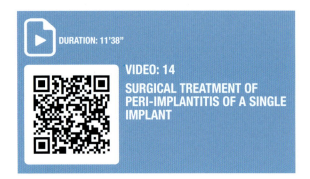

DURATION: 11'38"

VIDEO: 14
SURGICAL TREATMENT OF
PERI-IMPLANTITIS OF A SINGLE
IMPLANT

Regenerative technique and suturing

Regenerative techniques should be very simple. The use of a particulate graft of autologous bone harvested with a safe scraper within the same surgical site is indicated whenever possible. The particles are compacted within the defect without exceeding the bone margins, and then a resorbable collagen membrane is placed to protect the entire site. Biomaterials, such as deproteinized bovine bone, can also be used.

Overfilling should be avoided because a possible recurrence of infection could spread to the biomaterial particles left in the newly formed bone. Either interrupted sutures or Laurell-Gottlow sutures are used.

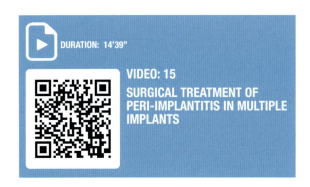

DURATION: 14'39"

VIDEO: 15
SURGICAL TREATMENT OF
PERI-IMPLANTITIS IN MULTIPLE
IMPLANTS

CLINICAL CASE 5

Implant removal and bone regeneration

A patient presented with peri-implantitis 7 years after bone regeneration surgery and the placement of an implant with an oxidized surface. Insertion of a periodontal probe into the implant sulcus in the site of the mandibular right central incisor zone showed pathologic probing depth and caused the emission of abundant purulent exudate and bleeding (**Figs 50 to 53**).

After several sessions of nonsurgical decontamination by means of Teflon ultrasonic inserts and perioflow applications of glycine powder, the clinical situation did not significantly improve, and a constant and spontaneous purulent exudate could still be observed, although the marginal soft tissues were less inflamed.

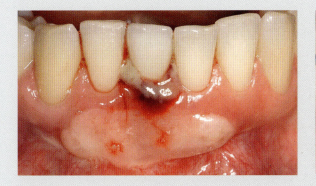

Fig 50 Purulent exudate is visible.

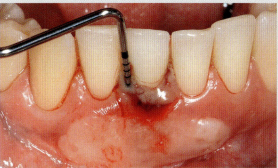

Fig 51 A probing depth of 10 mm is detected.

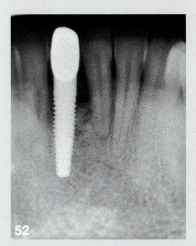

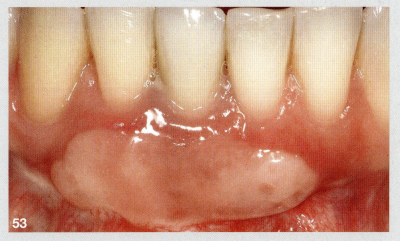

Fig 52 Preoperative periapical radiograph. **Fig 53** Bleeding after probing. The protuberance at the implant is due to an epithelial-connective graft performed during the first regenerative surgery.

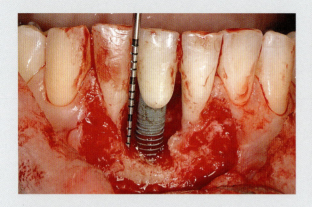

Fig 54 After the initial preparation, purulent exudate remains.

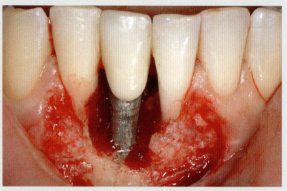

Fig 55 Buccal view after implant removal.

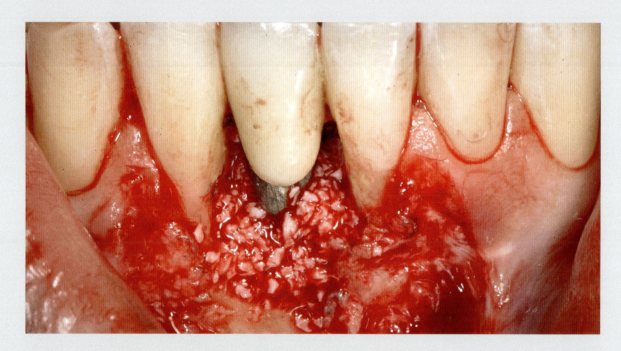

Fig 56 Filling the defect with bone of bovine origin.

Surgical therapy was indicated, aimed at the removal of the peri-implant granulation tissue, decontamination of the implant surface, and elimination of the rough implant surface. After the elevation of a buccal and lingual mucoperiosteal flap, the granulation tissue was removed. Because the residual bone defect had favorable characteristics, a regenerative technique was performed, and sutures were removed 15 days after surgery **(Figs 54 to 57)**. Follow-ups were performed at 1, 2, 4, and 6 months and at 1, 2, 3, and 7 years **(Figs 58 and 59)**. The inflammatory indices at 7 years were negative, and the closely observed results of treatment were definitely positive.

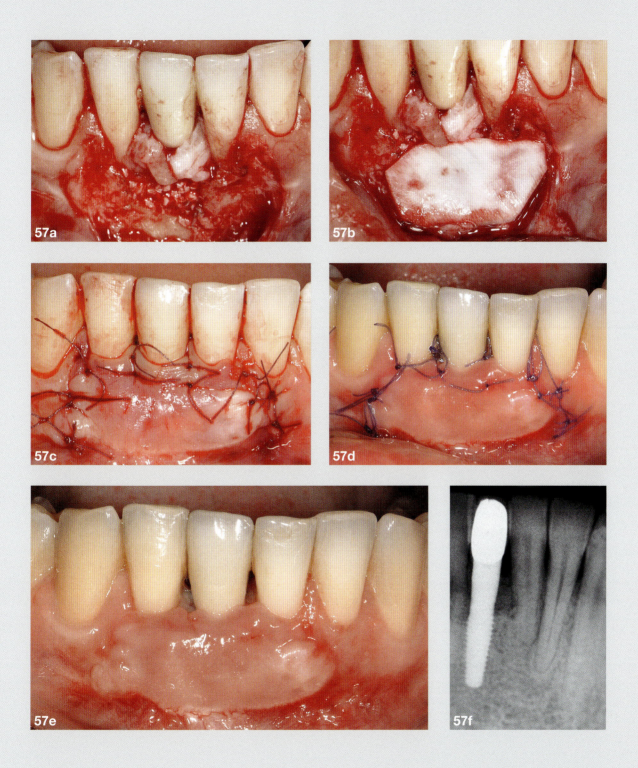

Fig 57 *(a)* Placement of a connective tissue graft, harvested by thinning the lingual mucosal flap. *(b)* Placement of a resorbable collagen membrane. *(c)* Interrupted resorbable 6-0 suture. *(d)* Before suture removal 15 days after surgery. *(e)* After suture removal 15 days after surgery. There is slight dehiscence of the papillae. *(f)* Radiograph 15 days after surgery.

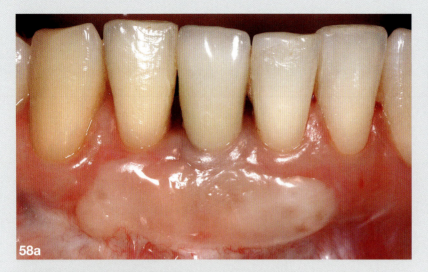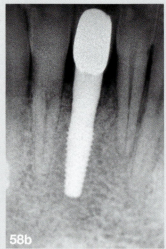

Fig 58 Clinical and radiographic images at 6 months.

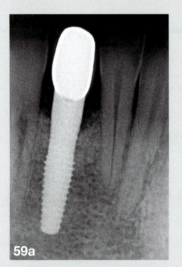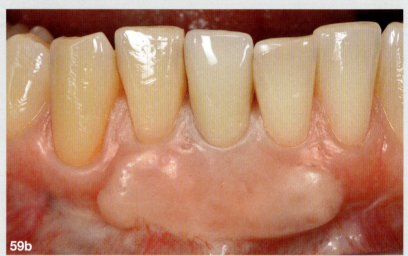

Fig 59 Radiographic and clinical images at 7 years.

CLINICAL CASE 6

Implant removal and bone regeneration

A patient who smoked more than 20 cigarettes per day and had a history of hypertension and psoriasis presented in 2011 with several implants affected by peri-implantitis and two teeth affected by periodontitis. He had received eight bilateral maxillary anodized implants in the sites of the first molar, second premolar, canine, and central incisor **(Fig 60a)**. The patient was poorly motivated and, despite attending follow-up visits, the management of home oral hygiene was not acceptable. By 3 years later, there were clear signs of peri-implantitis **(Fig 60b)**. Undergoing nonsurgical treatment did not seem to improve the clinical situation, and the patient continued to smoke heavily. Therefore, he underwent surgical removal of the implants in the sites of the maxillary right central incisor and maxillary left canine, as well as resective and regenerative peri-implant surgery according to the morphology of the bone defects around all the other implants **(Figs 61 to 64)**.

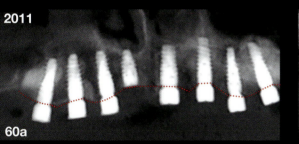

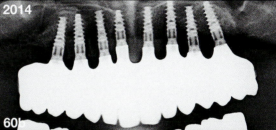

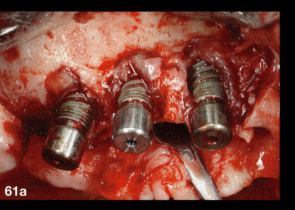

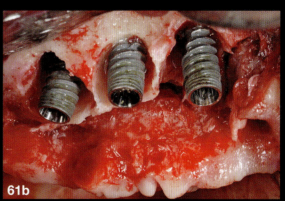

Fig 60 *(a)* Panoramic CBCT after the insertion of eight implants. The implant in the position of the maxillary right central incisor is the only one that is not loaded, due to poor primary stability. The implant in the position of the maxillary left canine is completely placed in regenerated bone. The red dotted line shows the crestal bone profile at the time of implant insertion. *(b)* Panoramic CBCT performed only 3 years after implant insertion, with generalized bone resorption evident at all implant sites. **Fig 61** *(a)* Intraoral photograph after the elevation of a mucoperiosteal flap from the maxillary right lateral incisor to the right first molar. The implant in the position of the central incisor was removed, and substantial bone resorption and the presence of granulation tissue can be seen around the other implants. *(b)* Bone morphology after removal of the granulation tissue.

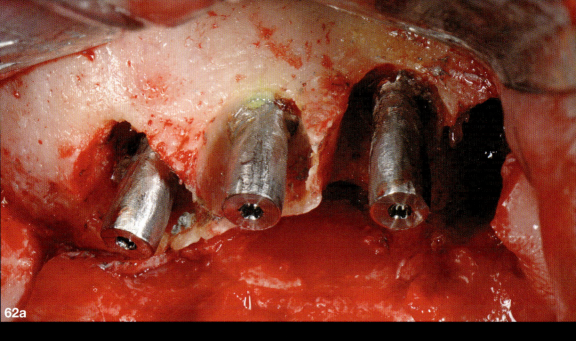

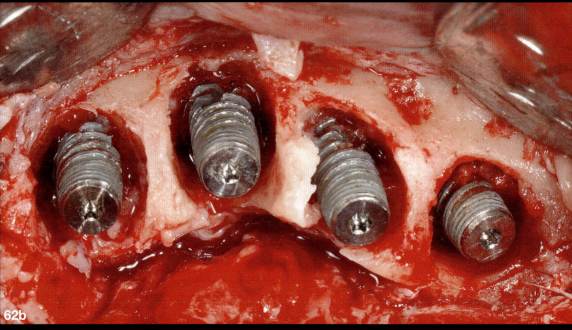

Fig 62 *(a)* View after implant removal. The positioning of the healing screws protects the prosthetic platform and implant neck from damage. *(b)* Intraoral view after the elevation of a mucoperiosteal flap from the maxillary left central incisor to the left first molar and removal of the granulation tissue.

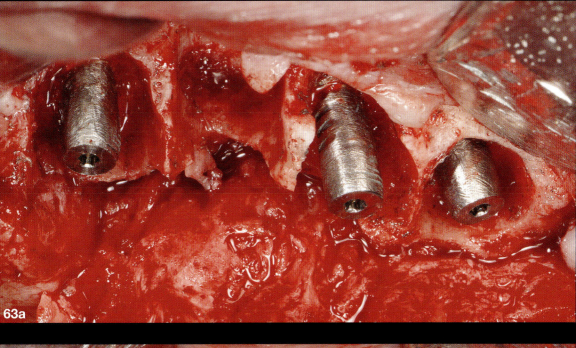

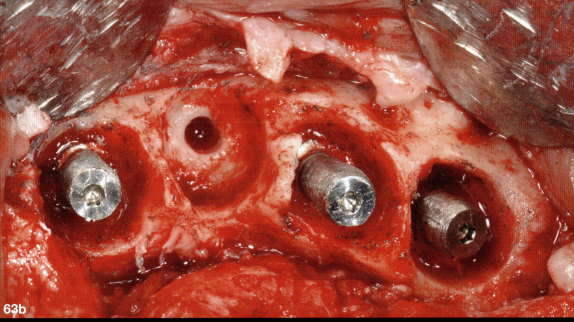

Fig 63 *(a and b)* Results after removal of the implant in the position of the maxillary left canine and
treatment of the other implants.

The patient was compliant with follow-ups and was provided supportive therapy, and from 2016 to 2019 a compromised situation was maintained (Figs 65 and 66).

Periodontitis, a history of peri-implantitis, smoking, poor home oral hygiene management, and rough implant surfaces played a key role in the onset of severe peri-implantitis in this case. Since 2016, although with severe impairment of peri-implant bone support, the clinical situation became stable, and the patient stopped smoking (due to the diagnosis of a lung tumor). He attended all follow-up appointments and learned to clean the exposed implant surfaces at home, which had no exposed threads and were less rough than at baseline.

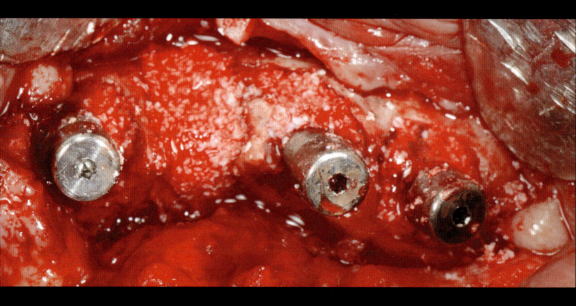

Fig 64 Peri-implant defects in the areas of the maxillary left central incisor, second premolar, and first molar are filled with heterologous biomaterial and amelogenins.

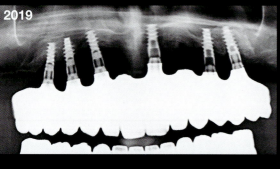

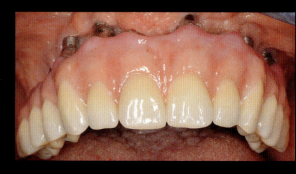

Fig 65 Panoramic CBCT 8 years after implant placement and after treatment of the peri-implant infectious disease. The full-arch prosthesis remains in function, even though the peri-implant bone support is greatly reduced.

Fig 66 Clinical image taken in 2019. The soft tissues show no signs of inflammation, although substantial recession is evident. The closely monitored patient maintained adequate oral hygiene, and the peri-implant pathology appears to be under control.

REFERENCES

1. Brånemark PI, Adell R, Albrektsson T, Lekholm U, Lundkvist S, Rockler B. Osseointegrated titanium fixtures in the treatment of edentulousness. Biomaterials 1983;4:25–28.

2. Astrand P, Ahlqvist J, Gunne J, Nilson H. Implant treatment of patients with edentulous jaws: A 20-year follow-up. Clin Implant Dent Relat Res 2008;10: 207–217.

3. Huynh-Ba, G. Thematic abstract review: Peri-implantitis: 'Tsunami' or marginal problem? Int J Oral Maxillofac Implants 2013;28:333–337.

4. Qian J, Wennerberg A, Albrektsson T. Reasons for marginal bone loss around oral implants. Clin Implant Dent Relat Res 2012;14:792–807.

5. Albrektsson T, Buser D, Chen ST, et al. Statements from the Estepona consensus meeting on peri-implantitis, February 2-4, 2012. Clin Implant Dent Relat Res 2012;14:781–782.

6. Sanz M, Lang NP, Kinane DF, Berglundh T, Chapple I, Tonetti MS. Seventh European Workshop on Periodontology of the European Academy of Periodontology at the Parador at La Granja, Segovia, Spain. J Clin Periodontol 2011;38(Suppl 11):1–2.

7. Berglundh T, Armitage G, Araujo MA, et al. Peri-implant diseases and conditions: Consensus report of workgroup 4 of the 2017 world workshop on the classification of periodontal and peri-implant diseases and conditions. J Periodontol 2018;89(Suppl 1):S313–S318.

8. Zitzmann NA, Berglundh T, Marinello CP, Lindhe J. Experimental peri-implant mucositis in man. J Clin Periodontol 2001;28:517–523.

9. Schwarz F, Mihatovic I, Golubovic V, Eick S, Iglhaut T, Becker J. Experimental peri-implant mucositis at different implant surfaces. J Clin Periodontol 2014;41:513–520.

10. Schwarz F, Becker J, Civale S, Hazar D, Iglhaut T, Iglhaut G. Onset, progression and resolution of experimental peri-implant mucositis at different abutment surfaces: A randomised controlled two-centre study. J Clin Periodontol 2018;45:471–483.

11. Derks J, Schaller D, Håkansson J, Wennström JL, Tomasi C, Berglundh T. Peri-implantitis - onset and pattern of progression. J Clin Periodontol 2016;43: 383–388.

12. Schwarz F, Derks J, Monje A, Wang HL. Peri-implantitis. J Periodontol 2018;89(Suppl 1):S267–S290.

13. Chung DM, Oh T-J, Shotwell JL, Misch CE, Wang H-L. Significance of keratinized mucosa in maintenance of dental implants with different surfaces. J Periodontol 2006;77:1410–1420.

14. Bouri A, Bissada N, Al-Zahrani MS, Faddoul F, Nouneh I. Width of keratinized gingiva and the health status of the supporting tissues around dental implants. Int J Oral Maxillofac Implants 2008;23:323–326.

15. Boynueğri D, Nemli SD, Kasko YA. Significance of keratinized mucosa around dental implants: A prospective comparative study. Clin Oral Implants Res 2013;24:928–933.

16. Adibrad M, Shahabuei M, Sahabi M. Significance of the width of keratinized mucosa on the health status of the supporting tis- sue around implants supporting overdentures. J Oral Implantol 2009;35:232–237.

17. Roccuzzo M, Grasso G, Dalmasso P. Keratinized mucosa around implants in partially edentulous posterior mandible: 10-year results of a prospective comparative study. Clin Oral Implants Res 2016;27:491–496.

18. Souza AB, Tormena M, Matarazzo F, Araujo MG. The influence of peri-implant keratinized mucosa on brushing discomfort and peri-implant tissue health. Clin Oral Implants Res 2016;27:650–655.

19. Lang NP, Berglundh T, Working Group 4 of Seventh European Workshop on Periodontology. Peri-implant diseases: Where are we now? Consensus of the Seventh European Workshop on Periodontology. J Clin Periodontol 2011;38(Suppl 11):178–181.

20. Schwarz F, Sahm N, Becker J. Impact of the outcome of guided bone regeneration in dehiscence-type defects on the long-term stability of peri-implant health: Clinical observations at 4 years. Clin Oral Implants Res 2012;23:191–196.

21. Jepsen S, Berglundh T, Genco R, et al. Primary prevention of peri-implantitis: Managing peri-implant mucositis. J Clin Periodontol 2015;42(Suppl 16): S152–S157.

22. Canullo L, Tallarico M, Radovanovic S, Delibasic B, Covani U, Rakic M. Distinguishing predictive profiles for patient-based risk assessment and diagnostics of plaque induced, surgically and prosthetically triggered peri-implantitis. Clin Oral Implants Res 2016;27: 1243–1250.

23. Dreyer H, Grischke J, Tiede C, et al. Epidemiology and risk factors of peri-implantitis: A systematic review. J Periodontol Res 2018;53:657–681.

24. Simion M, Gionso L, Grossi GB, Briguglio F, Fontana F. Twelve-year retrospective follow-up of machined implants in the posterior maxilla: Radiographic and peri-implant outcome. Clin Implant Dent Relat Res 2015;17(Suppl 2):e343d–e351.

25. Simion M, Nevins M, Rasperini G, Tironi F. A 13- to 32-year retrospective study of bone stability for machined dental implants. Int J Periodontics Restorative Dent 2018;38:489–493.

26. Ferrantino L, Tironi F, Pieroni S, Sironi A, Simion M. A clinical and radiographic retrospective study on 223 anodised surface implants with a 5- to 17-year follow-up. Int J Periodontics Restorative Dent 2019;39: 799–807.

27. Raes M, D'hondt R, Teughels W, Coucke W, guirynen M. A 5-year randomised clinical trial comparing minimally with moderately rough implants in patients with severe periodontitis. J Clin Periodontol 2018;45:711–720.

28. Esposito M, Murray-Curtis L, Grusovin MG, Coulthard P, Worthington HV. Interventions for replacing missing teeth: Different types of dental implants. Cochrane Database Syst Rev 2007;(4):CD003815.

29. Zitzmann NU, Berglundh T. Definition and prevalence of peri-implant diseases. J Clin Periodontol 2008;35(8 Suppl):286–291.

30. Leonhardt A, Berglundh T, Ericsson I, Dahlen G. Putative periodontal pathogens on titanium implants and teeth in experimental gingivitis and periodontitis in beagle dogs. Clin Oral Implants Res 1992;3:112–119.

31. Botero JE, González AM, Mercado RA, Olave G, Contreras A. Subgingival microbiota in peri-implant mucosa lesions and adjacent teeth in partially edentulous patients. J Periodontol 2005;76: 1490–1495.

32. Salvi GE, Furst MM, Lang NP, Persson GR. One-year bacterial colonization patterns of staphylococcus aureus and other bacteria at implants and adjacent teeth. Clin Oral Implants Res 2008;19:242–248.

33. Akagawa Y, Matsumoto T, Kawamura M, Tsuru H. Changes of subgingival microflora around single-crystal sapphire endosseous implants after experimental ligature-induced plaque accumulation in monkeys. J Prosthet Dent 1993;69:594–598.

34. Lang NP, Brägger U, Walther D, Beamer B, Kornman KS. Ligature-induced peri-implant infection in cynomolgus monkeys. I. Clinical and radiographic findings. Clin Oral Implants Res 1993;4:2–11.

35. Mombelli A, van Oosten MA, Schurch E Jr, Land NP. The microbiota associated with successful or failing osseointegrated titanium implants. Oral Microbiol Immunol 1987;2:145–151.

36. Pontoriero R, Tonelli MP, Carnevale G, Mombelli A, Nyman SR, Lang NP. Experimentally induced peri-implant mucositis. A clinical study in humans. Clin Oral Implants Res 1994;5:254–259.

37. Persson GR, Renvert S. Clusters of bacteria associated with peri-implantitis. J Periodontal Res 2016;51: 689–698.

38. De Boever AL, De Boever JA. Early colonization of non-submerged dental implants in patients with a history of advanced aggressive periodontitis. Clin Oral Implants Res 2006;17:8–17.

39. Quirynen M, De Soete M, van Steenberghe D. Infectious risks for oral implants: A review of the literature. Clin Oral Implants Res 2002;13:1–19.

40. Mombelli A, Maxer M, Gaberthuel T, Grunder U, Lang NP. The microbiota of osseointegrated implants in patients with a history of periodontal disease. J Clin Periodontol 1995;22:124–130.

41. Subramani K, Jung RE, Molenberg A, Hammerle CH. Biofilm on dental implants: A review of the literature. Int J Oral Maxillofac Implants 2009;24:616–626.

42. Charalampakis G, Rabe P, Leonhardt A, Dahlen G. A follow-up study of peri-implantitis cases after treatment. J clin Periodontol 2011;38:864–871.

43. Zitzmann NU, Abrahamsson I, Berglundh T, Lindhe J. Soft tissue reactions to plaque formation at implant abutments with different surface topography. An experimental study in dogs. J Clin Periodontol 2002;29:456–461.

44. Mombelli A, Décaillet F. The characteristics of biofilms in peri-implant disease. J Clin Periodontol 2011;38(Suppl 11):203–213.

45. Quirynen M, Vogels R, Peeters W, van Steenberghe D, Naert I, Haffajee A. Dynamics of initial subgingival colonization of 'pristine' peri-implant pockets. Clin Oral Implants Res 2006;17:25–37.

46. Simion M, Kim DM, Pieroni S, Nevins M, Cassinelli C. Bacterial biofilm morphology on a failing implant with an oxidized surface: A scanning electron microscope study. Int J Periodontics Restorative Dent 2016;36:485–488.

47. Gualini F, Berglundh T. Immunohistochemical characteristics of inflammatory lesions at implants. J Clin Periodontol 2003;30:14–18.

48. Berglundh T, Gislason O, Lekholm U, Sennerby L, Lindhe J. Histopathological observations of human periimplantitis lesions. J Clin Periodontol 2004;31: 341–347.

49. Carcuac O, Berglundh T. Composition of human peri-implantitis and periodontitis lesions. J Dent Res 2014;93:1083–1088.

50. Berglundh T, Gotfredsen K, Zitzmann NU, Lang NP, Lindhe J. Spontaneous progression of ligature-induced peri-implantitis at implants with different surface roughness: An experimental study in dogs. Clin Oral Implants Res 2007;18:655–661.

51. Carcuac O, Abrahamsson I, Albouy JP, Linder E, Larsson L, Berglundh T. Experimental periodontitis and peri-implantitis in dogs. Clin Oral Implants Res 2013;24:363–371.

52. Lindhe J, Meyle J. Peri-implant diseases: Consensus report of the Sixth European Workshzop on Periodontology. J Clin Periodontol 2008;35(Suppl 8):282–285.

53. Hakki SS, Tatar G, Dundar N, Demiralp B. The effect of different cleaning methods on the surface and temperature of failed titanium implants: An in vitro study. Lasers Med Sci 2017;32:563–571.

54. Mombelli A, Lang NP. Antimicrobial treatment of peri-implant infections. Clin Oral Implants Res 1992;3: 162–168.

BIOLOGIC PRINCIPLES OF GUIDED BONE REGENERATION

CHAPTER 14

Edited by Christer Dahlin and Massimo Simion

GUIDED TISSUE REGENERATION

In the early 1980s, a series of studies on the regenerative potential of periodontal tissues led to the development of guided tissue regeneration (GTR) techniques. These techniques are based on the principle that to maintain overall homeostasis within an organism, the healing of any tissue defect must occur via the migration of cells facing the defect. During healing, therefore, a migratory speed contest occurs between cells, with the fastest ones repopulating the defect area at the expense of the others, consequently determining the nature of healing.

To understand the mechanisms that regulate periodontal GTR, it is important to have a correct understanding of the concepts of periodontal reattachment versus new periodontal attachment. Periodontal reattachment refers to the reconnection of gingival connective tissue to a root surface on which viable periodontal cementum and periodontal ligament (PDL) are still present.[1] It does not imply periodontal regeneration.

The term new periodontal attachment describes gingival connective tissue connected to a root surface that was previously exposed to periodontal disease,[1] and it does imply periodontal regeneration. In 1976, Melcher[2] postulated that the cells that repopulate the root surface after a periodontal access flap is performed determine the nature of the attachment that will form. After the removal of granulation tissue and suturing of the gingival tissues, four basic types of cells face the exposed root **(Fig 1)**: (1) epithelial cells, (2) gingival connective tissue cells, (3) bone cells, and (4) PDL cells. A series of preclinical experimental studies[3–5] have shown that the epithelium is by far the fastest type of tissue to migrate along the root surface to the previous level of connective fiber attachment, forming a long epithelial attachment and preventing the complete regeneration of the periodontal structure.

To test whether the inhibition of the epithelium was sufficient to regenerate a new attachment that was more coronal than the previous one, Nyman et al[6] extracted roots that were partially compromised

Guided bone regeneration (GBR) is based on biologic principles that have been studied for over 30 years. Knowledge of these principles guides the choice of surgical technique and the selection of barrier instruments and biomaterials. Performing these sophisticated techniques requires a thorough knowledge of the biologic principles behind them.

Massimo Simion

by periodontal disease in beagle dogs and immediately submerged them below the mucosa, leaving them in contact with the bone in the deep part and in contact with the gingival connective tissue in the superficial part, thus excluding the epithelium. The histologic results after 3 months showed ankylosis and rhizolysis of the root portion previously exposed to periodontal disease, both where in contact with the bone and where in contact with the gingival connective tissue.

In contrast, the root portion still covered with PDL showed reattachment. This experiment demonstrated that granulation tissue derived from bone or gingival connective tissue is not able to regenerate a new attachment, and rather causes extensive root resorption.

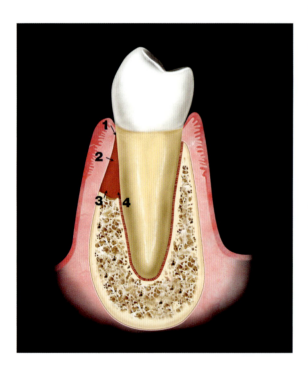

Fig 1 In an access flap, after removal of the granulation tissue and suturing of the gingival tissues, four types of cells face the root: (1) epithelial cells, (2) gingival connective tissue cells, (3) bone cells, and (4) PDL cells.

In light of these observations, a new study by Nyman et al[7] was performed to evaluate the possibility of regenerating a new periodontal attachment by excluding epithelium, gingival connective tissue, and bone from migrating to the root surface. This was achieved by using a Millipore filter (Merck) as a rudimentary membrane. After a u-shaped incision was made in the buccal fornix of monkeys, exposing the apical third of the root, and the cementum and PDL were removed from the root surface, the Millipore filters were placed as barriers to exclude unwanted cells and allow the migration of only cells from the PDL. After 3 months of healing, histologic examination revealed the presence of new cementum, new PDL, and new bone (ie, new periodontal attachment). This study demonstrated the potential of PDL cells to regenerate the periodontium in its entirety.

In another study,[8] extraction was indicated for a mandibular incisor with severe attachment loss in a 47-year-old man suffering from severe periodontitis. However, the tooth was treated with an access flap and thorough root planning, and a Millipore filter was applied with resin over the cementoenamel junction (CEJ), covering the defect like a curtain. The flap was then coronally repositioned, and interdental sutures were placed. The filter prevented both the connective tissue and the epithelium from migrating to the root surface. Histologic examination after 3 months showed regeneration of new cementum and new PDL up to 5 mm coronal to the previous position. This study demonstrated the possibility of regenerating a new periodontal attachment in humans on a root surface previously exposed to periodontal disease and showed that PDL cells are the only ones capable of achieving this.

A case series by Gottlow et al9 confirmed these results with Gore-Tex membranes **(Figs 2 and 3)**. After these studies, GTR was clinically implemented on a large scale for the treatment of periodontal defects.

DEVELOPMENT OF GUIDED BONE REGENERATION

A natural development of GTR has been the application of its biologic principles to guided bone regeneration (GBR) in defects associated with dental implants. The original techniques imply that a membrane should be placed over an alveolar defect to create a barrier between the rapidly growing soft tissue and the bone tissue. This creates a separate space within which only cells with osteogenic potential can migrate **(Fig 4)**.

The first preclinical study on GBR was performed by Dahlin et al[10] in rat mandibles. After the horizontal branch of the mandible was exposed, circular defects were drilled bilaterally into the bone. The defects were so large that they could not heal spontaneously. On the test side, the defects were covered both lingually and buccally with a Gore-Tex membrane, and on the control side, the defects were left without a membrane **(Figs 5 and 6)**.

After 9 weeks of healing, autopsy examination showed complete bone regeneration in the membrane-treated defects and minimal healing in the control sites **(Figs 7 and 8)**. Histologic examination confirmed complete bone regeneration in the test sites **(Figs 9 and 10)**.

A second study by Dahlin et al[11] was performed to evaluate use of the GBR technique around titanium implants placed in the tibia of rabbits with dehiscence-type defects **(Fig 11a)**. The test sites were covered with Gore-Tex membranes, whereas the control sites were allowed to heal spontaneously **(Fig 11b)**.

After 6 weeks, autopsy examination showed complete healing of the treated defects and minimal regeneration in the control sites **(Fig 12)**.

Histologic examination showed, for the first time, the neoformation of trabecular bone directly in contact with the implant surface **(Figs 13 and 15)**. In the early 1990s, the biologic principles of GBR were applied clinically on a large scale, and it is still a popular technique worldwide.[12] It is estimated that GBR is used with about 35% to 40% of implants placed every year.

Membranes for GBR

During the development phase of GBR, the first experimental studies were carried out using membranes alone, without graft or bone substitutes, to cover defects to create a favorable environment for the normal process of bone neoformation.[9,10,12–15]

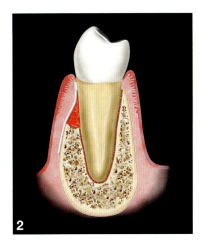
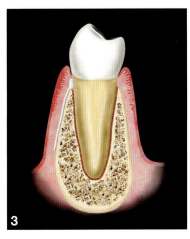

Fig 2 Placement of a Gore-Tex membrane to prevent the migration of gingival epithelial and connective tissue cells.[10]
Fig 3 PDL cells have regenerated cementum and PDL, and thus, the alveolar bone (ie, new periodontal attachment was achieved).

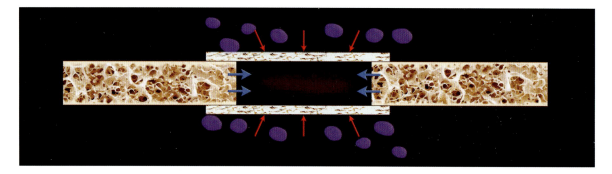

Fig 4 *Barrier membranes can be used to create a separate space in which only cells with osteogenic potential can migrate. (Figures 4 to 10 are reprinted with permission from Int J Oral Maxillofac Implants 1989;4:19–25.)*

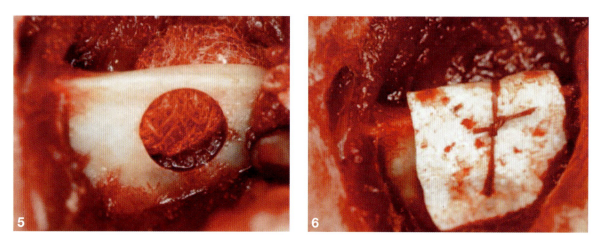

Fig 5 *Circular critical defects drilled bilaterally into the ascending ramus of a rat.* **Fig 6** *The defect was covered with a Gore-Tex membrane both lingually and buccally on the test side, whereas the control side was left untreated.*

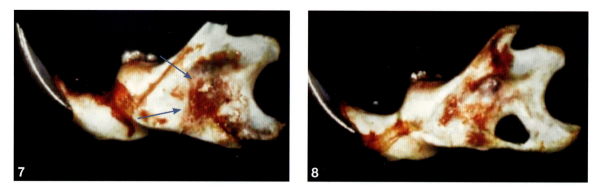

Fig 7 *Autopsy specimen of a test side. The bone defect appears completely healed with new bone.* **Fig 8** *On the control side, the defect shows minimal regeneration. (Figures 7 and 8 are reprinted with permission from Plast Reconstr Surg. 1988;81:672–6.)*

Any interaction between the membrane biomaterial and the host tissues must not interfere with bone regeneration in a clinically significant way. The material of choice for these membranes, expanded polytetrafluoroethylene (ePTFE), was used because it is inert and causes virtually no immune reaction, making it close to ideal. The material consists of chains of carbon and fluorine joined by a strong chemical bond. This gives ePTFE a very high chemical and hydrophobic stability that makes it extremely biocompatible with biologic tissues. Furthermore, ePTFE has been used extensively throughout the history of medicine in the fields of thoracic surgery and orthopedics. In subsequent years, titanium was added to reinforce membranes and prevent them from collapsing, improving membrane stability and ability to maintain adequate space, which are essential factors for bone regeneration.

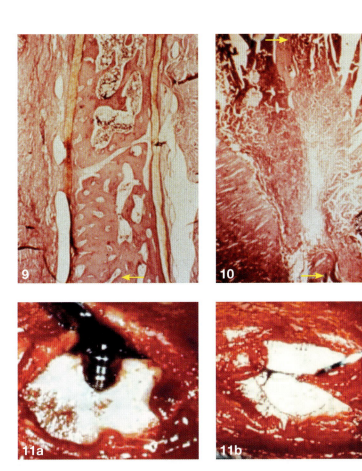

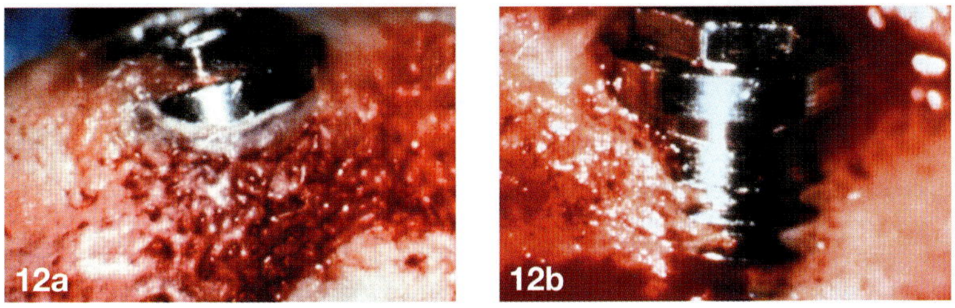

Fig 9 *Histologic preparation of the test side. The defect appears to be completely repopulated by new bone* (arrows).

Fig 10 *The control side showed complete invagination of connective tissue and muscle within the defect and minimal bone regeneration* (arrows). *(Figures 9 and 10 are reprinted with permission from Plast Reconstr Surg. 1988;81:672–6.)*

Fig 11 (a) *Implant inserted into a rabbit tibia with a dehiscence-type bone defect.* (b) *The test side was treated with a Gore-Tex membrane.*

Fig 12 (a) *Autopsy preparation after 6 weeks of healing showing a complete neoformation of bone up to the head of the implant.* (b) *Implant dehiscence is still present on the untreated side (Figures 11 and 12 are reprinted with permission from Int J Oral Maxillofac Implants. 1989;4:19–25.)*

Initial preclinical and clinical experimental studies have shown excellent results. A great deal of effort has been put into researching and understanding the dynamics of bone neoformation, with or without the addition of graft materials under the membrane. In an experimental study on surgically created ridge defects in the mandible of dogs, Schenk et al[13] showed that bone regeneration under the membranes takes place following the same sequence of events as natural bone regeneration. These findings were corroborated by Buser et al,[14] who used the same model in combination with titanium implants. An experimental study by Simion et al[15] compared the effectiveness of three different types of titanium-reinforced ePTFE membranes for bone regeneration. The first type was the standard commercially available membrane, consisting of a highly occlusive central portion and a more porous and permeable peripheral portion.

The second type was a membrane constructed with only the more porous and permeable peripheral portion. The third type was a prototype constructed with a totally impermeable inner layer and two extremely porous outer layers. Histologic results after 4 months showed maximum effectiveness with the prototype membrane. The rapid integration of this material led to bone regeneration even within the porous layer of the membrane itself **(Figs 16 to 18)**. This study demonstrates the negligible importance of a membrane's fluid permeability and the importance of its surface characteristics. However, the prototype studied was never used clinically because the excessive integration with the newly formed bone made its complete removal impossible. These studies in the development phase of GBR led to the conclusion that for a membrane to be used for alveolar ridge augmentation, it must meet the following requirements in addition to acting as a physical barrier:[16]

1. The membrane must be made of sufficiently biocompatible materials. The interaction between the material and the biologic tissue must not adversely affect the surrounding tissue, healing, or patient safety.

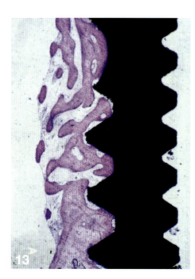 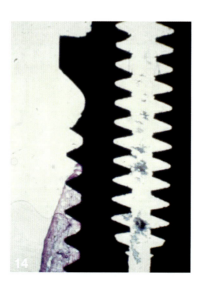 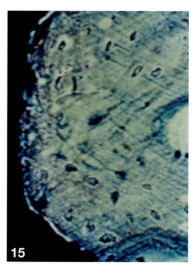

Fig 13 Histologic preparation of a test side specimen showing regenerated bone up to the head of the implant. **Fig 14** On the control side, regeneration appears minimal. **Fig 15** Histologic preparation of the test side. There is direct contact between the implant surface and the regenerated bone. (Figures 13 to 15 are reprinted with permission from Int J Oral Maxillofac Implants. 1989;4:19–25.)

2. The membrane must have an occlusive effect on the cells to prevent invasion by fibrous tissue adjacent to the bone surface and provide some protection from bacteria when exposed to the oral environment.

3. The membrane must be able to maintain sufficient space within which bone regeneration can take place. The space must provide the necessary volume and correct shape for functional reconstruction.

4. The membrane must be able to integrate or adhere to the surrounding tissues. Tissue integration helps stabilize the healing zone and creates a seal between the bone and the material to prevent connective tissue from penetrating into the defect and, in the case of exposure, to delay the migration of epithelium around the material.

5. The membrane must be easy to handle.

GBR membranes are currently used in combination with various bone substitute biomaterials.

The original idea behind this practice was that while the membranes isolate the bone defect from nonosteogenic soft tissue cells, the bone substitutes can function as a scaffold for the regeneration of new bone.[10–12] However, even after 30 years of clinical success with this technique, the cellular and molecular mechanisms that govern the sequence of biologic events during GBR and the role of membranes in modulating these events remain poorly understood.

Resorbable membranes

With the advent of cellular and molecular analysis techniques, correlative interpretations of the molecular and morphologic bases of GBR have recently emerged.

The need for a second surgical procedure for membrane removal and its difficulties and associated complications have increased interest in resorbable (biodegradable) membranes of natural origin, mainly collagen.

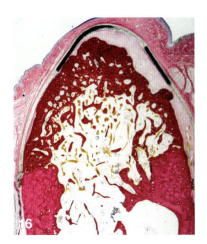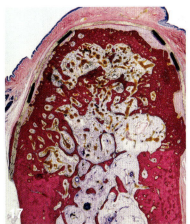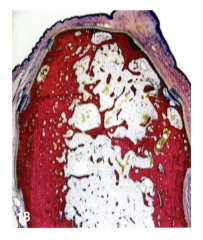

Fig 16 *Standard Gore-Tex membrane with bone regeneration up to the membrane surface, but separated by a connective tissue layer.* **Fig 17** *With the porous and permeable membrane, a thinner layer of connective tissue was found with areas of integration between the newly formed bone and the membrane. Toluidine blue and basic Fuchsin staining; ×2 magnification.* **Fig 18** *With the membrane prototype with a totally impermeable inner layer and two extremely porous outer layers, the regenerated bone appeared totally integrated with the membrane tissue, making it impossible to remove.*

Natural collagen membranes have received much attention in recent years not only because they are easy to use but also for their positive biologic effects, such as their low immunogenicity and the stimulating action of growth factors in the extracellular matrix (ECM) of collagen (including fibroblast growth factor 2 [FGF-2], which stimulate angiogenesis).[17,18]

These membranes are resorbed by enzymatic degradation, while synthetic polymers are degraded into lactic acid and water. By far the most documented resorbable material (Bio-Gide, Geistlich Biomaterials) is made up of native, non-cross-linked Type I and III collagen and consists of several functional layers. The membrane is hydrophilic, which allows for natural adhesion to the bone surface and thus greater ease of use.

With the adaptation of surgical techniques, resorbable membranes are the material of choice in most GBR applications today. Because of their lack of rigidity, collagen membranes are used in combination with grafting materials that maintain space for bone regeneration. However, in some clinical situations, such as extensive horizontal or vertical ridge augmentation, there is still a need for nonresorbable membranes to maintain the integrity of the area to be regenerated while it is under pressure from the surrounding tissues.[12]

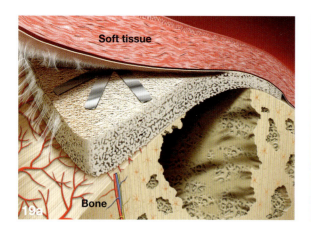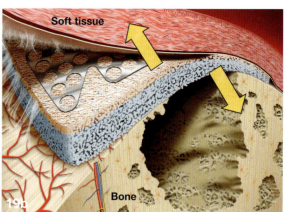

Fig 19 (a) *Characteristics of the original ePTFE membrane.* (b) *Characteristics of the new dual-surface membrane.*

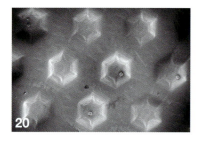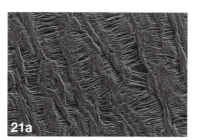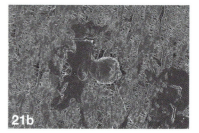

Fig 20 *Scanning electron microscope (SEM) image showing the surface characteristics of a dPTFE (cytoplast) membrane. ×100 magnification* **Fig 21** (a) *SEM image showing the surface characteristics of a multilayer, dual-surface ePTFE membrane. ×1,000 magnification.* (b) *Fibroblasts adhered to a multilayer, dual-surface ePTFE membrane*

Surgical techniques

After the period of preclinical research, which started in the second half of the 1980s under the leadership of Sture Nyman and Christer Dahlin,[10–15,19] the clinical use of GBR using ePTFE membranes was evaluated by several research groups worldwide. The first clinical studies, published in 1989 and the early 1990s,[20–25] were mainly concerned with the treatment of implants placed in extraction sites with three- to four-walled defects and the treatment of implant dehiscence defects and fenestrations. The results, while encouraging, nevertheless showed considerable problems with the effectiveness and reliability of the surgical technique. Complications were frequent and mainly involved the collapse of the membrane into the defect or its premature exposure with consequent infection of the deep tissues undergoing regeneration.

Thus, in 1990, began the period of developing a more suitable technique, which effectively ended in 1996. It was immediately understood that the membrane needed to be supported and stabilized to maintain an adequate space for bone regeneration. Support screws with particulate autologous bone grafts were used as both space maintainers and to stabilize the blood clot and provide an osteogenic effect. The addition of a graft material under the membranes made it possible to reduce healing times and increase the effectiveness of the regenerative technique.

In addition, ePTFE membranes with a thin, malleable titanium scaffold, which could be molded to predetermine the shape and size of the regenerated bone, were produced by a research group at Gore. The flap design used in the surgical technique was also modified to reduce the incidence of wound dehiscence and consequent premature exposure of the membrane. Full-thickness flaps were extended beyond the defect to at least one adjacent tooth element, and periosteal releasing incisions and horizontal mattress ePTFE sutures with a simple interrupted suture technique were also introduced.

By 1996, the refined surgical technique allowed for not only the treatment of small intraosseous or dehiscence-type defects but also for extensive horizontal and vertical bone regeneration in atrophic alveolar ridges.[26–33] Extraordinarily, the surgical technique remains the same today and has undergone only slight evolution aimed at reducing its invasiveness. The introduction of resorbable membranes made from collagen of animal origin and particulate bone grafts of homologous and heterologous origin have been the major changes.[28–30]

LONG-TERM STUDIES ON GBR

Since 1996, the focus of researchers and clinicians has been on evaluating the long-term effectiveness of GBR techniques via prospective and retrospective studies. Numerous long-term studies with follow-ups of more than 10 years have demonstrated the predictability of GBR techniques and its various indications. **Table 1** summarizes some of the significant literature.[34–40] The first long-term retrospective clinical study on vertical bone regeneration of atrophic alveolar ridges was published by Simion et al in 2001.[41] This multicenter study evaluated 123 Brånemark-style implants with machined surfaces placed in vertically regenerated bone in 49 patients with a follow-up of 1 to 5 years after prosthetic loading. The implants were allowed to protrude above the atrophic bone ridge from 2 to 7 mm and covered with a titanium-reinforced ePTFE membrane.

The patients were divided into three groups: In group A, the space under the membrane was filled with only the blood clot, in group B with demineralized freeze-dried bone allograft (DFDBA), and in group C with autologous bone particles. Upon removal of the membrane, group C showed the greatest amount of vertical bone regeneration, with bone levels often coronal to the implant head. The vertical marginal bone loss (MBL) in subsequent years was 1.35 mm for group A, 1.87 mm for group B, and 1.71 mm in group C. Only 1 out of 123 implants had not osseointegrated, and only 2 implants showed MBL exceeding the limits for success described by Albrektsson et al.[42] The authors concluded that vertically regenerated bone using GBR techniques responds to implant placement in the same way as native, nonregenerated bone.

Similar results were obtained in a study published in 2004 on 38 machined implants placed in atrophic alveolar ridges in the maxillary posterior sectors with vertical regeneration associated with sinus elevation.[43] At follow-ups of 1 to 7 years, the MBL was 1.68 mm. Along the same lines, a study by Urban et al[44] showed high success rates (94.7%) in 84 implants in vertical elevations with a follow-up of 12 to 72 months.

A recent retrospective study by Simion et al[36] reported the clinical and radiographic results of 91 machined implants placed in vertically regenerated bone in 33 patients with a follow-up of 13 to 21 years (average 15 years).

The patients included in the study were treated with vertical ridge augmentation between 1992 to 2000, with follow-up visits between April 2013 and December 2014. Analysis with periapical radiographs showed MBL of 1.02 mm, demonstrating great stability of the vertically regenerated bone. Only 9.9% of the implants showed moderate or slow bone resorption over the years, resulting in an implant survival rate of 94%.

THE FUTURE OF GBR

The application of a membrane to prevent soft tissue cells from entering the underlying bone defect is a well-established practice that has been successfully improved clinically.

In the future, the classic role of membranes acting as a passive barriers and mere graft containers may change so that they take on a more bioactive role and guide healing events during regeneration. Multilayer membranes with modified composition and structural characteristics are also being investigated.[45]

A careful review of GBR literature indicates that biologic events both on the membrane and in the underlying tissues are important for bone regeneration. Based on current trends and knowledge, future scientific developments focusing on specific membrane properties (eg, porosity, thickness, affinity to cells) can be expected.

Furthermore, structural differences that influence the regulation of cellular and molecular events within the membrane and in the protected area of the bone defect are being explored.

The authors foresee a renewed interest in and development of nonresorbable membranes, especially with regard to more advanced applications. The original nonresorbable membrane from WL Gore, which consisted of multilayer ePTFE with parallel fibrils, is no longer commercially available. Its successors are made of dense polytetrafluoroethylene (dPTFE), a material with a more solid structure in which pores are created for tissue retention. Recently, an ePTFE membrane with a unique surface on each side has been introduced both experimentally and clinically **(Figs 19 to 21)**. This material was compared with dPTFE in rat femur defects.

Preliminary results have shown many molecular differences between the two types of PTFE membranes, but the differences were more involved with the surrounding soft tissue rather than the bone within the defect.

For example, the expression of the FGF-2 and vascular endothelial growth factor (VEGF) genes in the overlying soft tissue was overregulated in only the ePTFE membranes with double surface area.[45]

Similarly, bone substitutes could be modified to trigger specific cellular and molecular events during bone regeneration. Another area of great potential is the possible application of mesenchymal cells to bone substitutes and membranes to stimulate healing.

GBR research will likely not develop with separate projects on membranes or bone substitutes. Recent findings suggest that they are closely intertwined throughout the healing phases and should therefore be considered together.[46,47]

Table 1 Studies on implants placed in regenerated bone (follow-ups of 10 or more years.

Article	Implant survival	Implant no.	Patient no.	Follow-up (y)	Mean Bone Loss MBL (mm)	Type of regeneration
Thoma et al (2019)[34]	100%	27	19	10.2	1.75 ± 1.11	Autogenous bone with collagen membrane and DBBM
Roccuzzo et al (2017)[35]	94.1%	68	34	10	0.43 ± 0.50 (patients with healthy periodontium) 0.78 ± 0.59 (patients with healthy periodontium)	Autogenous bone and articulate bone with/without titanium mesh
Simion et al (2016)[36]	96.7%	91	33	15	1.02 ± 1.47	Vertical guided bone regeneration with ePTFE membranes
Meijndert et al (2017)[37]	95.7%	93	93	10	0.48 ± 1.19 (mesial) 0.30 ± 1.24 (distal)	Augmentation with *(1)* chin bone with/without membrane and *(2)* bone substitute with membrane
Chappuis et al (2017)[38]	98.1%	52	38	10	0.17 ± 0.23 (maxilla) 0.09 ± 0.43 (mandible)	Autogenous bone with collagen membrane and DBBM
Roccuzzo et al (2014)[39]	100%	19	19	1	0.21 ± 0.42	Preservation of the alveolar ridge
Jung et al (2013)[40]	91.9% 92.6%	72	112 41	12.5	2.40 2.53	Collagen membrane with DBBM ePTFE with DBBM

MBL = marginal bone loss; DBBM = demineralized bovine bone.

C. Dahlin • M. Simion

CLINICAL CASE 1

Vertical bone regeneration in the sites of the maxillary right second premolar, first molar, and second molar in a periodontal patient with a 26-year follow-up

A 51-year-old patient who was in good health and did not smoke presented with severe periodontitis in 1992. The intraoral and radiographic examination revealed partial edentulism in the first quadrant associated with severe vertical atrophy of the bone crest, edentulousness of the third quadrant, and severe suprabony and infrabony defects spread over most of the dental elements. In particular, the maxillary left second premolar and first molar appeared to be irreparably compromised (Figs 22 and 23). After complete causal therapy and the extraction of the maxillary left second premolar and first molar, the patient underwent vertical ridge augmentation with GBR simultaneously with the placement of three machined implants in the positions of the maxillary right second premolar, first molar, and second molar. The implants were placed 7 mm supracrestal and were

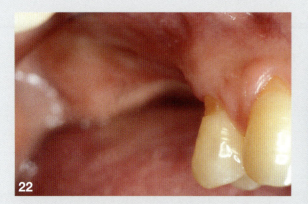
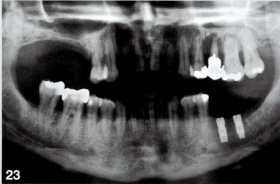

Fig 22 Severe vertical bone atrophy in the first quadrant. **Fig 23** Panoramic radiograph showing diffuse periodontal disease and minimal residual bone in the sites of the maxillary right second premolar and first and second molars.

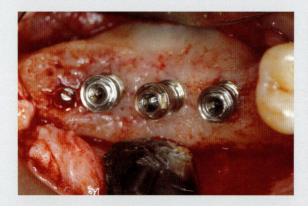
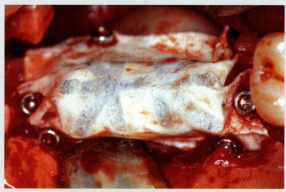

Fig 24 Three machined implants were placed in a 7-mm supracrestal position.

Fig 25 A titanium-reinforced ePTFE membrane was fixed with several mini-screws, and the space was filled with a blood clot.

covered with a titanium-reinforced ePTFE Gore-Tex membrane (**Figs 24 and 25**). The space below the membrane was filled with the patient's blood to develop an adequate blood clot without the addition of graft materials.

Healing took place without early or late complications (**Figs 26 and 27**). After 9 months, a full-thickness flap was elevated, and the membrane was removed, revealing partial vertical bone regeneration limited to half of the exposed part of the implant (**Figs 28 and 29**). On periapical radiographic examination, the limited regeneration caused by the lack of a particulate bone graft stimulating regeneration in such a large vertical defect was evident (**Fig 30**).

The patient was placed on a maintenance protocol for periodontitis with quarterly appointments. At the radiographic follow-up after 5 years, additional mineralization of the regenerated bone was evident both crestally and within the maxillary sinus (**Fig 31**). At the 21- and 26-year follow-ups, continued mineralization in the coronal direction could be observed, probably due to masticatory function with healthy peri-implant tissues (**Figs 32 and 33**).

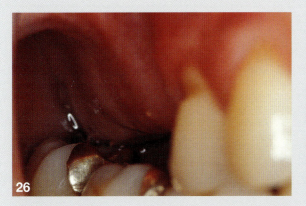
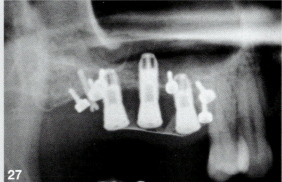

Fig 26 Healing occurred without any complications. **Fig 27** Postoperative radiograph. Note the titanium structure of the membrane and the fixation instruments.

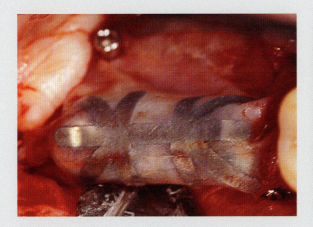
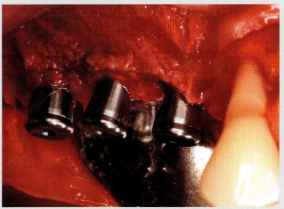

Fig 28 After 9 months of healing, the membrane was removed.

Fig 29 The implants appear partially covered by regenerated bone.

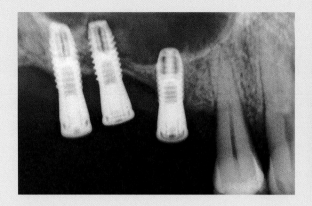

Fig 30 Periapical radiograph showing only partial bone regeneration due to the absence of graft material associated with the membrane.

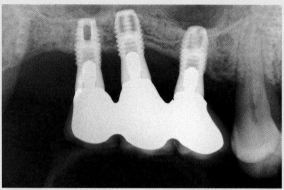

Fig 31 Radiographic control after 5 years of supportive therapy. Mineralization of the peri-implant bone, both crestal and within the maxillary sinus, can be seen.

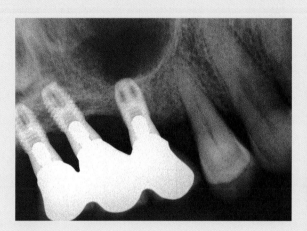

Fig 32 Radiograph after 21 years.

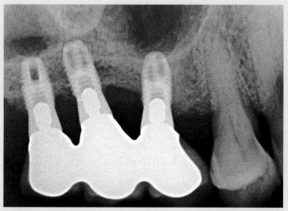

Fig 33 Radiograph after 26 years. A continuous mineralization process of the crestal bone over the years is evident, probably due to masticatory function in the presence of healthy peri-implant tissues.

CLINICAL CASE 2

Vertical bone regeneration from the site of the maxillary right incisor to the right first premolar with 22-year follow-up

A healthy, nonsmoking 21-year-old patient suffered a serious automobile accident in 1996. The accident resulted in the traumatic avulsion of the maxillary right central incisor, lateral incisor, and canine, associated with severe vertical alveolar bone loss **(Fig 34)**. The periapical radiograph showed that the maxillary right first premolar was fractured horizontally in the apical third **(Fig 35)**. The patient underwent GBR. Elevation of the flap revealed an 18-mm vertical bone defect from the mesial to the distal bone peak **(Fig 36)**. A palatal ePTFE membrane was secured with two titanium pins, and the defect was filled with autologous bone particles taken from the ascending ramus of the mandible **(Fig 37)**.

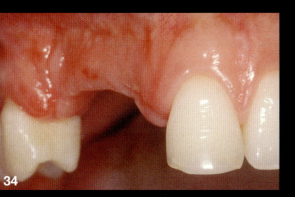
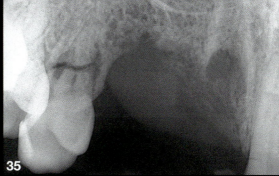

Fig 34 Atrophic alveolar ridge after an automobile accident. The maxillary right central incisor, lateral incisor, and canine are absent, and the severe ridge deficiency in both the horizontal and vertical directions is evident. **Fig 35** Periapical radiograph showing the bone defect and the horizontal fracture of the root of the first premolar.

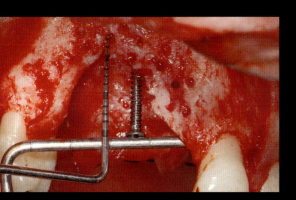
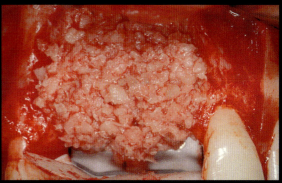

Fig 36 Intraoperative image of the 18-mm vertical bone defect from the mesial to the distal peak. A support screw for the reinforced membrane was placed.

Fig 37 A titanium-reinforced ePTFE membrane was fixed palatally with pins, and a particulate autologous bone graft was placed in the defect.

then, the membrane was secured with two buccal pins (Fig 38). After 1 month of healing without complications, the fractured first premolar was removed to avoid potential infection secondary to pulpal necrosis (Figs 39 and 40).

After an additional 6 months of healing, the membrane was removed, and three machined implants were placed in the position of the maxillary right central incisor, canine, and first premolar (Figs 41 and 42). In the same operation, a connective tissue graft was harvested from the palate and placed to increase soft tissue thickness (Figs 43 and 44).

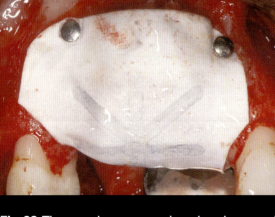

Fig 38 The membrane was closed and secured with buccal pins, avoiding the roots of adjacent teeth.

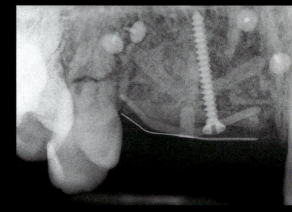

Fig 39 Postoperative periapical radiograph showing the graft, membrane, and fixation instruments.

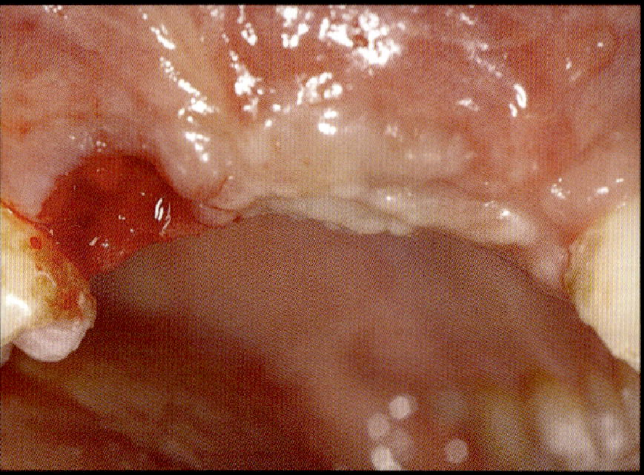

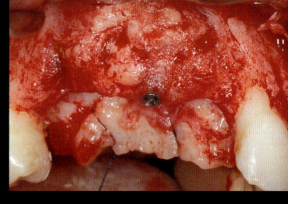

Fig 40 The fractured maxillary first premolar was extracted to avoid possible complications.

Fig 41 After 7 months of submerged healing, the membrane was removed. The regenerated bone tissue appears to be of good quality and coronal to the area of the premolar extracted without alveolar ridge preservation.

The implants remained submerged for 4 months. Then, the second phase of implant surgery was carried out to connect the prosthetic abutments.

The provisional prosthesis was left in place for 6 months, pending tissue maturation, when the definitive alumina and ceramic prosthesis was placed (Fig 45).

Follow-ups after 16 and 22 years showed a slight passive eruption and modest gingival recession at the level of the natural teeth but complete stability of the bone and mucosal levels at the implant sites in regenerated bone (Figs 46 to 49).

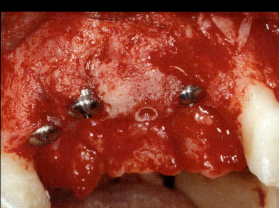

Fig 42 Three machined implants were placed in the locations of the maxillary right central incisor, canine, and first premolar.

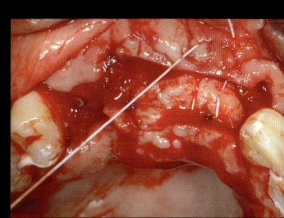

Fig 43 A connective tissue graft harvested from the palate was placed to increase soft tissue thickness.

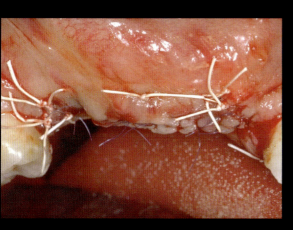

Fig 44 The flaps were sutured, and the implants were left to integrate in a submerged position for 4 months.

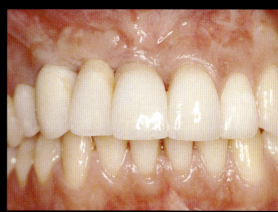

Fig 45 After the prosthetic abutments were connected and the tissue matured for 6 months with a provisional, a definitive alumina and ceramic prosthesis was placed. (Courtesy of Professor F. Zarone.)

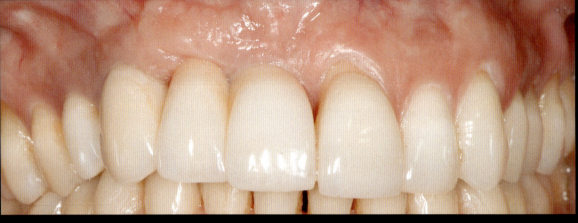

Fig 46 After 16 years of function, slight extrusion of the natural teeth and tissue stability at the implant sites can be seen.

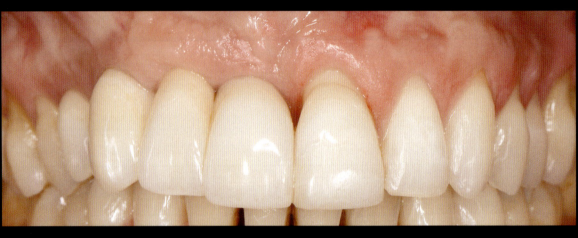

Fig 47 Clinical follow-up after 22 years. There is gingival recession at the level of the natural teeth, but the peri-implant soft tissue is stable and clinically healthy.

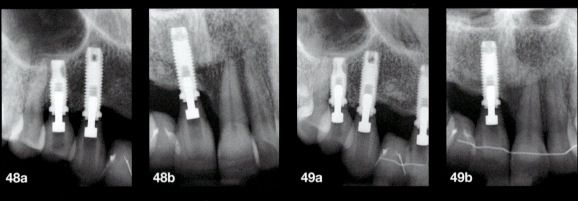

48a 48b 49a 49b

Fig 48 *(a and b)* Periapical radiographs after 16 years showing stability of the peri-implant bone margins. **Fig 49** *(a and b)* Periapical radiographs after 22 years showing the complete stability of the peri-implant bone tissue regenerated with GBR.

REFERENCES

1. Kalkworf Kl. Periodontal new attachment without the placement of osseous potentiating grafts. Periodontal Abstr 1974;22:53–62.

2. Melcher AH. On repair potential of periodontal tissues. J Periodontol 1976;47:256–260.

3. Caton J, Nyman S. Histometric evaluation of periodontal surgery I. The modified Widman flap procedure. J Clin Periodontol 1980;7:212–223.

4. Caton J, Nyman S, Zander H. Hisometric evaluation of periodontal surgery II. Connective tissue attachment levels after four regenerative procedures. J Clin Periodontol 1980;7:224–231.

5. Nyman S, Lindhe J, Karring T. Healing following surgical treatment and root demineralisation in monkeys with periodontal disease. J Clin Periodontol 1981;8:249–258.

6. Nyman S, Karring T, Lindhe J, Platén S. Healing following implantation of periodontitis-affected roots into gingival connective tissue. J Clin Periodontol 1980;7:394–401.

7. Nyman S, Gottlow J, Karring T, Lindhe J. The regenerative potential of the periodontal ligament. An experimental study in monkeys. J Clin Periodontol 1982;9:157–265.

8. Nyman S, Lindhe, Karring T, Rylander H. New attachment following surgical treatment of human periodontal disease. J Clin Periodontol 1982;9:290–296.

9. Gottlow J, Nyman S, Lindhe J, Karring T, Wennström J. New attachment formation in the human periodontium by guided tissue regeneration. Case reports. J Clin Periodontol 1986;13:604–616.

10. Dahlin C, Gottlow J, Linde A, Nyman S. Healing of bone defects by guided tissue regeneration. Plast Reconstr Surg 1988;81:672–676.

11. Dahlin C, Sennerby L, Lekholm U, Linde A, Nyman S. Generation of new bone around titanium implants using a membrane technique: An experimental study in rabbits. Int J Oral Maxillofac Implants 1989;4:19–25.

12. Retzepi M, Donos N. Guided bone regeneration: Biological principle and therapeutic applications. Clin Oral Implants Res 2010;21:567–576.

13. Schenk RK, Buser D, Hardwick R, Dahlin C. Healing pattern of bone regeneration in membrane-protected defects: A histologic and histomorphometric study in the mandible of dogs. Int J Oral Maxillofac Implants 1994;9:13–29.

14. Buser D, Ruskin J, Higginbottom F, Hardwick R, Dahlin C, Schenk R. Osseointegration of titanium implants in regenerated bone in membrane-protected defects. A histologic study in the canine mandible. Int J Oral Maxillofac implants 1995;10:666–681.

15. Simon M, Dahlin C, Blair K, Schenk R. Effect of 3 different types of titanium reinforced membranes on bone regeneration in surgically crated defects: A histological study in canine model. Clin Oral Implants Res 1999;10:73–84.

16. Hardwick R, Scantlebury T, Sanchez R, Whitley N, Ambruster J. Membrane design criteria for guided bone regeneration of the alveolar ridge. In: Buser D, Dahlin C, Schenk R (eds). Guided Bone Regeneration in Implant Dentistry. Quintessence, 1994:101–136.

17. Elgali I, Igawa K, Palmquist A, et al. Molecular and structural patterns of bone regeneration in surgically created defects containing bone substitutes. Biomaterials 2014;35:3229–3242.

18. Elgali I, Turri A, Xia W, et al. Guided bone regeneration using resorbable membrane and different bone substitutes: Early histological and molecular events. Acta Biomater 2016;29:409–423.

19. Simion M, Dahlin C, Rocchietta I, Stavropulos A, Sanchez R, Karring T. Vertical ridge augmentation with guided bone regeneration in association with dental implants: An experimental study in dogs. Clin Oral Implants Res 2007;18:8–94.

20. Jovanovic SA, Spiekermann H, Richter EJ. Bone regeneration around titanium implants in dehisced defect sites: A clinical study. Int J Oral Maxillofac Implants 1992;7:233–245.

21. Dahlin C, Lekholm U, Becker WB, Higuchi K, Callens A, van Steenberghe D. Treatment of fenestration and dehiscence bone defects around oral implants using the guided tissue regeneration technique: A prospective multicenter study. Int J Oral Maxillofac Implants 1995;10:312–318.

22. Simion M, Misitano U, Gionso L, Salvato A. Treatment of dehiscence and fenestrations around dental implants using resorbable and non-resorbable membranes associated with bone autografts: A comparative clinical study. In J Oral Maxillofac Implants 1997;12:159–167.

23. Buser D, Brägger U, Lang NP, Nyman S. Regeneration and enlargement of jaw bone using guided tissue regeneration. Clin Oral Implant Res 1990;1:22–32.

24. Buser D, Dula K, Belser U, Hirt HP, Bertold H. Localized ridge augmentation using guided bone regeneration prior to implant placement. Surgical procedure in the maxilla. Int J Periodontics Restorative Dent 1993;13:29–45.

25. Nevins R, Mellonig JT. The advantage of localised ridge augmentation prior to implant placement. A staged event. Int J Periodontics Restorative Dent 1994;14: 97–111.

26. Buser D, Dula K, Hirt HP, Schenk R. Lateral ridge augmentation using autografts and barrier membranes: A clinical study with 40 partially edentulous patients. J Oral Maxillofac Surg 1996;54:420–432.

27. Von Arx T, Buser D. Horizontal ridge augmentation using autogenous block grafts and the guided bone regeneration technique with collagen membranes: A clinical study with 42 patients. Clin Oral Implants Res 2006;17:359–336.

28. Hammerle CH, Jung RE, Yaman D, Lang NP. Ridge augmentation by applying bioresorbable membranes and deproteinized bovine bone mineral: A report of 12 consecutive cases. Clin Oral Implants Res 2008;19:19–25.

29. Urban IA, Nagursky H, Lozada JL. Horizontal ridge augmentation with a resorbable membrane and particulated autogenous bone with or without anorganic bovine bone-derived mineral: A prospective case series in 22 patients. Int J Oral Maxillofac Implants 2011;26:404–414.

30. Urban IA, Nagursky H, Lozada JL, Nagy K. Horizontal ridge augmentation with a collagen membrane and a combination of particulate autogenous bone and anorganic bovine bone-derived mineral: A prospective case series in 25 patients. Int J Periodontics Restorative Dent 2013;33:299–307.

31. Meloni SM, Jovanovic SA, Urban I, Canullo L, Pisano M, Tallarico M. Horizontal ridge augmentation using GBR with a native collagen membrane and 1:1 ratio of particulate xenograft and autologous bone: A 1-year prospective clinical study. Clin Implants Dent Relat Res 2017;19:38–45.

32. Simion M, Trisi P, Piattelli A. Vertical ridge augmentation using a membrane technique associated with osseointegrated implants. Int J Periodontics Restorative Dent 1994;14:496–511.

33. Simion M, Jovanovic SA, Trisi P, Scarano A, Piattelli A. Vertical ridge augmentation around dental implants using a membrane technique and autogenous bone or allografts in humans. Int J Periodontics Restorative Dent 1998;18:8–23.

34. Thoma DS, Bienz SP, Figuero E, Jung RE, Sanz-Martín I. Efficacy of lateral bone augmentation performed simultaneously with dental implant placement. A systematic review with meta-analysis. J Clin Periodontol 2019;46(Suppl 21):257–276.

35. Roccuzzo M, Savoini M, Dalmasso P, Ramieri G. Long-term outcomes of implants placed after vertical alveolar ridge augmentation in partially edentulous patients: A 10-year prospective clinical study. Clin Oral Implants Res 2017;28:1204–1210.

36. Simion M, Ferrantino L, Idotta E, Zarone F. Turned implants in vertical augmented bone: A retrospective study with 13 to 21 years follow-up. Int J Periodontics Restorative Dent 2016;36:309–317.

37. Meijndert CM, Raghoebar GM, Meijndert L, Stellingsma K, Vissink A, Meijer HJ. Single implants in the aesthetic region preceded by local ridge augmentation; A 10-year randomised controlled trial. Clin Oral Implants Res 2017;28:388–395.

38. Chappuis V, Cavusoglu Y, Buser D, Von Arx T. Lateral ridge augmentation using autogenous block grafts and guided bone regeneration: A 10-year prospective case series study. Clin Implant Dent Relat Res 2017;19: 85–96.

39. Roccuzzo M, Gaudioso L, Bunino M, Dalmasso P. Long-term stability of soft tissues following alveolar ridge preservation: 10-year results of a prospective study around nonsubmerged implants. Int J Periodontics Restorative Dent 2014;34:795–804.

40. Jung RE, Fenner N, Hämmerle CH, Zitzmann NU. Long-term outcome of implants placed with guided bone regeneration (GBR) using resorbable and non-resorbable membranes after 12-14 years. Clin Oral Implants Res 2013;24:1065–1073.

41. Simion M, Jovanovic SA, Tinti C, Benfenati SP. Long-term evaluation of osseointegrated implants inserted at the time or after vertical ridge augmentation. A retrospective study on 123 implants with 1-5 year follow-up. Clin Oral Implants Res 2001;12:35–45.

42. Albrektsson T, Zarb G, Worthington P, Eriksson AR. The long term efficacy of currently used dental implants: A review and proposal criteria of success. Int J Oral Maxillofac Implants 1986;1:11–25.

43. Simion M, Fontana F, Rasperini G, Maiorana C. Long-term evaluation of osseointegrated implants placed in sites augmented with sinus floor elevation associated with vertical ridge augmentation: A retrospective study of 38 consecutive implants with 1- to 7-year follow-up. Int J Periodontics Restorative Dent 2004;24:208–221.

44. Urban IA, Jovanovic SA, Lozada JL. Vertical ridge augmentation using guided bone regeneration (GBR) in three clinical scenarios prior to implant placement: A retrospective study of 35 patients 12 to 72 months after loading. Int J Oral Maxillofac Implants 2009;24:502–510.

45. Omar O, Trobos M, Johansson A, Emanuelsson L, Sahlin H, Dahlin C. Pr586: Molecular events in bone and soft tissue at different non-resorbable PTFE membranes during GBR. J Clin Periodontol 2018;9:320.

46. Omar O, Elgali I, Dahlin C, Thomsen P. Barrier membranes: More than the barrier effect? J Clin Periodontol 2019;46(Suppl 21):103–123.

47. Elgali I, Omar O, Dahlin C, Thomsen P. Guided bone regeneration: Materials and biological mechanisms revisited. Eur J Oral Sci 2017;125:315–337.

SURGICAL TECHNIQUES FOR GUIDED BONE REGENERATION

CHAPTER 15

Edited by Massimo Simion

INTRODUCTION

The only weakness of guided bone regeneration (GBR) is its complexity and the fact that it is extremely dependent on the skill of the clinician. This surgery requires delicacy and can be considered more similar to periodontal surgery than to oral or maxillofacial surgery. Although the surgical protocol is well standardized and has not undergone substantial change in decades,[1–3] countless variables can affect the course of this procedure, which requires experience and manual dexterity. The best surgeons not only make few mistakes but also manage unfavorable and unforeseen situations effectively.

Prior to surgery, the treatment of any periodontitis and the adequate control of bacterial plaque is essential to avoid intraoperative infections. Complete sterility should be ensured when preparing the operating field and instrumentation.

Mastering guided bone regeneration (GBR) techniques requires detailed knowledge of all the surgical steps and great care in their application. These are not techniques with which one can improvise. Techniques developed during 30 years of experience should be followed to the letter.

Massimo Simion

FLAP DESIGN

Flap designs for all GBR techniques share common features, both for one and two-stage surgeries. A general principle is to create flaps with a wide base for blood supply to avoid ischemic phenomena that may lead to marginal flap necrosis and premature membrane exposure. Because regenerative techniques always involve increasing the volume of bone beneath the flap, it is necessary to have the option of displacing the flaps coronally to cover the membrane and bone graft without causing tension at the time of suturing.

Flap design differs slightly depending on the area of the mouth that will be treated and whether the area is partially or completely edentulous. When performing crestal incisions, the position of the incision in interspersed or distal edentulous areas of the maxilla differs from that in the mandible. Whereas in the mandible both the buccal and lingual flaps can be repositioned coronally with a periosteal incision, in the maxilla, only the buccal flap can be released and moved in a coronal direction. This is due to the rigidity of the palatal flap, which does not have a lax submucosa.

Thus, crestal incisions in the maxilla are performed in a distinctly buccal position to compensate for the discrepancy between the flaps at the time of suturing. The complete flap design is comprised of two slightly divergent vertical incisions extending at least one tooth beyond the edentulous area, intrasulcular buccal and palatal incisions in the adjacent teeth, and a slightly buccal crestal incision. The vertical releasing incisions must have a golf club shape. From the buccal aspect, the clinician incises at the level of the interproximal space distal to the adjacent tooth by pointing at the papilla. Before reaching the vertex, the incision is redirected toward the gingival margin and continues intrasulcularly **(Fig 1)**. All incisions must be full-thickness. In the distal portion of the maxilla, flap design has the same characteristics except for the distal vertical incision which, of course, is made in the edentulous mucosa **(Fig 2)**. No vertical palatal incisions are made. In the mandible, flaps have the same design characteristics except that the crestal incision is made in the center of the residual keratinized mucosa so that only half of it is left on the buccal aspect and the remaining half is left on the lingual aspect

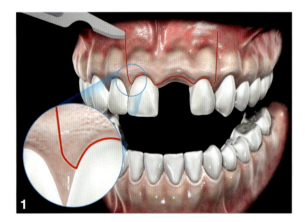 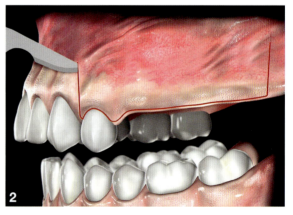

Fig 1 *Incision for GBR surgery in a single maxillary anterior edentulous site. Vertical releasing incisions one tooth beyond the defect with a golf club shape and a slightly buccal crestal incision and intrasulcular incisions are performed.* **Fig 2** *Incision for maxillary distal edentulous sites. The vertical incision is distally positioned in the alveolar mucosa.*

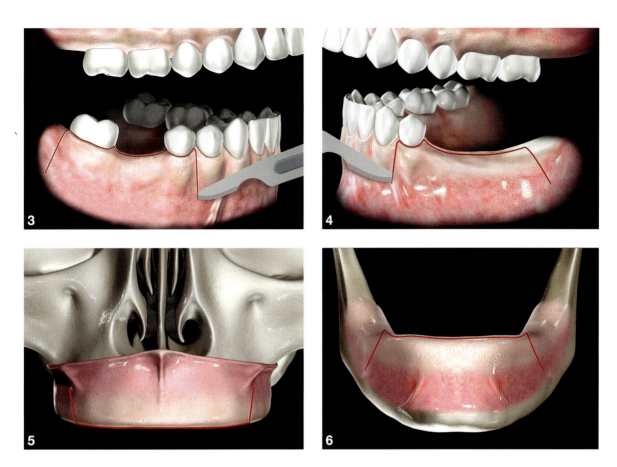

Fig 3 Incision for a mandibular edentulous span. Vertical incisions are used to release the mucosa one tooth beyond the golf club–shaped defect, along with a crestal incision in the center of the keratinized mucosa and intrasulcular incisions. *Fig 4* Incisions for distal mandibular edentulous spans are the same, with the distal vertical vestibular incision through the alveolar mucosa. *Fig 5* Flap design for GBR in a completely edentulous maxilla. *Fig 6* Flap design for a completely edentulous mandible.

(Figs 3 and 4). No vertical lingual incisions are made. In completely edentulous arches, the flap design is exactly the same as in cases of implants being placed without GBR techniques (see chapter 5) **(Figs 5 and 6).**

Periosteal releasing incisions

A key step for successful regenerative therapy is creating a periosteal releasing incision at the base of the flap to increase its elasticity and allow it to stretch in the coronal direction. In buccal and lingual flaps, the only inextensible anatomical structure is the periosteum, so by interrupting the connective fibers within it, the flaps can be extended easily to cover the membrane and bone graft without tension at the time of suturing. A single continuous incision must be made from the inside of the distal vertical incision to the inside of the mesial (or contralateral distal) incision **(Fig 7)**. Even a small portion of intact periosteum prevents adequate flap release.

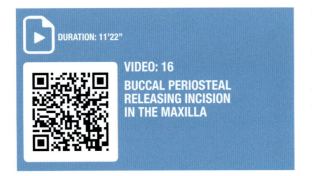

DURATION: 11'22"

VIDEO: 16
BUCCAL PERIOSTEAL
RELEASING INCISION
IN THE MAXILLA

In patients who have edentulous sites as a consequence of severe traumatic injuries and in patients with scars from previous operations, the periosteum may be thickened and the submucosal connective tissue may be extremely fibrous and rigid. In these cases, a simple incision at the periosteum may not be sufficient. The incision must be continued apically, with partial-thickness scoring with the scalpel performed until a normal, extensible submucosa is found. In all cases, after periosteal release, two surgical tweezers are used to pull the flap in all directions to stretch the collagen fibers **(Fig 8)**.

The posterolateral buccal and lingual areas of the mandible require special attention.

The emergence of the inferior alveolar nerve (IAN) from the mental foramen, typically situated between the two inferior premolars (see chapter 2), exposes the nerve to the risk of injury during the periosteal incision.

After emerging, the nerve divides into three separate branches that run into the alveolar mucosa immediately below the periosteum.

In this area, therefore, an upward loop must be performed with the scalpel to move away from the foramen, where the nerves are more superficial. As a precaution, cutting the periosteum directly can be avoided. Instead, it can be loosened by using the scalpel blade like a razor blade and simultaneously exerting traction on the flap with

surgical tweezers. This maneuver, referred to as "shaving the periosteum," results in the gentle defibration of the periosteum in a manner similar to stretching a nylon stocking, and it does not run the risk of injuring the nerve **(Figs 9 and 10)**.

The lingual periosteum of the posterolateral mandible is very delicate and can be released with great ease, but the presence of important nerve and vascular structures in the immediate vicinity (see chapter 2) means that this procedure must be performed with great care. From distal to mesial, two zones can be distinguished **(Fig 11)**. In the distal portion, the area of the retromolar trigone and the molars, the periosteum is easily dissected without sharp instruments; it is sufficient to exert traction on the flap and reflect it with a blunt periosteal elevator up to the insertion of the mylohyoid muscle.

To avoid injuring the lingual nerve, contact must never be lost between the periosteal elevator and the medial surface of the horizontal branch of the mandible **(Fig 12)**.

In the more mesial portion, the area of the premolars, canines, and incisors, the mylohyoid muscle inserts more deeply and the periosteum becomes more resistant, so in many cases, it is necessary to score it with the tip of the scalpel by turning the blade on the non-cutting side while at the same time exerting traction on the flap **(Figs 13 and 14)**.

DURATION: 09'03"

VIDEO: 17
BUCCAL AND LINGUAL
PERIOSTEAL INCISIONS
IN THE MANDIBLE

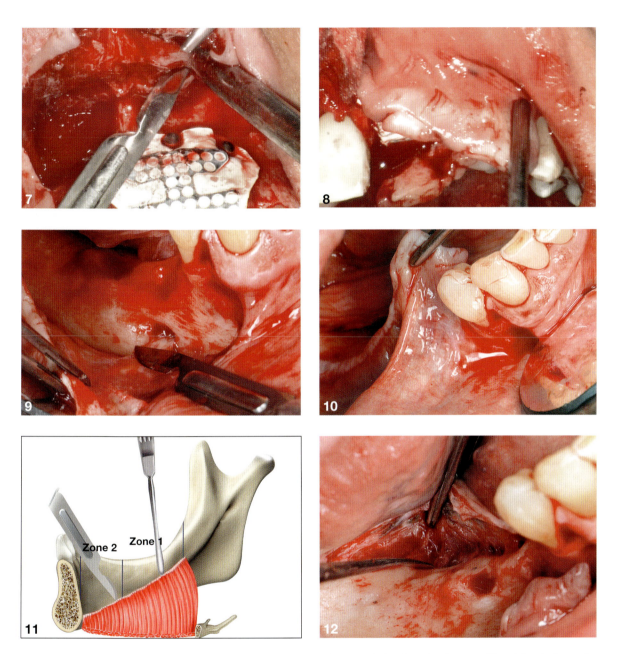

Fig 7 *Continuous periosteal releasing incision at the base of the flap in the maxilla.* **Fig 8** *Stretching the periosteum in all directions to stretch the connective fibers after the periosteal incision.* **Fig 9** *Release of the periosteum in the vicinity of the mental foramen. A loop is performed toward the coronal aspect, and the scalpel blade is used like a razor while exerting traction on the flap in a coronal direction.* **Fig 10** *Pulling the periosteum coronally and lingually to stretch the connective fibers after the periosteal incision.* **Fig 11** *Scoring of the lingual periosteum. In zone 1, where the periosteum is very thin and fragile, it is easily lacerated with a blunt scalpel by exerting coronal traction on the flap. In zone 2, which is more mesial and where the periosteum is stronger, it is necessary to scrape it with the tip of the scalpel, again exerting coronal traction.* **Fig 12** *Scoring the lingual periosteum in zone 1 with a blunt periosteal elevator adherent to the bone and coronal traction of the flap.*

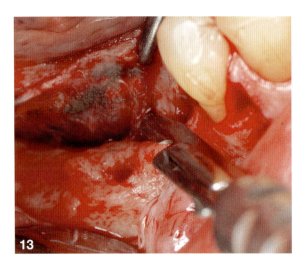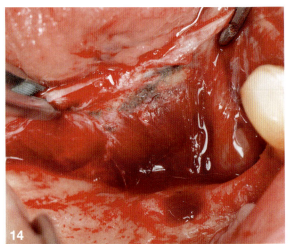

*Fig 13 Scoring the lingual periosteum in zone 2 by scraping it with the tip of the scalpel and exerting coronal traction on the flap. **Fig 14** Stretching the lingual flap in the coronal direction with two surgical tweezers.*

Some authors have proposed a digital technique of detaching the lingual flap without the use of cutting instruments to avoid any injury to the deep vascular-nervous structures.[4]

Releasing incisions at the periosteum can be made either at the beginning of the operation, after the flap has been elevated, or immediately before applying sutures. The disadvantage of an early incision is that the tissues tend to bleed profusely for a few minutes and thus obstruct the view during surgery. A late periosteal release has the advantages that sufficient lengthening or tensioning of the flaps can be checked directly before applying sutures and the graft and membrane having already been placed. On the other hand, profuse bleeding immediately before suturing may result in more extensive hematomas due to the sequestration of residual blood below the already closed flaps.

CHOOSING A MEMBRANE

There are fundamental properties that membranes used for GBR must have (see chapter 14):[5]

- biocompatibility
- occlusive effect on cells
- ability to integrate with tissues
- ability to maintain space
- easy to use

There are basically two classes of membranes that meet these qualifications—nonresorbable and resorbable membranes. They differ substantially from one another in their chemical, physical, and biologic characteristics and consequently in their indications.

Nonresorbable membranes

This material is not biodegradable but is extremely inert and has a very high biocompatibility. Once inserted into the body, it does not stimulate any

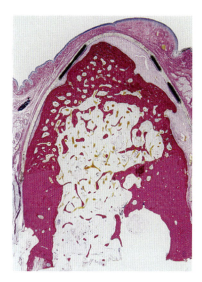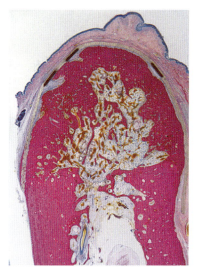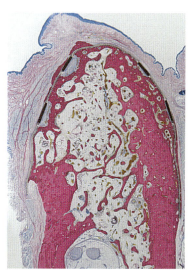

Fig 15 (a to c) *Histologic sections of three different titanium-reinforced ePTFE membranes. The titanium reinforcement within the membrane is evident. Toluidine blue and basic Fuchsin staining; ×2 magnification.*

inflammatory foreign body response. Most of the basic research on GTR/GBR was undertaken in the late 1980s by research groups supported by the WL Gore company, which funded a countless number of preclinical studies in its Flagstaff, Arizona, laboratories and prospective clinical studies in major universities around the world.[6–9] Gore's ePTFE membranes, now discontinued, consisted of a complex fibrillar structure capable of blocking the passage of connective tissue cells completely while allowing for the passage of fluids. They were, therefore, semiocclusive membranes capable of serving as barriers for GBR techniques. Their superficial fibrillar structure allowed for the integration of connective tissue external to the membrane, enabling good stabilization of the flaps during the healing process. In the early 1990s, problems with maintaining space for bone regeneration were solved by incorporating thin, malleable titanium structures that were bent and molded to predetermine the shape of the future alveolar ridge[8] **(Fig 15)**.

After the Gore-Tex membranes were withdrawn from the market for purely commercial reasons, new nonresorbable membranes with very similar characteristics made of dense PTFE (dPTFE), which has a non-fibrillar structure and is completely occlusive, have been available **(Fig 16)**. The clinical results obtained with dPTFE membranes are like those of their predecessors.[10,11] More recently, a new dual-surface, multilayer ePTFE membrane has been launched on the market **(Fig 17)**.

This membrane has elasticity and fibrillar surface characteristics similar to the original Gore-Tex membranes.

A common feature of all nonresorbable membranes is that they can be left in place indefinitely to allow for the regeneration of even very large volumes of bone and in critical situations from the point of view of regenerative potential, such as for vertical ridge augmentation.

A common disadvantage of these membranes, however, is that they are difficult to use and

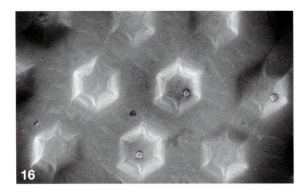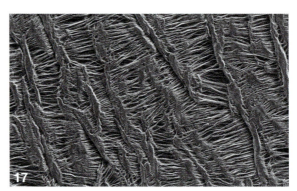

Fig 16 *Scanning electron microscope (SEM) image showing the surface characteristics of a dPTFE membrane (Cytoplast, Osteogenics). ×100 magnification.* Fig 17 *SEM image showing the characteristics of the dual-surface multilayer ePTFE membrane. ×1,000 magnification.*

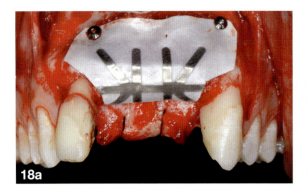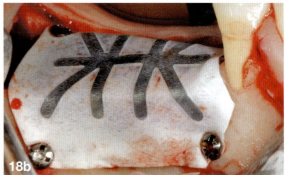

Fig 18 (a) *Correct positioning of an ePTFE membrane, trimmed and fixed with buccal and palatal titanium pins.* (b) *Membrane for posterolateral vertical mandibular augmentation fixed with mini-screws.*

require meticulous positioning and careful stabilization with mini-screws or fixation pins **(Fig 18)**. They also require a second operation for removal. Moreover, in the event of wound dehiscence and early exposure, their immediate removal is necessary to avoid rapid infection of the membrane and regenerating tissue. Given their maximum effectiveness, combined with their difficulty of use, nonresorbable membranes are currently indicated for the treatment of larger bone defects and in the most critical situations from the point of view of the regenerative potential of the site:

1. Extensive horizontal ridge augmentation
2. Vertical ridge augmentation

Resorbable membranes

In the second half of the 1990s, the need to simplify GBR and reduce its invasiveness led to the development of biodegradable membranes. These membranes combine greater ease of use with the ability to be resorbed within 1 to 2 months, thus eliminated the need for a second operation. Even in the case of early exposure, these membranes tend to reabsorb quickly without the risk of deep infection. Unfortunately, these tangible advantages are accompanied by lower efficacy, which means these membranes are contraindicated in larger defects and for vertical ridge augmentation. There are two main types of resorbable membranes:

- synthetic membranes (usually polylactic acid [PLA] and polyglycolic acid [PGA] or their polymers)
- type I collagen membranes of animal origin

PLA/PGA membranes are degraded into carbon dioxide and water during the Krebs cycle, but numerous studies have shown the presence of macrophages and multinucleated giant cells in the vicinity of the membrane during resorption.[12] Their use in clinical practice is currently limited, and membranes made of natural collagen (usually porcine) are preferred.

Collagen membranes have countless advantages, including ease of application, good biocompatibility, low antigenic response, hydrophilicity, and excellent integration, which makes them well-tolerated by the soft tissues **(Figs 19 and 20)**. In contrast, their efficacy is reduced due to their rapid enzymatic breakdown by macrophages and polymorphonuclear granulocytes and early resorption, which limits the barrier effect to the first month of healing.

To overcome this problem, collagen membranes treated with cross-linking technology were tested to prolong the resorption time. Cross-linking, obtained by applying ultraviolet radiation or performing treatment with alcohols or glutaraldehyde, increased the inflammatory response during the healing period and reduced its effectiveness in bone regeneration.[13] This is why cross-linked membranes are not used clinically.

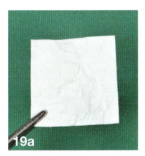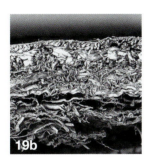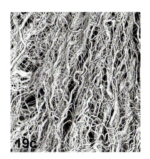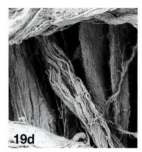

Fig 19 (a) *Resorbable porcine collagen membrane (Bio-Gide, Geistlich Biomaterials). (b) SEM image showing the two different layers of the membrane, superficial and deep (×750 magnification). (c) Higher magnification (×5,000) of the superficial portion. (d) Higher magnification (×5,150) of the deep portion.*

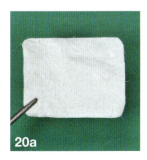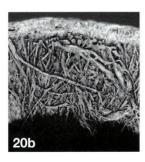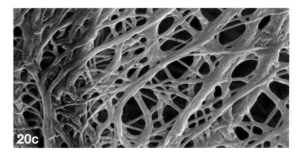

Fig 20 (a) *CellGro (Orthocell) porcine collagen resorbable membrane. (b) SEM image of a section (×750 magnification). (c) Higher magnification (×5,200).*

Another problem related to collagen membranes is their reduced mechanical resistance for maintaining space in non-containing defects. Bone and biomaterial grafts, which are the real agents of bone regeneration in these cases, are therefore of fundamental importance, with membranes playing a purely restraining and protective role during the initial healing phase.

Indications for collagen membranes are therefore limited to the regeneration of small peri-implant defects, limited horizontal ridge augmentation, and the coverage of lateral sinus wall ostectomies. Porcine collagen membranes do, however, remain the most frequently used membranes in daily practice and are indicated in the following situations:

- peri-implant bone defects, such as dehiscence and fenestrations
- residual peri-implant defects following extractions
- limited horizontal ridge augmentation

MEMBRANE FIXATION TOOLS

Because precise membrane positioning and stability are essential for successful final bone regeneration, tools for fixation have received great attention since the 1990s. Currently, self-tapping mini-screws of different lengths are available for securing nonresorbable PTFE membranes in the palatal cortical of the maxilla and in the mandible **(Fig 21)**.

Generally, mini-screws are not indicated with resorbable collagen membranes, which tend to become entangled during screw rotation. In these cases, titanium pins that are fixed with a carrier and a hammer are more suitable **(Fig 22)**. However, in the mandible, they must be inserted perfectly perpendicular to the surface of the cortical bone to avoid bending them.

BONE GRAFTS AND BIOMATERIALS

It was realized very early on in development phase of GBR techniques that the barrier effect in combination with the blood clot alone requires an excessive amount of time to regenerate even limited amounts of bone.

Therefore, as early as the early 1990s, researchers and clinicians began using autologous bone grafts, biomaterials, or a combination of the two to fill the space in bone defects under membranes. Depending on their origin and the way they are prepared, bone graft materials may be

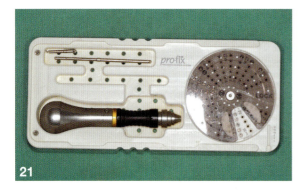
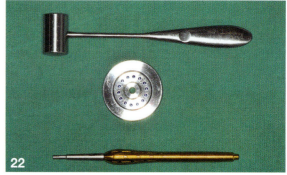

Fig 21 *Self-tapping mini-screw kit for securing nonresorbable membranes.* **Fig 22** *Titanium pin kit with hammer and carrier for resorbable and nonresorbable membranes.*

osteoconductive (capable of acting as a scaffold and support for the migration of osteogenic cells), osteoinductive (containing molecules capable of stimulating the action or differentiation of osteogenic cells), or osteogenic (capable of transferring cells for bone regeneration).

Bone grafts and their substitutes have significantly increased the effectiveness of GBR and reduced the waiting time for bone formation, contributing to the following:[14]

- stabilization of the blood clot
- support of the membrane to prevent it from collapsing
- guidance of osteoprogenitor cells
- transfer of cells or growth factors to the recipient site
- reduction of bone resorption in the long-term

In general, bone grafts are classified according to whether they are of human, animal, or synthetic origin. Classification is crucial for determining their biologic properties. The following types of grafts can be distinguished:

- autograft (autologous bone)
- allograft (homologous bone)
- xenograft (heterologous bone)
- alloplastic graft

Autologous bone grafts

Autologous bone grafts are derived from the same individual that they are placed in, so they are characterized by maximum biocompatibility and are the gold standard graft.

They can be used as blocks or as particles and combine all the biologic properties useful for bone integration and regeneration. They are osteoconductive, osteoinductive, and osteogenic.

Osteoconductivity is guaranteed by the presence of hydroxyapatite, a solid material with high mechanical properties, which contributes to the stabilization of the clot and acts as a bridge during the migration of osteogenic cells. Autologous bone contains several growth factors that are transferred to the donor site and stimulate bone neoformation.

These include bone morphogenetic proteins (BMPs), transforming growth factor beta (TGF-β), insulin-like growth factors (IGFs) I and II, platelet-derived growth factors (PDGFs), and fibroblast growth factors (FGFs) A and B.

The number of growth factors largely depends on individual patient characteristics, such as age, the presence of metabolic or systemic diseases (such as osteoporosis), and the type of bone grafted (whether cortical or trabecular and particulate or block). The release mechanism of growth factors can be traced back to the action of osteoclasts, which reabsorb the portions of bone recognized as unsuitable while simultaneously exposing growth factors that stimulate osteogenic cells to begin the neoattachment phase of bone growth (see chapter 3). The greater the exposed surface area of the graft is, the faster resorption and the release of growth factors takes place (meaning particulate grafts allow for greater osteogenic stimulus than blocks).

Alongside these undisputed advantages, autologous grafts have a greater tendency to resorption and thus less dimensional stability than heterologous and alloplastic grafts.

Disadvantages include the invasiveness of graft harvesting, which often requires a second surgical site, and their limited availability at the intraoral level, which limits their use to the treatment of small or medium-sized defects.

Usually, particulate bone grafts are used in GBR techniques **(Fig 23)**. This is due to their greater ease of harvesting and adaptability to the spaces under the membrane.

On the other hand, the membrane itself limits their tendency to resorb by excluding competition from connective cells and withstanding the pressure of the overlying soft tissues.

Block grafts, when secured with fixation screws, provide maximum mechanical support during the regeneration phases and are slowly replaced by means of the shear cone mechanism (see chapter 3). However, the resorption and replacement process is extremely slow and can last for years, which results in the presence of large portions of nonviable bone in the regenerated bone[15] **(Fig 24)**, which can suffer volume losses of up to 60% in the first 6 months[16,17] **(Fig 25)**.

Intraoral bone graft harvesting techniques

lìThis discussion on graft harvesting techniques is limited to intraoral autologous bone grafting techniques because extraoral techniques are now extremely rare and limited to cases of major reconstructive surgery.

Chin symphysis

lThe chin symphysis is the harvesting site that allows for the greatest amount of bone to be collected at the intraoral level.

The procedure is rather simple because of the easy access and the wide view of the surgical field. A full-thickness horizontal incision is made in the mandibular fornix from canine to canine, approximately 10 mm apical to the mucogingival junction of the anterior teeth.

The mucosa is dissected full-thickness apically until reaching the tip of the chin and laterally to gently visualize the chin foramen.

Bone harvesting can be performed with trephine burs of various diameters with confluent osteotomies **(Fig 26)** to facilitate the removal of bone fragments with a Molt curette or a lever.

Before suturing, a collagen sponge is placed at the harvest site to improve hemostasis, and suturing is performed with continuous interlaced stitches **(Fig 27)**.

The collected bone fragments are then reduced to small chips (1- to 2 mm) with a bone grinder **(Fig 28)**.

Alternatively, in the case of block grafts, the osteotomy is performed with a piezoelectric ultrasonic handpiece **(Fig 29a)**, and the blocks are removed with small chisels.

Part of the spongiosa can be removed with alveolar spoons **(Fig 29b)**.

Chin harvesting is not void of complications, though the complications that do arise are generally transitory and not serious. In the postoperative period, edema and hematomas in the chin and neck region are common, sometimes even conspicuous, and resolve spontaneously within 15 days. Hypoesthesia at the level of the mandibular incisors, which is felt by patients as insensitivity to pressure and thermal stimuli, is also very common. Neurologic complications to the skin caused by stretching the IAN at the level of its emergence from the mental foramen are rare.

Hypoesthesia is generally well tolerated by patients and resolves completely within a month. Finally, with large harvests from the chin, permanent bone deficits may remain, which, although asymptomatic, may complicate further harvests or future implant treatments **(Fig 30)**.

Retromolar trigone and lateral wall of the posterior mandible

The retromolar trigone and lateral wall of the posterior mandible is currently the most commonly used site for bone harvesting due to the relative simplicity of the procedure and the low incidence of postoperative complications. A full-thickness incision is made at the mandibular external oblique line at a distance of about 5 mm from the mucogingival junction. The incision may be extended distally along the ascending ramus. A full-thickness incision is made in the apical direction to expose the mandibular external oblique line, and the mucosa is protected by inserting a Minnesota retractor.

Harvesting can be performed with a 4- to 6-mm diameter trephine **(Fig 31)**, bone scrapers **(Fig 32a)**, or piezoelectric handpieces **(Fig 32b)**.

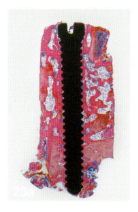
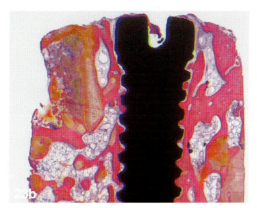

Fig 23 *Histologic sections of mini-implants used for vertical ridge augmentation via GBR with autologous bone particles. The particles are surrounded by newly formed bone. Hematoxylin and eosin (H&E) staining; ×10 magnification (a) and ×20 magnification (b).*

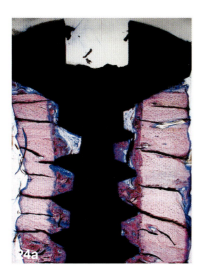
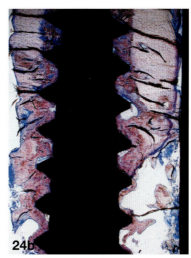

Fig 24 *Histologic section of a titanium fixation screw in a cortical bone block. The regeneration of new bone along the screw surface is evident. (a) Coronal portion. (b) Apical portion.[15]*

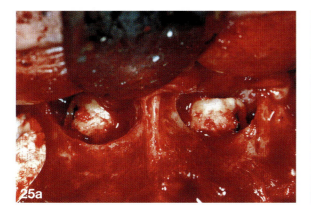
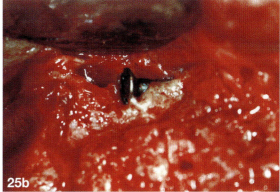

Fig 25 *(a) Cortical block grafts taken from the chin placed for elevation of the nasal fossae. (b) After 6 months of healing, more than 60% of the volume has resorbed.*

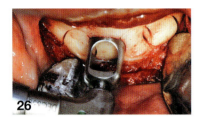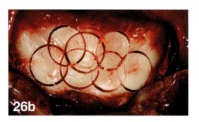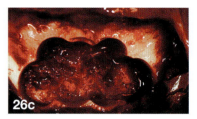

Fig 26 (a) *Extensive bone graft harvesting from the chin along two lines using 8-mm trephine burs.* (b) *The preparations are overlapped to facilitate removal.* (c) *The bone was harvested with a lever and ground with a bone grinder.*

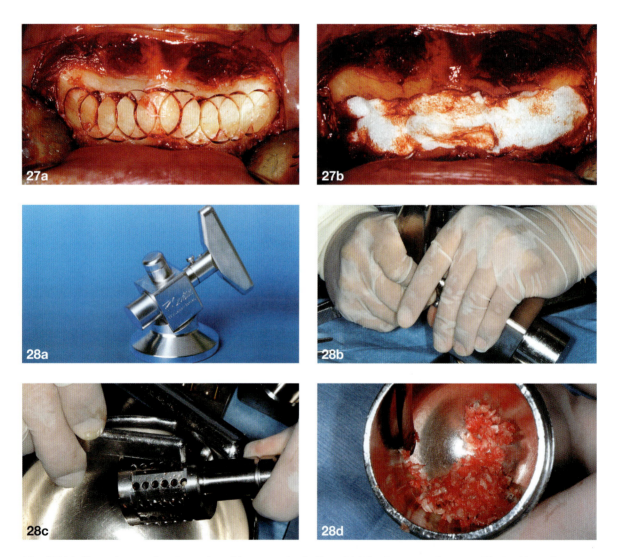

Fig 27 (a) *Bone harvesting from the chin on a single line.* (b) *The harvest site was filled with collagen to limit bleeding and subsequent postoperative hematoma.* **Fig 28** (a) *Quetin bone mill.* (b) *The harvested bone blocks are placed, pressed against the inner blade, and ground by hand.* (c) *The blade is cleaned to collect all bone fragments.* (d) *The ground bone accumulates in a special container screwed to the mill.*

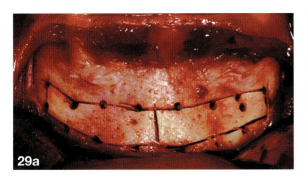 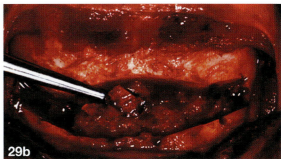

Fig 29 (a) *Osteotomies to harvest two block grafts from the chin.* (b) *The blocks are removed, and the bone marrow is harvested with a special bone spoon.*

The latter have the advantage of directly delivering thin bone chips of the correct size without the need for additional grinding instruments. Using bone scrapers excludes the risk of nerve or vascular injury while performing a superficial harvest. When harvesting block grafts, the osteotomy is performed with a piezoelectric ultrasonic handpiece on the lateral wall of the mandible apical to the external oblique line **(Fig 33)**.

If used improperly, trephine burs used to harvest block grafts expose the patient to the risk of IAN injury.

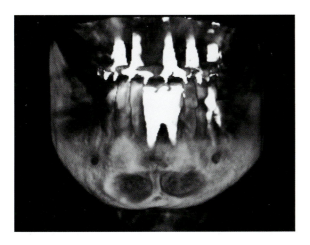

Fig 30 *Residual bone defects 18 years after graft harvesting from the chin.*

Anterior nasal spine

In patients with a large vertical dimension of the maxilla, small harvests of autologous bone can be performed near the anterior nasal spine. Typically, 4-mm-diameter trephines are used with plenty of irrigation without going beyond the palatal bone plate **(Fig 34)**. A CBCT is used to assess the thickness of the maxillary bone at the sampling point and the position of the tooth apices to avoid accidental devitalization.

Maxillary tuberosity

Small amounts of graft can be harvested from the retromolar tuberosity of the maxilla, but generally the quality of the bone is not ideal due to the strong presence of yellow marrow, which is rich in adipose tissue and poorly mineralized **(Fig 35)**.

Homologous bone grafts

Homologous bone grafts are derived from the same species as the recipient but from different individuals.

There are three main families of homologous bone grafts: fresh homologous bone grafts, freeze-dried bone allografts (FDBAs), and demineralized freeze-dried bone allografts (DFDBAs).

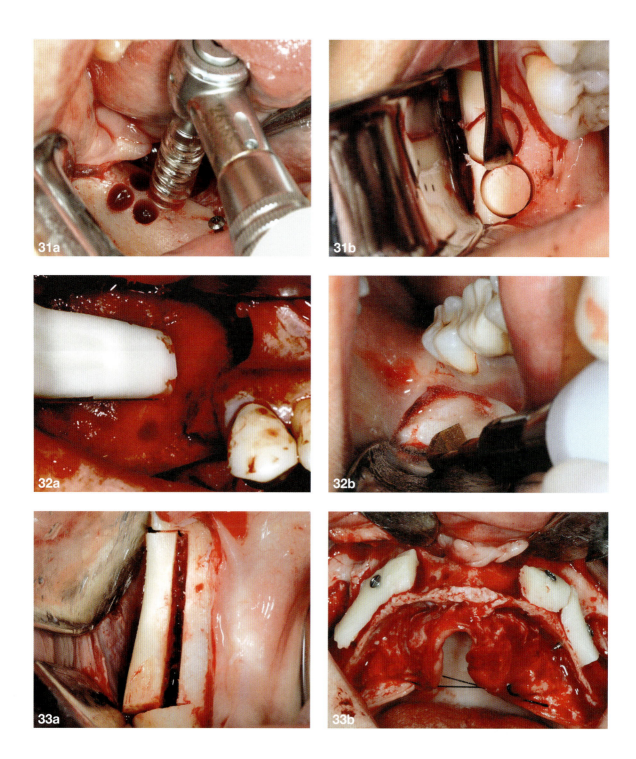

Fig 31 (a) *Bone harvesting from the mandibular retromolar trigone with a self-retentive trephine.* (b) *Bone harvesting with a traditional trephine and lever.* **Fig 32** *Bone harvesting using bone scraper* (a) *and a piezoelectric handpiece* (b). **Fig 33** *Block graft removal from the lateral wall parallel to the external oblique line.* (a) *The osteotomy is performed with a piezo handpiece, and the block is removed with chisels.* (b) *Blocks placed in an edentulous maxilla.*

Fresh homologous bone grafts originate from individuals who undergo bone removal, such as from the femoral head, for therapeutic reasons. The grafts are sterilized, frozen, and stored in bone banks. Their efficacy is highly controversial because they retain their antigenic power and may cause unwanted immune responses.[18,19] Their use is therefore very limited in GBR techniques.

In addition to being osteoconductive materials, FDBAs and DFDBAs have been shown to contain osteoinductive molecules, such as BMPs.[20–22] The concentration of these molecules, however, is very limited and varies depending on the donor and how the product is prepared. Thus, the clinical relevance of these osteoinductive capabilities is questionable.

In DFDBAs, the bone is treated with acids to remove the inorganic component and expose more BMPs, but demineralization drastically worsens the graft material's biomechanical characteristics, making it unsuitable for use in GBR. Remineralization occurs over a very long period of time through the precipitation of calcium salts in small, roundish corpuscles (Yamashita nuclei) that tend to merge together over time[23–25] **(Fig 36)**.

Homologous bone grafts are used on a large scale in the United States for both periodontal and implant applications, whereas European regulations on organ harvesting severely limit their clinical use.

Heterologous bone grafts

The most studied and clinically used bone substitute today is deproteinized bovine bone mineral (DBBM).[26] DBBM is a biocompatible and osteoconductive material with the same macroscopic and microscopic characteristics as human spongy bone **(Fig 37)**. The inorganic component is removed by heat and/or chemical treatment to eliminate the antigenic power and the risk of transmission of diseases such as bovine spongiform encephalopathy (mad cow syndrome).

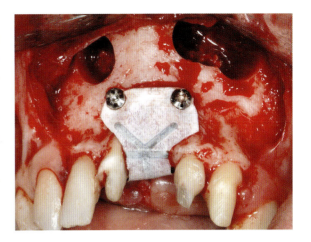

Fig 34 *Bone harvesting from the anterior nasal spine with a 4-mm trephine.*

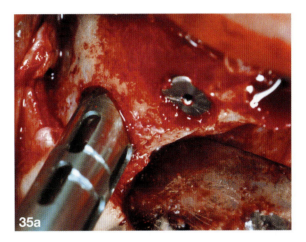

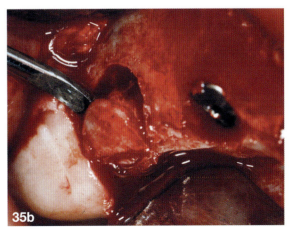

Fig 35 (a) *Bone harvesting from the maxillary tuberosity with a trephine.* (b) *The block is removed with a lever.*

Because it consists of only calcium hydroxyapatite, DBBM contributes significantly to improving the biomechanical characteristics of regenerated bone, which is an essential feature for achieving good primary implant stability. Moreover, DBBM is resorbed very slowly and incompletely via osteoclastic activity.

This process is so slow that a study with human biopsies showed the presence of residual DBBM particles 10 years after the performance of maxillary sinus elevations.[27,28] Although this slow and incomplete resorption was considered a negative feature for many years (as biomaterials should resorb completely so replacement with new bone can take place), it is now considered a positive characteristic because it contributes to the long-term dimensional stability of the regenerated bone (Figs 38 and 39).

Alloplastic bone grafts

Alloplastic grafts consist of bone of synthetic origin. Their greatest advantage lies in their wide availability and the complete absence of the risk of transmitting infectious diseases.

They are biocompatible and osteoconductive materials with a composition and structure similar to the inorganic component of bone. There are essentially three alloplastic materials: calcium hydroxyapatite, beta tricalcium phosphate (ß-TCP), and bioglass.

Despite the considerable advances in the production technology of these materials, their macrostructure and microstructure still differ from the inorganic matrix of natural bone (Fig 40), which presents limitations.

Differences between alloplastic grafts and natural bone in porosity and surface roughness reduce the osteoconductive capabilities of grafts, making them second-rate materials. Hydroxyapatite of synthetic origin is also practically nonresorbable, whereas TCP resorbs too quickly, before the bone has time to regenerate and replace it.

SUTURE TECHNIQUES

Tension-free suturing techniques are of paramount importance to avoid wound dehiscence and membrane exposure. Suture material must be moderately elastic, inert, nonresorbable, and

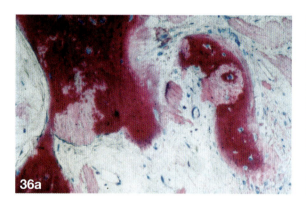
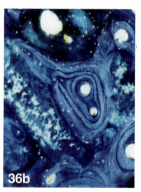
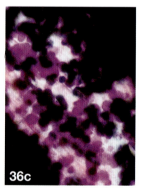

Fig 36 (a) *Histologic preparation showing the mineralization cores (Yamashita nuclei) of a DFDBA graft after 8 months of healing. H&E staining; ×10 magnification.* (b and c) *Mineralization cores are still present 4 years after surgery. H&E staining; ×20 (b) and ×40 (c) magnification. (Reprinted with permission from Int J Periodontics Restorative Dent 1996;16:338–347.)*

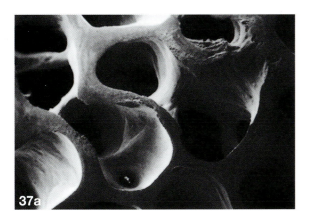
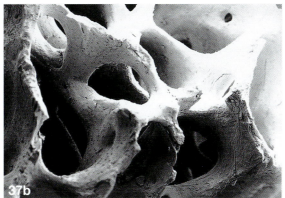

Fig 37 (a) *SEM image of human spongy bone.* (b) *Deproteinized bovine spongy bone. ×40 magnification.*

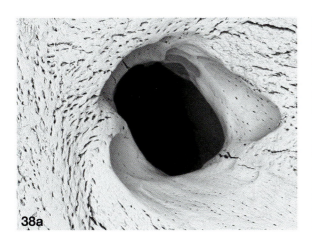
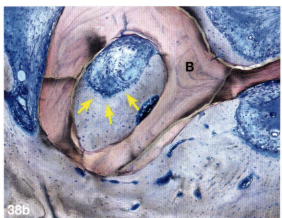

Fig 38 (a) *SEM image of DBBM trabecula (×2,540 magnification).* (b) *Histologic preparation showing bone regeneration within DBBM trabecula. The osteoblastic rim in the process of bone matrix deposition is visible (Toluidine blue staining; ×20 magnification). (Reprinted with permission from Int J Periodontics Restorative Dent 1996;16:338–347).*

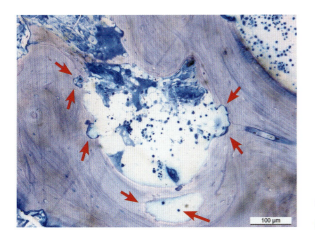

Fig 39 *Histologic image of osteoclastic resorption gaps in DBBM particles.*

monofilament. Elasticity is important because it cushions against any excessive knot tension that could strangle the tissue and cause marginal necrosis. Biologic inertness and nonresorbability prevent inflammatory foreign body reactions and uncontrolled early suture loss. Monofilaments reduce plaque accumulation during the delicate healing phase. The only materials that meet all of these requirements are Teflon, in either its expanded (ePTFE) or dense (dPTFE) forms, and Prolene (Ethicon). Two lines of sutures are placed, a deeper horizontal mattress suture line and a more superficial simple interrupted suture line. The horizontal mattress sutures are placed first to achieve eversion of the flaps that must interface with their deep connective surface. This avoids overlapping the two margins and subsequently causing contact between the epithelium of the underlying flap and the connective tissue of the flap above. Eversion of the flaps also significantly increases the contact surface area for healing. The mattress sutures must engage fairly large portions of tissue to prevent the

thread from cutting through the tissue. The 4-mm rule should be observed: the distance between the needle penetration from the edge of the flap must be 4 mm on both the buccal and lingual aspects and also on the return from lingual to buccal penetration, 4 mm in the distal direction **(Fig 41)**. Size 4-0 PTFE suture material is always used for this.

Simple sutures are placed between the mattress sutures, 2 to 3 mm from the wound margin. In esthetic areas, for simple sutures only, it is important to use a finer suture to perfect the approximation of the flap margins and reduce scar formation. Synthetic threads, such as Prolene 6-0, are indicated for this. Lastly, simple 4-0 PTFE sutures are applied to the mesial and distal vertical incisions and the papillae of the adjacent teeth are sutured with Prolene 6-0.

After suturing, light pressure is applied with wet gauze to reduce the residual blood clot under the flap and an antiseptic hyaluronic acid gel (Hobagel Plus, Hobama) is applied **(Fig 42)**. Sutures are removed after 12-15 days.

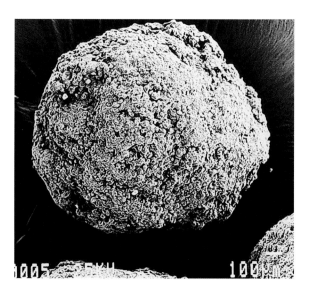

Fig 40 *SEM image of a TCP particle (×1,000 magnification).*

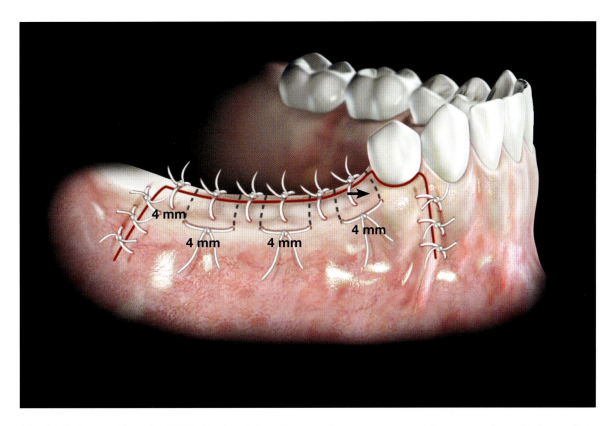

Fig 41 *Suture pattern for GBR. Horizontal mattress sutures are spaced 4 mm apart, and intermediate simple sutures are placed along the crestal incision and the buccal vertical incisions.*

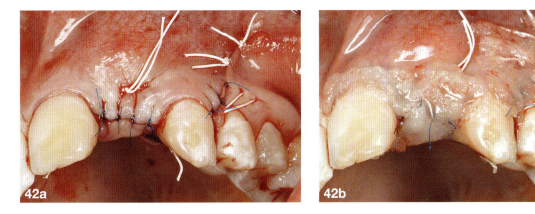

Fig 42 (a) *Horizontal ePTFE mattress sutures and simple interrupted Prolene sutures.* (b) *Final application of Hobagel hyaluronic acid antiseptic gel.*

REFERENCES

1. Simion M, Trisi P, Piattelli A. Vertical ridge augmentation using a membrane technique associated with osseointegrated implants. Int J Periodontics Restorative Dent 1994;14:496–511.

2. Simion M, Jovanovic SA, Trisi P, Scarano A, Piattelli A. Vertical ridge augmentation around dental implants using a membrane technique and autogenous bone or allografts in humans. Int J Periodontics Restorative Dent 1998;18:8–23.

3. Simion M, Rocchietta I. Guided bone regeneration for vertical ridge augmentation: Past, present and future. In: Buser D. 20 years of Guided Bone Regeneration in Implant Dentistry. Quintessence, 2009:231–253.

4. Pistilli R, Checchi V, Sammartino G, Simion M, Felice P. Safe new approach to the lingual flap management in mandibular augmentation procedures: The digitoclastic technique. Implant Dent 2017;26:790–795.

5. Hardwick R, Scantlebury T, Sanchez R, Whitley N, Ambruster J. Membrane design criteria for guided bone regeneration of the alveolar ridge. In: Buser D, Dahlin C, Schenk R (eds). Guided Bone Regeneration in Implant Dentistry. Quintessence, 1994:101–136.

6. Schenk RK, Buser D, Hardwick R, Dahlin C. Healing pattern of bone regeneration in membrane-protected defects: A histologic and histomorphometric study in the mandible of dogs. Int J Oral Maxillofac Implants 1994;9:13–29.

7. Buser D, Ruskin J, Higginbottom F, Hardwick R, Dahlin C, Schenk R. Osseointegration of titanium implants in bone regenerated in membrane-protected defects. A histologic study in the canine mandible. Int J Oral Maxillofac Implants 1995;10:666-681.

8. Simion M, Dahlin C, Blair K, Schenk R. Effect of 3 different types of titanium reinforced membranes on bone regeneration in surgically crated defects: A histological study in canine model. Clin Oral Implants Res 1999;10:73–84.

9. Simion M, Dahlin C, Rocchietta I, Stavropulos A, Sanchez R, Karring T. Vertical ridge augmentation with guided bone regeneration in association with dental implants: An experimental study in dogs. Clin Oral Implants Res 2007;18:86–94.

10. Urban IA, Lozada JL, Jovanovic SA, Nagursky H, Nagy K. Vertical ridge augmentation with titanium-reinforced, dense-PTFE membranes and a combination of particulated autogenous bone and anorganic bovine bone-derived mineral: A prospective case series in 19 patients. Int J Oral Maxillofac Implants 2014;29: 185–193.

11. Ronda M, Rebaudi A, Torelli L, Stacchi C. Expanded vs. dense polytetrafluoroethylene membranes in vertical ridge augmentation around dental implants: A prospective randomized controlled clinical trial. Clin Oral Implants Res 2014;25:859–866.

12. Piattelli A, Scarano A, Coraggio F, Matarasso S. Early tissue reactions to polylactic acid resorbable membranes: A histological and histochemical study in rabbit. Biomaterials 1998;19:889–896.

13. von Arx T, Broggini N, Jensen SS, Bornstein MM, Schenk RK, Buser D. Membrane durability and tissue response of different bioresorbable barrier membranes: A histologic study in the rabbit calvarium. Int J Oral Maxillofac Implants 2005;20:843–853.

14. Storgard Jensen S, Bosshardt DD, Buser D. Bone grafts and bone substitute materials. In: Buser D. 20 years of Guided Bone Regeneration in Implant Dentistry. Quintessence, 2009:71–96.

15. Rocchietta I, Simion M, Hoffmann M, Trisciuoglio D, Benigni M, Dahlin C. Vertical bone augmentation with an autogenous block or particles in combination with guided bone regeneration: A clinical and histological preliminary study in humans. Clin Implants Dent Relat Res 2016;18:19–29.

16. Widmark G, Andersson B, Ivanoff CJ. Mandibular bone graft in the anterior maxilla for single-tooth implants. Int J Oral Maxillofac Surg 1997;26:106–109.

17. Johanson B, Grepe A, Wannfors K, Hirsch GM. A clinical study of changes in the volume of bone grafts in the atrophic maxilla. Dentomaxillofac Radiol 2001;30: 157–161.

18. Chiapasco M, Colletti G, Coggiola A, Di Martino G, Anello T, Romeo E. Clinical outcome of the use of fresh frozen allogeneic bone grafts for the reconstruction of severely resorbed alveolar ridges: Preliminary results of a prospective study. Int J Oral Maxillofac Implants 2015;30:450–460.

19. Dellavia C, Giammattei M, Carmagnola D, Musto F, Canciani E, Chiapasco M. Iliac Crest fresh-frozen allografts versus autografts in oral pre-prosthetic bone reconstructive surgery: Histologic and histomorphometric study. Implant Dent 2016;25: 731–738.

20. Reddi AH, Wientroub S, Muthukumaran N. Biologic principles of bone induction. Orthop Clin North Am 1987;18:207–212.

21. Schwartz Z, Weesner T, van Dijk S, et al. Ability of deproteinized cancellous bovine bone to induce new bone formation. J Periodontol 2000;71:1258–1269.

22. Boyan BD, Ranly DM, McMillan J, Sunwoo M, Roche K, Schwartz Z. Osteoinductive ability of human allograft formulations. J Periodontol 2006;77:1555–1563.

23. Simion M, Dahlin C, Trisi P, Piattelli A. Qualitative and quantitative comparative study on different filling materials used in bone tissue regeneration: A controlled clinical study. Int J Periodontics Restorative Dent 1994;14:198–215.

24. Simion M, Trisi P, Piattelli A. GBR with an e-PTFE membrane associated with DFDBA: Histologic and histochemical analysis in a human implant retrieved after 4 years of loading. Int J Periodontics Restorative Dent 1996;16:338–347.

25. Fontana F, Santoro F, Maiorana C, Iezzi G, Piattelli A, Simion M. Clinical and histologic evaluation of allogeneic bone matrix versus autogenous bone chips associated with titanium-reinforced e-PTFE membrane for vertical ridge augmentation: A prospective pilot study. Int J Oral Maxillofac Implants 2008;23: 1003–1012.

26. Simion M, Fontana F. Autogenous and xenogeneic bone grafts for the bone regeneration. A literature review. Minerva Stomatol 2004;53:191–206.

27. Piattelli M, Favero GA, Scarano A, Orsini G, Piattelli A. Bone reactions to anorganic bovine bone (Bio-Oss) used in sinus augmentation procedures: A histologic long-term report of 20 cases in humans. Int J Oral Maxillofac Implants 1999;14:835–840.

28. Simion M, Fontana F, Rasperini G, Maiorana C. Vertical ridge augmentation by expanded polytetrafluoroethylene membrane and a combination of intraoral autogenous bone graft and deproteinized anorganic bovine bone (Bio Oss). Clin Oral Implants Res 2007;18:620–629.

HORIZONTAL ALVEOLAR RIDGE AUGMENTATION

CHAPTER 16

Edited by Massimo Simion and Stefano Pieroni

INTRODUCTION

The presence of adequate bone volume around implants is an essential factor for the long-term success of implant-supported restorations.[1] In the early 1990s, the first experiments in guided bone regeneration (GBR) led to the development of techniques to increase the thickness of deficient alveolar ridges, both with simultaneous implant placement[2–6] and in two-stage procedures.[7–10]

Early GBR procedures were performed with membranes alone, without any tools to maintain the space required for bone regeneration and with the membrane itself collapsing against the defect. Very early on, however, support screws, autologous bone particles, and biomaterials, or a combination of these, were used. Today, the details of the technique are well-documented and supported by a vast number of articles and systematic reviews with meta-analyses.[11,12] Horizontal bone regeneration is a very broad topic that encompasses countless different situations. Depending on the morphology and severity of the defect, two major types of procedure can be distinguished:

Anyone performing implant surgery must be able to use horizontal bone regeneration techniques to correct at least small exposures of the implant surface through the bone. In most cases, these techniques are simple and predictable.

Massimo Simion

- one-stage techniques, in which the implant is placed within the bone defect and the regenerative technique is performed during the same surgery;
- two-stage techniques, which involve regeneration of the bone first and then implant placement.

ONE-STAGE REGENERATIVE TECHNIQUES

The indication for the treatment of small areas of implant dehiscence or fenestration has been the subject of constant debate since the advent of osseointegrated implantology. In a 2017 study, Jung et al[13] compared clinical values of peri-implant health in a series of sites with areas of implant dehiscence less than 5 mm in size, with or without regenerative therapy. The probing depth, bleeding on probing, and plaque index measured at 18 months were similar in both groups and compatible with good peri-implant health. The difference highlighted by the authors concerned the average peri-implant bone resorption, which was higher in the sites not treated with regenerative techniques. Another consideration has to do with the exposure of rough implant surfaces outside the bone crest, a condition that favors bacterial biofilm accumulation and thus predisposes the patient to the development of peri-implantitis. A clinical study by Schwartz et al[14] evaluated the impact of residual implant dehiscence after regenerative techniques on peri-implant tissue health after a 4-year observation period.

The results showed an increased risk of developing peri-implantitis when the areas of residual dehiscence were greater than 1 mm. This and other studies demonstrate the need for the complete submergence of the implant surface below the bone margin to maintain long-term implant stability and peri-implant health. The challenge of working with bone deficits consists in placing and stabilizing implants in a prosthetically correct position in bone of reduced quantity with altered anatomical characteristics. Performance of a regenerative technique, fortunately, is not particularly difficult because the volume of bone to be regenerated is generally small. Immediate implant placement in alveolar ridges with bone deficits can result in three different types of peri-implant defects: dehiscence, fenestration, and residual peri-implant defects from previous extractions.

1. Implant dehiscence is a defect characterized by the exposure of the coronal portion of the implant surface outside the bone crest **(Fig 1)**. These defects can be buccal or palatal/lingual. They occur in alveolar processes that are thin in the crestal portion and increase in thickness in the apical direction, or in the presence of residual bone defects from previous extractions.

2. Fenestrations are exposures of the middle and/or apical third of the implant surface when the crestal bone is of adequate thickness **(Fig 2)**. They are generally buccal and occur in cases of concavities present in the apical portion of the alveolar process.

3. Peri-implant defects are usually residual from previous extractions and can be categorized as two-, three- or four-walled bone defects **(Fig 3)**.

To use a one-step technique, the following characteristics must be present:

- The quality of the soft tissue and its maturation must allow for healing by primary intention and the submergence of implant and membrane throughout the healing period.
- Sufficient quantity and quality of bone must be present to achieve adequate primary implant stability.
- It must be possible to place the implant in a prosthetically correct position to meet both functional and esthetic requirements (see chapter 18.

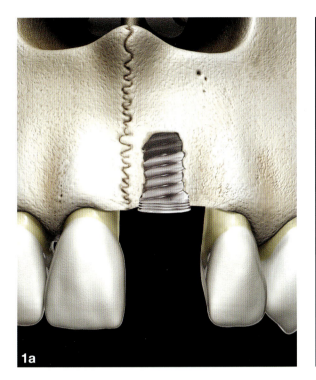
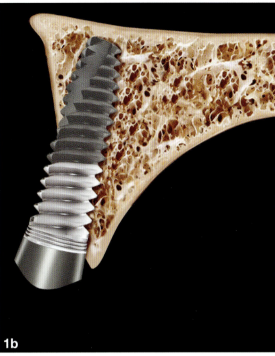

Fig 1 *Implant dehiscence. The coronal portion of the implant is exposed outside the bone crest. (a) Frontal view. (b) Sectional view.*

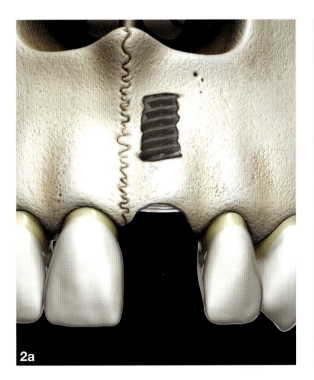
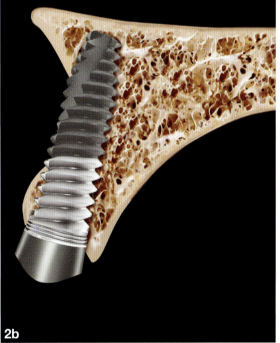

Fig 2 *Implant fenestration. The middle and/or apical third of the implant is exposed outside the bone crest. (a) Frontal view. (b) Sectional view.*

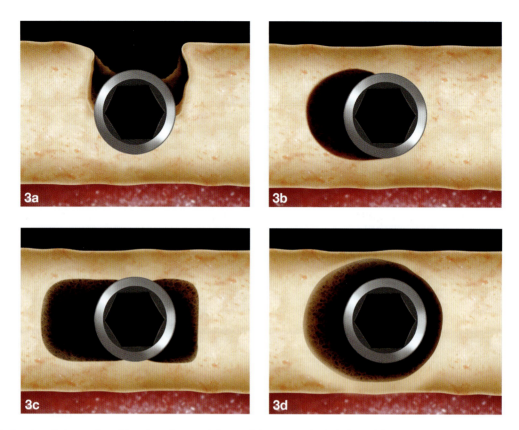

Fig 3 *Occlusal view of peri-implant bone defects:* (a) *two-walled defect,* (b) *three-walled defect,* (c) *double three-walled defect,* (d) *four-walled/circumferential defect.*

In the 1990s, these types of defects were treated with autologous particulate bone and expanded polytetrafluorethylene (ePTFE) membranes secured with titanium pins.[2-6] This technique was characterized by high reliability, but it required considerable expertise on the part of the clinician to avoid complications such as infection and early exposure of the membranes (see chapter 22).

Today, resorbable collagen membranes are preferred in the vast majority of cases. Collagen membranes allow for easier application and are less prone to complications in the immediate postoperative period.[6,15,16] On the other hand, their complete resorption within 30 to 40 days limits their effectiveness as a barrier in the initial stages of bone regeneration, reducing predictability. This is why indications for resorbable membranes are limited to implant dehiscence involving exposure of the implant body outside the bone structure no greater than 2 mm in the horizontal direction.

After perforating the surrounding cortical, the dehiscence areas and defects are filled with a mixture of 50% autologous and 50% heterologous bone particles and covered with collagen membranes. In cases of increased exposure of the implant surface outside the bone, membrane fixation with titanium pins is recommended. Bone regeneration occurs within 4 to 6 months of submerged healing.

CLINICAL CASE 1

Treatment of multiple areas of implant dehiscence in the maxilla

A 41-year-old patient, who had previously undergone a series of apicoectomies with incongruous retrograde amalgam fillings, presented with diffuse infections and fistulas from the maxillary right canine to the maxillary left canine and edentulousness at the site of the maxillary right second premolar. The teeth were extracted, and the sockets were curetted to completely remove all granulation tissue.

After 3 months of healing **(Fig 4a)**, a full-thickness flap was lifted, which revealed the complete loss of the buccal bone plate at the level of all involved teeth **(Figs 4b and 5a)**. Because there was an adequate amount of bone apical to the remaining defects, it was possible to place five machined implants at the sites of the maxillary right second premolar, first premolar, and canine, as well as in the sites of the maxillary left lateral incisor and canine.

The absence of the buccal plate resulted in a large areas of dehiscence-type implant exposures 10 to 12 mm in size **(Fig 5b)**. The defects were treated with two ePTFE membranes and autologous particulate bone harvested from the anterior nasal spine at the same surgical site **(Figs 5c and 5d)**. The flap was sutured with horizontal mattress sutures and 4-0 ePTFE simple interrupted sutures **(Fig 6a)**.

After 6 months, a full-thickness flap was elevated, revealing that the membranes were integrated perfectly with the underlying tissue with no signs of inflammation **(Fig 6b)**. After delicate removal of the membranes, complete regeneration of the buccal plate with adequate bone thickness was revealed **(Figs 7a and 7b)**. The definitive metal-ceramic prosthesis **(Fig 7c)** was placed after 6 months of tissue conditioning with an acrylic provisional. Periapical radiographs after 22 years confirmed the stability of the regenerated bone **(Fig 8)**.

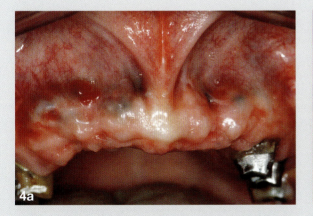
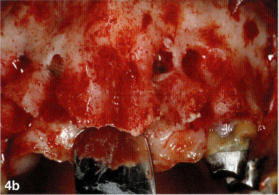

Fig 4 *(a)* Clinical image after 3 months of healing after extraction of the teeth from the maxillary right canine to the maxillary left canine. *(b)* A full-thickness flap was elevated, revealing the bony defects and the total absence of the buccal bone plate.

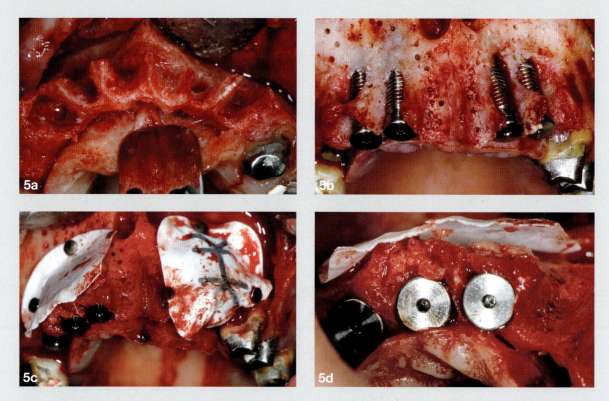

Fig 5 *(a)* Occlusal view of the bony defects and the complete absence of the buccal bone plate. *(b)* The placement of five implants with machined surfaces resulted in areas of buccal dehiscence from 10 to 12 mm in size. *(c)* Dehiscence was treated with two ePTFE membranes and autologous particulate bone taken from the anterior nasal spine. *(d)* The particulate graft under the membrane.

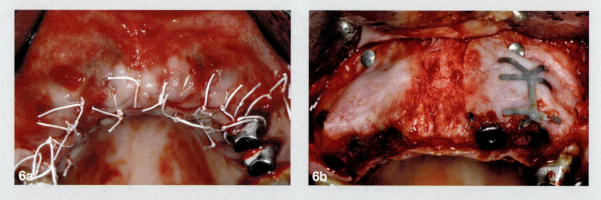

Fig 6 *(a)* The flaps were sutured with horizontal mattress sutures and simple ePTFE sutures. *(b)* After 6 months of healing, the membranes were removed, revealing complete healing of the defects with newly formed bone.

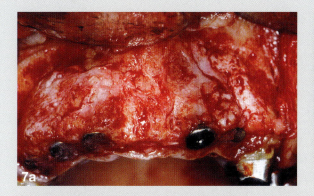
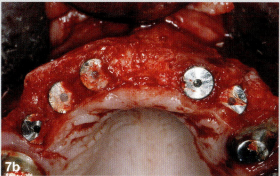
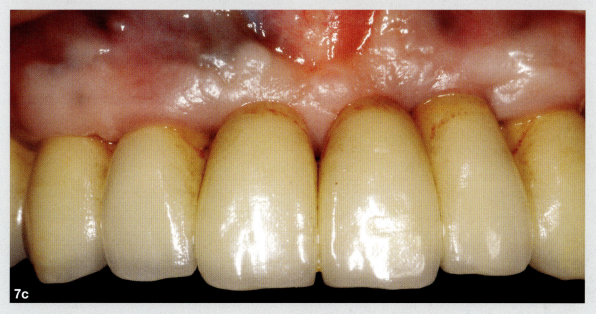

Fig 7 The complete healing of defects with newly formed bone. *(a)* Buccal view. *(b)* Occlusal view. *(c)* The patient was rehabilitated with a fixed metal-ceramic prosthesis.

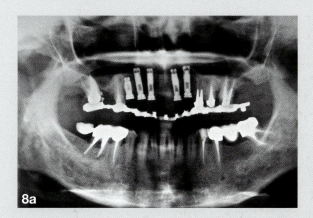
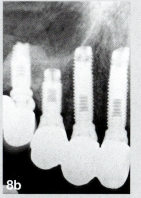
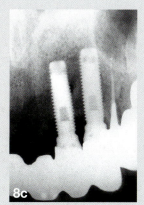

Fig 8 *(a)* Panoramic radiograph after 6 months of healing. *(b and c)* Periapical radiographs after 22 years showing the stability of the regenerated bone.

CLINICAL CASE 2

Treatment of implant dehiscence and fenestrations in a completely edentulous patient

A 58-year-old patient who was completely edentulous in the maxilla expressed the wish to receive a fixed complete implant-supported prosthesis. Clinical examination and CBCT imaging showed adequate vertical alveolar bone height but a maximum alveolar bone thickness of only 3.5 to 4 mm. The placement of implants resulted in areas of dehiscence and fenestrations on both the buccal and palatal aspects. The preparation of the implant sites was particularly difficult because it is essential to position the implant exactly in the center of the ridge to minimize the exposure of the threaded surface. Inserting an implant in a dehiscence-type defect also presents a number of difficulties, as the implant tends to slip out of the preparation, which lacks a bone wall, and risks compromising the integrity of the recipient site.

Treating bone defects with the GBR technique, however, did not present any particular difficulties. In this case, after creating perforations in the buccal and palatal plates, a first layer of autologous particulate graft was placed in direct contact with the exposed implant surfaces, and a second layer of deproteinized bovine bone (DBBM) was placed on top of it **(Fig 9)**.

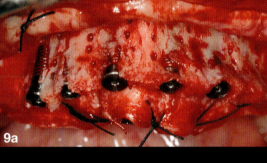
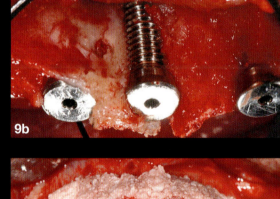
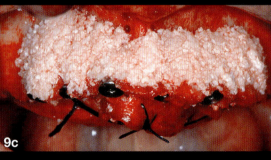
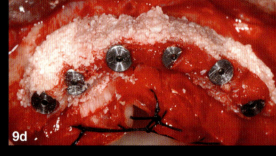

Fig 9 Buccal *(a)* and palatal *(b)* dehiscence and fenestration in a patient with an atrophic and completely edentulous alveolar ridge. A layer of autologous bone particles was placed to cover the exposed implant surfaces, and a second layer of deproteinized bovine bone (DBBM) was placed to cover the autologous bone. Buccal *(c)* and occlusal *(d)* views.

Finally, four resorbable collagen membranes were placed to cover both the buccal and palatal defects without the need for fixation instruments, as the volume of bone to be regenerated was very limited (Figs 10a and 10b). Upon reopening after 6 months, all implants appeared to be surrounded by an abundance of buccal and palatal bone (Figs 10c and 10d). The patient was rehabilitated with a fixed removable implant-supported prosthesis (Figs 10e and 10f).

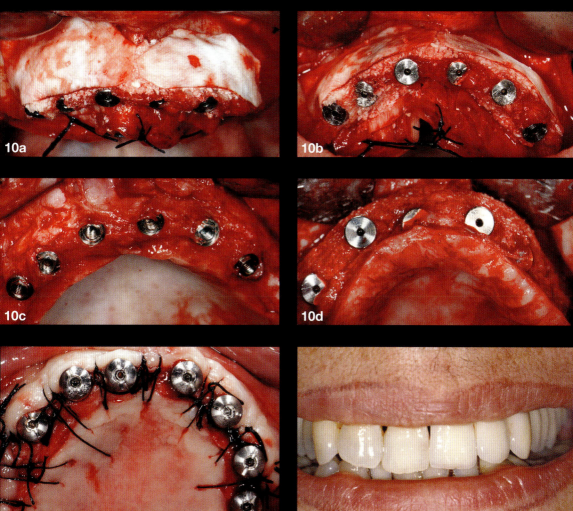

Fig 10 Two buccal and two palatal porcine collagen membranes were placed to cover the graft. (a) Frontal view. (b) Occlusal view. Upon reentry after 6 months, the implants appear to be surrounded by an abundance of bone both buccally (c) and palatally (d). (e) The healing abutments were connected with a partial-thickness flap and apically repositioned to increase the proportion of keratinized mucosa. (f) The patient was rehabilitated with a fixed/removable complete implant-supported prosthesis.

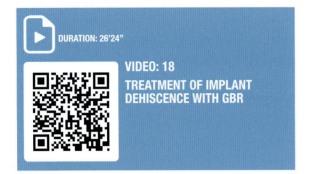

DURATION: 26'24"

VIDEO: 18
TREATMENT OF IMPLANT
DEHISCENCE WITH GBR

TWO-STAGE REGENERATIVE TECHNIQUES

Two-stage horizontal regenerative techniques are used when the alveolar ridge is of adequate vertical dimension but so thin that the implant cannot be inserted and stabilized in a suitable position.

Regenerative techniques with nonresorbable membranes

Larger defects are treated with nonresorbable PTFE membranes using surgical steel screws to support the membrane and to predetermine the thickness of bone to be regenerated.

The membrane, appropriately cut and shaped, is attached with two titanium pins or mini-screws to the palatal or lingual wall of the defect to create a containing wall and facilitate placement of the particulate graft. The defect walls are perforated with a round bur to expose the medulla and facilitate clot formation. The graft material of choice is a mixture of 70% particulate autologous bone and 30% heterologous bone.

After placement of the graft, the membrane is adapted buccally and secured with two to three titanium pins or mini-screws to create a tenting effect and stabilize the graft particles. Before suturing, it is always necessary to make a periosteal releasing incision at the base of the flap.

Suturing is performed at two levels. First, horizontal mattress sutures with PTFE are applied to achieve proper flap eversion, then simple interrupted sutures are placed between each mattress suture. Healing by primary intention and complete submergence of the membrane over a period of 6 to 8 months, depending on the size of the defect, is essential (**Figs 11 to 20**).

Regenerative techniques with resorbable membranes

Due to the greater ease of use and lower incidence of complications with resorbable collagen membranes, most clinicians favor them for the treatment of larger horizontal defects.[17–19] To achieve bone regeneration of adequate thickness, it is essential to use several titanium pins to create a kind of pouch inside which excess graft material is placed to achieve a certain tension in the overlying membrane.

The material of choice in these cases is a mixture of 70% autologous particulate bone and 30% DBBM. After the bone graft is placed, the membrane is wetted, stretched mesially, and secured with additional titanium pins.

The suturing technique is the same as for techniques with nonresorbable membranes. A single, continuous periosteal releasing incision is made at the base of the flap, and a two-level suture is applied, consisting of horizontal mattress sutures interspersed with simple interrupted 4-0 PTFE sutures. Sutures are removed after 12 to 15 days, and a 6-month healing period is required before implant placement (**Figs 49**).

CLINICAL CASE 3

Horizontal maxillary ridge augmentation with a nonresorbable membrane

A 61-year-old patient, who smoked 5 to 6 cigarettes per day, underwent extraction of the maxillary right lateral incisor, canine, and first premolar and removal of a large maxillary cyst. After 3 months of healing, the soft tissue appeared to be in good condition, but a severe horizontal bone defect that was incompatible with immediate implant placement was present (**Fig 11**). CBCT revealed a thin, blade-like alveolar ridge with a perforation of the palatal bone plate (**Fig 12**). A full-thickness incision was made at the crest, with a slight buccal offset, with intrasulcular extension to the adjacent elements and oblique j-shaped vertical incisions mesially at the right central incisor and distally at the second premolar. The flap was extensively reflected to full thickness (**Fig 13**). To prevent the membrane from collapsing, two oblique osteosynthesis screws were placed to provide support in both the horizontal and vertical directions (**Fig 14**).

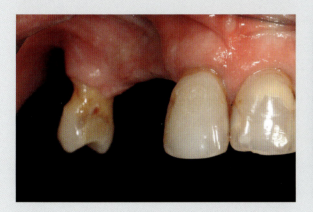

Fig 11 Severe horizontal residual defect after removal of a maxillary cyst in the location of the maxillary right lateral incisor to the maxillary right first premolar.

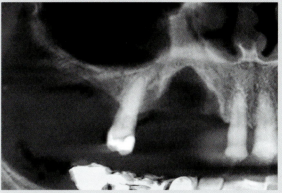

Fig 12 CBCT showing the extremely thin ridge and fenestration of the palatal bone plate.

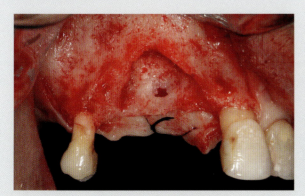

Fig 13 Elevation of the palatal flap makes visible the horizontal bone defect that is incompatible with immediate implant placement.

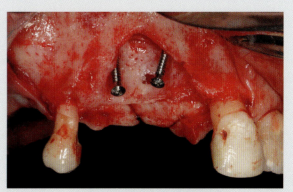

Fig 14 Frontal view of two surgical steel screws placed obliquely to support the membrane both horizontally and vertically.

A nonresorbable dense PTFE (dPTFE) membrane was cut and adapted to the defect, then secured palatally with two fixation pins. The wall of the defect was perforated with a round bur. Autologous bone was harvested at the level of the mandibular outer oblique line with a bone safe scraper. Autologous bone particles were mixed with DBBM (70% and 30%, respectively) and applied to the defect **(Fig 15)**. Then the membrane was adapted buccally and fixed apically with slight tension using three titanium pins **(Fig 16a)**.

After flap passivation with a single, continuous periosteal incision, horizontal mattress sutures were placed first at the crestal level with 4-0 ePTFE sutures. Nonresorbable crestal simple interrupted sutures with 6-0 Prolene (Ethicon) were placed next, and then simple sutures in 4-0 ePTFE were placed at the vertical incisions, with 6-0 Prolene used at the papillary area **(Fig 16b)**.

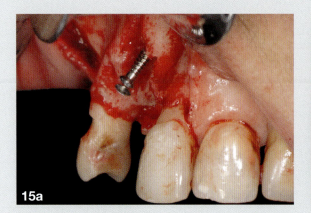
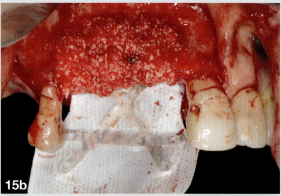

Fig 15 *(a)* Lateral view of two surgical steel screws placed obliquely to support the membrane both horizontally and vertically. *(b)* A titanium-reinforced dPTFE membrane was cut to fit the defect and fixed palatally with two pins. A particulate graft with 70% autologous bone and 30% DBBM was placed to fill the defect.

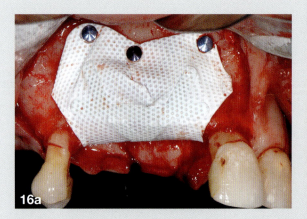
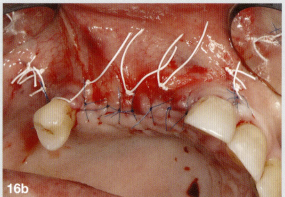

Fig 16 *(a)* The membrane was fixed buccally with three titanium pins. *(b)* After the periosteal releasing incision, the flaps were sutured with 4-0 ePTFE mattress sutures and 6-0 Prolene simple sutures.

The operation to remove the membrane and place the implants was performed after 7 months of healing, during which the patient was kept under strict hygienic control. Upon reentry, a similar incision was performed but without involving the marginal tissues of the central incisor. The membrane was adhered well to the underlying regenerated tissue, and there were no signs of contamination or infection in the adjacent tissues **(Fig 17a)**. After removal of the membrane, regenerated tissue of adequate thickness and vertical dimension was revealed **(Fig 17b)**, and two hybrid surface implants were inserted in the positions of the canine and first premolar, leaving the lateral incisor as an extension for esthetic reasons **(Fig 18)**. The flap was sutured in the same manner as described previously **(Fig 19a)**. After 4 months of healing **(Fig 19b)**, a partial-thickness flap was performed with palatal access to reposition an abundant portion of keratinized mucosa buccal to the implants **(Fig 19c)**.

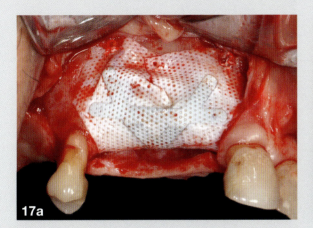
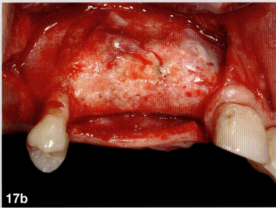

Fig 17 *(a)* After 7 months of submerged healing, a new full-thickness flap was elevated to expose the membrane and fixation instruments. *(b)* The membrane was removed, exposing the regenerated bone tissue.

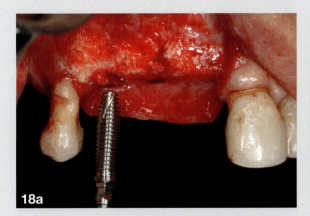
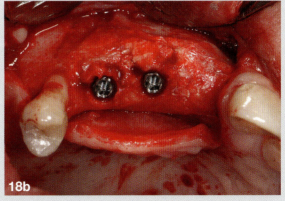

Fig 18 *(a)* Two iMAX hybrid implants (iRES) were placed in the sites of the maxillary right canine and first premolar. *(b)* The lateral incisor was left as a mesial extension for esthetic reasons.

A connective tissue graft was placed around the healing abutments and buccally to increase the thickness of the peri-implant soft tissue and promote the development of adequate emergence profiles for the final prosthesis (Figs 19d to 19f).

The provisional prosthesis was left for 6 months to achieve complete tissue maturation, and then the final metal-ceramic prosthesis was placed (Fig 20).

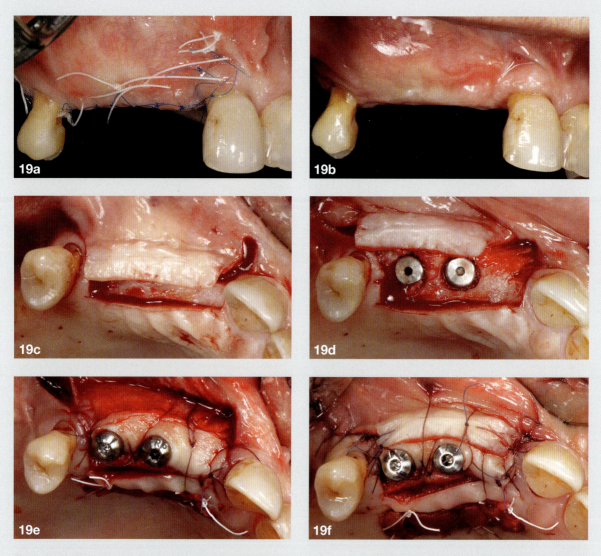

Fig 19 *(a)* The flaps were sutured with mattress sutures and simple sutures. *(b)* The implants were left submerged for 4 months to await osseointegration and maturation of the regenerated bone. *(c)* Upon reopening, a partial-thickness flap was elevated with palatal access to reposition an abundant portion of keratinized mucosa buccal to the implants. *(d)* The implants were uncovered, and the cover screws were removed. *(e)* Healing abutments were screwed in, and a connective tissue graft harvested from the palate was placed to increase soft tissue thickness. *(f)* The buccal flap was sutured to partially cover the graft, and the palatal flap was coronally advanced.

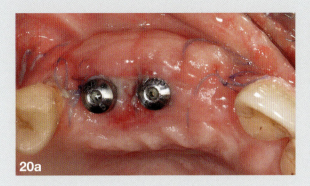

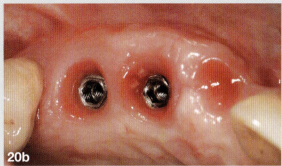

Fig 20 Healing after 15 days. *(a)* Note the considerable thickness of the mucosal tissue. *(b)* Development of the emerging mucosal contours after 6 months of conditioning with the provisional.

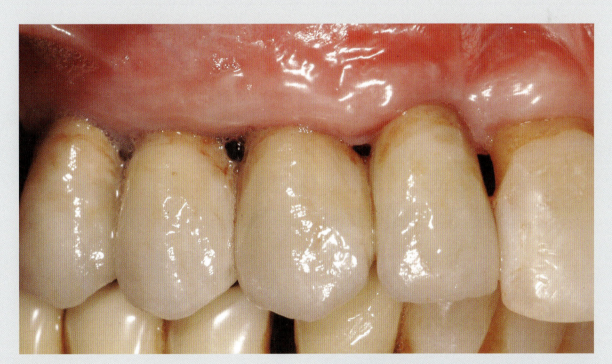

Fig 20c Final ceramic prosthesis.

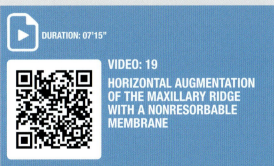

DURATION: 07'15"

VIDEO: 19

HORIZONTAL AUGMENTATION OF THE MAXILLARY RIDGE WITH A NONRESORBABLE MEMBRANE

CLINICAL CASE 4

Horizontal bone augmentation in a partially edentulous distal mandibular ridge

A 48-year-old, nonsmoking patient presented with partial edentulism in the third quadrant, missing the mandibular left first and second molars.

Upon examination **(Figs 21a and 21b),** the mandibular left second premolar, which was rotated by 90 degrees, showed a loss of attachment in the distal portion. The second premolar showed no signs of pathologic periodontal probing or bleeding on probing. The lack of a bone distal to the second premolar made vertical bone regeneration impossible. CBCT imaging **(Figs 21c and 21d)** showed a considerable horizontal defect in the area of the first and second molars, which if regenerated, would make the insertion of two 8-mm implants possible.

This case required horizontal bone augmentation of the residual ridge by means of a resorbable porcine native collagen membrane.

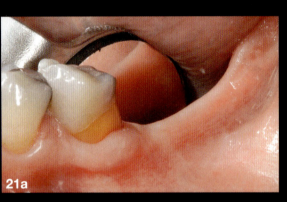

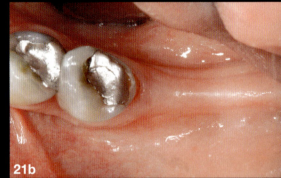

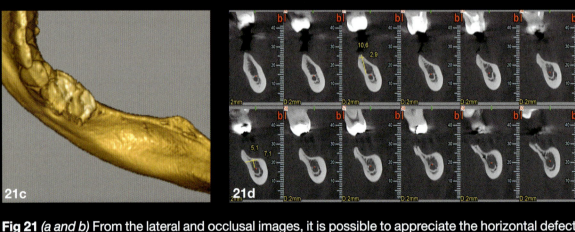

Fig 21 *(a and b)* From the lateral and occlusal images, it is possible to appreciate the horizontal defect caused by long-term edentulousness. One can also see the loss of attachment in the distal portion of the mandibular left first premolar, which appears to be rotated. *(c and d)* On 3D radiographic examination, the horizontal defect of the hard tissue is evident, with only the lingual component of the alveolar process still present.

Performing vertical bone regeneration would have allowed for the placement of longer implants but would have required the extraction of the second premolar to exploit the distal bone peak at the site of the first premolar.

Careful exposure **(Fig 22)** of the blade-like bone ridge made it possible to isolate the mental foramen. Careful curettage of the bone surface and root of the second premolar was performed to prepare the sites adequately for grafting.

The collagen membrane was first secured with four pins (three crestal pins on the lingual side and one distobuccal pin) and then protected during the execution of the cortical perforations performed with a round bur mounted on a straight handpiece **(Fig 23)**. At this point, an adequate amount of graft material, which in this case consisted of a mixture of 40% DBBM and 60% autologous bone harvested from the mandibular ramus with a bone scraper, was placed under the membrane.

To stabilize the graft correctly, several more titanium pins were then placed on the buccal aspect from distal to mesial, with care taken to achieve perfect stabilization of the graft **(Fig 24a to 24c)**.

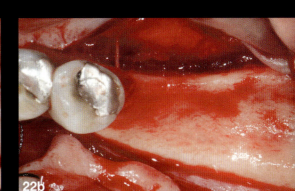

Fig 22 *(a and b)* After elevation of the buccal and lingual flaps, the bone defect that is incompatible with correct immediate implant placement can be seen.

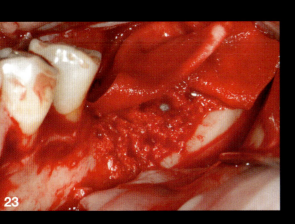

Fig 23 A resorbable collagen membrane was initially fixed on the lingual side and the distal portion, thus creating a sort of container to hold the bone graft, which was composed of 40% DBBM and 60% autologous bone harvested from the mandibular ramus with a bone scraper.

The surgery concluded with soft tissue passivation steps by means of a continuous incision at the buccal periosteum with a loop at the level of the mental foramen to move away from the emergence of the inferior alveolar nerve (IAN) and avoid causing injury to the proximal aspect of the vascular-nervous bundle. The lingual flap was gradually passivated by means of blunt instruments to allow for the gentle release of the fibers of the mylohyoid muscle. Finally, a two-layer suture method with internal horizontal mattress sutures and single interrupted sutures in the ridge allowed for flap closure for healing by primary intention **(Fig 24d)**.

Removal of the sutures at 14 days and subsequent follow-ups attested to the adequate soft tissue management maneuvers and the proper healing of the surgical wound without exposure and without signs of inflammation or infection **(Fig 25a and 25b)**.

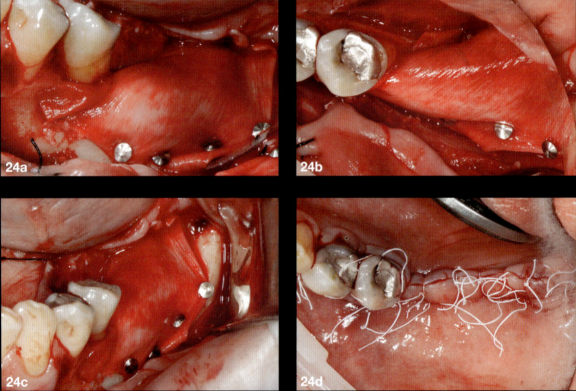

Fig 24 *(a)* The membrane was subsequently fixed in the buccal and mesial areas to create tension to stabilize the underlying graft. *(b)* Occlusal view of the fixed membrane. *(c)* One can appreciate the 3D structure of the reconstruction given by the graft contained within the membrane. *(d)* Deeper internal horizontal mattress sutures and simple interrupted sutures.

The surgical reentry for the placement of two implants with a hybrid surface took place 8 months later, and as can be seen from the 3D radiographic **(Fig 25c)** and clinical images **(Fig 26a)**, the horizontal defect was adequately regenerated. Once inserted, the implants were entirely surrounded by bone of good quality **(Figs 26b and 26c)**. Suturing was performed with 4-0 silk sutures, and the implants were submerged.

The reopening procedure at 4 months included the restoration of an adequate band of adherent gingiva by means of an epithelial-connective tissue graft harvested from the palate **(Figs 26d and 27a)**. Finally, a provisional screw-retained prosthesis made of polymethyl methacrylate (PMMA) bonded to titanium cylinders was fabricated, followed by two screw-retained monolithic zirconia crowns **(Figs 27b and 27c)**.

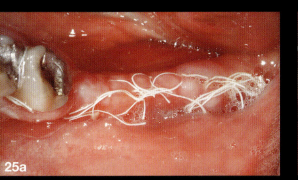

25a

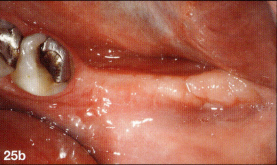

25b

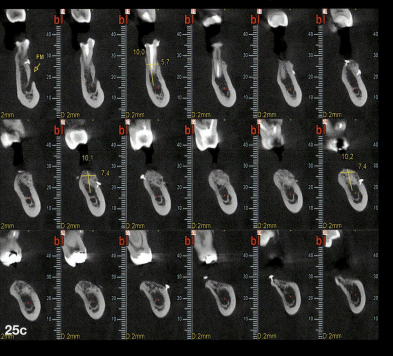

25c

Fig 25 *(a)* Healing 2 weeks after suture removal. *(b)* Healing via primary intention is noted 1 month after surgery. *(c)* CT imaging at 8 months shows the new bone volume with the correction of the horizontal defect, as well as the good integration of the graft, which shows no areas of radiolucency.

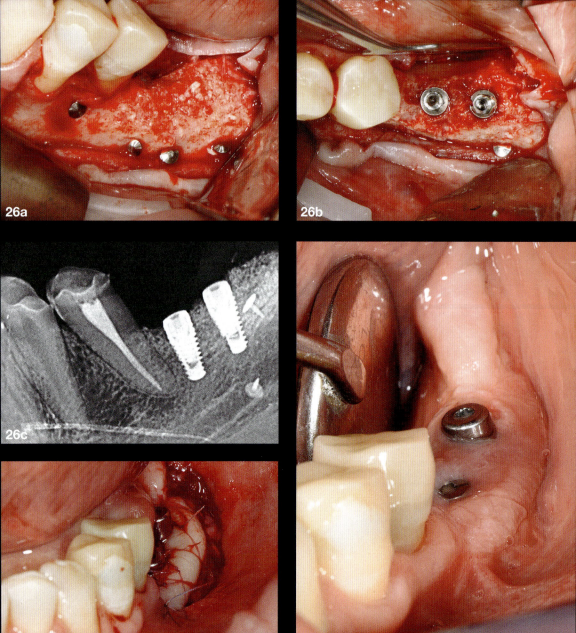

Fig 26 *(a)* Upon reentry for implant placement, the considerable amount of regenerated bone can be appreciated. *(b)* The regenerated bone volume allowed for the placement of two implants in a prosthetically guided position with 2 mm of residual buccal bone. *(c)* Postoperative radiographic control. *(d)* Upon reopening, an apically repositioned flap was performed to restore the fornix associated with placement of a free epithelial-connective tissue graft to restore an adequate keratinized mucosal portion. *(e)* After healing, the restored fornix and the adequate width of the keratinized mucosal band can be appreciated.

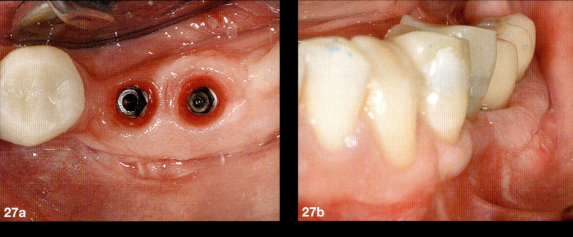

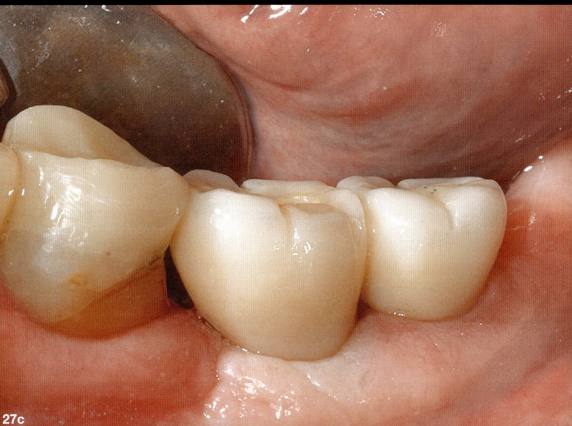

Fig 27 *(a)* Occlusal view showing the horizontal bone regeneration achieved. *(b)* Screw-retained PMMA provisional elements. *(c)* The definitive restoration with screw-retained monolithic zirconia crowns.

CLINICAL CASE 5

Horizontal bone augmentation in an edentulous maxilla

A 44-year-old, nonsmoking woman presented with an edentulous anterior sector of the maxilla. The patient had a history of a sinus neoplasm followed by a series of invasive treatments that led the patient to neglect her oral health. Given the patient's age, the aim was to place implants in a prosthetically guided position to create a prosthesis without a flange and with teeth of adequate size and morphology. As can be seen from the clinical images, exposure of the alveolar ridge revealed the remaining defects after the extractions (**Figs 28 to 30**). Bone loss was predominantly horizontal. Given the esthetic considerations of the case, a two-stage approach was opted for, involving first a horizontal bone regeneration procedure and then implant placement. Due to the extent of the defect, two collagen membranes were used, secured with several titanium pins (**Fig 31**).

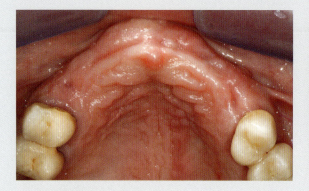

Fig 28 The edentulous area in the anterosuperior sector.

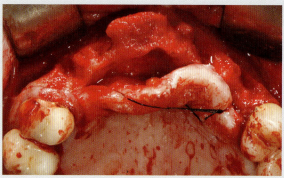

Fig 29 Occlusal view of the bone ridge showing horizontal bone defects.

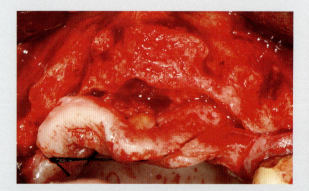

Fig 30 From a frontal view, it is evident that it is impossible to place implants in a prosthetically favorable position due to the bone deficit.

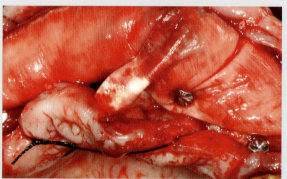

Fig 31 Two native collagen membranes were fixed to the bone with several titanium pins. In this way, the bone graft, composed of 50% autologous bone and 50% DBBM, was stabilized.

The membranes were fixed tightly to immobilize the underlying graft as much as possible. Bone grafting was performed with a mix of autologous bone harvested from the nasal spine (50%) and heterologous bone of bovine origin (50%).

The double-layered PTFE sutures (**Fig 32**) were removed after 14 days, and the good passivation of the buccal flap allowed for healing by primary intention.

Upon surgical reentry after 8 months, four implants were placed in a prosthetically guided position without further bone augmentation (**Figs 33 to 36**). At the same time, a porcine collagen membrane was placed buccal to each implant with the aim of achieving an increase in soft tissue thickness (**Figs 37 and 38**). A screw-retained PMMA provisional prosthesis was inserted 4 months later (**Fig 39**), which was eventually replaced with a final metal-ceramic prosthesis (**Figs 40 and 41**).

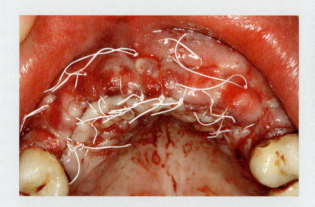

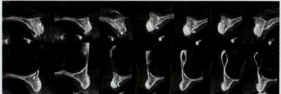

Fig 33 CBCT performed 8 months later showing the good integration of the graft and the volume of bone regeneration achieved.

Fig 32 A two-layer closure is planned with deep horizontal mattress sutures and more superficial simple interrupted sutures.

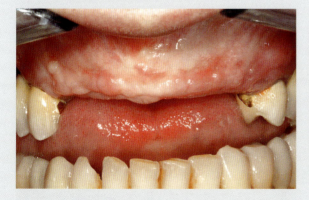

Fig 34 The soft tissues, healed by primary intention, show no signs of inflammation 8 months after surgery.

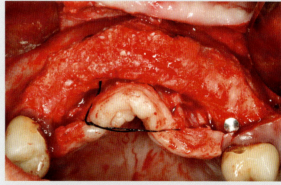

Fig 35 Upon reopening to insert the implants, the quality and volume of the regenerated bone can be observed.

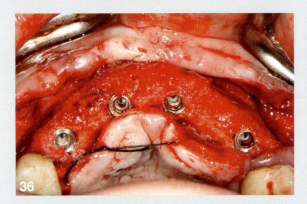
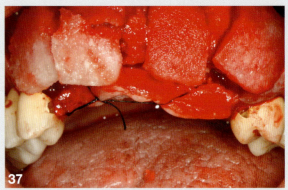

Fig 36 The bone volume allowed for prosthetically guided placement of the implants, which were entirely surrounded by more than 2 mm of bone thickness. **Fig 37** To augment the soft tissue thickness, a tissue matrix made of porcine collagen (Fibro-Gide) was used.

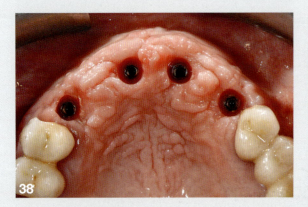
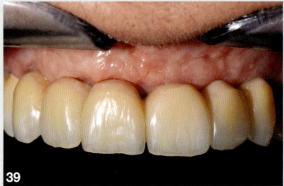

Fig 38 After reopening 4 months after implant placement, the volume of soft tissue obtained can be appreciated. **Fig 39** The provisional was kept in place for about 1 year to achieve good soft tissue conditioning.

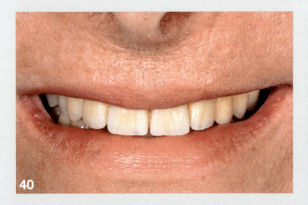
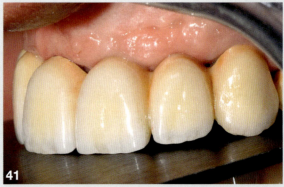

Fig 40 The patient's smile at the end of treatment. **Fig 41** Tissue 3 years after reconstructive surgery.

CLINICAL CASE 6

Horizontal bone augmentation in a completely edentulous maxilla

A 58-year-old nonsmoking patient presented with a completely edentulous maxilla and expressed the wish to receive an implant-supported fixed prosthesis. Objective examination **(Fig 42)** and CBCT imaging **(Fig 43)** revealed severe horizontal bone atrophy, giving a blade-like shape to the entire alveolar ridge, and a lack of vertical dimension in the posterolateral sectors could be observed. The treatment plan involved horizontal bone augmentation with a resorbable membrane, along with bilateral maxillary sinus elevation.

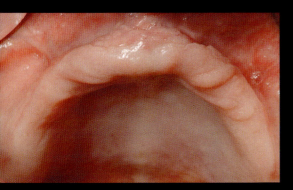

Fig 42 Completely edentulous alveolar ridge with clear signs of horizontal atrophy. The mucosa appears hypertrophied and fluctuating.

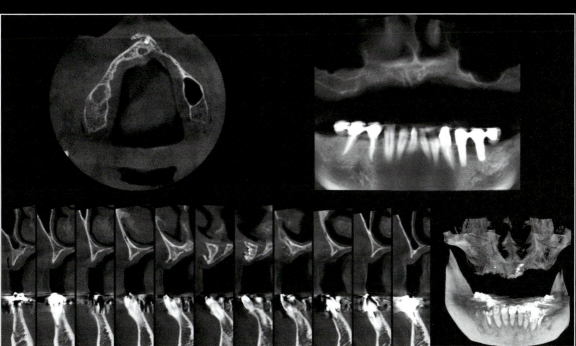

Fig 43 CBCT showing severe horizontal and vertical atrophy.

A full-thickness flap was elevated to expose the atrophic alveolar ridge and maxillary sinuses. The bone surface was carefully smoothed with a back-action chisel, and the inside of the nasopalatine canal was completely denuded of soft tissue with alveolar spoons **(Fig 44a)**. After performing an osteotomy on the lateral wall of the maxillary sinuses, the sinus membranes were gently elevated, creating space for the particulate bone graft. The buccal plate was completely perforated with a low-speed round bur, and the obtained bone particles were left in situ **(Fig 44b)**. Two porcine collagen membranes were fixed to the palatal surface of the bone ridge, adapted and fixed buccally with titanium pins, leaving a buccal and mesial opening to allow for the introduction of a particulate mixture of 70% autologous bone, harvested from the mandibular ascending ramus, and 30% DBBM. The mesial opening was then closed with additional pins **(Fig 44c)**.

Fig 44 *(a)* After the full-thickness flaps were elevated, the bladelike coronal portion of the ridge became evident. *(b)* The buccal cortical was perforated, and the bone particles produced were left in situ. *(c)* Two porcine collagen membranes were fixed palatally with titanium pins and adapted and fixed buccally, leaving an opening for filling with 70% autologous and 30% particulate bone graft. The mesial opening was then closed with additional pins. *(d)* After generous release of the flap by means of a continuous periosteal incision, horizontal and alternating simple sutures were applied.

The flap was extensively released with a periosteal incision, and two-level suturing with horizontal mattress and simple interrupted ePTFE sutures was performed **(Fig 44d)**.

The sutures were removed after 12 days, and the patient was unable to wear the prosthesis for 3 weeks. The waiting period for the bone neoformation was 6 months, during which no adverse events occurred.

At the time of implant placement surgery, the mucosa appeared pink and without signs of infection or inflammation **(Fig 45a)**. CBCT imaging showed a bone-like tissue, more radiopaque due to the inorganic component of the xenograft, with sufficient vertical and horizontal dimensions for implant placement **(Fig 45b)**. A full-thickness flap elevation confirmed a significant increase in the volume of the alveolar ridge **(Fig 46)**.

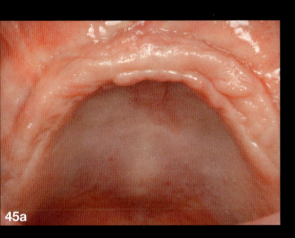

45a

Fig 45 *(a)* Healing after 6 months. The mucosa appears pink and without signs of inflammation. *(b)* CBCT shows the regenerated tissue, which is extremely radiopaque due to the presence of heterologous bone particles.

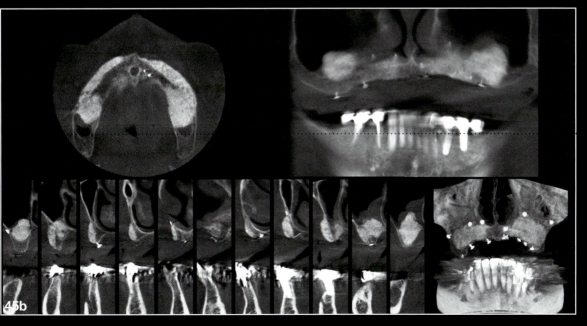

45b

Six slightly tapered hybrid surface iMAX (IRES) implants were inserted bilaterally in the sites of the maxillary second premolars, first premolars, and canines (Fig 47), and the flap was sutured with 4-0 silk sutures (Fig 48).

After an additional 4 months of submerged healing, the prosthetic abutments and the provisional acrylic denture were attached. Finally, after 3 months of tissue maturation, the final screw-retained zirconia and ceramic prosthesis was placed (Fig 49).

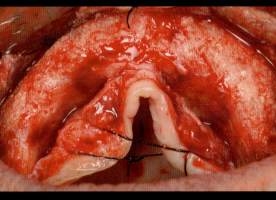

Fig 46 After elevation of the full-thickness flaps, the abundant quantity and good quality of the newly formed bone is evident.

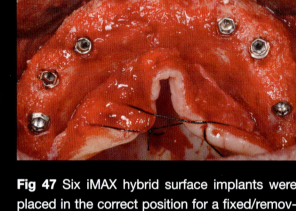

Fig 47 Six iMAX hybrid surface implants were placed in the correct position for a fixed/removable prosthesis. Bone thickness of more than 2 mm was maintained buccally to compensate for any resorption.

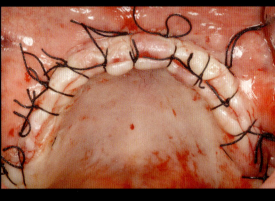

Fig 48 The flaps were sutured with alternating mattress and simple silk sutures.

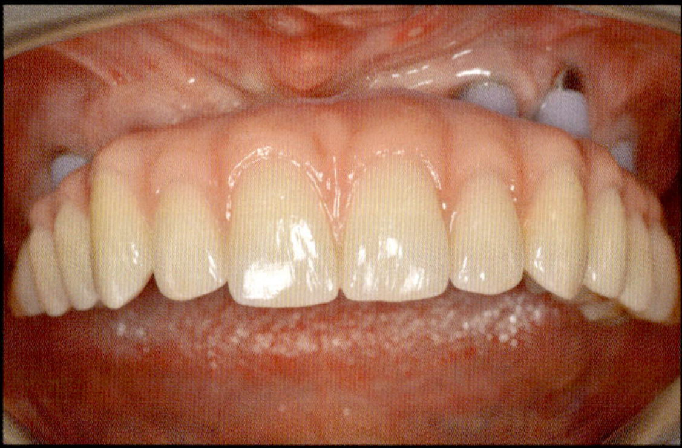

Fig 49 After 4 months of submerged healing, a provisional was used for an additional 3 months, and then the final screw-retained zirconia and ceramic prosthesis was placed.

REFERENCES

1. Albrektsson T, Zarb G, Worthington P, Eriksson AR. The long-term efficacy of currently used dental implants: A review and proposal criteria of success. Int J Oral Maxillofac Implants 1986;1:11–25.

2. Dahlin C, Anderson L, Linde A. Bone augmentation at fenestrated implants by an osteopromotive membrane technique. A controlled clinical study. Clin Oral Implants Res 1991;2:159–165.

3. Dahlin C, Lekholm U, Linde A. Membrane-induced bone augmentation at titanium implants. A report of 10 fixtures followed from 1 to 3 years after loading. Int J Periodontics Restorative Dent 1991;11:273–281.

4. Jovanovic SA, Spiekermann H, Richter EJ. Bone regeneration around titanium implants in dehisced defect sites: A clinical study. Int J Oral Maxillofac Implants 1992;7:33–245.

5. Dahlin C, Lekholm U, Becker W, Higuchi K, Callens A, van Steenberghe D. Treatment of fenestration and dehiscence bone defects around oral implants using the guided tissue regeneration technique: A prospective multicenter study. Int J Oral Maxillofac Implants 1995;10:312–318.

6. Simion M, Misitano U, Gionso L, Salvato A. Treatment of dehiscence and fenestrations around dental implants using resorbable and non-resorbable membranes associated with bone autografts: A comparative clinical study. Int J Oral Maxillofac Implants 1997;12:159–167.

7. Buser D, Bragger U, Lang NP, Nyman S. Regeneration and enlargement of jaw bone using guided tissue regeneration. Clin Oral Implants Res 1990;1:22–32.

8. Buser D, Dula K, Belser U, Hirt HP, Bertold H. Localized ridge augmentation using guided bone regeneration prior to implant placement. Surgical procedure in the maxilla. Int J Periodontics Restorative Dent 1993;13:29–45.

9. Nevins R, Mellonig JT. The advantage of localised ridge augmentation prior to implant placement. A staged event. Int J Periodontics Restorative Dent 1994;14:97–111.

10. Buser D, Dula K, Hirt HP, Schenk R. Lateral ridge augmentation using autografts and barrier membranes: A clinical study with 40 partially edentulous patients. J Oral Maxillofac Surg 1996;54:420–32.

11. Thoma DS, Bienz SP, Figuero E, Jung RE, Sanz-Martín I. Efficacy of lateral bone augmentation performed simultaneously with dental implant placement. A systematic review and meta-analysis. J Clin Periodontol 2019;46 (Suppl 21):257–276.

12. Naenni N, Lim HC, Papageorgiou SN, Hämmerle CHF. Efficacy of lateral ridge augmentation prior to implant placement: A systematic review and meta-analysis. J Clin Periodontol 2019;46(Suppl 21):287–306.

13. Jung RE, Herzog M, Wolleb K, Ramel CF, Thoma DS, Hämmerle CH. A randomized controlled clinical trial comparing small buccal dehiscence defects around dental implants treated with guided bone regeneration or left for spontaneous healing. Clin Oral Implants Res 2017;28: 348–354.

14. Schwartz F, Sahm N, Becker J. Impact of the outcome of guided bone regeneration in dehiscence-type defects on the long-term stability of peri-implant health: Clinical observations at 4 years. Clin Oral Implants Res 2012;23:191–196.

15. Von Arx T, Buser D. Horizontal ridge augmentation using autogenous block grafts and the guided bone regeneration technique with collagen membranes: A clinical study with 42 patients. Clin Oral Implants Res 2006;17:359–366.

16. Hämmerle CH, Jung RE, Yaman D, Lang NP. Ridge augmentation by applying bioresorbable membranes and deproteinized bovine bone mineral: A report of 12 consecutive cases. Clin Oral Implants Res 2008;19:19–25.

17. Urban IA, Nagursky H, Lozada JL. Horizontal ridge augmentation with a resorbable membrane and particulated autogenous bone with or without anorganic bovine bone-derived mineral: A prospective case series in 22 patients. Int J Oral Maxillofac Implants 2011;26:404–414.

18. Urban IA, Nagursky H, Lozada JL, Nagy K. Horizontal ridge augmentation with a collagen membrane and a combination of particulate autogenous bone and anorganic bovine bone-derived mineral: A prospective case series in 25 patients. Int J Periodontics Restorative Dent 2013;33:299–307.

19. Meloni SM, Jovanovic SA, Urban I, Canullo L, Pisano M, Tallarico M. Horizontal ridge augmentation using GBR with a native collagen membrane and 1:1 ratio of particulate xenograft and autologous bone: A 1-year prospective clinical study. Clin Implant Dent Relat Res 2017;19:38–45.

VERTICAL ALVEOLAR RIDGE AUGMENTATION

CHAPTER 17

Edited by Massimo Simion

INTRODUCTION

Vertical alveolar ridge augmentation using guided bone regeneration (GBR) is the most sophisticated and complex of implant surgery techniques, as well as the most fascinating. At the beginning of the 1990s, the possibility of regenerating bone in a vertical direction was far from the common imagination of practitioners, but three visionary clinicians, Massimo Simion, Carlo Tinti, and Sascha Jovanovic, simultaneously and independently developed a technique for vertical alveolar ridge augmentation using virtually identical membranes.[1-5] The advent of vertical ridge augmentation has significantly altered implant treatment planning by extending its indications to a large number of patients who were previously excluded due to a lack of vertical ridge dimension. The typical indications for vertical ridge augmentation are for patients with insufficient bone height in the lateral sectors of the mandible and maxilla, for patients with mucosa-supported skeletal prostheses, and for the rehabilitation of the anterior maxilla in patients with severe bone deficits caused by trauma or periodontal disease.

Performing vertical bone regeneration techniques requires considerable experience and should be reserved for those primarily involved in periodontal and implant surgery.

Massimo Simion

There is a current trend of using increasingly short-er dental implants[6] in an attempt to avoid complex vertical regeneration techniques and to reduce the invasiveness of treatment. However, using short implants to rehabilitate alveolar ridges with vertical atrophy has a number of limitations, which are often insurmountable.

First, using short implants in anterior sectors with esthetic value is contraindicated because short implants correspond to prostheses with long clinical crowns and unacceptable esthetic results. Short implants can therefore be used only in limited cases in posterolateral sectors, when structures such as the inferior alveolar nerve (IAN) and maxillary sinus are unlikely to be damaged.

Imagine, for example, that implants must be inserted in the sites of the mandibular premolars and molars in a ridge with vertical atrophy. Implants considered reasonably short have a length of 6 mm. As a basic rule of caution, 2 mm should be maintained between the apex of the implant and the IAN. In the absence of regenerative techniques, therefore, this limits the treatment of atrophic mandibles with short implants to ridges with a vertical dimension of at least 8 mm from the crestal plate to the IAN.

Finally, the considerable length of the prosthetic crowns is also often associated with a shallow fornix depth, which hampers proper home cleaning of the prosthesis and peri-implant tissues.

On the other hand, as with horizontal bone regeneration, numerous preclinical animal studies have confirmed the biologic basis of vertical bone regeneration. In 1991, Schmid et al[7] published a study in which domed implants were placed in rabbit calvaria and allowed to protrude a few millimeters. The implants were covered with an expanded polytetrafluoroethylene (ePTFE) membranes and left to heal in a submerged position. After 3 months of healing, it was possible to demonstrate bone neoformation under the membranes and osseointegration at the interface between the titanium and the regenerated bone. Similar results were obtained by Linde et al,[8] who used dome-shaped ePTFE membranes in rat calvaria. In 1995, Jovanovic et al[2] presented a study on five dogs, in which a surgical protocol similar to that used in the first clinical trials in humans was used. The implants were allowed to protrude 2.7 mm, covered with an ePTFE membrane, reinforced with a titanium framework, and left to heal in a submerged position for 4 months. Histologic examination of the block sections demonstrated complete bone regeneration down to the most coronal portion of the implant.

A similar study published by Simion et al[9] described the pattern of vertical bone regeneration in the mandibles of four dogs with a surgical protocol identical to that used in humans.

The implants on the test side were allowed to protrude from the mandibular bone crest by 4 mm (**Fig 1**) and were covered with a titanium-reinforced ePTFE membrane.

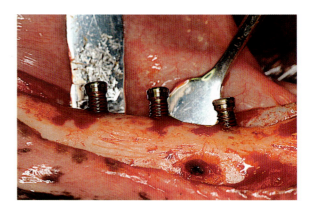

Fig 1 *Three implants with machined surfaces were inserted and allowed to protrude 4 mm above the edentulous bone crest. (Figures 1 to 4 reprinted with permission from Clin Oral Implants Res 2007;18:86–94.)*

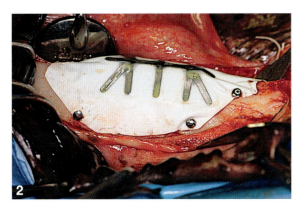 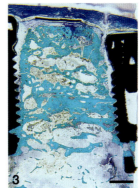 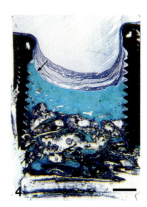

Fig 2 The implants were covered with a titanium-reinforced ePTFE membrane, and the defect was filled with a blood clot. *Fig 3* Histologic preparation showing almost complete bone regeneration of a test site after 6 months of healing. Mesiodistal section. Tetrachromic staining: Sudan black, Toluidine blue, basic Fuchsin, and light green; ×4 magnification. *Fig 4* Histologic preparation of a control site. Without the presence of a membrane, the soft tissue collapsed within the defect, preventing bone regeneration. Mesiodistal section. Tetrachromic staining: Sudan black, Toluidine blue, basic Fuchsin, and light green; ×4 magnification.

Venous blood was then injected beneath the membrane to achieve adequate clot formation **(Fig 2)**. On the control side, the implants were allowed to protrude to the same extent without the application of the membrane. After 6 months of submerged healing without complications, the test sites showed complete bone regeneration up to the lower surface of the membrane, whereas in the control sites there was complete soft tissue collapse around the implants and minimal bone regeneration.

Histologic evaluation showed that regeneration occurred via osteoblastic proliferation from the native crestal bone facing the defect **(Figs 3 and 4)**.

The first clinical and histologic study in humans on vertical ridge augmentation with the GBR technique was published by Simion et al in 1994.[1]

Five patients were treated with a total of 10 implants, which were left protruding 4 to 7 mm above the atrophic ridge **(Fig 5)** and covered with an ePTFE membrane secured with several miniscrews. The space below the membrane was filled carefully with blood to obtain a stable clot **(Fig 6)**. An additional mini-implant with a diameter of 1.6 mm was placed at each site for subsequent histologic evaluation. This important work demonstrated for the first time the possibility of using GBR to regenerate up to 4 mm of bone vertically in humans without the aid of bone grafts **(Fig 7)**. Histologic evaluation of the samples obtained from the mini-implants removed with core drills showed that the regenerated bone was able to integrate with the implant surface with contact percentages (bone-to-implant contact [BIC]) of about 42% **(Fig 8)**. A similar surgical protocol was described by Tinti et al[3] with the addition of autologous bone particles to fill the defect under the membrane. This study, on 16 implants placed in six patients, demonstrated the possibility of regenerating up to 7 mm of bone vertically.

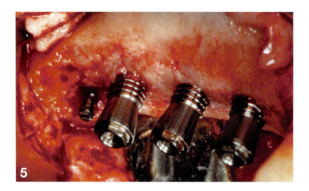
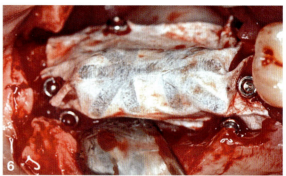

Fig 5 *Three machined implants were allowed to protrude 7 mm in a supracrestal position in the sites of the maxillary right second premolar, first molar, and second molar. (Figures 4 to 8 reprinted with permission from Int J Periodontics Restorative Dent 1994;14:496–511.)* **Fig 6** *A titanium-reinforced ePTFE membrane was secured with six mini-screws, and the space underneath was filled with a blood clot.*

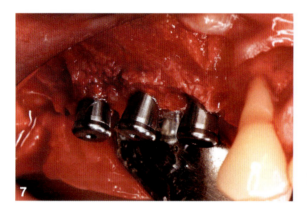
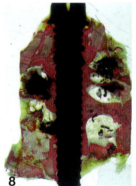

Fig 7 *Upon removal of the membrane after 9 months of healing, the implants were covered two-thirds with regenerated bone.* **Fig 8** *The histologic examination of the titanium pin showed partly woven and partly lamellar bone in direct contact with the implant.*

Another clinical and histologic study by Simion et al,[4] which included 20 patients and 56 implants, confirmed these results. The membrane technique was combined with autologous bone chips or freeze-dried and demineralized human bone particles (DFDBA) **(Figs 9 to 20)**. The histologic results showed BIC percentages ranging between 39.1% and 63.2% **(Fig 21)**. Similar results were obtained by Tinti and Parma-Benfenati,[5] confirming the effectiveness of combining autologous bone particles with nonresorbable ePTFE membranes. The GBR technique for vertical ridge

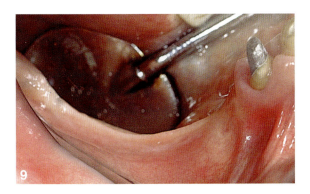
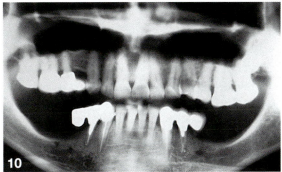

Fig 9 *Mandibular right distal edentulous ridge with severe vertical atrophy. (Figures 9 to 21 reprinted with permission from Int J Periodontics Restorative Dent 1998;18:8–23.)* **Fig 10** *Panoramic radiograph showing bilateral mandibular atrophy at the sites of the mandibular second premolars, first molars, and second molars. The mandibular canal runs 4 mm apical to the bone crest.*

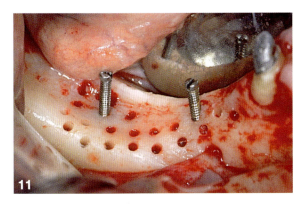
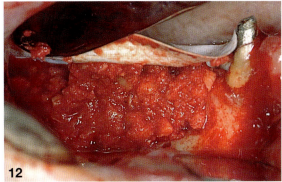

Fig 11 *Two full-thickness flaps, one vestibular and one lingual, were elevated. Two titanium pins were inserted, and the cortical bone plate was perforated with a round bur. The IAN at the exit of the mental foramen is visible.* **Fig 12** *An ePTFE membrane was secured lingually with two mini-screws, and a particulate graft of autologous bone was placed to fill the defect.*

augmentation has been successfully used by many clinicians worldwide, and numerous publications have confirmed its effectiveness, while also emphasizing the complexity of the technique,[10–15] which was standardized as far back as 1996, in the publications of Simion, Jovanovic, and Tinti. In the years that followed development of the technique, important long-term evidence was obtained by means of prospective and retrospective studies that demonstrated the stability of the regenerated bone over time and the high percentage of implant survival, with follow-ups from 5 to 22 years.[16–23]

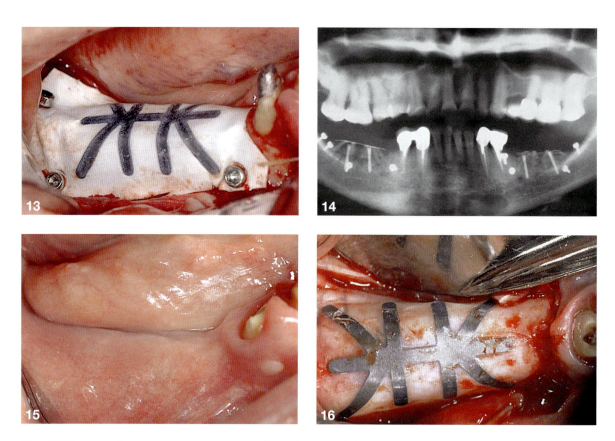

Fig 13 *The membrane was secured buccally with two mini-screws.* **Fig 14** *Postoperative panoramic radiograph showing the membrane and fixation instruments.* **Fig 15** *Healing occurred without complications for 6 months, until the membrane was removed.* **Fig 16** *The membrane was exposed with a new flap, and the fixation screws were removed.*

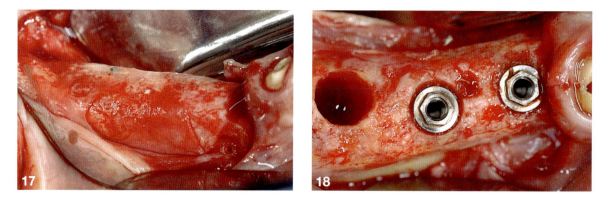

Fig 17 *After removal of the membrane, abundant bone regeneration is visible.* **Fig 18** *Two machined implants were inserted, and the distal pin was cored with a trephine for histologic examination.*

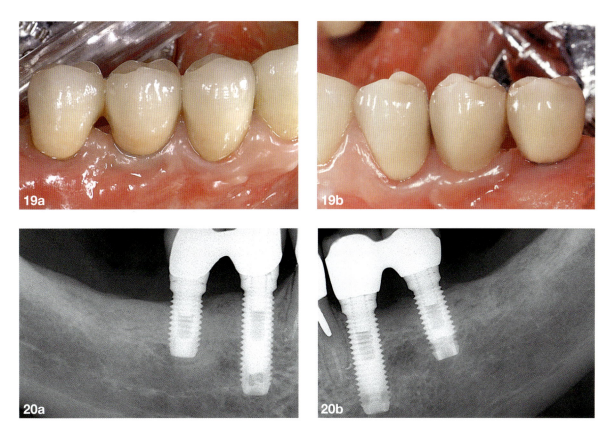

Fig 19 *Final prosthetic restoration after 4 months of submerged implant integration.* (a) *Right side.* (b) *Left side.* **Fig 20** *Periapical radiographs after 1 year.* (a) *Right side.* (b) *Left side.*

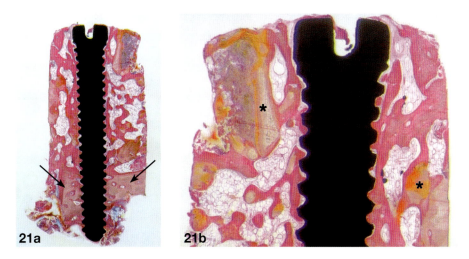

Fig 21 (a) *Histologic preparation showing native cortical bone* (arrow) *and regenerated bone in direct contact with the titanium pin. Hematoxylin and eosin (H&E) staining; ×4 magnification.* (b) *At higher magnification (×10), the grafted bone particles integrated with the newly formed bone are visible* (asterisk).

INDICATIONS FOR VERTICAL ALVEOLAR RIDGE AUGMENATION

The indications for vertical ridge augmentation naturally include all cases of vertical bone atrophy in which it is not possible to opt for short implants without compromising long-term implant success, esthetics, or peri-implant tissue hygiene, and when surgery cannot be performed without risking injury to important anatomical structures such as the IAN or maxillary sinuses.

Patient selection must be performed on the basis of well-defined decision-making parameters such as the following:

- the patient's oral health status
- characteristics of the soft tissue
- bone peaks around adjacent teeth
- quantity of residual alveolar/basal bone
- adjacent prosthetic margins
- adjacent third molars

Oral health status of the patient

The health of the periodontal tissues and remaining teeth must be evaluated during the clinical examination because both implant therapy and GBR techniques are contraindicated in patients with active periodontal disease.

In periodontal patients, complete causal therapy must be completed before proceeding with regenerative techniques.

The presence of apical granulomas adjacent to the defect also constitutes a significant risk because surgical trauma may stimulate the formation of latent peri-apical abscesses involving the regenerative site.

An accurate evaluation of the occlusal relationship between the arches must also be performed to identify and, if necessary, correct any malocclusion, particularly deviations of the curve of Spee that may reduce the interocclusal dimension and thus prevent adequate prosthetic rehabilitation

of the area to be regenerated. Finally, the level of patient motivation and compliance should be considered.

Soft tissue characteristics

A careful examination of the soft tissue characteristics at the surgical site and adjacent teeth is essential to avoid complications in the postoperative period. Thin, delicate tissues and a lack of keratinized mucosa are not an absolute contraindication to vertical ridge augmentation, but they are predisposed to wound dehiscence and consequent early exposure of the membrane. Compression decubitus caused by prosthetic elements, incompletely healed extraction sites, and tissue clefts resulting from traumatic extractions contraindicate surgery. Tissue clefts **(Fig 22a)** should be treated beforehand with connective tissue grafts, and extraction sites should be left for 2 to 3 months until the soft tissue has completely healed **(Fig 22b)**.

Bone peaks around adjacent teeth

The level of periodontal attachment and bone peaks of adjacent elements are fundamental for determining the vertical dimension of bone that can be regenerated. In fact, the presence of bone peaks is indispensable to support membranes in the vicinity of other teeth and to provide adequate blood supply and osteogenic cells to the tissues being regenerated **(Fig 23)**.

In the diagnostic phase, CBCT imaging and periodontal probing of the elements adjacent to the defect are essential.

Vertical ridge augmentation coronal to the bone peaks is possible but not predictable and is extremely difficult to achieve.

Its predictability and success rates have yet to be determined with long-term longitudinal studies, and its use is limited to areas of important esthetic value. It is discussed later in this chapter.

Amount of residual alveolar/basal bone

The possibility of adequately stabilizing an implant at the time of its insertion should be evaluated when considering either a one-stage operation, in which the bone around already inserted implants is regenerated, or a two-stage operation, in which the alveolar ridge is first regenerated and then the implants are inserted. In the single-stage procedure, the submerged healing time varies from 6 to 8 months, depending on the volume of bone to be regenerated. In the two-stage procedure, 6 to 8 months are allowed for bone neoformation before inserting the implants and letting them integrate in the submerged position for an additional 4 months.

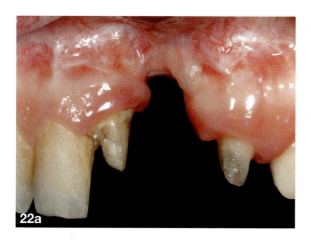 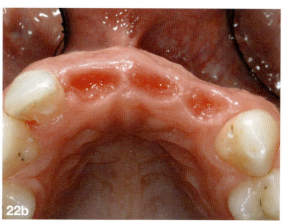

Fig 22 (a) *Tissue clefts following traumatic avulsion of the maxillary left central incisor.* (b) *Extraction sites after 1 month of healing. The mucosa is not yet fully mature for regenerative intervention.*

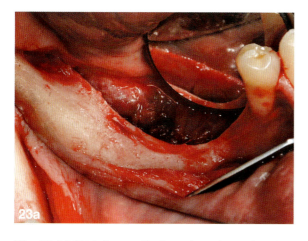 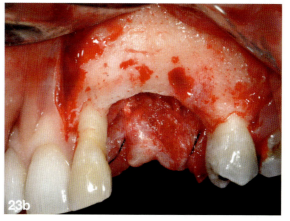

Fig 23 (a) *Distal mandibular edentulous alveolar ridge with vertical atrophy. The ideal bone peaks for vertical bone regeneration are present.* (b) *Atrophic intercalated edentulous ridge complicated by loss of attachment on the maxillary left central incisor resulting in the absence of a mesial bone peak.*

Assuming an approximate bone regeneration rate of 1 mm per month, a healing period of 8 to 12 months is required for vertical bone regeneration of more than 7 mm.

A further decision criterion for choosing between a one- or two-stage operation is the esthetic value of the site.

Two-stage surgery is more appropriate in the anterior maxilla, where the esthetic result is decisive for the success of the operation. A two-stage surgical protocol also provides more opportunities to intervene with soft tissue augmentation techniques (see chapter 19).

Adjacent prosthetic margins

The presence of implant-supported adjacent prosthetic crowns with incongruous margins is a serious risk factor for postoperative infections caused by bacterial colonization of the interface between the prosthetic margin and the abutment. Incongruous crowns must be replaced with provisionals that can be removed during surgery. Because there is no real periodontal attachment, the presence of implants adjacent to the area to

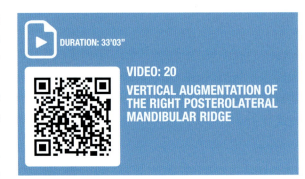

DURATION: 33'03"

VIDEO: 20
VERTICAL AUGMENTATION OF THE RIGHT POSTEROLATERAL MANDIBULAR RIDGE

be regenerated also contraindicates vertical ridge augmentation because the implant surface provides a conduit for bacteria to reach deep into the membrane surface.

Adjacent third molars

In partially edentulous posterior sectors, the presence of third molars, especially if they are inclined mesially, considerably complicates the technical surgical procedure. Coronal repositioning of the flaps tends to result in excessive submergence of the distal element, predisposing the surgical site to infections. Therefore, removal of the third molars 2 months prior to surgery is indicated.

CLINICAL CASE 1

Vertical ridge augmentation in the area of the mandibular incisors

A 40-year-old, nonsmoking patient in good health was involved in a serious car accident and suffered a fracture of the horizontal branch of the mandible and traumatic avulsion of the mandibular incisors with the alveolar process (Fig 24). The idea of rehabilitating the patient with short implants and very long prosthetic teeth was discarded due to esthetic reasons, as well as the difficulty of maintaining proper oral hygiene. A one-stage vertical ridge augmentation technique was therefore opted for, given the possibility of adequately stabilizing the implants.

After a crestal incision in the center of the residual keratinized mucosa, extensive buccal and lingual flaps were elevated, extending as far as the premolars (Fig 25). The osteosynthesis plates were removed, and three machined surface implants were inserted (Fig 26). The implant heads were positioned 3 mm apical to the cementoenamel junction (CEJ) of the two adjacent canines. As a result, the implants protruded above the bone crest by 6 to 8 mm (Fig 27). A bone graft was harvested from the chin with a trephine, ground to particles of less than 1 mm, and placed around the implants to fill the bone defect. A nonresorbable titanium-reinforced ePTFE membrane was secured buccally (Fig 28) and then adapted and secured palatally (Fig 29). After the releasing incision was performed at the periosteum, the flaps were sutured with horizontal mattress sutures alternating with simple ePTFE sutures.

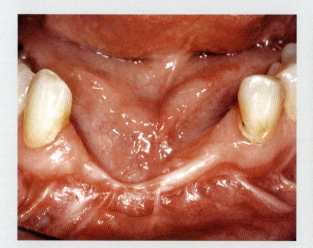

Fig 24 A patient with partial edentulism and severe vertical bone atrophy in the area of the mandibular incisors following a car accident.

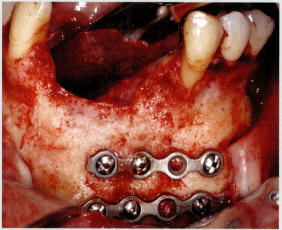

Fig 25 After the elevation of full-thickness flaps, the bony defect and the osteosynthesis plates used to stabilize the fracture of the horizontal branch of the mandible are visible.

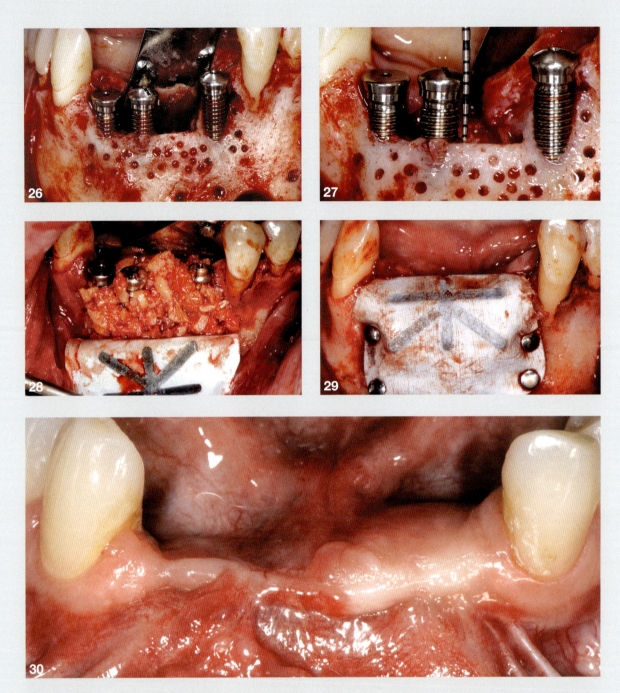

Fig 26 The osteosynthesis plates were removed, and three machined implants were inserted in a supracrestal position. The bone was perforated, and a bone graft was harvested from the same site with a trephine. **Fig 27** The implant heads were positioned 3 mm apical to the CEJ of the adjacent teeth, resulting in an implant body exposure of 6 to 8 mm. **Fig 28** A reinforced ePTFE membrane was secured buccally with two pins, and bone samples were crushed and placed in the defect. **Fig 29** The membrane was adapted lingually and secured with additional buccal and lingual pins. **Fig 30** Healing occurred without complications.

Healing occurred without complications (**Fig 30**), and after 6 months of submerged healing, the membrane was removed, revealing total bone regeneration up to the head of the implants (**Fig 31**). Healing abutments were applied and, after 1 month, a free gingival graft was placed to increase the amount of keratinized mucosa (**Fig 32**). The final ceramic crowns were delivered after 3 months of provisional prosthesis use (**Fig 33**).

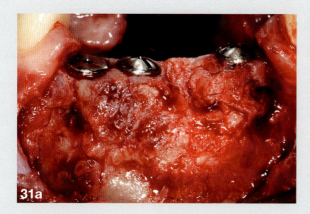
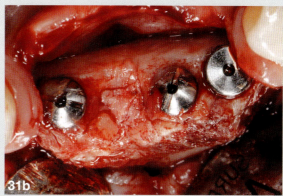

Fig 31 *(a and b)* After 6 months, the membrane was removed, revealing the regenerated bone around the implants.

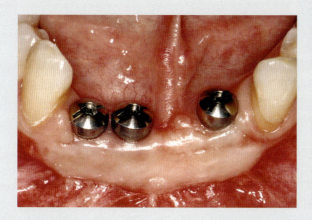
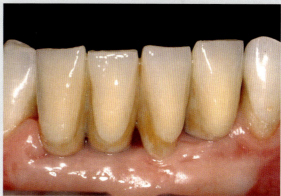

Fig 32 After 1 month, a free gingival graft was placed to increase the amount of keratinized mucosa.

Fig 33 Finally, the patient received the definitive restorations.

CLINICAL CASE 2

Vertical ridge augmentation beyond the bone peaks in an esthetic zone

A 25-year-old, nonsmoking patient in good health underwent surgical removal of an epidermoid mucosal carcinoma in the area of the maxillary left lateral incisor and canine. The operation resulted in the loss of the two teeth and created a large residual bone defect (**Fig 34**). CBCT imaging showed a defect encompassing the entire alveolar process and the basal bone involving the floor of the nasal cavity and the left maxillary sinus (**Fig 35**). A full-thickness flap was extended to the adjacent incisor and premolar. The periosteum was elevated up to the inside of the nasal cavity and maxillary sinus to completely isolate the defect. The distal root portion of the maxillary left central incisor and the mesial root portion of the maxillary left first premolar appeared to be affected by the bone defect, with an attachment loss of approximately 5 and 3 mm, respectively. The total vertical dimension of the defect was 20 mm (**Fig 36**).

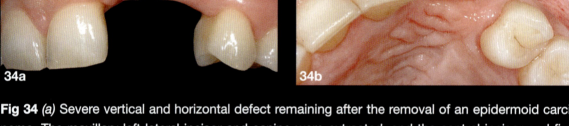

Fig 34 *(a)* Severe vertical and horizontal defect remaining after the removal of an epidermoid carcinoma. The maxillary left lateral incisor and canine were extracted, and the central incisor and first premolar suffered a loss of periodontal attachment on the distal and mesial surfaces respectively. *(b)* From the palatal view, horizontal loss of bone volume is evident.

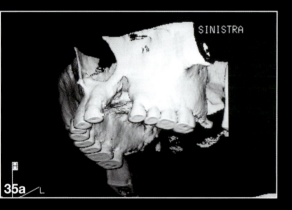
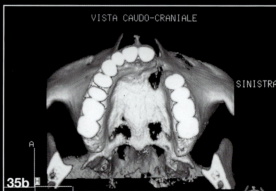

Fig 35 *(a and b)* CBCT showing a huge bony defect extending to the basal bone and involving the floor of the nasal cavity and the left maxillary sinus.

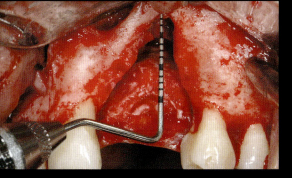

Fig 36 An extensive full-thickness flap was elevated, revealing a vertical bone defect of 20 mm and the loss of attachment of 5 mm on the distal aspect of the root of the central incisor and 3 mm on the mesial aspect of the first premolar.

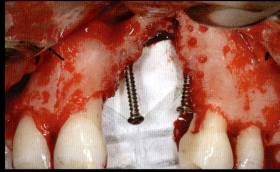

Fig 37 Two support screws were fixed obliquely to the mesial and distal walls of the defect, and a titanium-reinforced ePTFE membrane was secured palatally with two pins.

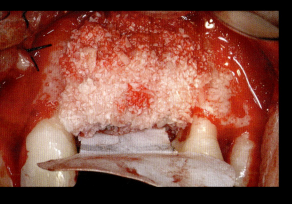

Fig 38 The exposed root portions were treated with amelogenins, and a particulate bone graft with 80% autologous bone and 20% DBBM was placed in the defect and against the root surfaces.

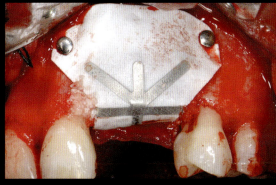

Fig 39 The membrane was secured buccally with two additional titanium pins so that it wouldn't come into contact with the adjacent roots.

Because no bone roof was present, the two screws supporting the membrane were anchored obliquely to the mesial and distal walls of the defect. A titanium-reinforced ePTFE membrane was appropriately cut and secured palatally with two mini-screws **(Fig 37)**. The exposed root surfaces were treated with amelogenins and ethylenediaminetetraacetic acid (EDTA) for 3 minutes before placement of a particulate graft with 80% autologous bone and 20% deproteinized bovine bone mineral (DBBM) (Bio-Oss, Geistlich Biomaterials) **(Fig 38)**. The membrane was then closed buccally and secured with two pins so that the bone graft was in contact with the root surfaces without the membrane margins touching the roots **(Fig 39)**.

The periosteum of the buccal flap at the defect was elevated in a partial-thickness flap (Fig 40) and anchored 4 mm below the palatal flap (Fig 41). The buccal flap was sutured with horizontal mattress sutures and simple interrupted sutures (Fig 42). Healing occurred without complications and with partial crown coverage of the adjacent teeth (Fig 43).

After 8 months of healing, the membrane was removed, and two implants with machined surfaces were placed in the sites of the maxillary left lateral incisor and canine (Fig 44). The site was then covered with a layer of particulate DBBM (Bio-Oss) (Fig 45) and a resorbable collagen membrane (Bio-Gide, Geistlich Biomaterials) (Fig 46) and sutured with the same technique to achieve healing by primary intention. After an additional 4 months (Fig 47), the implants were connected to the healing abutments and a provisional was placed. The final ceramic prosthesis was placed after 6 months to await tissue maturation (Fig 48).

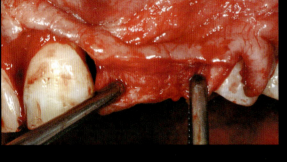

Fig 40 The periosteum of the buccal flap at the defect was elevated partial thickness and rotated palatally.

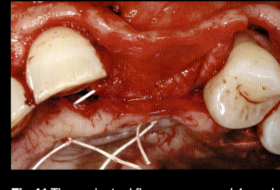

Fig 41 The periosteal flap was secured 4 mm below the palatal flap.

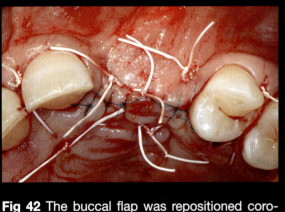

Fig 42 The buccal flap was repositioned coronally and sutured to the palatal flap with horizontal ePTFE mattress sutures and simple Prolene (Ethicon) sutures.

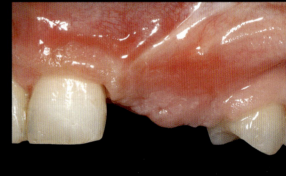

Fig 43 After 15 days of healing without complications, the tissues partially covered the crowns of the adjacent teeth.

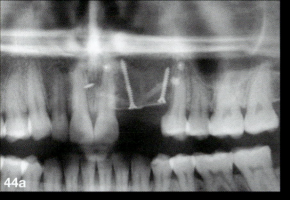

44a

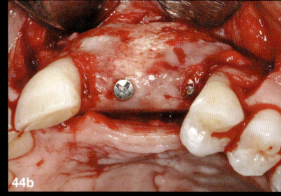

44b

DURATION: 21'00"

VIDEO: 21

VERTICAL RIDGE AUGMENTATION BEYOND THE BONE PEAKS IN AN ESTHETIC ZONE

Fig 44 *(a)* Panoramic radiograph after 8 months of healing. *(b)* The membrane has been removed, revealing bone regeneration in relation to the root surfaces. A thin layer of connective tissue covers the newly formed bone. *(c)* Two machined implants were placed in the sites of the maxillary right lateral incisor and canine.

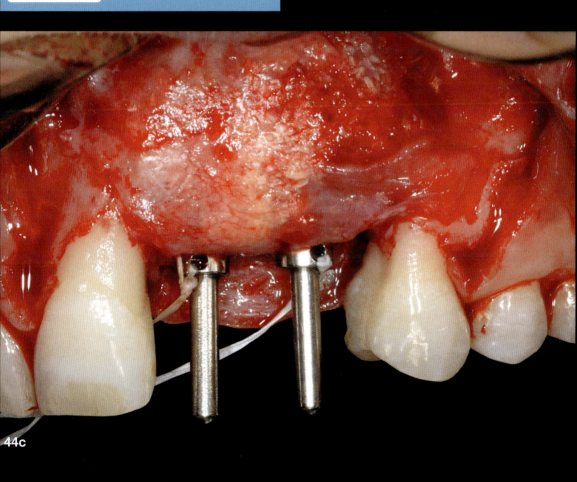

44c

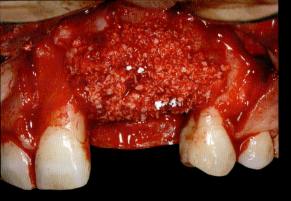

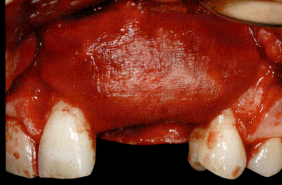

Fig 45 A layer of DBBM was placed to cover the regenerated bone.

Fig 46 The biomaterial was covered with a re-sorbable collagen membrane, and the flaps were sutured.

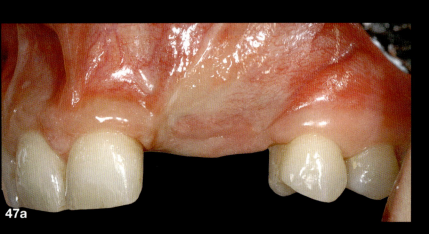
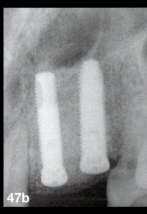

47a

47b

Fig 47 The implants were submerged for 4 months to wait for sufficient osseointegration. *(a)* Clinical image. *(b)* Periapical radiograph.

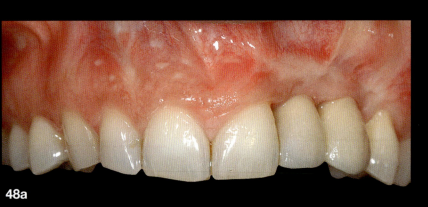
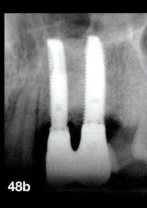

48a

48b

Fig 48 *(a)* Definitive ceramic prosthesis after 1 year of function. *(b)* Radiograph after 1 year. The bone margin appears stable.

CLINICAL CASE 3

Vertical ridge augmentation beyond the bone peaks in an esthetic zone

A 25-year-old, nonsmoking woman in good health was suffering from bilateral agenesis of the maxillary lateral incisors and had been treated with two implants of unknown design and surface type. A series of postoperative complications led to the early failure of the implant in the site of the right lateral incisor, with severe bone and periodontal attachment loss on the adjacent canine and central incisor **(Fig 49)**.

The implant in the site of the right lateral incisor was removed immediately, and the bone defect was curetted **(Fig 50)**.

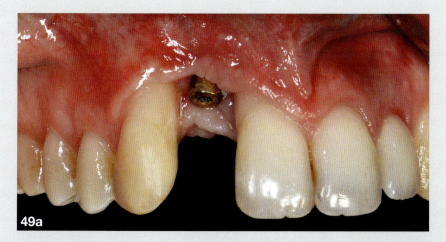
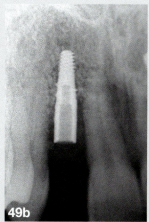

Fig 49 *(a and b)* Clinical image of the implant in the site of the maxillary right lateral incisor. The implant caused severe vertical bone resorption, attachment loss, and recession of the gingival tissues around the right canine and central incisor. (b) Radiograph showing the implant and the bone defect.

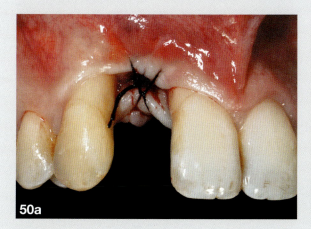
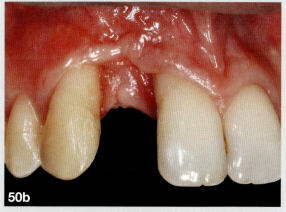

Fig 50 *(a and b)* The biomaterial was covered with a resorbable collagen membrane, and the flaps were sutured.

The implant in the site of the left lateral incisor also showed signs of mobility and loss of osseointegration and was removed (**Fig 51**). Before proceeding, a waiting period of 6 months was observed to allow for healing to achieve sufficient maturation of the tissues, which appeared inflamed and rich in scar tissue (**Fig 52**). CBCT imaging after 6 months showed severe bone loss around the adjacent natural teeth (**Fig 53**).

The traditional treatment plan would have involved bilateral extraction of the maxillary canines and central incisors with vertical ridge augmentation from the mesial bone peaks to the first premolars, which appeared healthy. However, because the patient was very young and all the teeth to be extracted were completely healthy, an alternative treatment plan was formulated: vertical bone regeneration above the bone peaks and in contact with the root surfaces. The right site, being the most compromised, was treated first.

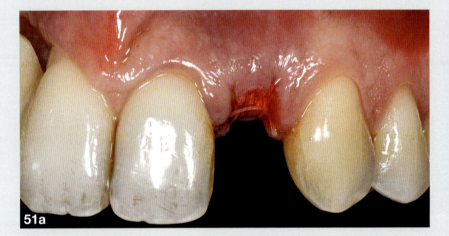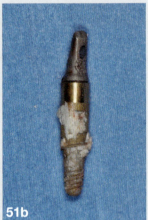

Fig 51 *(a)* The implant in the site of the maxillary left lateral incisor, which was not integrated, was also removed. *(b)* The implant with abundant calculus deposits and cement residue.

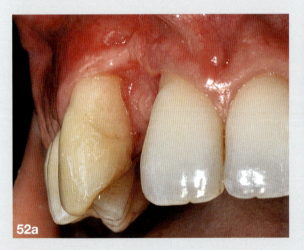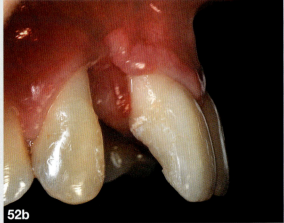

Fig 52 The tissues after 6 months of healing still appear inflamed and rich in scar tissue. *(a)* Right side view. *(b)* Left side view.

A full-thickness flap was elevated through a crestal buccal incision to exclude the fibrous scar tissue present on the edentulous ridge. The incision was extended intrasulcularly to the adjacent canine and central incisor and connected with two vertical j-shaped incisions at the level of the fornix. The palatal incision also excluded crestal scar tissue, which was removed so that only healthy, well-vascularized tissue was available. The exposed roots were carefully planed, sparing the millimeter of connective attachment still present near the bone crest (**Fig 54**).

Because it was considered too risky and perhaps impossible to regenerate 12 mm of vertical bone in the total absence of bone peaks, a partial bone regeneration of 6 mm was opted for, and the remaining height was compensated for with connective tissue grafts. Then, a membrane support screw was inserted in a 6-mm crestal position (**Fig 55**), and a titanium-reinforced ePTFE membrane was appropriately trimmed and fixed palatally with two pins (**Fig 56**).

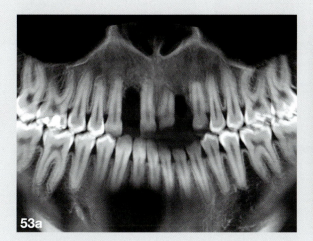
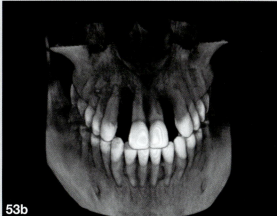

Fig 53 CBCT imaging showing severe bone loss at the sites of the maxillary central incisors, right canine, and left lateral incisor. *(a)* Panoramic view. *(b)* 3D view.

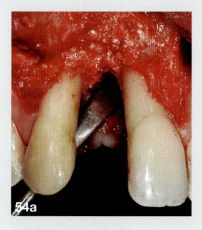
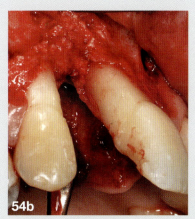
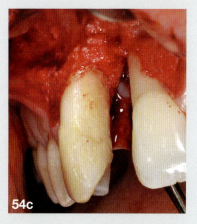

Fig 54 Full-thickness buccal and palatal flaps were elevated, and the tooth roots were planed, sparing the millimeter of vital fibers near the bone margin. *(a)* Frontal view. *(b)* Right lateral view. *(c)* Left lateral view.

The exposed roots were conditioned for 3 minutes with EDTA and treated with amelogenin before a particulate graft of 80% autologous bone and 20% DBBM was placed (**Fig 57**). The membrane was adapted buccally and secured with two additional pins, carefully avoiding contact with the roots of adjacent teeth (**Fig 58**).

A connective tissue graft harvested from the palate was positioned on the crest and buccally (**Fig 59**). Healing occurred without complications (**Fig 60**).

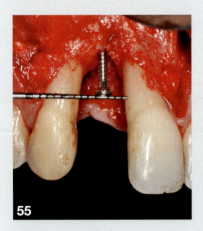
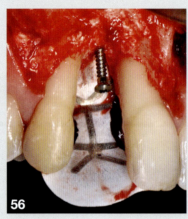
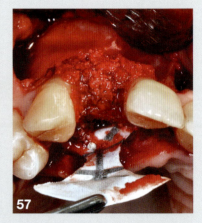

Fig 55 A support screw for the membrane was placed, allowing it to protrude from the bone crest by 6 mm. **Fig 56** A reinforced ePTFE membrane was cut and secured with two palatal pins. The roots were conditioned for 3 minutes with EDTA and treated with amelogenins. **Fig 57** A particulate graft of 80% autologous bone and 20% DBBM was placed in the defect in contact with the root surfaces.

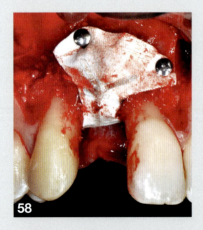
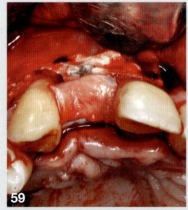
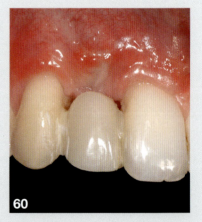

Fig 58 The membrane was stabilized buccally with two pins so that it had no contact with the roots of the adjacent teeth. **Fig 59** A connective tissue graft harvested from the palate was placed on the crest and buccally. **Fig 60** Healing occurred without complications.

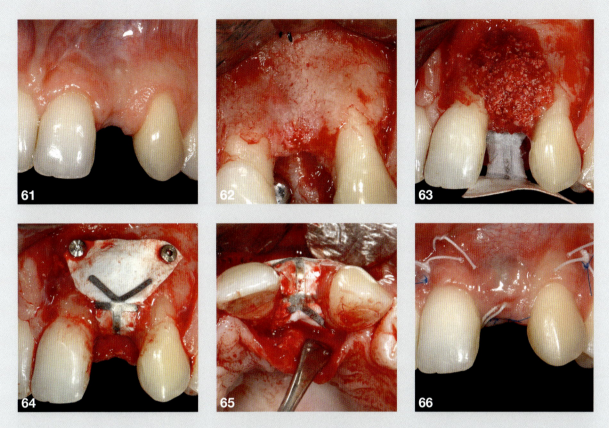

Fig 61 The site of the maxillary left lateral incisor 6 months after implant extraction. **Fig 62** Treatment similar to that for the right lateral incisor, with full-thickness buccal and palatal flaps. **Fig 63** Palatal membrane placement, root treatment with amelogenins, and placement of the particulate composite graft. **Fig 64** Membrane stabilization. **Fig 65** Stabilization of the membrane buccally and with sutures. **Fig 66** Healing after 15 days without complications.

On the contralateral side, where the situation was less severe, a similar, though less difficult, operation was performed (**Figs 61 to 66**), and CBCT imaging confirmed the correct position of the two membranes (**Fig 67**).

After 8 months of healing (**Fig 68**), the membranes were removed by tunnelling into the mucosa without opening a flap to avoid exposing the delicate newly formed bone tissue. Two horizontal buccal access incisions were made in the fornix, and two palatal incisions were made to remove the fixation pins at the two sites. The membranes were removed by elevating two tunneled flaps and gently peeling them off with a scalpel. The two supporting crestal screws were unscrewed through a small incision in the mucosa (**Fig 69**).

After intrasulcular incisions were made in the adjacent teeth to interrupt the periodontal attachment apparatus, the crestal mucosa was pushed coronally to create space for two connective tissue grafts harvested from the palate and placed on the ridge by pulling two sutures inserted through the crestal incision (**Fig 70**).

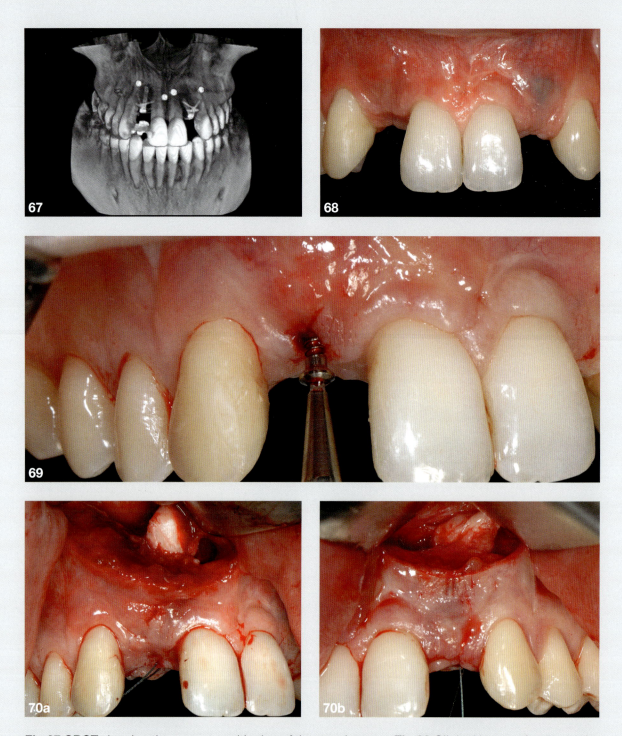

Fig 67 CBCT showing the correct positioning of the membranes. **Fig 68** Clinical image after 8 months of recovery without complications. **Fig 69** After 8 months of healing, the membrane support screws were removed through a small opening in the mucosa. **Fig 70** *(a and b)* Two bilateral full-thickness horizontal incisions were made, one buccal and one palatal, with intrasulcular incisions around both maxillary canines and central incisors. The membranes were removed through the buccal incision, and two additional connective grafts were inserted under the crestal mucosa.

The horizontal incisions were sutured with 6-0 Vicryl resorbable sutures (Ethicon) (**Fig 71**). This procedure corrected the vertical dimension of the edentulous area and the gingival recession of the adjacent natural teeth. After 1 month of healing, two machined iMAX (iRES) implants were placed with a flapless technique. The first drill was used with a surgical guide obtained with CBCT (**Fig 72**). The implants remained in a transmucosal position to integrate for 4 months before two provisional crowns were placed (**Fig 73**). After 6 months of soft tissue conditioning with the provisionals, the two final crowns were fitted (**Fig 74**). Periapical radiographs confirmed the satisfactory level of bone tissue (**Fig 75**). At the 6-year follow-up, the bone levels on radiographs (**Fig 76**) and the gingival margins (**Fig 77**) appeared stable.

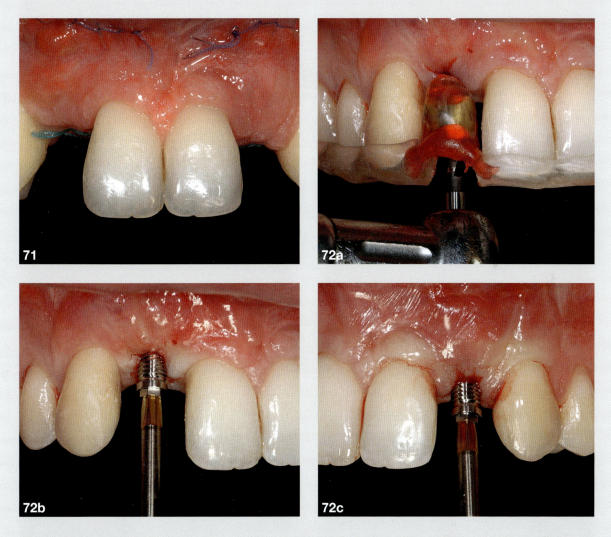

Fig 71 Healing showed satisfactory vertical and horizontal dimension of the edentulous ridges and almost complete root coverage at the level of the adjacent teeth. **Fig 72** *(a)* After 1 month of healing, two machined iMAX implants were inserted according to the flapless technique with a surgical guide. Manual insertion of the right *(b)* and left *(c)* implants.

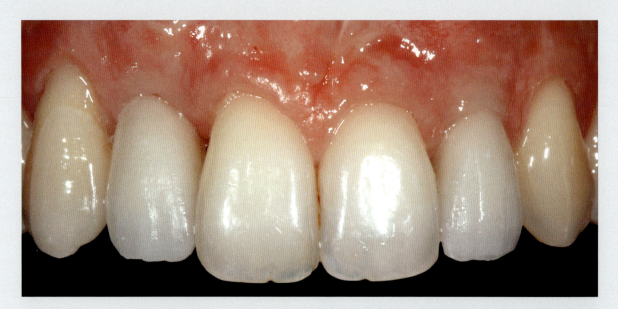

Fig 73 The provisional restorations for the lateral incisors were maintained for 6 months for soft tissue conditioning and maturation.

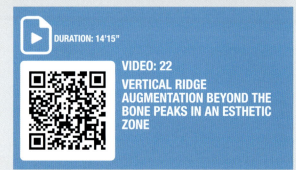

DURATION: 14'15"

VIDEO: 22

VERTICAL RIDGE AUGMENTATION BEYOND THE BONE PEAKS IN AN ESTHETIC ZONE

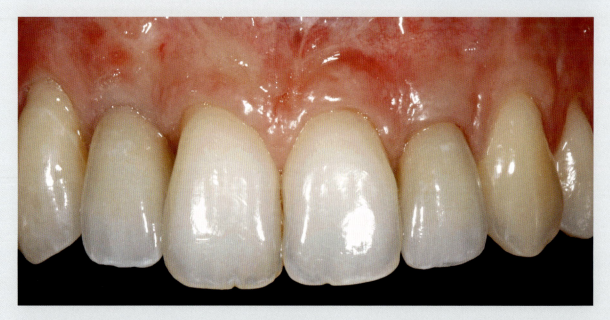

Fig 74 The definitive prostheses after 1 year of function. Modest gingival recession has recurred around the implant in the site of the maxillary right canine, but the other tissues appear stable.

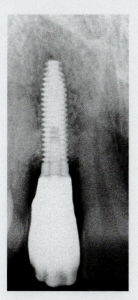 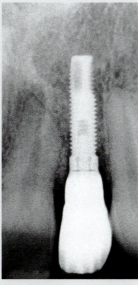 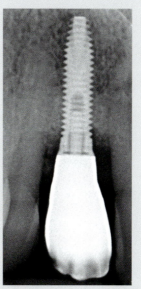 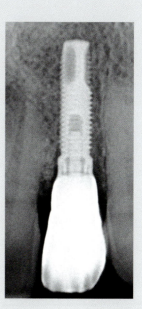

Fig 75 Radiograph after 1 year of function. The bone margins appear stable.

Fig 76 Radiograph after 6 years, showing perfect stability of the bone margins.

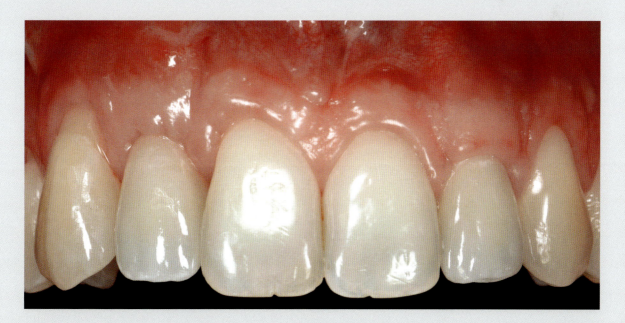

Fig 77 Clinical follow-up image after 6 years. The gingival margins are stable and clinically healthy.

REFERENCES

1. Simion M, Trisi P, Piattelli A. Vertical ridge augmentation using a membrane technique associated with osseointegrated implants. Int J Periodontics Restorative Dent 1994;14:496–511.

2. Jovanovic SA, Schenk RK, Orsini M, Kenney EB. Supracrestal bone formation around dental implants: An experimental dog study. Int J Oral Maxillofac Implants 1995;10:23–31.

3. Tinti C, Parma-Benfenati S, Polizzi G. Vertical ridge augmentation: What is the limit? Int J Periodontics Restorative Dent 1996;16:220–229.

4. Simion M, Jovanovic SA, Trisi P, Scarano A, Piattelli A. Vertical ridge augmentation around dental implants using a membrane technique and autogenous bone or allografts in humans. Int J Periodontics Restorative Dent 1998;18:8–23.

5. Tinti C, Parma-Benfenati S. Vertical ridge augmentation: Surgical protocol and retrospective evaluation of 48 consecutively inserted implants. Int J Periodontics Restorative Dent 1998;18:434–443.

6. Felice P, Pistilli R, Barausse C, Piattelli M, Buti J, Esposito M. Posterior atrophic jaws rehabilitated with prostheses supported by 6-mm-long 4-mm-wide implants or by longer implants in augmented bone. Five-year post-loading results from an within-person randomised controlled trial. Oral Implantol (Berl) 2019;12:57–72.

7. Schmid J, Hämmerle CH, Stich H, Lang NP. Supraplant, a novel implant system based on the principle of guided bone generation. A preliminary study in the rabbit. Clin Oral Implants Res 1991;2:199–202.

8. Linde A, Thorén C, Dahlin C, Sandberg E. Creation of new bone by an osteopromotive membrane technique: An experimental study in rats. J Oral Maxillofac Surg 1993;51:892–897.

9. Simion M, Dahlin C, Rocchietta I, Stavropulos A, Sanchez R, Karring T. Vertical ridge augmentation with guided bone regeneration in association with dental implants: An experimental study in dogs. Clin Oral Implants Res 2007;18:86–94.

10. Merli M, Bernardelli F, Esposito M. Horizontal and vertical ridge augmentation: A novel approach using osteosynthesis microplates, bone grafts, and resorbable barriers. Int J Periodontics Restorative Dent 2006;26:581–587.

11. Simion M, Fontana F, Rasperini G, Maiorana C. Vertical ridge augmentation by expanded-polyytetrafluoroethylene membrane and a combination of intraoral autogenous bone graft and deproteinized anorganic bovine bone (bio oss). Clin Oral Implants Res 2007;18:620–629.

12. Fontana F, Santoro F, Maiorana C, Iezzi G, Piattelli A, Simion M. Clinical and histologic evaluation of allogeneic bone matrix versus autogenous bone chips associated with titanium-reinforced e-PTFE membrane for vertical ridge augmentation: A prospective pilot study. Int J Oral Maxillofac Implants 2008;23:1003–1012.

13. Merli M, Moscatelli M, Mariotti G, Rotundo R, Bernardelli F, Nieri M. Bone level variation after vertical ridge augmentation: Resorbable barriers versus titanium-reinforced barriers. A 6-year double-blind randomised clinical trial. Int J Oral Maxillofac Implants 2014;29:905–913.

14. Urban IA, Iozada JL, Jovanovic SA, Nagursky H, Nagy K. Vertical ridge augmentation with titanium-reinforced, dense-PTFE membranes and a combination of particulated autogenous bone and anorganic bovine bone-derived mineral: A prospective case series in 19 patients. Int J Oral Maxillofac Implants 2014;29:185–193.

15. Ronda M, Rebaudi A, Torelli L, Stacchi C. Expanded vs. dense polytetrafluoroethylene membranes in vertical ridge augmentation around dental implants: A prospective randomized controlled clinical trial. Clin Oral Implants Res 2014;25:859–866.

16. Simion M, Jovanovic SA, Tinti C, Benfenati SP. Long-term evaluation of osseointegrated implants inserted at the time or after vertical ridgeaugmentation. A retrospective study on 123 implants with 1-5 year follow-up. Clin Oral Implants Res 2001;12:35–45.

17. Simion M, Fontana F, Rasperini G, Maiorana C. Long-term evaluation of osseointegrated implants placed in sites augmented with sinus floor elevation associated with vertical ridge augmentation: A retrospective study of 38 consecutive implants with 1- to 7-year follow-up. Int J Periodontics Restorative Dent 2004;24:208–221.

18. Canullo L, Malagnino VA. Vertical ridge augmentation around implants by e-PTFE titanium-reinforced membrane and bovine bone matrix: A 24- to 54-month study of 10 consecutive cases. Int J Oral Maxillofac Implants 2008;23:858–866.

19. Keestra JA, Barry O, Jong LD, Wahl G. Long-term effects of vertical bone augmentation: A systematic review. J Appl Oral Sci 2016;24:3–17.

20. Simion M, Ferrantino L, Idotta E, Zarone F. Turned implants in vertical augmented bone: A retrospective study with 13 to 21 years follow-up. Int J Periodontics Restorative Dent 2016;36:309–317.

21. Urban IA, Monje A, Lozada JL, Wang HL. Long-term evaluation of peri-implant bone level after reconstruction of severely atrophic edentulous maxilla via vertical and horizontal guided bone regeneration in combination with sinus augmentation: A case series with 1 to 15 years of loading. Clin Implant Dent Relat Res 2017;19:46–55.

22. Roccuzzo M, Savoini M, Dalmasso P, Ramieri G. Long-term outcomes of implants placed after vertical alveolar ridge augmentation in partially edentulous patients: A 10-year prospective clinical study. Clin Oral Implants Res 2017;28:1204–1210.

23. Elnayef B, Monje A, Gargallo-Albiol J, Galindo-Moreno P, Wang HL, Hernández-Alfaro F. Vertical ridge augmentation in the atrophic mandible: A systematic review and meta-analysis. Int J Oral Maxillofac Implants 2017;32:291–312.

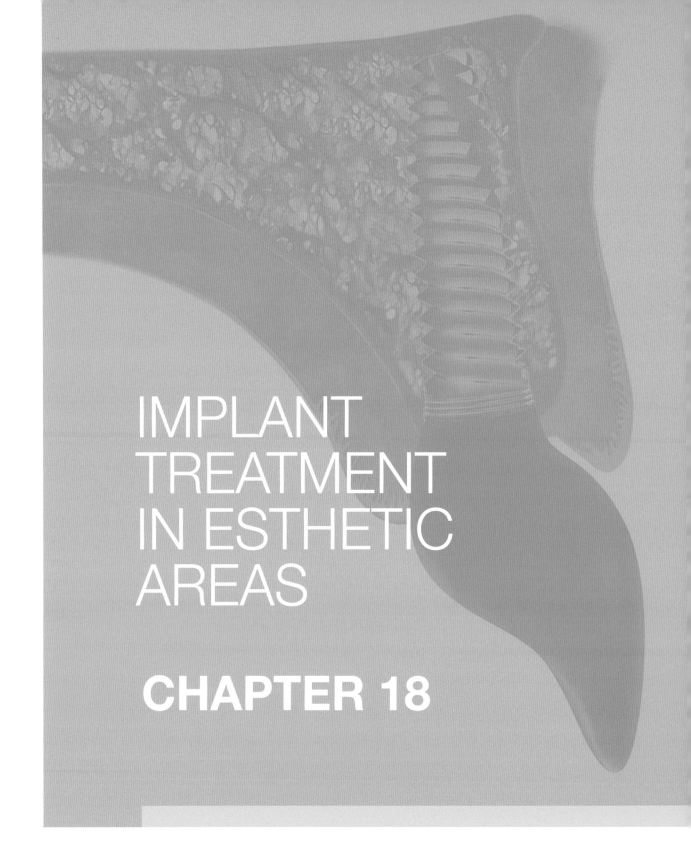

IMPLANT TREATMENT IN ESTHETIC AREAS

CHAPTER 18

Edited by Massimo Simion and Michele Maglione

INTRODUCTION

Rehabilitating esthetic areas with implants involves rules that are different than those for other areas of the mouth, and it deserves a chapter of its own. Whereas small discrepancies in tooth and peri-implant tissue shape, size, or color can be tolerated in the posterolateral zones of the maxilla and mandible, in the esthetic zones, from maxillary premolar to premolar, lack of perfect harmony between the different dental elements can lead to disastrous results.[1]

The size of an implant, which differs completely from that of the root of a natural tooth, heavily conditions the characteristics of the emergence profile and morphology of the prosthetic restoration. Crowns up to 8 to 10 mm wide are often attached to an implant platform with a diameter of about 4 mm. Also fundamental are the anatomical and pathologic characteristics of the edentulous site to be rehabilitated.

Tooth extractions in the anterior areas of the maxilla lead to natural bone resorption of 1 to 2 mm vertically and 40% to 50% horizontally in the first 3 to 6 months.[2–6] Traumatic avulsions can result in even greater resorption.

In every case of implant rehabilitation in esthetic areas, a somewhat complex regenerative technique involving hard tissue, soft tissue, or both is required to achieve a satisfactory result.

The rehabilitation of esthetic areas is undoubtedly the most complex procedure in implant dentistry and requires the utmost skill and experience in both hard and soft tissue management.

Massimo Simion

ANATOMICAL CONSIDERATIONS FOR ESTHETIC IMPLANT-SUPPORTED RESTORATIONS

As with natural teeth, the harmony of implant-supported restorations, although also influenced by the phenotype of the patient (whether ectomorph, endomorph, or mesomorph), is dependent on general anatomical characteristics that must be considered[7] (Fig 1):

1. **Midline of the maxillary central incisors.** The midline should coincide with the midline of the face and, if possible, that of the mandibular central incisors. Ideally, the anterior teeth should be mesially inclined at the incisal level and distally inclined at the apical level. This axis inclination is accentuated as one moves from the central incisors toward the canines.

2. **Position of the gingival margin.** The gingival margin should be more apical at the canines than at the central incisors, while the lateral incisors have a more coronal margin than the central incisors.

3. **Zenith position of the gingival contours.** The zenith of the gingival contours should always be off-center toward the distal to give the gingival parabolas an asymmetric appearance.

4. **Shape of the crowns and their proportions.** Crowns can be triangular, rounded, or square, with a width-to-length ratio ranging from 75% to 80%. The central incisors of men are generally larger than those of women.

5. **Proportions of the crowns to one another.** From a frontal view, the central incisor should appear 60% wider than the lateral incisor, and in turn, the lateral incisor should appear wider than the canine by the same amount.

6. **Closure of interdental spaces.** The absence of diastemas and the presence of interdental papillae that completely close the interproximal spaces are essential for acceptable esthetics.

7. **Position of interdental contact areas.** Interdental contact should occur more apically between canines and lateral incisors, becoming progressively more coronal between lateral and central incisors and between the two central incisors.

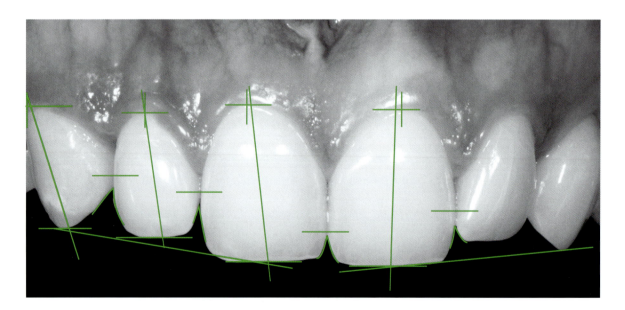

Fig 1 *General anatomical factors influencing esthetics in implant rehabilitations.*

8. **Interincisal angles.** Interincisal angles should be more open between the canines and lateral Incisors, gradually closing up between the lateral and central incisors and between the two central incisors.

9. **Incisal edge position.** The incisal edge should be more coronal in canines and central incisors and slightly more apical in lateral incisors.

10. **Smile line.** A high smile line that reveals a large amount of gingiva constitutes a major challenge in esthetic rehabilitations.

11. **Shape of the incisal edges.** Incisal edges have mamelons that tend to disappear early in adolescence.

12. **3D implant positioning.** Even minimal errors in the apicocoronal, buccopalatal, and mesiodistal positions can dramatically affect the final esthetic results.

13. **Ceramic color.** Color is characterized by hue, chroma, value, translucency, and surface characterizations. Lateral incisors generally have the same hue as central incisors but a slightly lower value. The canines usually have a higher chroma, appearing visibly darker.

14. **Surface characteristics.** The microstructure of implant surfaces is determined by horizontal microgrooves, and the macrotexture is characterized by lobes that break up the buccal face of the crown. These features tend to disappear with age.

INDICES FOR THE ESTHETIC EVALUATION OF IMPLANT REHABILITATIONS

In addition to the general anatomical characteristics that affect restoration esthetics, there are specific characteristics that relate to the rehabilitation of an implant site that are used in research for objective assessments of esthetic results. These characteristics have been described with various numerical indices, such as the Jemt papillary index,[8] the implant crown esthetic index,[9] the pink esthetic score (PES),[10] the pink and white esthetic score,[11] and the complex esthetic index.[12] Despite the limitations inherent in these indices, which attempt to transform an essentially subjective assessment, esthetics, into an objective evaluation, they allow attention to be focused on each detail that characterizes the final esthetic results of an implant rehabilitation.

Without falling into excessive complexity, the index that most comprehensively describes the characteristics that determine esthetics is the implant crown esthetic index,[9] which takes into account nine fundamental characteristics **(Fig 2)**:

1. **Mesiodistal dimensions of the crown.** The size of a residual edentulous space may not coincide with the size of the contralateral reference tooth/teeth due to dental malpositioning/collapses, previous diastemas, or long-standing edentulism. Crowns that differ in size from reference teeth are not esthetically acceptable, and it is necessary to intervene with orthodontic or reconstructive therapy or with veneers or composites to change the size of the adjacent tooth.

2. **Position of the incisal edge of the crown.** Naturally, the incisal edge of the crown should be identical to that of the reference tooth. However, malpositioning of the opposing mandibular incisors can cause interferences in centric occlusion or in eccentric protrusive and lateral movements that jeopardize the stability of the implant. Therefore, especially in cases of immediate loading, the use of provisionals without centric or protrusive occlusal contacts is indicated, even at the cost of temporarily unesthetic results.

3. **Buccal convexity of the crown.** Convexity is necessary to distinguish the buccal surface of the clinical crown from the convexity of the transmucosal emergence profile. If the latter is too convex, resulting compression on the soft

tissues may cause recession of the gingival margin. This is why a concave emergence profile must be constructed in many cases.

4. **Color and translucency of the prosthetic crown.** These depend not only on the expertise of the technician but also on the thickness of the ceramic crown itself and the type of abutment that is used. Zirconia abutments or full-ceramic crowns are increasingly being used for this purpose.[13]

5. **Surface and texture of the crown.** A successful crown surface is dependent solely on the expertise of the prosthodontist and technician.

6. **Margin and shape of the gingival contour.** These factors depend equally on the surgeon and the prosthodontist. The surgeon must obtain a sufficient amount of peri-implant soft tissue and ideal 3D implant positioning, and the

prosthodontist must condition the soft tissue to obtain adequate emergence profiles.

7. **Conformity of the interdental papillae.** The interdental papillae are the most difficult structures to maintain and also to regenerate when lost. Their presence depends both on the work of the surgeon, who must obtain sufficient bone support and adequate interproximal soft tissue thickness, and on the prosthodontist, who can condition the interdental papillae with the emergence crown profiles.

8. **Peri-implant mucosal contour.** The mucosal contour depends on the thickness of the bone and buccal mucosa around the implant. In most cases there are deficits caused by trauma, periodontal disease, or long-standing avulsions, and it is the surgeon's responsibility to restore the lost volumes.

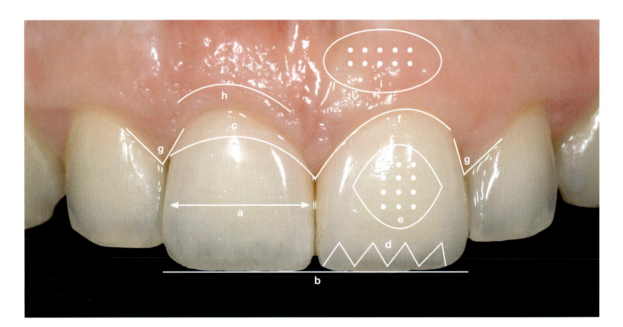

Fig 2 The nine fundamental points considered as part of the implant crown esthetic index: (a) mesiodistal crown dimension, (b) incisal edge position, (c) convexity of the crown, (d) crown color and translucency, (e) crown surface and texture, (f) margin and shape of the gingival contour, (g) conformity of the interdental papillae, (h) peri-implant mucosa contour, (i) buccal mucosa color and surface characteristics.

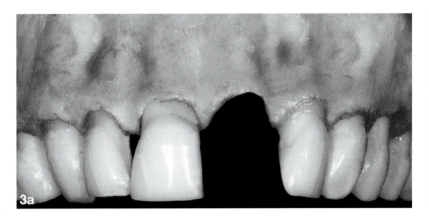
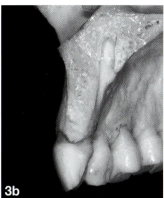
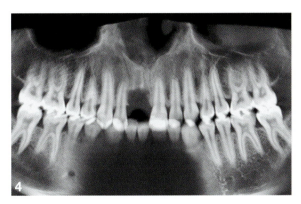
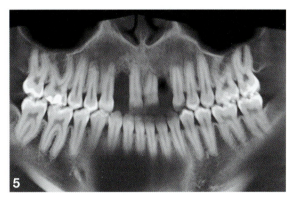

Fig 3 Dry skull reconstruction showing the bony peaks responsible for the retention of the interproximal papillae after the loss of a single tooth. (a) Frontal view. (b) Lateral view. *Fig 4* CBCT imaging showing severe bone defects in the extraction site of the maxillary right central incisor with adjacent bone peaks present. *Fig 5* CBCT showing osseous defects in the sites of the maxillary lateral incisors with periodontal attachment loss and interproximal bone peaks.

9. **Color and surface of the buccal mucosa.** The presence of amalgam tattoos from previous apicoectomies with incongruous retrograde fillings is the most frequent cause of unsightly pigmentation of the buccal mucosa. A lack of tissue thickness (less than 3 mm of combined bone and soft tissue) can also cause the appearance of dark implant titanium through the buccal mucosa.[14]

RESTORATIONS FOR SINGLE TEETH

When rehabilitating single edentulous sites adjacent to teeth with normal periodontal attachment, it is possible to achieve near-perfect results, even in the presence of severe bone defects.

This is because the interdental papillae are supported by the bone peaks **(Fig 3)** and connective fibers inserted into the cementum of the adjacent teeth.

This allows for effective bone regeneration to take place from mesial to distal bone peaks without involving the exposed root surface **(Fig 4)**.

In the presence of periodontal attachment loss in the teeth adjacent to the defect, the probability of esthetic success is drastically reduced. This is because the papillae are absent and their regeneration is very difficult, if not impossible **(Fig 5)**. In fact, guided bone regeneration (GBR) with standard techniques does not allow for vertical bone regeneration coronal to the level of the bone peaks, although there are some case reports in the literature demonstrating the possibility of obtaining bone neoformation adjacent to exposed root surfaces through the use of growth factors (see chapter 20).[15,16]

RESTORATIONS FOR ADJACENT EDENTULOUS SITES

The rehabilitation of two adjacent missing teeth presents additional challenges. While the lateral papillae are supported by the bony peaks of the natural teeth, the papilla interproximal to the two implants tends to be flat, as a consequence of bone resorption following tooth extraction **(Fig 6)**. Hard and/or soft tissue augmentation techniques must be used to obtain a well-shaped papilla. The most complex cases involve replacement of the central incisors due to the high visibility of the

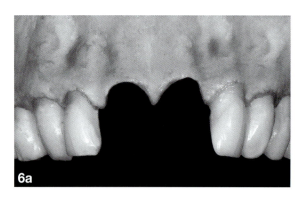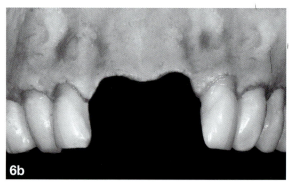

Fig 6 *Dry skull reconstruction showing the presence of the bone peaks at the level of the adjacent natural teeth. The interproximal peak* (a), *however, is completely resorbed 6 months after the extraction of the two central incisors* (b).

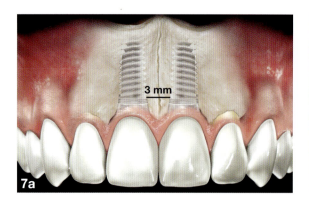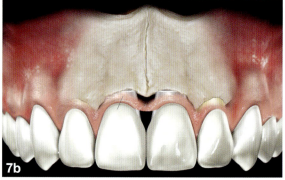

Fig 7 *Peri-implant distance between the two central incisors. The minimum distance is 4 mm. A distance of 3 mm* (a) *leads to resorption of the interproximal bone peak, which in turn leads to a loss of the interdental papilla* (b).

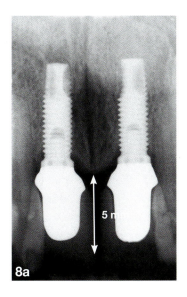
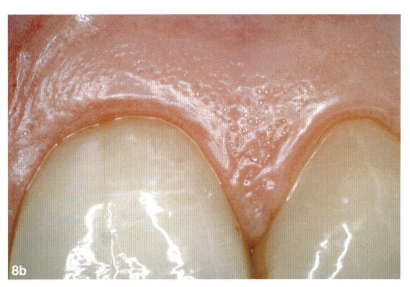

Fig 8 Correlation of the distance between the bone ridge and the contact point between two teeth with papillae. (a and b) *When the distance is 5 mm or less, the interdental papilla is present and well formed.*

interproximal space. Rehabilitating a central and lateral incisor or a lateral incisor and canine also present particular difficulties due to the reduced mesiodistal space, which limits the interimplant distance and therefore the availability of bone support for the interdental papilla.[17]

Alveolar bone preservation and immediate implant placement techniques in extraction sites are particularly useful to prevent bone resorption that occurs in the 3 to 6 months following extractions (see chapter 7).

Maintaining an appropriate interimplant distance is essential for obtaining an adequate interdental papilla that can completely close the interproximal space and avoid interproximal black triangles. A study by Tarnow et al[18] on 36 patients each receiving two adjacent implants showed that the minimum distance between two implants must be greater than 3 mm to maintain sufficient bone support for the papilla. The explanation for this clinical observation lies in the small (about 1.5 mm) bone defect that forms apically and laterally around the platform of implants after the connection of the prosthetic abutments.[19] If the interimplant distance is 3 mm or less, the two adjacent defects converge, leading to a reduction in the vertical dimension of the interproximal bone peak of about 1 mm. The interdental papilla is also affected accordingly **(Fig 7)**.

Another clinical study by Tarnow et al[20] on 30 patients correlated the distance between the bone ridge and the contact point between two teeth with the presence or absence of the interproximal papilla. The results showed that when this distance was 5 mm or less, the papilla was present and complete in almost 100% of sites **(Fig 8)**. When the distance was 6 mm (only 1 mm more), the papilla was present in only 56% of the sites, and when the distance was 7 mm or more, only 27% of the sites had a well-formed papilla.

In esthetic areas, therefore, it is necessary to regenerate the alveolar bone as coronally as possible and to position the interdental contact area as apically as possible, without compromising the morphology of the crowns and the harmony of the prosthesis.

3D IMPLANT POSITIONING

Correct implant positioning is the basis for success in esthetic rehabilitations. All too often, even minor errors in positioning cause poor esthetic results, even in sites that are ideal from an anatomical point of view or previously treated with effective regenerative techniques.

Three essential positions must be carefully considered when preparing the implant site:

- apicocoronal position
- buccopalatal position and angulation
- mesiodistal position

Apicocoronal position

When placing bone-level implants, the implant platform must be located 3 mm apical to the imaginary horizontal line passing through the zenith of the gingival parabola of the reference element (**Fig 9**). If, for example, a central incisor is being replaced, the gingival zenith of the adjacent central incisor is the reference point. If a lateral incisor is being replaced, the gingival margin of the contralateral tooth is used. The need for this distance

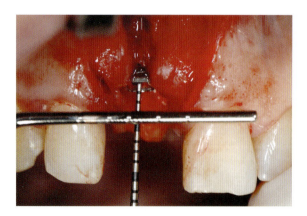

Fig 9 *Correct apicocoronal position of an implant in the site of the maxillary right central incisor. The probes indicate a distance between the implant platform and the gingival margin of the adjacent element of 3 mm in the apical direction.*

is due to the dimensional increase that the emergence profile must undergo when passing from the 4-mm-diameter implant platform to the 8- to 9-mm diameter of the prosthetic crown at the gingival margin.

A distance of less than 3 mm would lead to the development of an emergence profile that is too convex and compressive on the soft tissue. A greater distance, although better tolerated, would lead to a peri-implant sulcus that is too deep and, consequently, difficulty to clean. Respecting this rule during implant insertion means disregarding the position of the residual bone crest as a reference point for the apicocoronal position. If the bone crest is more apical than 3 mm, it must be regenerated vertically; if it is more coronal, the implant platform is placed apical to it.

Buccopalatal position and angulation

Positioning errors in the buccopalatal direction are the most common and the ones that compromise esthetic results the most. Inexperienced clinicians tend to position the long axis of the implant according to the long axis of the adjacent tooth or the previously extracted tooth, and this results in an overly buccal position and angulation. The position of the implant should must be more palatal than the root of the tooth, and its axis must be angled in such a way that it protrudes slightly palatal to the incisal edge (**Fig 10**). Another fundamental requirement is that at least 2 mm of bone thickness remains buccal to the coronal third of the implant (**Fig 11**). This is for three very important reasons:

1. To avoid the gray appearance of implant titanium through the tissues. An in vitro study by Jung et al14 showed that when the total thickness of the buccal bone and soft tissues at the implant is less than 3 mm, the mucosa takes on a dark red color due to the color of titanium showing through the tissues. This reddish discoloration gives the

prosthetic restoration a false inflammatory and unesthetic appearance. If the thickness of the buccal bone plate at the implant is at least 2 mm, a thickness of even only 1 mm of mucosa ensures a color that matches with the surrounding tissue.

2. If the thickness of the buccal bone plate is at least 2 mm, the physiologic angular defect occurring with an average diameter of 1.5 mm around the implant platform **(Fig 12)** remains confined within the thickness of the bone and does not cause recession of either the bone or the gingival margins **(Fig 13)**. If, on the other hand, the thickness is less than 2 mm, the small defect causes implant dehiscence in the coronal third of the implant, with consequent gingival margin recession[21] **(Fig 14)**.

3. Bone recession around the implant head inevitably leads to exposure of the implant surface and the consequent increased susceptibility of the implant to peri-implantitis, especially in the presence of rough implant surfaces up to the implant platform.[22]

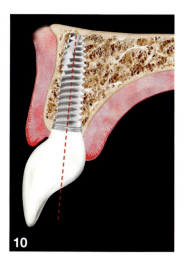

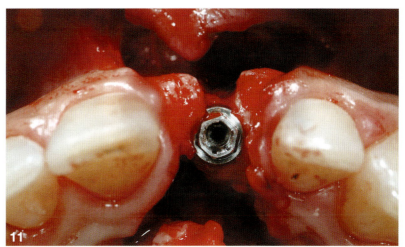

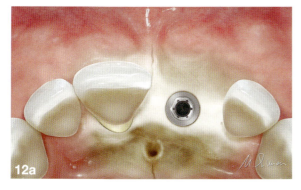

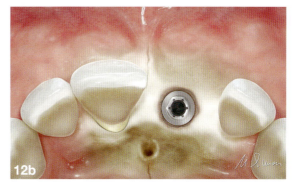

Fig 10 The position of the implant should be more palatal than the tooth root, and the long axis should protrude palatal to the incisal edge. *Fig 11* Corrected implant position with 2 mm buccal bone thickness. The small bone defect must be regenerated with a GBR technique. *Fig 12* Peri-implant angular defect forming around osseointegrated implants. (a) Occlusal view at the time of implant insertion. (b) View 6 months after connection of the prosthetic abutment, when the circumferential defect has already formed.

Mesiodistal position

The gingival contours of the teeth in the anterior maxilla, from canine to canine, is asymmetric, with the zenith always located slightly distal to the center of the tooth. A crown with a symmetric, rounded parabola or, worse still, an asymmetric parabola in the mesial direction, appears strongly unnatural.

Therefore, to facilitate a prosthetic rehabilitation with asymmetric emergence profiles and gingival margins, it is necessary to decentralize the implant slightly in a distal direction **(Fig 15)**. At the level of the central incisors, proper positioning also avoids the partial invasion of the nasopalatine canal present on the midline.

Development of emergence profiles

At the time of the second implant surgical phase for the connection of the prosthetic abutments, certain anatomical conditions must be present

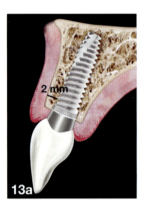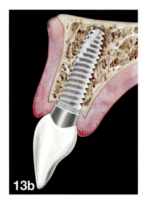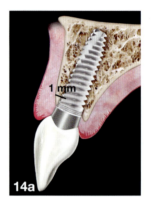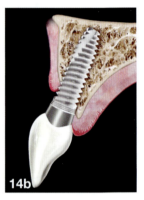

Fig 13 Correct implant positioning within the bone crest. (a) There is 2 mm of bone thickness buccal to the head of the implant. (b) The 1.5-mm-thick circumferential angular defect remains confined within the present bone. *Fig 14* (a) Insufficient bone thickness (< 2 mm) buccal to the implant head. (b) The angular defect led to a dehiscence of the buccal implant surface and subsequent gingival recession.

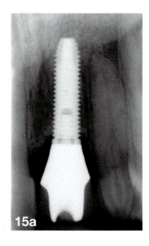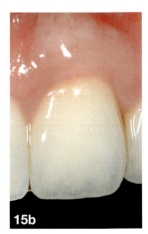

Fig 15 Periapical radiograph showing the correct mesiodistal position of the implant. (a) The position is slightly off-center in the distal direction. (b) The prosthetic crown in turn has a naturally asymmetric gingival parabola in the distal direction.

that are indispensable for the correct development of the emergence profiles that condition the position and shape of the gingival contours and the morphology of the interdental papillae:

- The mucosal thickness must be greater than 5 mm in the apicocoronal direction **(Fig 16)**.
- Considering the inevitable recession of the marginal soft tissues during the development of the emergence profiles with the provisional prosthesis, a mucosal tunnel of 5 to 6 mm is ideal for a final peri-implant sulcus depth of approximately 3 mm.
- Before placement of the provisional, the position of the mucosal margin must be at least 3 mm coronal to that of the adjacent reference tooth **(see Fig 16)** to compensate for the marginal recession that inevitably occurs when going from a diameter of about 4 mm of the healing abutment to the 7 to 9 mm diameter of the final crown.
- The horizontal mucosal thickness must be greater than 2 mm to maintain an adequate gingival contour **(Fig 17)**.

The development of the emergence profile through the action of the provisional should occur progressively as the tissues mature over a period of 6 months. The direct placement of a provisional with a definitive emergence profile would lead to a sudden change in diameter from 4 mm to between 7 and 8 mm, along with a consequent immediate compression of the peri-implant soft tissues. Ischemia, caused by compression, would cause uncontrolled and unpredictable recession of the marginal tissues. For this reason, modifications to the emergence profile must be performed in small, successive steps so that only slight compression, well tolerated by the tissues, occurs and to achieve a progressive and controlled recession of the gingival margin.

In particular, one must be aware that the greater the compression at the level of the interproximal spaces is, the greater is the tendency of the papillae to grow coronally, and the greater the compression of the buccal transmucosal pathway is, the greater the tendency for apical recession of the gingival margin **(Fig 18)**.

To obtain an asymmetric shape of the parabola, it is therefore necessary to compress the distobuccal portion of the transmucosal pathway more **(Figs 19 and 20)** to achieve a greater recession of the distobuccal margin than the mesiobuccal margin. The compression by the provisional must be extremely moderate at each step and cause only slight soft tissue ischemia, which tends to resolve spontaneously in no more than 4 to 5 minutes.

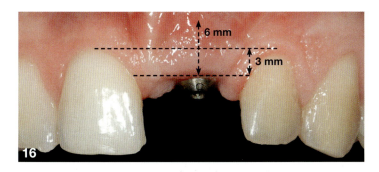
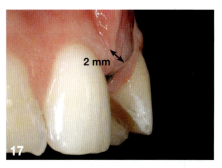

Fig 16 Apicocoronal thickness of the peri-implant mucosa of 6 mm and the position of the gingival margin 3 mm coronal to that of the adjacent reference tooth before placement of the provisional. *Fig 17* The horizontal thickness of the buccal mucosa must be greater than 2 mm.

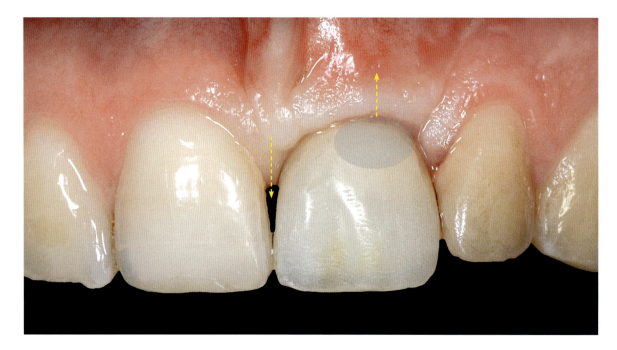

Fig 18 *Slight ischemia of the gingival margin indicates moderate compression by the emergence profile of the provisional. The greater the compression of the interproximal spaces is, the greater the coronal growth of the papillae will be. The greater the buccal compression is, the greater the recession of the gingival margin will be.*

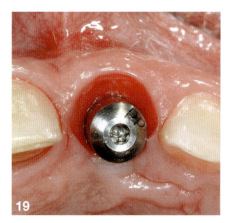

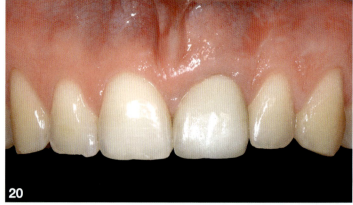

Fig 19 *Clinical image showing the change in the emergence profile compared to the shape of the original healing abutment after 6 months of conditioning with the provisional.* **Fig 20** *Final prosthetic restoration. The complete closure of the interproximal spaces by the papillae and the distally asymmetric shape of the gingival contour can be seen.*

CLINICAL CASE 1

Replacing a single tooth and treating a vertical bone defect (with Dr M. Maglione)

A 30-year-old, nonsmoking man in good health was treated with an implant to replace the right central incisor, which had been lost as a result of trauma. At the first visit, the peri-implant tissues were noticeably inflamed **(Fig 21)** and palpation caused purulent discharge from the buccal sulcus **(Fig 22)**. Periodontal probing of the adjacent teeth was normal. CBCT imaging revealed a large peri-implant bone defect and residual radiopaque material, probably hydroxyapatite, buccally at the defect **(Fig 23)**. The treatment plan involved removal of the implant, placement of an epithelial-connective tissue graft, vertical ridge augmentation, and subsequent placement of a new implant. Upon implant removal, the ceramic crown showed a yellowish deposit, probably consisting of excess cement, calculus, and hydroxyapatite residue **(Fig 24)**.

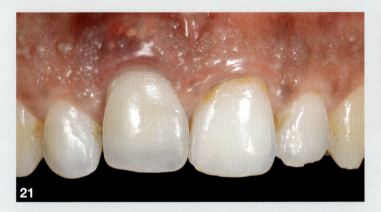
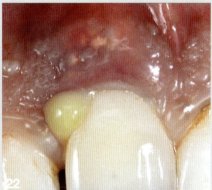

Fig 21 Maxillary right central incisor with untreatable peri-implantitis. The mucosa appears hyperemic and edematous. **Fig 22** Purulent secretion from the peri-implant sulcus.

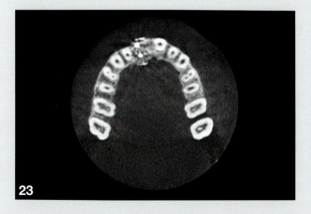
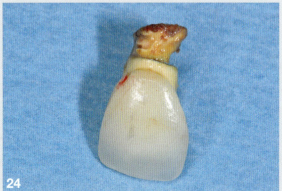

Fig 23 CBCT showing the extent of the bone defect. Residual biomaterial is present at the buccal margins of the defect. **Fig 24** Ceramic crown removed from the site. Cement mixed with calculus and hydroxyapatite is adhered to the edge of the crown.

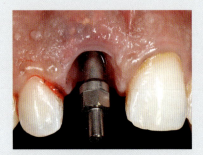

Fig 25 The implant is removed with a reverse-torque instrument.

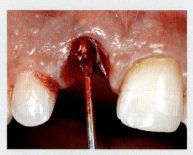

Fig 26 Curettage of the defect walls to remove all granulation tissue and hydroxyapatite residues.

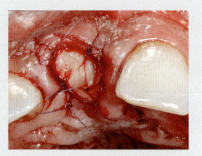

Fig 27 An epithelial-connective tissue graft was sutured in placed to close the defect.

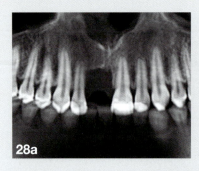

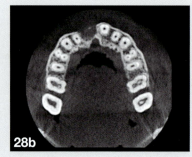

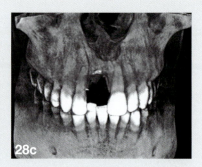

Fig 28 CBCT showing the morphology of the bone defect. The buccal and palatal plates are completely resorbed, but the bone peaks of the adjacent teeth are preserved. Some hydroxyapatite residue is evident. Panoramic *(a)*, axial *(b)*, and 3D *(c)* views.

The implant was removed with a reverse-torque instrument **(Fig 25)**, and the socket was carefully curetted to remove all granulation tissue and residual infected biomaterial **(Fig 26)**. Finally, an oval-shaped epithelial-connective tissue graft was harvested from the palate, deepithelialized in the peripheral areas, and tunneled buccally and palatally to close the soft tissue **(Fig 27)**. CBCT revealed the presence of normal bone peaks on the adjacent teeth and an almost complete removal of hydroxyapatite residues **(Fig 28)**. The patient was temporarily rehabilitated with a resin-bonded prosthesis.

After 2 months of healing, a full-thickness flap was elevated with a slightly buccal crestal incision and extended to the two adjacent teeth. The bone surface, soft tissues, and roots of the adjacent teeth were carefully planed to remove all residual biomaterial, and a support screw was placed, with its head matching the position of the bone peaks **(Fig 29)**. The defect was filled with a 70% autologous particulate graft harvested from the mandibular ascending ramus and 30% DBBM (Bio-Oss, Geistlich Biomaterials). It was then covered with a titanium-reinforced expanded polytetrafluoroethylene (ePTFE) membrane **(Fig 30)**. After incising the buccal periosteum, the flaps were sutured with horizontal ePTFE mattress sutures and simple 6-0 Prolene sutures (Ethicon). Healing occurred without complications by 8 months **(Fig 31)**.

Next, the membrane was removed to place a new implant. The flap was designed with the same characteristics as that in the first operation: full-thickness and extended to the two adjacent teeth. The membrane appeared to be strongly adhered to the underlying tissue, a sign of successful bone regeneration (Fig 32). The fixation pins were removed, and the membrane was lifted out with the help of tweezers and a periosteal elevator.

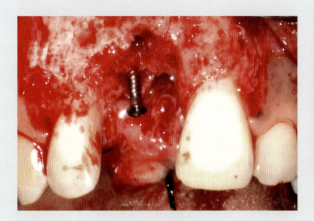

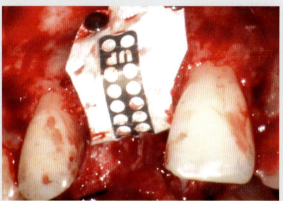

Fig 29 The surgical site shows the bone defect completely freed of granulation tissue and hydroxyapatite remnants. A support screw was placed to determine the position of the membrane at the level of the bone peaks.

Fig 30 Particulate bone graft with 70% autologous bone and 30% DBBM was placed and covered with an ePTFE Neoss membrane fixed with two buccal and two palatal pins.

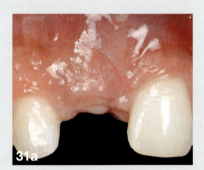
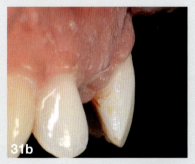
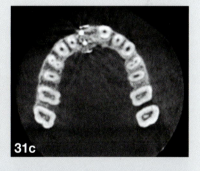

Fig 31 Soft tissue healing after 8 months. The vertical *(a)* and horizontal *(b)* bone dimensions appear adequate. *(c)* CBCT shows the defect fill.

DURATION: 18'35"

VIDEO: 23
VERTICAL BONE DEFECT TREATMENT FOR THE REPLACEMENT OF A SINGLE TOOTH

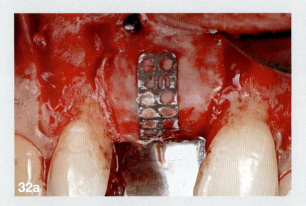 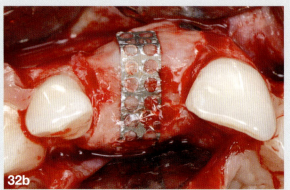

Fig 32 Upon removal, the membrane appears adhered to the underlying regenerated tissue. Frontal *(a)* and occlusal *(b)* views.

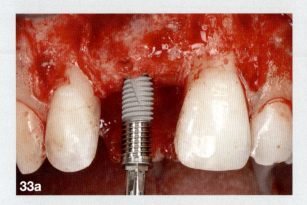 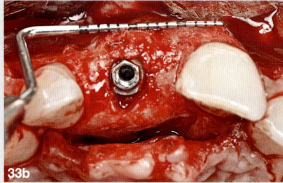

Fig 33 *(a)* An iMAX hybrid surface implant was placed slightly distal to facilitate the development of a suitable emergence profile of the future crown. *(b)* Bone thickness of more than 3 mm was maintained both buccally and palatally.

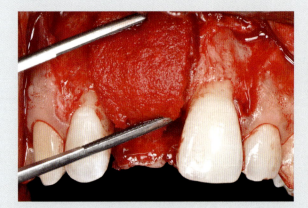 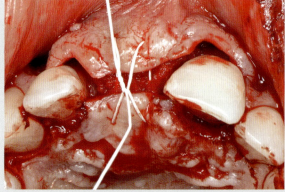

Fig 34 Porcine collagen matrix (Fibro-Gide) placed on the crest and buccally to increase the soft tissue thickness.

Fig 35 The flaps were sutured with a Laurell-Gottlow suture and simple sutures.

Hard, bleeding tissue appeared, into which a hybrid surface implant (iMAX, iRES) was inserted, maintaining a bone thickness of more than 3 mm both buccally and palatally **(Fig 33)**.

To increase the thickness of the soft tissue, a porcine collagen matrix (Fibro-Gide, Geistlich Biomaterials) was placed **(Fig 34)**, and the buccal flap was released again to achieve tension-free wound closure **(Fig 35)**. The site was allowed to heal for an additional 4 months **(Fig 36)**, and then a mucosal punch was performed, and a healing abutment with a length slightly less than the thickness of the mucosa and of the same diameter as the implant platform was inserted **(Fig 37)**.

The provisional crown was kept in place for 6 months, during which time the soft tissue was conditioned with progressive modifications **(Fig 38)** to develop an adequate emergence profile and correct gingival contours **(Fig 39)**. The final prosthesis was constructed of zirconia and ceramic **(Fig 40)**.

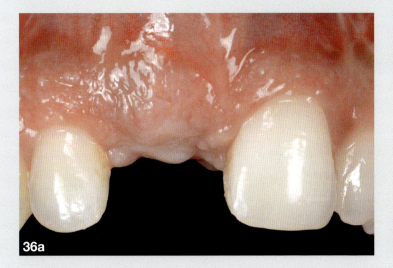
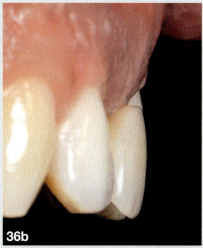

Fig 36 Soft tissue healing after 4 months. The vertical *(a)* and horizontal *(b)* thickness is adequate.

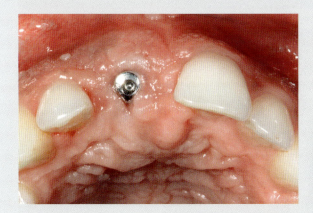
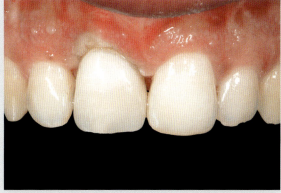

Fig 37 Mucosal punch for the insertion of a healing abutment.

Fig 38 Provisional crown for the development of the emergence profile. The slight distobuccal compression of the mucosal margin is evident.

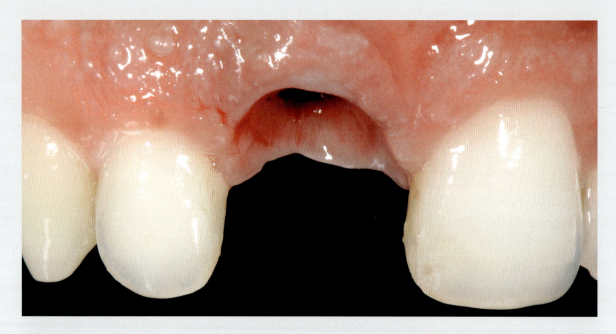

Fig 39 Morphology of the emerging profile after 6 months.

Fig 40 Final zirconia and ceramic crown. *(a)* The gingival contour and interdental papillae are adequate. *(b)* Occlusal view of the gingival contour. *(c)* Periapical radiograph after 1 year of prosthetic loading. The implant appears to be osseointegrated, and the bone margins are normal.

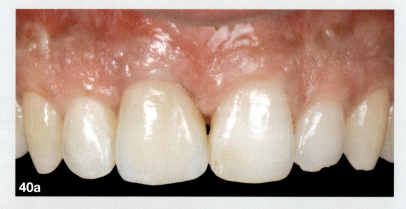

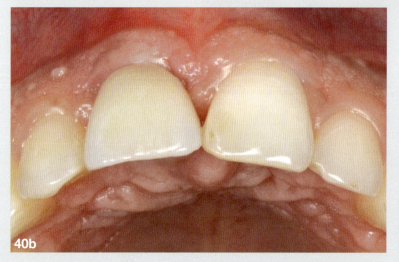

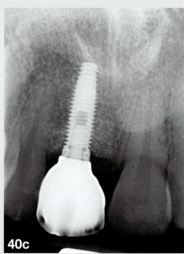

CLINICAL CASE 2

Vertical ridge augmentation above the bone peaks when replacing two adjacent teeth

A 27-year-old, nonsmoking patient suffered traumatic avulsion of the maxillary central incisors in a car accident. On clinical examination, the edentulous ridge appeared severely atrophic, with both vertical and horizontal bone resorption. The two distally inclined lateral incisors showed a clear loss of periodontal attachment and gingival recession at the level of the mesial interproximal papillae (**Fig 41**). In these clinical situations, several unfavorable factors coexist that complicate reconstructive therapy: *(1)* The need to insert two adjacent implants, which makes it difficult to develop an adequate interimplant bone peak to support a well-shaped interproximal papilla; *(2)* the lack of space between the two lateral incisors, which reduces the interimplant distance; *(3)* the severe vertical and horizontal bone atrophy; and *(4)* the loss of periodontal attachment and bone peaks on the mesial papillae of the adjacent elements, which compromises the development of the interproximal papillae between the central and lateral incisors. The treatment plan in this case included horizontal and vertical bone regeneration beyond the bone peaks in contact with the root surfaces and simultaneous orthodontic therapy on the lateral incisors.

A full-thickness trapezoidal flap was excised with vertical j-shaped intrasulcular and crestal incisions distal to the lateral incisors. After elevation up to the nasal fossae, a very thin, bladelike bony ridge was evident, with a vertical bone loss of about 5 mm and 7 mm at the mesial root surface of the right lateral incisor (**Fig 42**). The connective pedicle of the nasopalatine canal was severed, and the canal was emptied of soft tissue. After careful root planing, sparing the vital periodontal ligament (PDL) fibers present 1 mm from the bony margin, three supporting screws were placed: one vertical, protruding beyond the bony peaks by 4 mm, and two horizontal, protruding by 7 mm (**Fig 43**). A titanium-reinforced ePTFE membrane was cut and secured with two palatal screws (**Fig 44**). The cortical was perforated, and the exposed roots were conditioned with ethylenediaminetetraacetic acid (EDTA) for 3 minutes and treated with amelogenins.

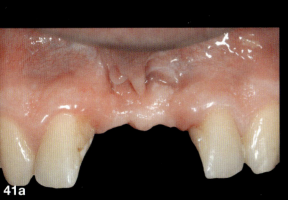
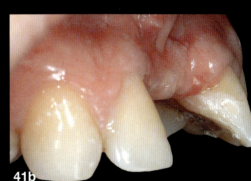

41a

41b

Fig 41 Edentulism in the sites of the maxillary central incisors caused by a vehicle accident. *(a)* The severe vertical and horizontal bone deficiency and loss of attachment on the mesial surfaces of both laterals is evident. *(b)* Lateral view emphasizing the horizontal loss of bone volume.

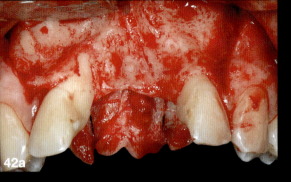
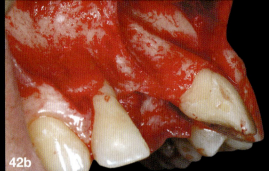

Fig 42 *(a)* After flap elevation, a bladelike residual bone ridge and the loss of the normal bone peaks mesial to the lateral incisors are visible. *(b)* Lateral view showing the severe lack of bone tissue.

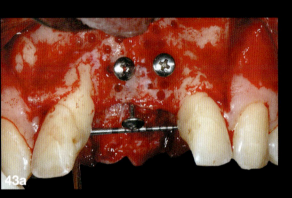
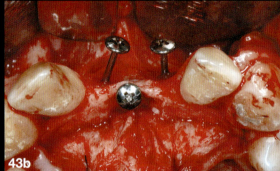

Fig 43 *(a)* A vertical support screw was placed protruding 4 mm above the bony peaks. *(b)* Two support screws were placed horizontally, protruding 7 mm buccal to the buccal bone plate.

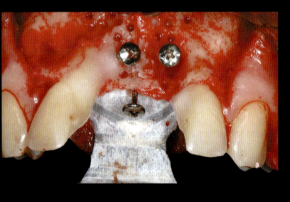
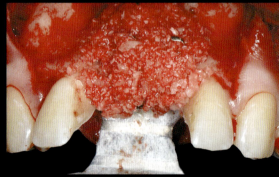

Fig 44 The buccal cortical was perforated, and a titanium-reinforced ePTFE membrane was trimmed and secured palatally with two pins. The roots of the lateral incisors were planed, conditioned with EDTA, and treated with amelogenins.

Fig 45 An 80% autologous and 20% DBBM particulate graft (Bio-Oss) was placed to fill the defect in excess.

A particulate autologous graft mixed with 20% DBBM (Bio-Oss, Geistlich Biomaterials) was placed in the defect and on the treated roots **(Fig 45)**, and the membrane was adapted to cover the graft and secured buccally with two titanium pins so that it did not touch the tooth roots **(Fig 46)**.

The periosteum of the buccal flap was elevated partial thickness **(Fig 47)** and anchored under the palatal flap. An epithelial-connective tissue graft was harvested from the palate and placed on the exposed periosteum and, above it, the buccal flap was repositioned coronally and sutured to the palatal flap with horizontal mattress simple sutures with ePTFE **(Fig 48)**.

After 15 days, healing appeared very good, with soft tissue partially covering the lateral incisors **(Fig 49)**. After 8 months **(Fig 50)**, surgery was performed to remove the membrane and place the implants. Flap elevation, following the design previously described, revealed a membrane perfectly integrated with the underlying tissues and no clinical signs of inflammation or infection **(Fig 51)**.

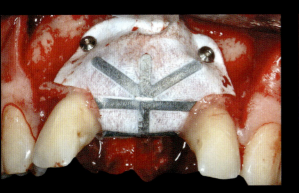

Fig 46 The membrane was closed buccally to cover the graft and anchored with two pins. The graft is in contact with the root surfaces, but the membrane margins are 1 mm apart.

Fig 47 The periosteum of the buccal flap was elevated partial thickness and sutured under the palatal flap.

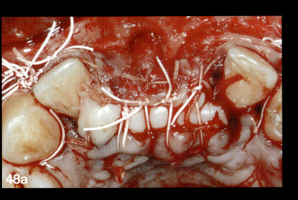
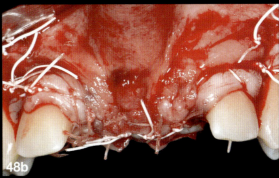

Fig 48 An epithelial-connective tissue graft was harvested from the palate and placed over the periosteum. The buccal flap was sutured to the palatal flap with vertical mattress simple sutures with ePTFE. Occlusal *(a)* and frontal *(b)* views.

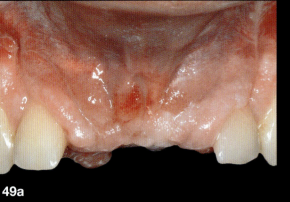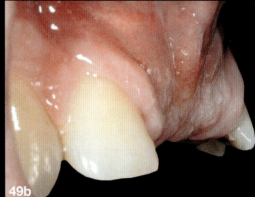

Fig 49 Healing after 2 weeks was very good. *(a)* The crowns of the lateral incisors appear to be partially covered by soft tissue. *(b)* Lateral view of healing. The considerable vertical and horizontal increase can be appreciated.

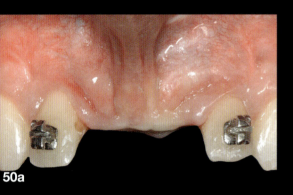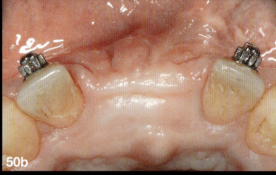

Fig 50 After 8 months, the soft tissues have partially contracted and appear perfectly healed. Frontal *(a)* and palatal *(b)* views.

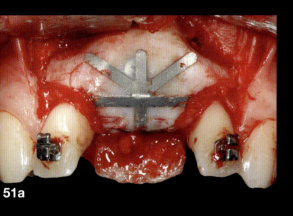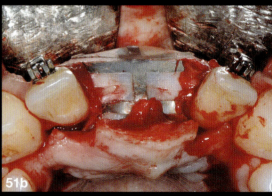

Fig 51 A flap similar to the previous one was elevated to expose the membrane and anchoring instruments. Frontal *(a)* and palatal *(b)* views.

After its removal, regenerated bone tissue appeared, covered by a thin layer of periosteum-like connective tissue **(Fig 52)**. Two implants with a diameter of 3.5 mm and a length of 13 mm were placed, while attempting to respect the minimum interimplant distance of 4 mm **(Fig 53)**, and a thick connective tissue graft harvested from the palate was placed on the ridge to increase the soft tissue thickness **(Fig 54)**. The periosteum was released with a continuous incision, and the buccal flap was sutured to the palatal flap with horizontal mattress and simple sutures **(Fig 55)**.

After 4 months of submerged integration, the mucosa appeared to be in a healthy state, but with considerable displacement of the mucogingival junction caused by the previous coronally repositioned flaps **(Fig 56)**. Soft tissue punches were used so the provisional abutments could be screwed in **(Fig 57)**, and a partial-thickness flap was elevated from the mucogingival junction and repositioned apically in the fornix to gain keratinized mucosa and correct the position of the mucogingival junction **(Fig 58)**. The periosteum was covered with a collagen matrix (Mucograft, Geistlich Biomaterials) sutured to the surrounding tissues **(Fig 59)**. After 1 month, the keratinized mucosa appeared to be of sufficient width **(Fig 60)**, and the prosthetic reconstruction phase could be continued **(Fig 61)**.

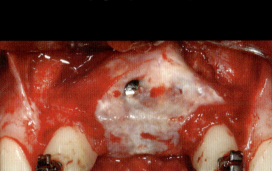
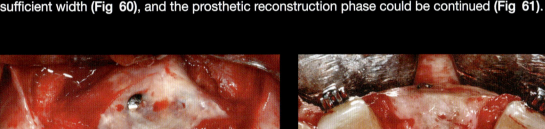

Fig 52 The membrane has been removed. A thin layer of periosteum-like connective tissue covers the regenerated bone. Frontal *(a)* and palatal *(b)* views.

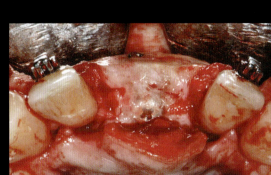

Fig 53 Two implants with a diameter of 3.5 mm were placed in the sites of the maxillary central incisors. The buccal bone thickness appears sufficient.

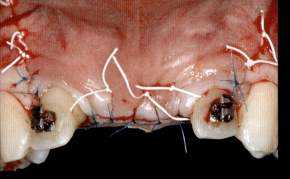

Fig 55 After release of the periosteum, the flaps were sutured with horizontal mattress sutures in ePTFE and simple interrupted sutures in Prolene.

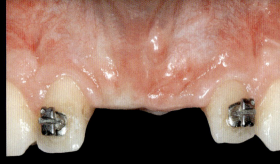

Fig 56 Healing occurred smoothly. After 4 months, a coronal deviation of the mucogingival junction became evident.

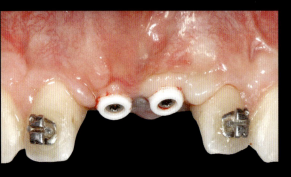

Fig 57 The implants were connected to the healing abutments.

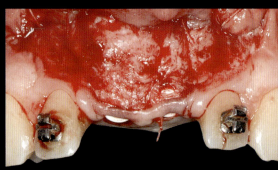

Fig 58 To correct the position of the mucogingival junction, a buccal partial-thickness flap was elevated.

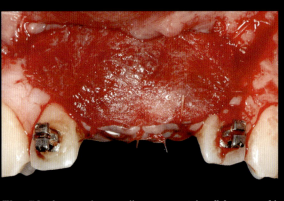

Fig 59 A porcine collagen matrix (Mucograft) was used to protect the periosteum.

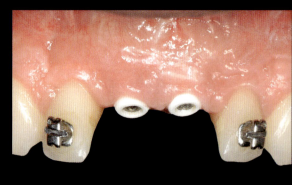

Fig 60 Healing after 1 month. The position of the mucogingival junction has been restored to its original level.

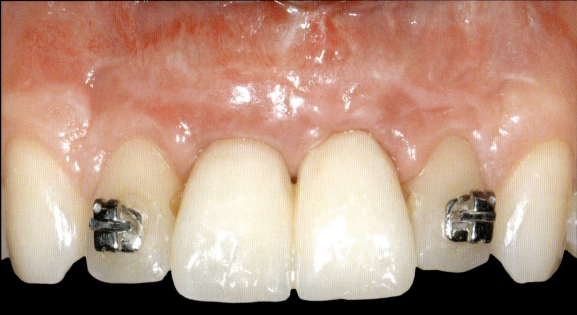

61a

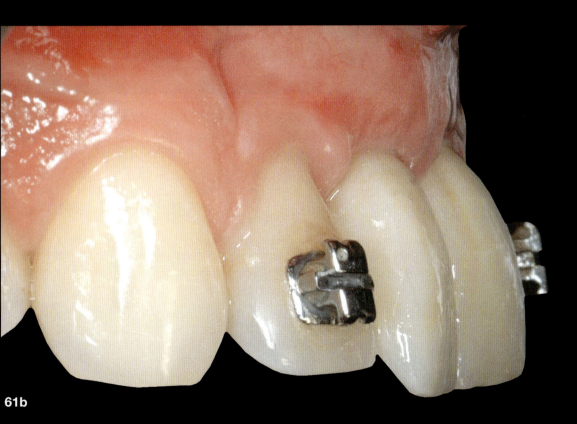

61b

Fig 61 *(a and b)* Final prosthesis. The gingival contours and interproximal papillae are visible.

CLINICAL CASE 3

Vertical ridge augmentation for the replacement of two adjacent teeth in two separate sites in a periodontal (with Dr M. Maglione)

A 26-year-old, nonsmoking patient in good health presented with severe periodontal disease, with gingival recessions of 5 to 7 mm in the area of the maxillary central incisors, left canine, and left first premolar (**Fig 62**). The probing depth indicated a loss of periodontal attachment up to the apex of the aforementioned teeth and deep pockets in the maxillary and mandibular molars. The panoramic radiograph confirmed almost complete loss of bone support around the same teeth (**Fig 63**). After causal therapy, which included creating a periodontal chart, taking a complete set of periapical radiographs, patient motivation to perform proper oral hygiene, and full-mouth disinfection, the

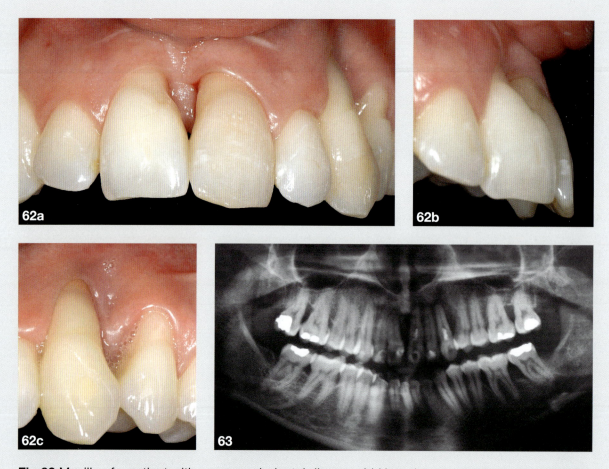

Fig 62 Maxilla of a patient with severe periodontal disease. *(a)* Note the severe gingival recession in the areas of the central incisors, canine, and left first premolar. *(b)* The severe hard and soft tissue deficiency in the interincisal area is evident. *(c)* In the area of the left canine and first premolar, the serious lack of gingiva and volume at the buccal level can be observed. **Fig 63** Panoramic radiograph showing almost total loss of bone support at the central incisors, canine, and first premolar and severe defects in the molar region.

treatment plan was drawn up. The challenged when rehabilitating periodontal patients with severe gum recession is the lack of soft tissue, which makes covering and healing by primary intention of any bone grafts with membranes difficult. Therefore, the treatment plan initially included the extraction of the central incisors, left canine, and left first premolar, with DBBM graft and epithelial-connective tissue harvested from the palate to restore an adequate amount of keratinized mucosa, and only then vertical augmentations with GBR.

The teeth were extracted, the sockets carefully curetted (**Fig 64**), and a Bio-Oss Collagen graft (Geistlich Biomaterials) inserted up to 1 mm from the residual gingival margin of the socket (**Fig 65**). Four oval-shaped epithelial-connective tissue grafts were harvested from the palate, deepithelialized in the peripheral areas, and inserted under the buccal and palatal mucosa to cover the defect (**Figs 66 and 67**).

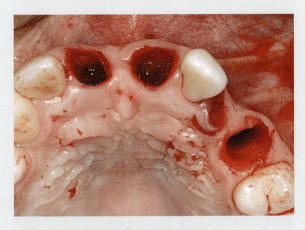

Fig 64 Extraction of the central incisors, left canine, and first premolar and alveolar curettage to remove all inflammatory tissue.

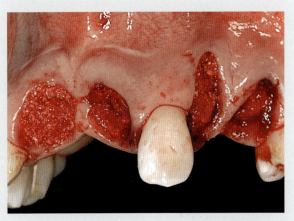

Fig 65 A DBBM graft (Bio-Oss Collagen) was inserted into the sockets to support the epithelial-connective tissue graft.

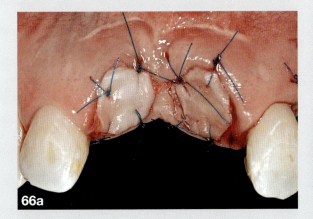

66a

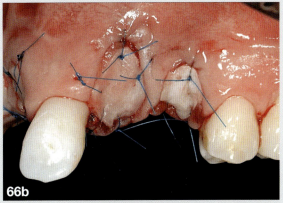

66b

Fig 66 After deepithelialization of the peripheral portion, the grafts were inserted under the buccal and palatal mucosa of the sockets and sutured with 6-0 Prolene. *(a)* Central incisors. *(b)* Canine and first premolar.

After 4 months of healing, vertical ridge augmentation was performed with GBR. A full-thickness flap was elevated from distal to the maxillary right canine to distal to the maxillary left second premolar, and the alveolar bone and tooth roots were carefully planed (Fig 68a). The nasopalatine canal was completely emptied (Fig 68b).

Two titanium-reinforced ePTFE membranes were trimmed to fit the anatomy of the defects and secured with tacks to the palatal surface in the sites of the central incisors, left canine, and left first premolar. Using the membranes as matrices, the defects were filled with a particulate graft of 70% autologous bone and 30% DBBM (Bio-Oss) (Fig 69).

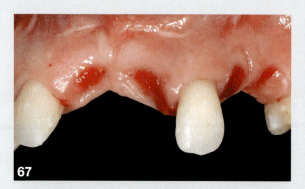

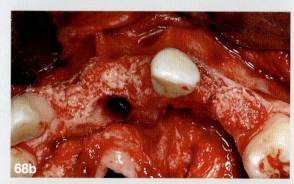

Fig 67 Healing of the grafts after 1 month.
Fig 68 After 4 months, a full-thickness flap from the right canine to the left first premolar was elevated, and the bone defects were exposed. *(a)* Remarkable lack of vertical dimension. *(b)* Occlusal view. The lack of residual bone thickness is noticeable. The nasopalatine canal was carefully emptied of connective tissue for treatment as a four-walled bone defect.

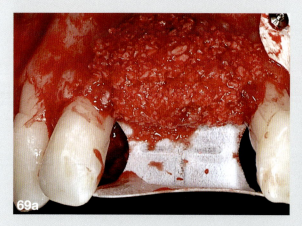

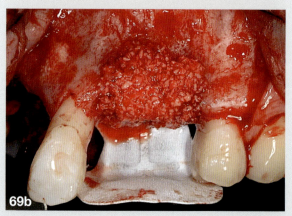

Fig 69 A membrane was fixed palatally, and a particulate bone graft was placed to fill the defect. (a) Area of the central incisors. (b) Area of the left canine and first premolar.

The membranes were then adapted buccally and secured with two pins each so that they did not touch the roots of the adjacent teeth (**Figs 70 and 71**). The periosteum was released via a single incision at the base of the buccal flap, and horizontal mattress sutures in 4-0 ePTFE and simple sutures in 6-0 Prolene were applied.

Healing occurred without any adverse events (**Fig 72**).

After 8 months (**Fig 73**), a flap with similar characteristics to the first one was elevated (**Fig 74**), and the membranes were removed (**Fig 75**). The volume of regenerated bone appeared to be sufficient in both the horizontal and vertical dimensions for the placement of four implants. Implants with a machined surface were then inserted, strictly observing a minimum distance of 4 mm between them (**Fig 76**). To further increase bone volume and to protect the regenerated, still immature bone, a new layer of DBBM was placed (**Fig 77**) and covered with two resorbable collagen membranes (Bio-Gide, Geistlich Biomaterials) (**Fig 78**). CBCT confirmed the correct positioning of the implants (**Fig 79**).

After 4 months of healing to achieve osseointegration (**Fig 80**), another procedure was performed to increase the volume of the soft tissue.

A partial-thickness flap was elevated (**Fig 81**), and a porcine collagen matrix (Mucograft) was inserted (**Fig 82**).

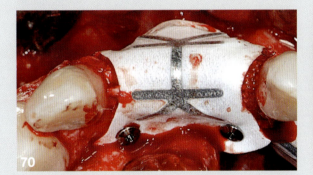
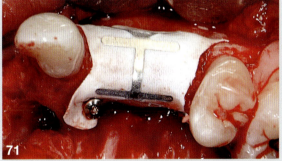

Fig 70 Membrane stabilized with two pins in the sites of the central incisors. **Fig 71** Membrane stabilized with two pins in the sites of the left canine and first premolar.

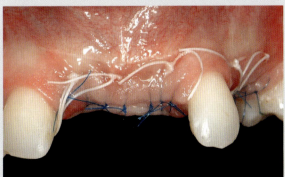
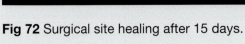

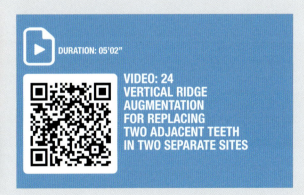

DURATION: 05'02"

VIDEO: 24
VERTICAL RIDGE AUGMENTATION FOR REPLACING TWO ADJACENT TEETH IN TWO SEPARATE SITES

Fig 72 Surgical site healing after 15 days.

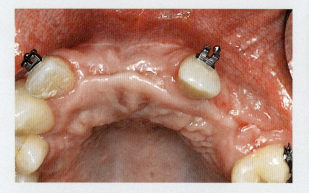

Fig 73 Appearance of the soft tissue 8 months after surgery.

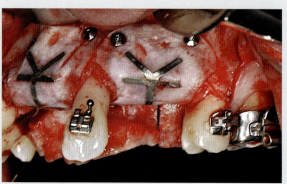

Fig 74 At the time of removal, the membranes appeared to be perfectly integrated with the underlying tissues.

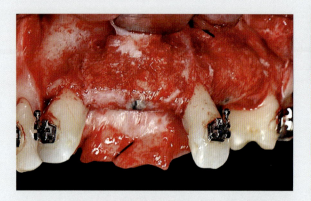

Fig 75 Clinical appearance of regenerated bone after membrane removal. The bone ridge has been completely reconstructed.

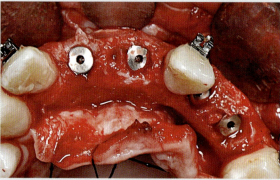

Fig 76 Four machined-surface iMAX implants were placed in the locations of the central incisors and the left canine and first premolar. An interimplant distance of 4 mm was well respected.

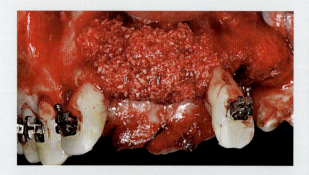

Fig 77 A DBBM graft (Bio-Oss) was layered to protect the regenerated bone to further increase the volume of the site.

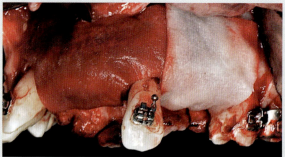

Fig 78 The DBBM graft was covered with a collagen membrane (Bio-Gide).

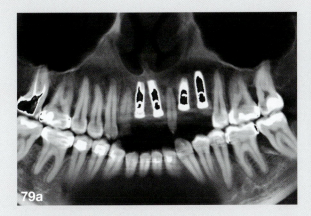
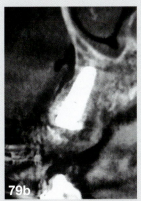

Fig 79 CBCT showing the correct position of the implants. *(a)* Panoramic view. *(b)* Cross-sectional view showing sufficient bone thickness buccal to the implants.

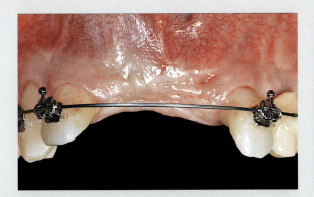

Fig 80 The edentulous ridge after 4 months of healing. The slight lack of soft tissue volume is evident around the central incisors, as well as orthodontic therapy on the natural teeth.

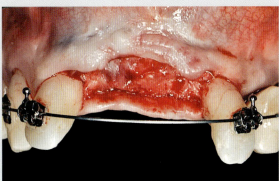

Fig 81 View of a partial-thickness flap extended intrasulcularly to the lateral incisors.

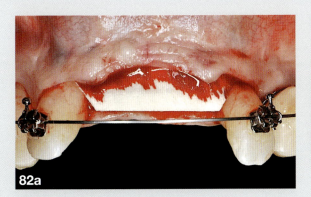
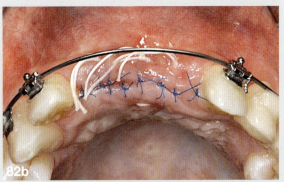

Fig 82 *(a)* A porcine collagen matrix (Mucograft) was inserted to increase the thickness of the crestal connective tissue. *(b)* The flap was sutured with horizontal ePTFE mattress sutures and simple 6-0 Prolene sutures.

At the same time, the patient underwent orthodontic therapy to realign the natural teeth that had drifted buccally due to periodontal disease, and the provisional prostheses were anchored to the orthodontic arch. After 1 month of healing, the implants were uncovered and provisionals were placed for a period of 6 months **(Fig 83)**. When the emergence profiles and gingival contours were sufficiently conditioned, a new impression was taken **(Fig 84)**, and the definitive restoration in zirconia and ceramic was delivered **(Fig 85)**.

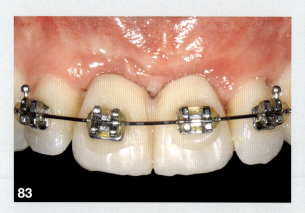

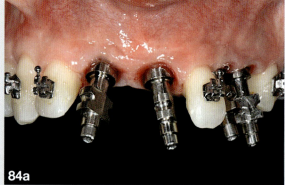

Fig 83 After 1 month of healing, the implants were uncovered and connected to provisional crowns. The provisional crowns were used as anchorage for the final stages of orthodontic therapy. **Fig 84** *(a)* Positioning of the transfers for the final impression. *(b)* Polyether impression with the transfers inserted. **Fig 85** Final zirconia and ceramic crowns. The interproximal papillae are well formed.

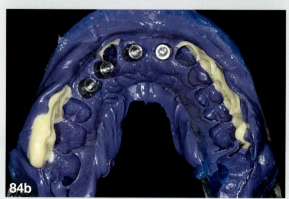

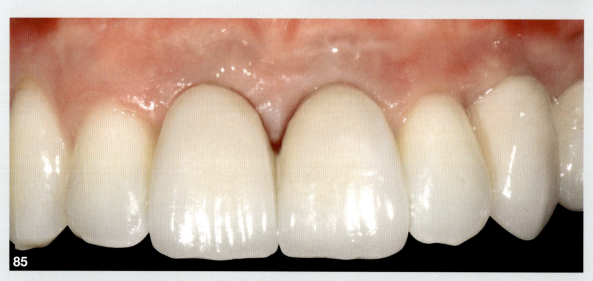

CLINICAL CASE 4

Vertical ridge augmentation for the replacement of three adjacent
(with Dr M. Maglione)

A 20-year-old, nonsmoking patient in good health suffered the traumatic avulsion of the two maxillary central incisors and the left lateral incisor in a car accident (Fig 86). The panoramic and periapical radiographs showed a considerable vertical and horizontal bone defects in the traumatized area and a residual root piece in the site of the left lateral incisor (Fig 87). Removal of the ill-fitting provisional prosthesis revealed the severe bone volume deficit in the edentulous area, which was not compatible with an esthetically adequate final prosthesis (Fig 88). The treatment plan involved two-stage vertical bone augmentation and the subsequent placement of two implants in the sites of the right central incisor and left lateral incisor, leaving the site of the left central incisor for a pontic.

A full-thickness flap was reflected from the right lateral incisor to the left canine with a slightly buccal crestal incision. The root surfaces of the adjacent teeth were planed, and the bone was carefully cu-retted to remove residual connective tissue (Fig 89), and the root residue in the site of the left lateral incisor was removed (Fig 90).

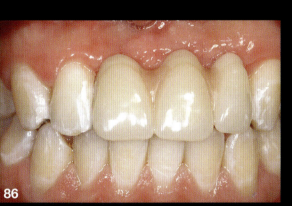

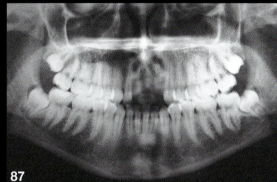

Fig 86 The patient's ill-fitting resin-bonded provisional after the trauma that resulted in the avulsion of the central incisors and left lateral incisor. **Fig 87** Panoramic radiograph showing the vertical bone defect and the root remnant in the site of the maxillary left lateral incisor.

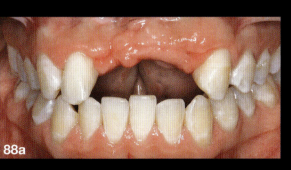

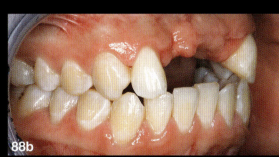

Fig 88 Edentulous ridge with vertical bone volume deficiency *(a)* and horizontal bone volume deficiency observable from a lateral view *(b)*.

Two screws were placed to support the membrane at the level of the bone peaks **(Fig 91)**. A titanium-reinforced ePTFE membrane was fixed palatally with two screws, and an autologous particulate bone graft mixed with 30% DBBM was placed over the defect **(Fig 92)**. The membrane was then repositioned buccally and tensioned with two titanium pins to provide maximum stability without touching the roots of the adjacent teeth **(Figs 93 and 94)**. The base of the buccal flap was released with a continuous incision at the periosteum, and horizontal mattress sutures in 4-0 ePTFE and simple sutures in Prolene 6-0 were applied **(Fig 95)**. After 12 days, the sutures were removed **(Fig 96)**.

After 8 months of healing, the tissues appeared healthy and mature **(Fig 97)**, and the panoramic radiograph showed an adequate amount of bone tissue **(Fig 98)**. Upon removal of the membrane **(Fig 99)**, dense and good quality regenerated bone tissue appeared **(Fig 100)**.

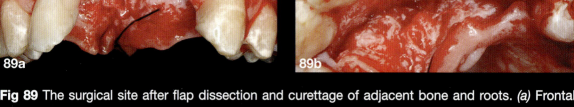

Fig 89 The surgical site after flap dissection and curettage of adjacent bone and roots. *(a)* Frontal view. *(b)* Palatal view.

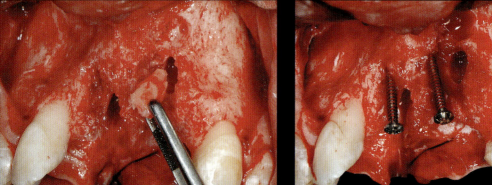

Fig 90 The residual root fragment of the maxillary left lateral incisor was removed.

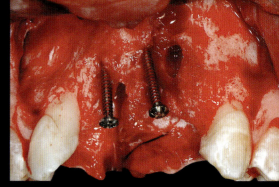

Fig 91 Two screws were placed to support the membrane at the level of the bony peaks of the adjacent teeth.

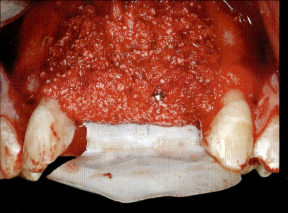

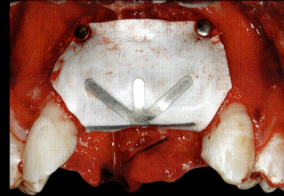

Fig 92 The palatally fixed titanium-reinforced ePTFE membrane was used a matrix for the placement of a particulate graft made of 70% autologous bone and 30% Bio-Oss.

Fig 93 The membrane was closed buccally and secured with two pins.

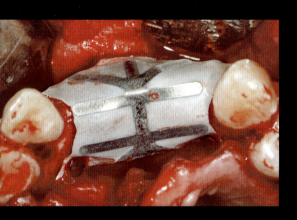

Fig 94 Palatal view of the membrane. Note the distance of approximately 1 mm from the membrane margin to the surface of the natural teeth.

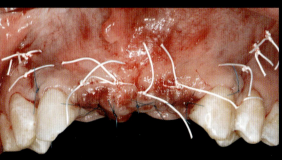

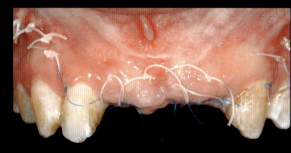

95

96

Fig 95 After release of the buccal flap with a periosteal incision, the flaps were sutured with horizontal mattress and simple sutures. **Fig 96** Flap healing after 12 days at the time of suture removal.

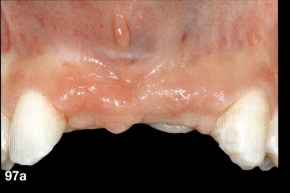
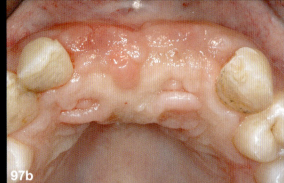

Fig 97 Edentulous ridge after 8 months of healing. *(a)* Frontal view. *(b)* Occlusal view.

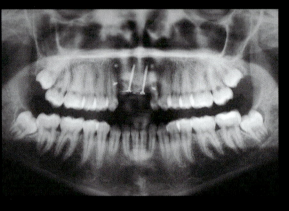

Fig 98 Panoramic radiograph showing regenerated bone and membrane fixation tools.

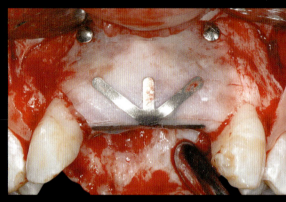

Fig 99 Appearance of the membrane at removal. It appears to be perfectly adhered to the underlying regenerated tissue.

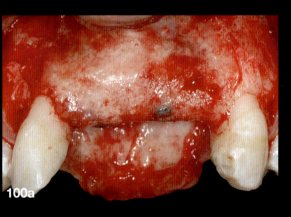
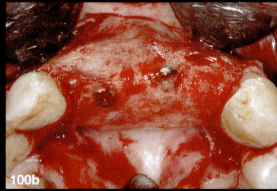

Fig 100 *(a)* After membrane removal, regenerated bone of good quality and correct vertical dimension is visible. *(b)* From an occlusal view, the thickness also appears sufficient.

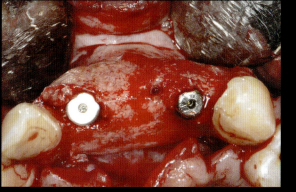

Fig 101 Two implants were placed. Note the correct interimplant distance to maintain space for a pontic.

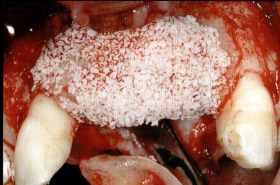

Fig 102 The site was covered with a layer of Bio-Oss and a collagen Bio-Gide membrane to protect the newly formed bone.

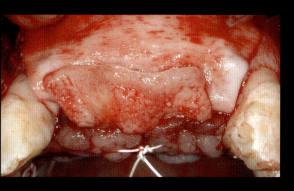

Fig 103 A connective tissue graft harvested from the palate was placed on the ridge and sutured to the palatal flap to increase the thickness of the mucosa.

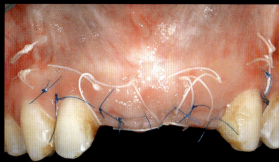

Fig 104 Healing of the site after 12 days.

In the same operation, two implants were placed, a 3.75-mm-diameter, 13-mm-long iMAX implant in the location of the maxillary right central incisor and a 3.3-mm-diameter iMAX implant of the same length in the location of the left lateral incisor **(Fig 101)**.

The implants and the newly formed bone tissue were covered with a layer of DBBM **(Fig 102)** and a collagen membrane (Bio-Gide), and a connective tissue graft harvested from the palate was placed on the ridge and secured with a horizontal mattress suture to the palatal mucosa **(Fig 103)**.

The buccal flap was released again, and suturing was performed in the same manner as described previously **(Fig 104)**.

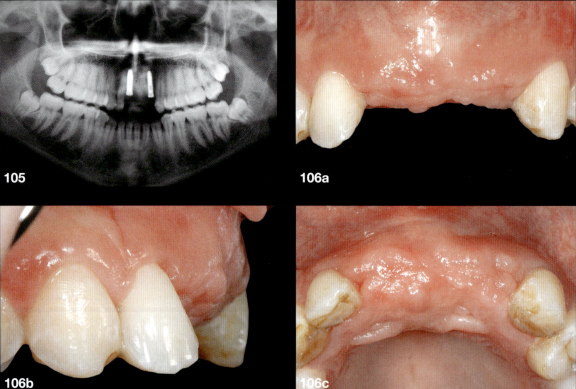

Fig 105 Panoramic radiograph showing the correct position of the implants in the regenerated bone.
Fig 106 lAìppearance of the edentulous ridge 4 months after implant placement. Frontal *(a)*, lateral *(b)*, and palatal *(c)* views The vertical and horizontal dimensions of the ridge are adequate.

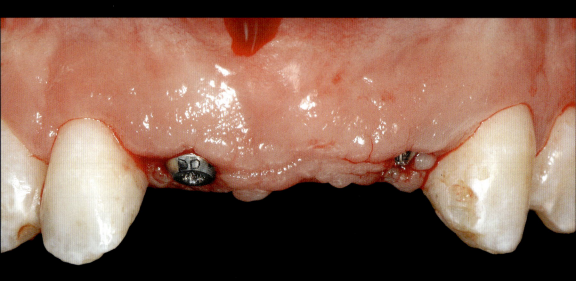

Fig 107 Uncovering the implants for the insertion of healing abutments. Note their small diameter and length so as not to compress or protrude beyond the thickness of the mucosa.

After an additional 4 months of healing, the edentulous ridge appeared sufficiently wide in both the vertical and horizontal dimensions **(Figs 105 and 106)**, and the implants were uncovered to screw in a healing abutment with a length equal to the mucosal thickness and a diameter equal to the implant platforms **(Fig 107)**. Two successive provisional restoration were designed to condition an adequate emergence profile at the level of both the implant and pontic elements **(Fig 108)**.

The placement of the two provisionals in a succession of 3 months resulted in progressive compression over 6 months until the tissues were fully matured and adequate emergence profiles were developed **(Fig 109)**. The final prosthesis was fabricated from zirconia and ceramic **(Figs 110 and 111)**.

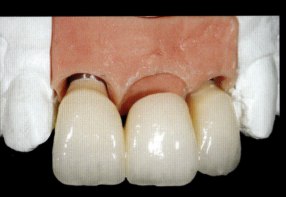

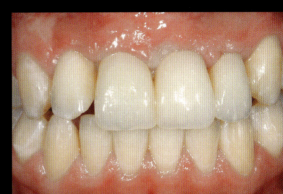

Fig 108 Second provisional prosthesis fabricated after 3 months. The emergence profiles and gingival contours are modelled to achieve a suitable shape for the final crowns.

Fig 109 The provisional prosthesis generates interproximal compression to evert the incisive papilla.

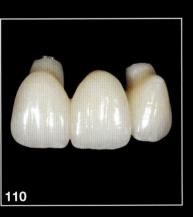

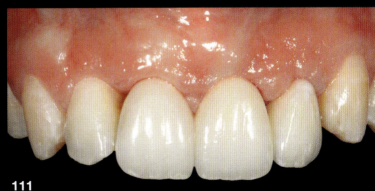

110

111

Fig 110 Final zirconia and ceramic prosthesis modelled on the basis of the emergence profiles and gingival contours obtained with the provisionals. **Fig 111** Definitive prosthesis in place.

CLINICAL CASE 5

Vertical ridge augmentation in a growing patient
(with Dr R. Cocconi)

A 10-year-old boy was kicked by a horse, resulting in the traumatic avulsion of the maxillary left lateral incisor, canine, and first premolar, gingival recession around the left central incisor, and severe bone loss in the left hemimaxilla (**Fig 112**). The trauma also caused buccal flaring of the incisors and an unbalanced growth of the maxillary jaw, with the right hemimaxilla being more developed than the left (**Fig 113**). The treatment of growing patients with GBR techniques is always unpredictable because, while it is known that implant treatment should be performed only at the end of growth, there is no experience regarding the ideal period to undertake regenerative techniques. In this case, it was decided to perform bone regeneration immediately and postpone implant placement until the age of 18. The resolution of this complex case required a multi-disciplinary approach in multiple stages, which lasted a total of 10 years and including specialists in orthodontics, dental hygiene, periodontics, and prosthodontics, as well as a laboratory technician.

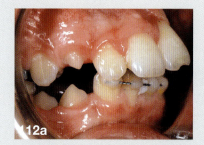 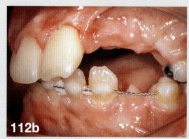 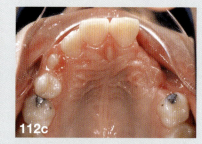

Fig 112 Traumatic avulsion of the maxillary left lateral incisor, canine, and first premolar in a 10-year-old patient. *(a)* Right lateral view. *(b)* From the left lateral view, the gingival recession on the maxillary left central incisor and the atrophic edentulous ridge around the maxillary left lateral incisor, canine, and first premolar can be appreciated. *(c)* Occlusal view.

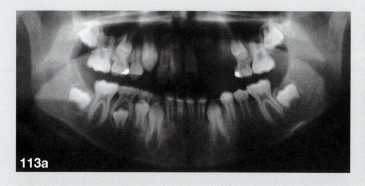 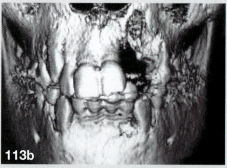

Fig 113 *(a)* Panoramic radiograph showing the severe vertical defect in the areas of the left lateral incisor to the first premolar and the mixed dentition. *(b)* 3D CBCT showing the bony defect and the overdevelopment of the right hemimaxilla compared to the left.

Phase I: GBR

After a few sessions to motivate the patient and teach him the correct techniques for home oral hygiene, a full-thickness flap extended to the adjacent teeth was performed **(Fig 114)**. The bone was carefully curetted and perforated to expose the trabecular bone and stimulate the formation of a suitable blood clot, and two support screws were then placed in a vertical position **(Fig 115)**. A titanium-reinforced ePTFE membrane was fixed palatally, and the defect was filled with 70% particulate autologous bone and 30% DBBM (Bio-Oss) **(Fig 116)**. The membrane was then closed buccally and stabilized, in tension, with two pins **(Figs 117 and 118)**. The buccal flap was released and sutured with horizontal mattress simple sutures to the palatal flap.

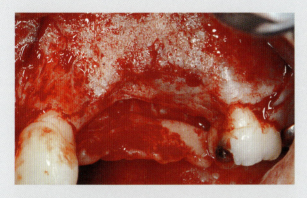

Fig 114 A full-thickness flap was elevated to expose the vertical bone defect.

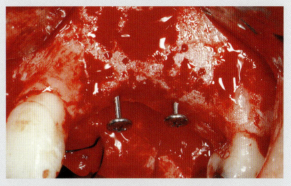

Fig 115 Two membrane support screws were placed in the ridge.

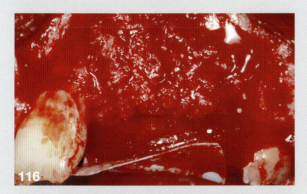

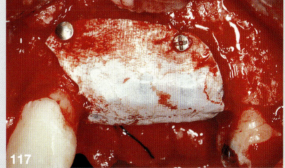

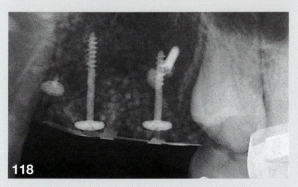

Fig 116 A titanium-reinforced ePTFE membrane was fixed palatally, and an autologous particulate bone graft mixed with 30% DBBM was placed to fill the defect. **Fig 117** The membrane was stabilized buccally with two titanium pins. **Fig 118** Periapical radiograph. The membrane and graft are in the correct position. The maxillary left second premolar is still erupting.

Fhase II: Removal of the membrane, placement of an implant in the center of the palate for orthodontic anchorage, and grafting

After 6 months of submerged healing, the membrane was removed by means of a full-thickness flap without including the adjacent teeth. Due to the young age of the patient and the resulting high regenerative potential, the membrane appeared partially covered by a thin layer of newly formed bone **(Fig 119)**. The underlying bone was of excellent quality **(Fig 120)**. To hinder the growth of the right hemimaxilla and to stimulate the left hemimaxilla, it was decided to extract the germ of the maxillary right second premolar, which had not yet erupted, and to re-implant it in the left hemimaxilla as a substitute for the canine. The deciduous tooth **(Fig 121a)** was then extracted to gain access to the definitive maxillary right first premolar **(Fig 121b)**. The latter was gently extracted with the entire follicle, and the root apex appeared still open and not fully formed **(Fig 121c)**.

In the regenerated bone at the site of the maxillary left canine, a cavity large enough to accommodate the extracted right second premolar and the follicle was created **(Fig 122)**, and the latter was immediately inserted and submerged with the soft tissue **(Figs 123 and 124)**. Finally, a flat Onplant (Nobel Biocare) **(Fig 125)** was placed through a narrow full-thickness tunnel in the palatal flap in the center of the palate for orthodontic anchorage and allowed to heal in a submerged position **(Fig 126)**.

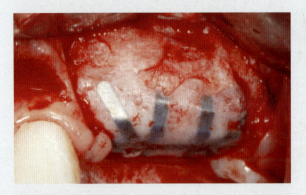 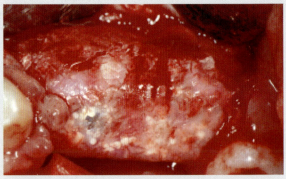

Fig 119 Removal of the membrane after 6 months of submerged healing. The membrane is covered by a thin layer of newly formed bone.

Fig 120 The newly formed bone appears to be of good quality.

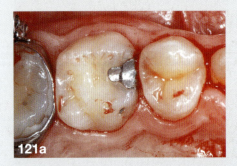 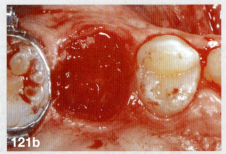 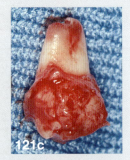

Fig 121 *(a and b)* The deciduous tooth was extracted to access the follicle of the maxillary right second premolar to be transplanted to the site of the left canine. (c) Extracted right second premolar with its follicle. The root apex is still open.

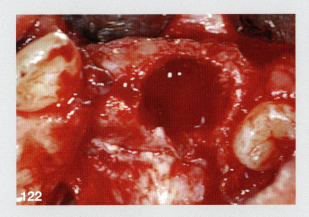 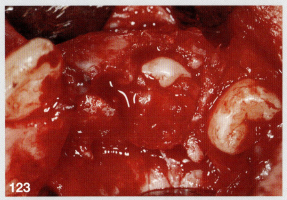

Fig 122 Dental transplant recipient site preparation. **Fig 123** Maxillary right second premolar inserted into the position of the left canine.

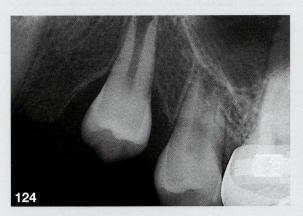 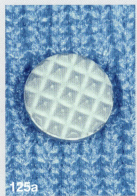 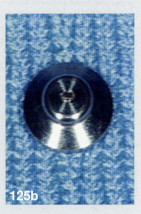

Fig 124 Radiograph of the dental transplant. **Fig 125** Onplant for orthodontic anchorage. *(a)* Lower surface. *(b)* Upper portion.

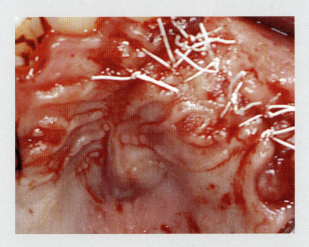

Fig 126 The Onplant was inserted through a submucosal tunnel in the center of the palate, and the flaps were sutured with ePTFE sutures.

Phase III: Implant uncovering and orthodontic therapy

After 4 months of integration, the Onplant was uncovered (**Fig 127**) and used as maximum anchorage for an orthodontic appliance (**Fig 128**). Orthodontic therapy continued for the next 3 years, during which the transplanted element in the site of the maxillary left canine was brought into the arch and all dental elements were aligned (**Figs 129 to 133**).

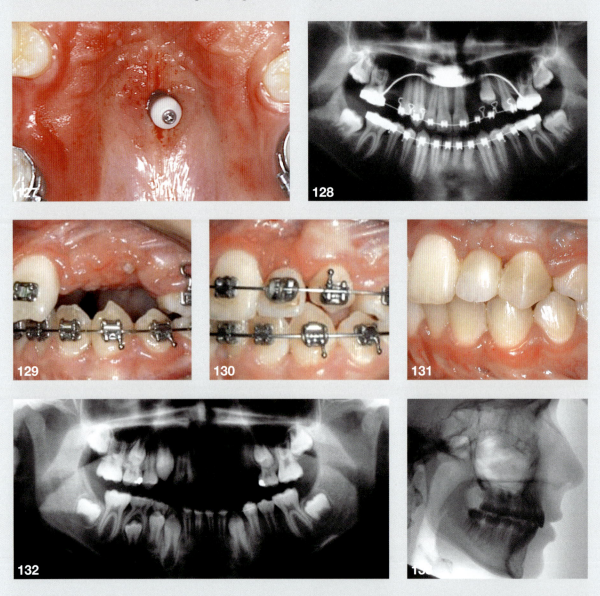

Fig 127 Mucosal punch and connection of the healing abutment on the Onplant after 4 months of healing. **Fig 128** Panoramic radiograph showing the orthodontic appliance anchored to the Onplant. **Fig 129** Start of orthodontic therapy for dental and skeletal realignment. **Fig 130** The maxillary right second premolar transplanted into the position of the left canine is gradually reaching the occlusal plane. **Fig 131** The premolar in the place of the canine has correctly reached the occlusal plane. **Fig 132** Panoramic radiograph at the end of orthodontic therapy. **Fig 133** Lateral teleradiograph showing the correct intermaxillary ratios.

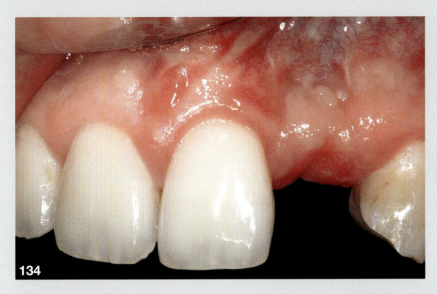

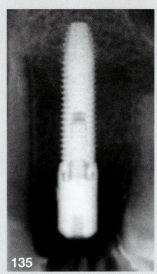

Fig 134 Condition of the edentulous span when the patient is 18 years old. The regenerated bone has maintained its trophism by continuing to grow together with the adjacent native bone.
Fig 135 A 3.3-mm-diameter implant was placed in the site of the maxillary left lateral incisor.

Phase IV: End of orthodontic therapy and maintenance until the age of 18 years
Phase V: Placing the implant in the site of the maxillary left lateral incisor
At the age of 18, the patient had an optimal orthodontic and dental situation. The maxillary right second premolar transplanted into the site of the left canine retained the vitality of both pulp and periodontium, with no ankylosis or root resorption, and the regenerated bone at the level of the edentulous ridge maintained its trophism by continuing to grow together with the adjacent native bone (**Fig 134**). An implant with a diameter of 3.3 mm and a length of 13 mm was then inserted in the site of the maxillary left lateral incisor without any further intervention on the hard or soft tissues (**Fig 135**).

Phase VI: Placement of the provisional and final prostheses
After 4 months, provisional crowns on the left lateral incisor and canine transplant were placed and maintained for 6 months to condition the soft tissue and to obtain an adequate emergence profile (**Fig 136**).
At the time of definitive prosthesis placement, a gingivectomy was performed from the maxillary left lateral incisor to the right central incisor and the left canine to harmonize the gingival contours, with a gingivoplasty on the maxillary left lateral incisor to remove the residual scars on the buccal gingival margin (**Fig 137**). The final prostheses were made of zirconia and ceramic (**Fig 138**).

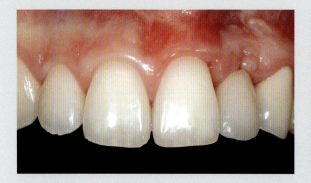

Fig 136 Provisional prostheses on the maxillary left lateral incisor and canine.

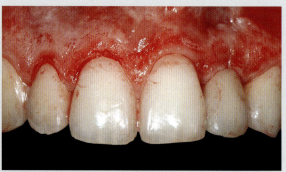

Fig 137 Gingivectomy on the maxillary right lateral incisor, right central incisor, left central incisor, and left canine and gingivoplasty on the left lateral incisor.

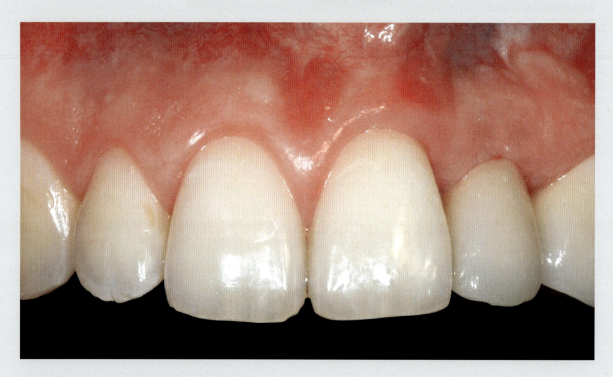

Fig 138 Final zirconia and ceramic prostheses.

REFERENCES

1. Rocchietta I, Ferrantino L, Simion M. Vertical ridge augmentation in the esthetic zone. Periodontol 2000 2018;77:241–255.

2. Araújo MG, Lindhe J. Dimensional ridge alterations following tooth extraction. An experimental study in the dog. J Clin Periodontol 2005;32:212–218.

3. Araújo MG, Wennström JL, Lindhe J. Modeling of the buccal and lingual bone walls of fresh extraction sites following implant installation. Clin Oral Implants Res 2006;17:606–614.

4. Chappuis V, Engel O, Shahim K, Reyes M, Katsaros C, Buser D. Soft tissue alterations in esthetic postextraction sites: A 3-dimensional analysis. J Dent Res 2015;94(9 Suppl):187S–193S.

5. Hämmerle CHF, Araújo MG, Simion M. Evidence-based knowledge on the biology and treatment of extraction sockets. Clin Oral Implants Res 2012;23 (Suppl 5):80–82.

6. Araújo MG, Hämmerle CHF, Simion M. Extraction sockets: Biology and treatment options. Clin Oral Implants Res 2012;23(Suppl 5):iv.

7. Fradeani M, Barducci G. Aesthetic Rehabilitation in Fixed Prosthetics. Vol. 2. Quintessence Italy, 2008.

8. Jemt T. Regeneration of gingival papillae after single-implant treatment. Int J Periodontics Restorative Dent 1997;17:326–333.

9. Meijer HJA, Stellingsma K, Meijndert L, Raghoebar GM. A new index for rating aesthetics of implant-supported single crowns and adjacent soft tissues—The implant crown aesthetic index. Clin Oral Implants Res 2005;16:645–649.

10. Furhauser R, Florescu D, Benesch T, Haas R, Mailath G, Watzek G. Evaluation of soft tissue around single-tooth implant crowns: The pink esthetic score. Clin Oral Implants Res 2005;16:639–644.

11. Belser UC, Grütter L, Vailati F, Bornstein MM, Weber H-P, Buser D. Outcome evaluation of early placed maxillary anterior single-tooth implants using objective esthetic criteria: A cross-sectional, retrospective study in 45 patients with a 2- to 4-year follow-up using pink and white esthetic scores. J Periodontol 2009;80:140–151.

12. Juodzbalys G, Wang H-L. Esthetic index for anterior maxillary implant-supported restorations. J Periodontol 2010;81:34–42.

13. Jung RE, Holderegger C, Sailer I, Khraisat A, Suter A, Hämmerle CH. The effect of all-ceramic and porcelain-fused-to-metal restorations on marginal peri-implant soft tissue staining: A randomised controlled clinical trial. Int J Periodontics Restorative Dent 2008;28:357–365.

14. Jung RE, Sailer I, Hämmerle CH, Attin T, Schmidlin P. In vitro colour changes of soft tissues caused by restorative materials. Int J Periodontics Restorative Dent 2007;27:251–257.

15. Simion M, Ferrantino L, Idotta E, Maglione M. The association of guided bone regeneration and enamel matrix derivative for suprabony reconstruction in the esthetic area: A case report. Int J Periodontics Restorative Dent 2015;35:767–772.

16. Simion M, Rocchietta I, Monforte M, Maschera E. Three-dimensional alveolar bone reconstruction with a combination of recombinant human platelet-derived growth factor bb and guided bone regeneration: A case report. Int J Periodontics Restorative Dent 2008;28:239–243.

17. Buser D, Martin W, Belser UC. Optimizing esthetics for implant restorations in the anterior maxilla: Anatomic and surgical considerations. Int J Oral Maxillofac Implants 2004;19(Suppl):43–61.

18. Tarnow DP, Cho SC, Wallace SS. The effect of inter-implant distance on the height of inter-implant bone crest. J Periodontol 2000;71:546–554.

19. Adell R, Lekholm U, Rockler B, Brånemark PI. A 15-year study of osseointegrated implants in the treatment of the edentulous jaw. Int J Oral Surg 1981;10:387–416.

20. Tarnow DP, Wagner AW, Fletcher P. The effect of the distance from the contact point to the crest of bone on the presence or absence of the interproximal dental papilla. J Periodontol 1992;63:935–996.

21. Grunder U, Gracis S, Hair M. Influence of the 3-d bone-to-implant relationship on esthetics. Int J Periodontics Restorative Dent 2005;25:113–119.

22. Schwarz F, Sahm N, Becker J. Impact of the outcome of guided bone regeneration in dehiscence-type defects on the long-term stability of peri-implant health: Clinical observations at 4 years. Clin Oral Implants Res 2012;23:191–196.

PERI-IMPLANT SOFT TISSUE MANAGEMENT

CHAPTER 19

Edited by Massimo Simion and Giovanni Zucchelli

INTRODUCTION

In the pioneering days of osseointegration, the focus of researchers and clinicians was almost exclusively on bone and its relationship to the implant surface. Very early on, however, the fundamental importance of the quality and quantity of soft tissue for both esthetic reasons and peri-implant health was understood. Dr Peter Whorle has likened harmonious soft tissues to a symphony, with the bone determining the tone. Bone and soft tissue are inextricably linked, and there can be no adequate implant rehabilitation when the quality of either is lacking.

KERATINIZED MUCOSA

For many years, the importance of an adequate band of keratinized mucosa around implant rehabilitations has been questioned, with a number of studies showing contradictory results.[1-4] Recently, an increasing number of studies have shown a higher incidence of biologic complications, such as increased plaque accumulation, mucosal recession,[5] and peri-implantitis,[6] in the absence of at least 2 mm of keratinized mucosa.

Other clinical studies have shown greater peri-implant bone resorption with mucosal thicknesses less than 2 mm.[7,8]

Soft tissue management, whether around teeth or implants, is almost an art form. It is more related to periodontics and esthetic dentistry than oral surgery itself. However, to consider it from only an esthetic point of view is limiting and inappropriate. The biologic implications of soft tissue management are enormous.

Massimo Simion

There is currently broad consensus among researchers and clinicians on the importance of a sufficient band of keratinized mucosa in peri-implant soft tissue.

Epithelial tissue differentiation in the oral cavity

To understand surgical techniques aimed at modifying both the thickness and characteristics of the oral mucosa, it is necessary to know the mechanisms that regulate epithelial differentiation. In a preclinical histologic study in primates, Karring et al[9] surgically moved the adherent keratinized gingiva apically within the alveolar mucosa, which itself was repositioned coronally in contact with the teeth **(Fig 1a)**.

After 4 months of healing, the apically displaced gingiva retained its keratinization characteristics, and a thin zone of new keratinized gingiva, originating from the connective attachment and the periodontal ligament (PDL), was formed close to the teeth.

The alveolar mucosa was interposed between the repositioned gingiva and the new keratinized gingiva **(Fig 1b)**. In another study, Karring et al[10]

prepared two recipient sites in the alveolar mucosa of primates for the placement of two different grafts. The first graft consisted of connective tissue derived from the alveolar mucosa, and the second was connective tissue from the keratinized gingiva.

In this way, the newly formed epithelium could only be derived from the surrounding nonkeratinized epithelium **(Fig 2a)**. After healing, the site that received the graft from the adherent gingiva showed a normally keratinized epithelium, whereas the epithelium of the other site had an appearance quite similar to that of nonkeratinized alveolar mucosa **(Fig 2b)**. These observations were confirmed histologically.

These two studies unequivocally demonstrated that the characteristics of the gingival epithelium are determined by the genetic factors of the underlying connective tissue.

The clinical implication of this discovery is enormous. If the characteristics of the gingival epithelium must be modified, the underlying connective tissue, and not the epithelium itself, must be dealt with first.

In other words, if connective tissue capable of modifying the specificity of the epithelium above is

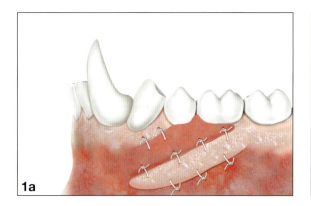
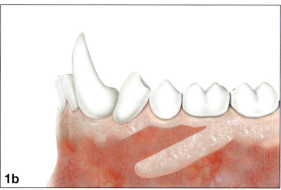

Fig 1 (a) *The adherent gingiva was displaced apically, and the alveolar mucosa was repositioned in contact with the natural teeth. (b) After healing, the ectopic adherent gingiva retained its keratinization characteristics. A small band of adherent gingiva from the PDL was formed in the vicinity of the teeth.*[9]

not inserted first, keratinization cannot be obtained with any type of intervention. The gingival and connective tissue grafting techniques available today are based on this information.

Techniques for autologous connective and epithelial-connective tissue harvesting

Since the late 1960s, various epithelial-connective tissue and purely connective tissue harvesting techniques have been proposed for covering gingival recessions or for increasing the mucosal thickness of edentulous alveolar ridges treated with implants.

The techniques basically fall into two categories: those involving superficial harvesting, the epithelial-connective tissue graft,[11–13] and those involving deep harvesting, the subepithelial tissue graft.[14,15]

Both techniques can be used either for root coverage or to increase the amount of adherent gingiva around natural teeth and implants, or to increase the mucosal thickness around an implant.

In the latter case, epithelial-connective tissue grafts must be carefully deepithelialized for submerged use. Both kinds of grafts have their particular advantages and disadvantages, and choosing which graft to use depends on various factors, such as the required thickness of the connective tissue and, above all, the preference of the clinician.

Superficial epithelial-connective tissue graft harvesting from the palate

Superficial epithelial-connective tissue grafts from the palate are richer in connective tissue and have low glandular and adipose components.[16–18] The disadvantage with these grafts is the creation of a superficial wound that is prone to postoperative bleeding and requires healing by secondary intention. For thick grafts, the postoperative period can last up to 15 days and be quite painful. This type of graft is particularly suitable for use in mucogingival periodontal surgery when connective tissue thicknesses must be minimal (< 1 mm).

Surgical technique

1. A partial-thickness flap should be designed in the palate with a no. 15C Bard-Parker blade. The depth of the flap depends on the thickness of tissue that will be harvested **(Fig 3a)**. The ideal harvest area extends distally from the second premolars to the second molars because the submucosa in this area is poor in glandular

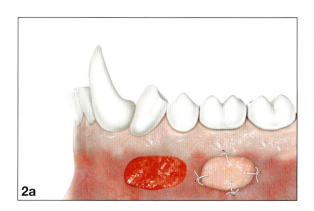
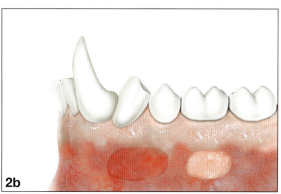

Fig 2 (a) *A piece of connective tissue from the adherent gingiva was grafted into the alveolar mucosa, and as a control, the same amount of connective tissue from the alveolar mucosa was grafted into an adjacent area.* (b) *After healing, the connective tissue derived from the adherent gingiva was covered with keratinized epithelium.*[10]

and adipose tissue. For thicker grafts, it is necessary to pay attention to the palatal artery that emerges from the greater palatine foramen between the first and second molars. The area around the first premolars, canines, and incisors should be avoided whenever possible due to the presence of palatal rugae, salivary glands, and thick layers of adipose tissue in the submucosa.

2. With the same blade, an incision is made parallel to the surface of the palate with a distal to mesial movement at a depth of less than 1 mm for periodontal indications and a significantly greater depth for the augmentation of edentulous ridges **(Figs 3b and 3c)**. The size of the graft should be approximately 20% greater than the final size that is required to compensate for the contraction of the elastic fibers that occurs at the time of harvest and the dimensional reduction that occurs during healing.

3. The excision is completed by lifting the free flap with atraumatic surgical tweezers **(Figs 3d and 3e)**. For submerged indications, the epithelium is removed with a no. 15C Bard-Parker scalpel.

4. Prior to suturing with crossed mattress compressive sutures, a collagen sponge trimmed to the size of the donor site is placed. The collagen is compressed against the wound with sutures **(Fig 3f)**. Finally, it is useful to apply an antiseptic healing gel based on hyaluronic acid (eg, Hobagel Plus, Hobama).

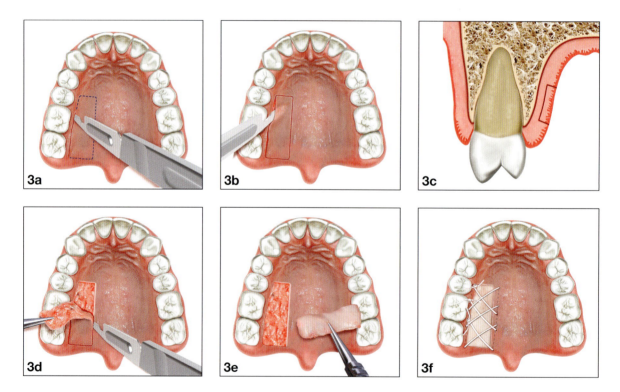

Fig 3 *Technique for harvesting an epithelial-connective tissue graft. (a) A scalpel is used to make an incision of the desired shape and size that is approximately 1 mm deep. (b) With the same blade, an incision is made parallel to the surface of the palate in a distal to mesial movement. (c) Area and depth of the harvest. (d and e) The graft is detached with surgical tweezers. (f) A collagen hemostatic sponge and a cross-mattress sutures are applied.*

Subepithelial connective tissue graft harvesting from the palate

Subepithelial tissue grafts have the advantage of maintaining the integrity of the epithelial surface of the palate, allowing for more effective suturing to prevent postoperative bleeding, making it more suitable for harvesting very thick connective tissue grafts to increase the thickness of edentulous alveolar ridges.

The disadvantage is that these grafts are harvested from the deeper portion of the submucosa, which is rich in salivary glands and adipose tissue that undergo complete resorption during the healing phase. In many cases, the thin mucosa of the palate undergoes partial or total necrosis after suturing due to poor vascularization.

Surgical technique

1. An incision is made parallel to the surface of the palate in a distal to mesial direction with a no. 15C Bard-Parker blade. The incision should be sufficiently extended to compensate for the contraction of the elastic fibers at the time of harvesting and the reduction in graft size that occurs during healing **(Fig 4a)**. The initial incision should be approximately 1 mm thick and then deepened obliquely in a medial direction **(Fig 4b)**.

2. With the superficial portion of the palatal mucosa elevated with surgical tweezers, three incisions are made: one mesial, one distal, and one medial up to the periosteum to draw a rectangular free connective flap **(Fig 4c)**.

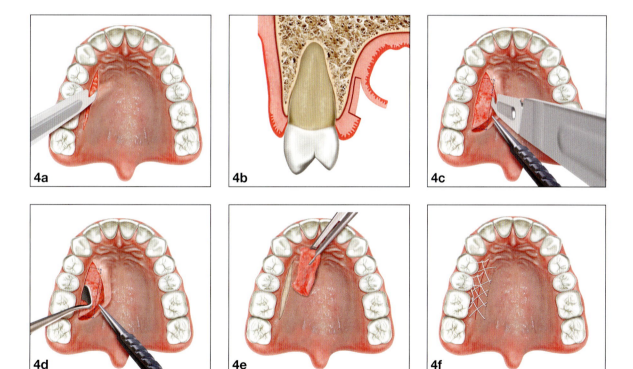

Fig 4 Technique for harvesting a subepithelial graft. (a) *A scalpel is used to make an incision that is approximately 1 mm thick parallel to the surface of the palate in a distal to mesial direction.* (b) *The connective tissue portion of the palate being harvested.* (c) *By elevating the palatal mucosa, the desired shape of the graft is designed.* (d and e) *The connective tissue is removed with a Kramer-Nevins scalpel and surgical tweezers.* (f) *The palatal mucosa is sutured with crossed mattress sutures.*

M. Simion • G. Zucchelli

3. The free connective flap is removed with a back-action chisel or a Kramer-Nevins scalpel **(Figs 4d and 4e)**.
4. The palatal mucosa is sutured with crossed mattress compressive sutures **(Fig 4f)**.

Subepithelial connective tissue graft harvesting from the retromolar tuberosity

The retromolar tuberosity is the harvest site of choice when a graft of considerable thickness but limited extension is required. The retromolar tuberosity site is rarely available because the presence of the third molars reduces the amount of connective tissue that is available. The connective tissue of the tuberosity is generally denser and less vascularized than that of the palate and has a lesser tendency to reduce in volume over time. In many cases, there is a hyperplastic response after healing that can lead to an unesthetic appearance.[20] Use of this technique is therefore limited to increasing the thickness of edentulous alveolar ridges, and it is not recommended in mucogingival therapy.

Surgical technique
1. A V-shaped incision that is approximately 1 mm deep is drawn with a no. 15C Bard-Parker blade distal to the last molar with the vertex

pointing distally. Two incisions are then made parallel to the epithelial surface, one buccal and one palatal **(Fig 5a)**.
2. The periodontal attachment distal to the last tooth is dissected with a Kramer-Nevins scalpel, and a somewhat triangular sample is isolated.
3. The graft is removed with a Kramer-Nevins scalpel and surgical tweezers **(Fig 5b and 5c)**, and the remaining epithelium is removed with the no. 15C blade.
4. The two flaps are sutured with simple or cross-mattress sutures **(Fig 5d)**.

SOFT TISSUE INTERVENTIONS BEFORE IMPLANT PLACEMENT
Epithelial-connective tissue grafts used in extraction sites to correct soft tissue deficits (cases 1 and 2)

After tooth extraction, bone remodeling phenomena occur. After 6 months, this bone remodeling leads to an average loss in bone of 3 to 4 mm horizontally and about 1.2 mm vertically. There is also a serious soft tissue deficit. In addition to performing alveolar ridge preservation by filling the alveolus with particulate biomaterials, it is essential to use epithelial-connective tissue grafts to treat

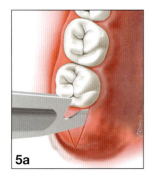 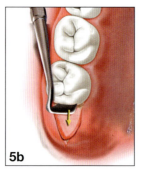 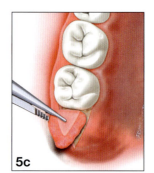 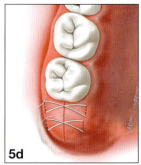

Fig 5 *Connective tissue graft harvesting technique from the retromolar tuberosity.* (a) *After a 1-mm-deep V-shaped incision is made, a connective wedge is designed distal to the last maxillary molar. The wedge is detached from the tooth and the underlying periosteum with a Kramer-Nevins scalpel* (b) *and the aid of surgical tweezers* (c). (d) *The two flaps are then sutured with cross-mattress sutures.*

the soft tissue deficit, especially in esthetic areas. On the one hand, these grafts prevent biomaterial from escaping from the alveolus, and on the other, they restore an adequate amount of keratinized mucosa. Coronal repositioning of the flaps is contraindicated because this deforms the mucogingival line and thus reduces the amount of keratinized mucosa. To overcome this problem, small connective tissue grafts or epithelial-connective tissue grafts harvested from the palate have been proposed for closing the mucosal component of the extraction socket.[16]

Periosteal flaps (case 3)

In cases of major horizontal and vertical bone defects, especially in edentulous spans of limited extent, such as in the area of the maxillary lateral incisors, tension-free suturing of the flaps can be challenging due to insufficient amounts of mucosal tissue. This is particularly true when regeneration must take place beyond the bony peaks of adjacent teeth (see chapter 17).

Flap tension inexorably leads to necrosis of the marginal tissues and premature exposure of the membrane.

To overcome this problem, Triaca et al described the periosteal flap (or periostioplasty) in 2001.[17] With this technique, the buccal flap is lengthened and a simultaneous increase in the thickness of the crestal soft tissue is achieved.

Surgical technique

1. A normal periosteal releasing incision is made with a no. 15C Bard-Parker blade at the base of the flap, extending from the right to the left vertical incision **(Fig 6a)**.
2. Two accessory vertical incisions are made at the edentulous ridge to form a quadrangular periosteal flap **(Fig 6b)**.
3. With the primary flap pulled coronally, a partial-thickness periosteal flap is elevated with two tweezers **(Fig 6c)**.

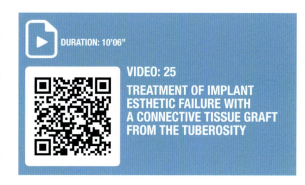

DURATION: 10'06"

VIDEO: 25
TREATMENT OF IMPLANT ESTHETIC FAILURE WITH A CONNECTIVE TISSUE GRAFT FROM THE TUBEROSITY

4. The periosteal flap is sutured under the palatal flap 3 to 4 mm from its margin with horizontal mattress sutures, leaving the knot on the outer aspect of the palate **(Fig 6d)**.
5. The primary buccal flap is sutured over the periosteum to the palatal flap with horizontal mattress and simple sutures **(Fig 6e)**.

INTERVENTIONS DURING THE FIRST STAGE OF IMPLANT SURGERY AND DURING SUBMERGED

Bilaminar connective tissue grafts for immediate implants

Bilaminar grafts are widely used to increase mucosal thickness at the buccal emergence profile in cases of immediate implant placement. Although there is not definitive support of their efficacy in the literature, they are strongly recommended for patients with thin gingival phenotypes and heavily scalloped gingival margins.

Connective tissue grafts to increase soft tissue thickness around submerged implants (cases 4 and 5)

In most cases, interventions to increase soft tissue thickness are aimed at allowing for the development of an adequate mucosal emergence profile. Insufficient peri-implant mucosa thickness can also lead to increased peri-implant bone resorption in posterolateral areas.[7,8]

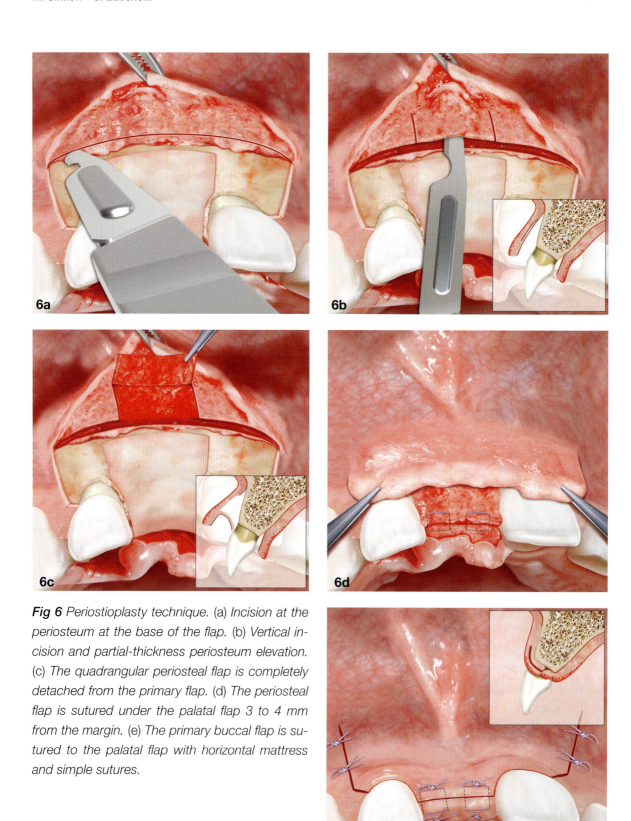

Fig 6 Periostioplasty technique. (a) Incision at the periosteum at the base of the flap. (b) Vertical incision and partial-thickness periosteum elevation. (c) The quadrangular periosteal flap is completely detached from the primary flap. (d) The periosteal flap is sutured under the palatal flap 3 to 4 mm from the margin. (e) The primary buccal flap is sutured to the palatal flap with horizontal mattress and simple sutures.

INTERVENTIONS DURING OR AFTER THE SECOND STAGE OF IMPLANT SURGERY

Second stage of implant surgery and connection of the healing abutments (cases 6–8)

Two-stage implant surgery with a submergence period offers clinicians the advantage of being able to operate on the soft tissues during different phases. The second surgical stage offers the opportunity to manage the quality and quantity of keratinized mucosa. Interventions after the second stage are mostly corrective surgeries following complications occurring after the application of the prosthesis, such as recession of the mucosal margin or deficiencies in the keratinized tissue.

Epithelial-connective tissue grafts during the second stage of implant surgery (case 9)

In both partially and completely edentulous arches, a deficiency of keratinized mucosa is very common. Particularly in the posterolateral sectors, tooth loss and the consequent atrophy almost always lead to a drastic reduction in keratinized mucosa, especially when vertical ridge augmentation procedures with regenerative techniques are required. Coronal repositioning and suturing with flap eversion further reduces the keratinized component of mucosa. The ideal time for the restoration of keratinized mucosa is the second phase of implant surgery for the connection of healing abutments. The graft of choice is the epithelial-connective tissue graft.

Connective or epithelial-connective tissue grafts after the second stage of implant surgery

Soft tissue interventions after the connection of healing abutments or the placement of a restoration are generally aimed at resolving esthetic or inflammatory complications. A deficiency in keratinized mucosa predisposes patients to peri-implantitis and recession of the mucosal margins.[5,6]

Treatment of peri-implant soft tissue dehiscence (case 10)

Recession of the buccal mucosal margin is referred to as peri-implant soft tissue dehiscence. Whereas with natural dentition the definition of gingival recession is universally understood as the apical displacement of the gingival margin relative to the cementoenamel junction (CEJ), there is no consensus on the definition of peri-implant soft tissue dehiscence (due to the lack of a fixed reference point).

Some authors use the mucosal margin at the time of the final restoration as a reference.

Others consider it to be the exposure of the metal surface of the implant or prosthetic abutment. These definitions, however, are not entirely appropriate because they do not take into account the gingival margin of the natural homologous tooth.

A prosthetic crown that is longer than the homologous tooth is often the first reason for patient dissatisfaction with esthetics.

For this reason, we define peri-implant soft tissue dehiscence as any apical migration of the peri-implant mucosal margin in relation to its esthetically ideal position, which is represented by the gingival margin of the natural contralateral tooth **(Fig 7)**. In some cases, the homologous tooth is also restored, or its gingival margin may not be in the correct position either due to gingival recession or altered passive eruption.

In these cases, it is important to define the esthetically ideal position of the homologous tooth before proceeding to treat the peri-implant soft tissue dehiscence.

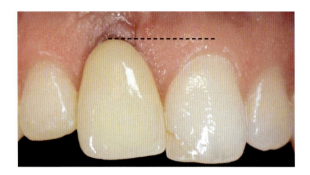

Fig 7 *Comparison of the peri-implant mucosal margin and the gingival margin of the homologous tooth.*

The onset of peri-implant soft tissue dehiscence depends on the thickness of the soft tissue at the level of the transmucosal pathway. Eventual exposure of the implant surface that should be osseointegrated is the clinical manifestation of soft tissue dehiscence progression, and it can occur only in the absence of an intact buccal bone wall. It is not fully understood why implants develops soft tissue dehiscence on the buccal aspect. There are anatomical/predisposing factors (eg, a buccal implant position, buccal bone dehiscence, inadequate keratinized soft tissue, thin gingival phenotype, muscle insertions, coronal frenum pull) and pathologic/precipitating factors (eg, plaque-induced inflammation, trauma induced by improper brushing or flossing) that contribute to the apical migration of the soft tissue margin.

The objective of treating peri-implant soft tissue dehiscence around osseointegrated implants is to achieve complete dehiscence coverage, with the reference point being the gingival margin of the healthy natural homologous tooth **(Fig 8)**. Achieving complete dehiscence coverage will restore soft tissue harmony and significantly improve the esthetics of an implant-supported prosthesis. To facilitate complete dehiscence coverage and to prevent the implant color from showing through the mucosal tissue, the soft tissue thickness must be increased, transforming a medium/thin phenotype into a thick one.

This is especially important in the most coronal millimeters (ie, the transmucosal pathway) **(Fig 9)**, where the soft tissues are not supported by underlying bone. The aim of the treatment is to modify the patient's site-specific gingival phenotype to achieve a marginal soft tissue thickness of at least 2 mm that is vertically maintained for 3 to 4 mm.

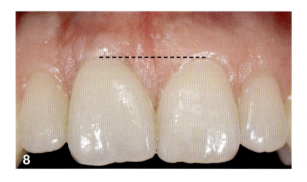

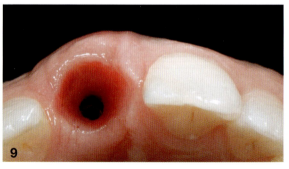

Fig 8 *Complete coverage of the dehiscence with alignment of the gingival contours.* Fig 9 *Transmucosal pathway with surgically increased thickness.*

CLINICAL CASE 1

Epithelial-connective tissue graft to close the mucosal defect in an extraction site

A 26-year-old, nonsmoking, healthy patient presented with internal root resorption of the maxillary right central incisor caused by trauma experienced some years earlier. The tooth had a pinkish appearance around the collar and showed signs of internal hemorrhage (**Fig 10**).

After extraction, the alveolus was curetted to remove all the granulation tissue (**Figs 11 and 12**), and both the palatal and buccal mucosa were elevated 3 to 4 mm to reveal two internal pouches. The alveolus was then filled with deproteinized bovine bone (DBBM) (Bio-Oss, Geistlich Biomaterials) up to the level of the bone margin (**Fig 13**).

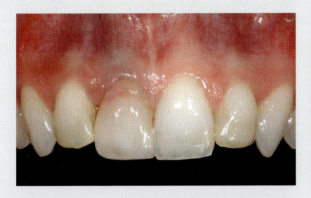

Fig 10 The right maxillary central incisor severely compromised by trauma. The pink pigmentation at the cervical area is evident.

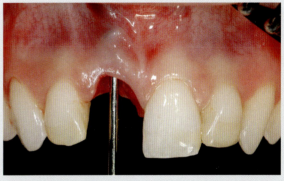

Fig 11 The tooth was extracted, and the socket was curetted with an alveolar spoon to remove all the granulation tissue.

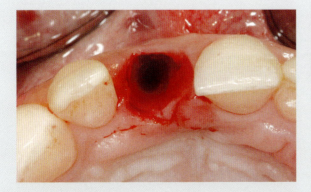

Fig 12 Occlusal view of the extraction site.

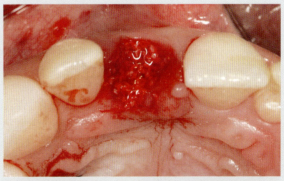

Fig 13 The alveolus was filled with DBBM up to the bony margin, and the buccal and palatal mucosa were tunneled to obtain two pouches.

An oval-shaped epithelial-connective tissue graft was harvested from the palate and deepithelialized in the peripheral portion, leaving a central epithelial island that was the shape and size of the mucosal defect (**Fig 14**).

The deepithelialized portions were inserted into the palatal and buccal areas of the socket, leaving only the central portion with the epithelium exposed (**Figs 15 and 16**). The graft was held in place without sutures by a resin-bonded provisional bridge with slight compression.

After 6 months of healing (**Fig 17**), an implant was inserted via a flapless technique with a surgical guide obtained with digital software and CBCT (**Fig 18**), and a prefabricated provisional was placed (**Fig 19**). After another 6 months of tissue maturation, the final ceramic crown was placed (**Figs 20 and 21**).

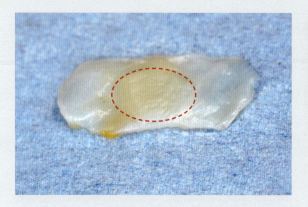

Fig 14 An oval-shaped epithelial-connective tissue graft was harvested from the palate and deepithelialized in the peripheral portion, with an island of epithelium left in the center (dotted oval) at the area that will remain exposed.

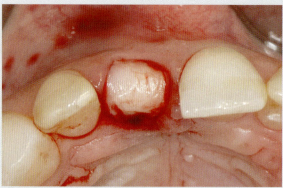

Fig 15 The graft was placed to close the socket by inserting the deepithelialized margins within the buccal and palatal pouches.

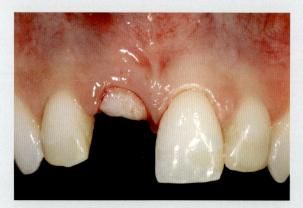

Fig 16 Buccal view of the graft placement.

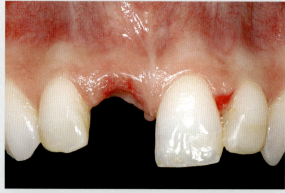

Fig 17 Healing of the alveolus after 6 months. The mucosal volume and maturation are ideal.

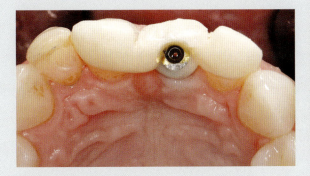

Fig 18 On the basis of CBCT, A surgical guide was fabricated for implant placement according to a flapless technique.

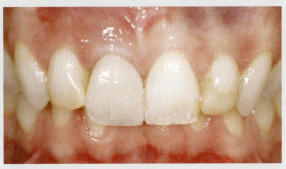

Fig 19 The provisional was kept in place for 6 months to await development of an adequate emergence profile and tissue maturation.

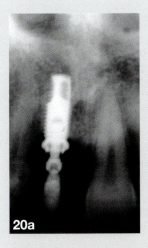
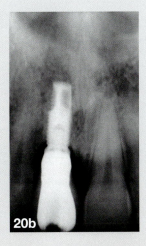

Fig 20 *(a)* Radiograph of the provisional at 6 months. *(b)* Radiograph at 1 year.

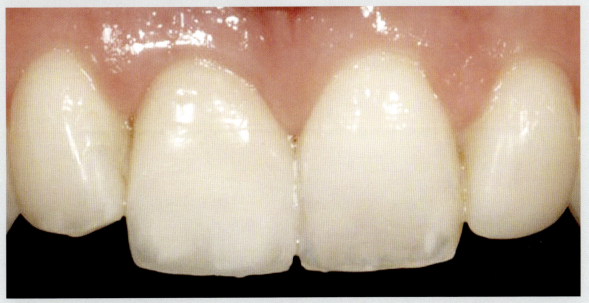

Fig 21 Final ceramic prosthesis.

CLINICAL CASE 2

Epithelial-connective tissue graft to correct severe soft tissue deficiency in preparation for GBR

A 23-year-old patient presented with an incongruous implant in the site of the maxillary right canine. Subsequent infection had resulted in the complete loss of periodontal attachment on the distal surface of the adjacent lateral incisor **(Fig 22)**. Extraction of the canine and lateral incisor resulted in a large bone defect associated with a severe soft tissue deficit **(Fig 23)**. The treatment plan involved an initial operation to restore the integrity of the mucosa and then subsequent GBR.

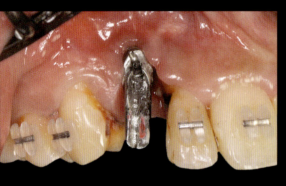

Fig 22 Unsatisfactory implant in the site of the maxillary right canine affecting the periodontium of the right lateral incisor.

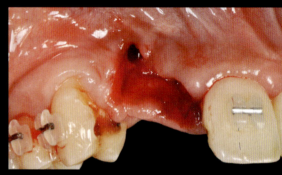

Fig 23 The canine and lateral incisor were extracted, resulting in a severe bone and soft tissue defect.

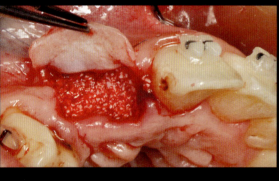

Fig 24 The bone defect was filled with DBBM, and a large epithelial-connective tissue graft with deepithelialized margins was inserted buccally and palatally under the mucosa.

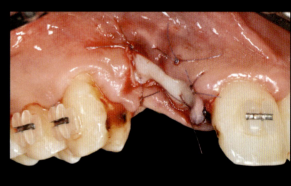

Fig 25 The graft was sutured with simple 6-0 Prolene sutures (Ethicon).

At the time of extraction, the bone defect was filled with DBBM to form a support base for an epithelial-connective tissue graft harvested from the palate (**Fig 24**). A large graft was harvested and deepithelialized for 3 mm near the margins, leaving an epithelial island similar in shape to the mucosal defect. The deepithelialized margins were then sutured with 6-0 sutures under the margins of the defect (**Fig 25**).

After 4 months of healing (**Figs 26 and 27**), the site was ready for GBR of the vertical and horizontal bone defects (**Figs 28 and 29**). The membrane and bone graft remained submerged for 8 months, and then two implants were placed in the sites of the maxillary right canine and lateral incisor (**Figs 30 to 35**). After another 4 months of healing (**Fig 37**), the healing abutments were connected (**Fig 38**), and the patient was able to return to her dentist for fabrication of the prosthesis.

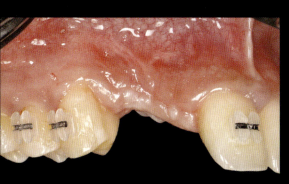
Fig 26 Healing after 4 months. The mucosal defect has been corrected.

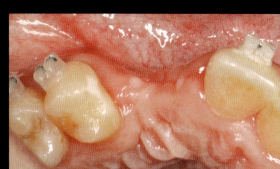
Fig 27 Occlusal view of the corrected defect.

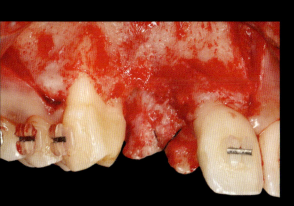
Fig 28 A full-thickness flap was elevated to reveal the vertical and horizontal bone defects.

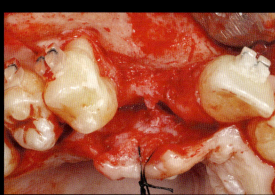
Fig 29 Occlusal view. The severe horizontal bone defect is evident.

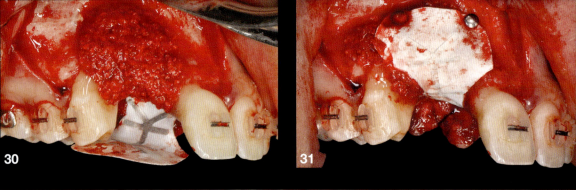

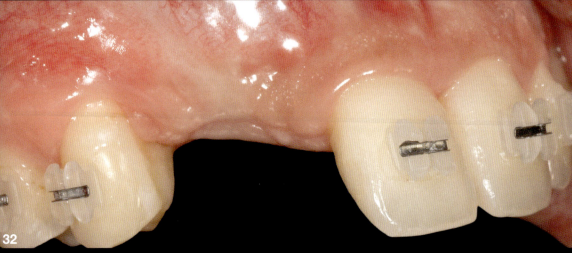

Fig 30 A titanium-reinforced expanded polytetrafluorethylene (ePTFE) membrane was secured palatally, and an autologous and heterologous particulate graft was placed over the defect. **Fig 31** The membrane was secured buccally with two pins. **Fig 32** Healing after 7 months. The volume of hard and soft tissue has been restored. **Fig 33** At the time of its removal, the membrane appeared to be perfectly integrated with the underlying regenerated tissue.

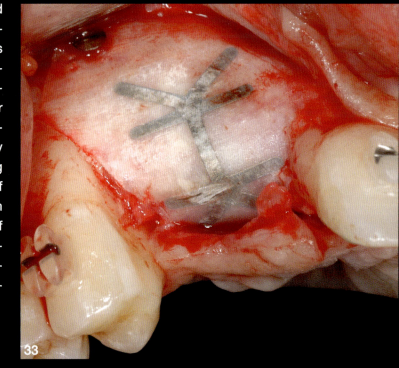

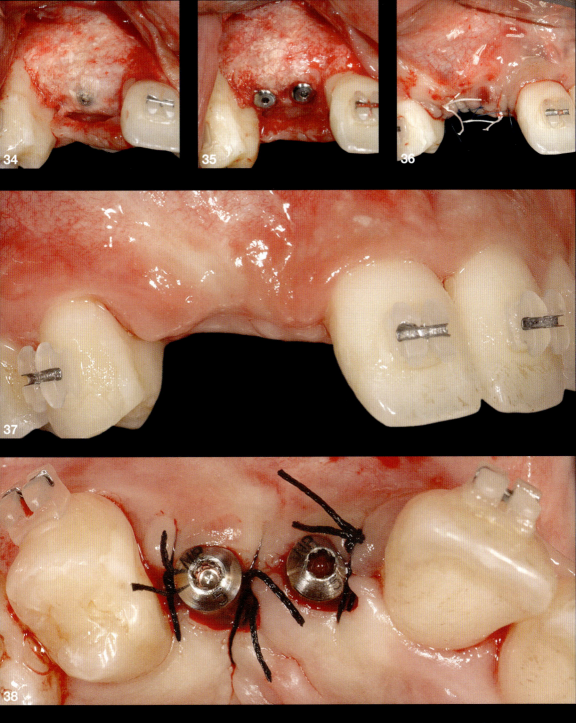

Fig 34 After membrane removal, dense, mature bone was revealed. **Fig 35** Two hybrid implants were inserted in the sites of the maxillary right canine and lateral incisor. **Fig 36** The flaps were sutured with horizontal mattress and simple sutures. **Fig 37** Healing after 4 months. **Fig 38** The implants have been connected to the healing abutments, and the patient can return to her dentist for fabrication of the prosthesis.

CLINICAL CASE 3

Treatment of agenesis of the right lateral incisor with GBR and a periosteal flap

A 31-year-old woman in good health required implant treatment for the loss of her deciduous maxillary right lateral incisor, which was suffering from severe root resorption. The adjacent central incisor and canine were mesially and distally inclined, respectively, reducing the interradicular space. In both teeth, there was a modest loss of attachment and gingival recession facing the edentulous area, with loss of the interproximal papillae **(Fig 39)**. A lateral view showed a buccal bone volume deficit **(Fig 40)**. It was decided to intervene with horizontal and vertical ridge augmentation beyond the bony peaks. The flap was performed according to protocol, with two vertical golf club–shaped incisions mesial to the central incisor and distal to the canine associated with intrasulcular incisions and a slightly buccal crestal incision. A full-thickness flap was elevated, revealing loss of the interproximal bone peaks and a residual bone defect after extraction of the deciduous tooth **(Figs 41 and 42)**. An expanded polytetrafluorethylene (ePTFE) membrane was placed palatally and then secured buccally

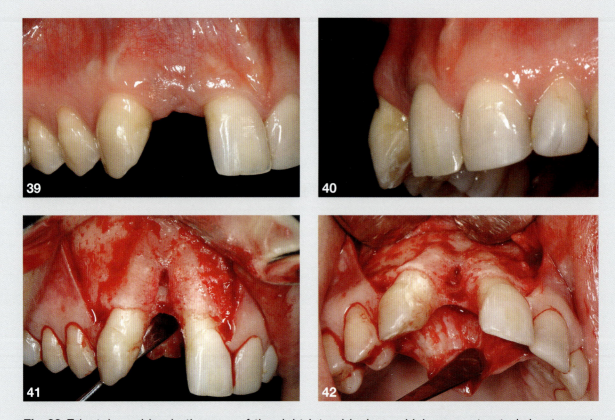

Fig 39 Edentulous ridge in the area of the right lateral incisor, which was extracted due to posttraumatic root resorption. The adjacent canine and central incisor are inclined distally and mesially, respectively, and show a modest loss of attachment and flattening of the papillae. **Fig 40** Lateral view showing the horizontal deficit in bone volume. **Fig 41** After flap detachment, the vertical bone defect and the loss of the interproximal bone peaks are evident. **Fig 42** Occlusal view showing the horizontal bone defect.

to protect a particulate graft of 80% autologous bone and 20% DBBM (**Figs 43 and 44**). To facilitate tension-free flap closure and to increase the crestal soft tissue thickness, a periosteal flap was performed. After the traditional incision of the periosteum at the base of the flap, from the mesial to the distal vertical incision, two half-thickness vertical incisions were made in the periosteum at the edentulous ridge. With the aid of tweezers and a no. 15C Bard-Parker blade, the periosteum was dissected at partial thickness from apical to crestal for approximately 7 to 8 mm (**Fig 45**) and was sutured with mattress sutures below the palatal flap (**Fig 46**). The primary flap was then sutured to the palatal flap with horizontal ePTFE mattress sutures and simple 6-0 Prolene sutures (Ethicon) (**Fig 47**). In this way, closure took place over two layers of tissue, increasing the thickness of the soft tissue and allowing for flap closure without tension. The patient underwent orthodontic therapy (**Fig 48**), and after 8 months, the membrane was removed to place a 3.3-mm-diameter hybrid implant (**Figs 49 and 50**). The provisional crown was maintained for a period of 6 months, during which orthodontic therapy was completed. The patient was then provided with a definitive crown in the site of the maxillary right lateral incisor and ceramic veneers on the central incisor and the left lateral incisor (**Figs 51 and 52**).

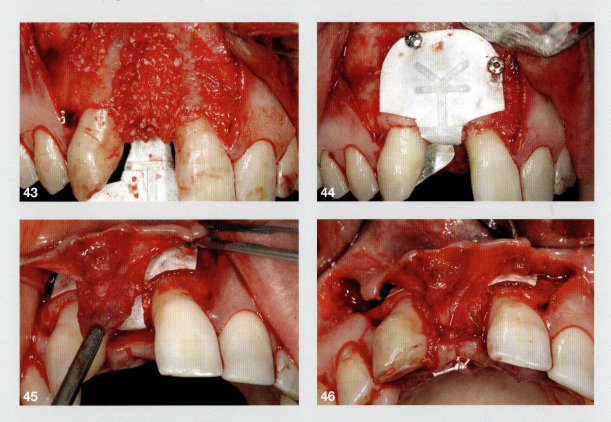

Fig 43 A titanium-reinforced ePTFE membrane was trimmed and secured palatally, and an autologous particulate bone graft mixed with DBBM was placed over the defect. **Fig 44** The membrane was secured buccally. **Fig 45** After the periosteal releasing incision was made, a pedicled periosteal flap was reflected at the defect site to facilitate flap closure without tension and to increase soft tissue thickness simultaneously. **Fig 46** The periosteal flap was sutured under the palatal flap with a horizontal mattress suture.

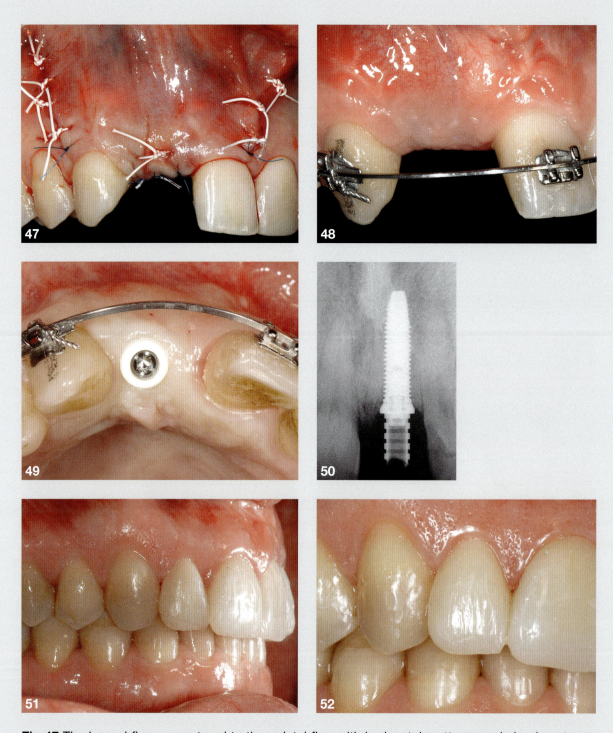

Fig 47 The buccal flap was sutured to the palatal flap with horizontal mattress and simple sutures. **Fig 48** After 7 months of healing, the bone deficit appeared to be corrected. **Fig 49** Occlusal image at the time of uncovering the hybrid implant placed upon removal of the membrane. **Fig 50** Periapical radiograph of the implant with the provisional in place. **Fig 51** Provisional prosthesis for the right lateral incisor and veneers on both the central incisors and the left lateral incisor after 6 months. **Fig 52** Final ceramic crown on the maxillary right lateral incisor.

CLINICAL CASE 4

Connective tissue graft placement at the time of implant placement

A 59-year-old hypertensive patient who smoked required implant rehabilitation to replace a maxillary left central incisor lost due to periodontal reasons. After causal periodontal therapy with full-mouth disinfection, the site showed modest horizontal and vertical bone deficits. The adjacent elements showed atrophic interproximal papillae **(Figs 53 and 54)**, but the patient did not have high esthetic demands. It was decided to treat the horizontal bone deficit with a DBBM graft and resorbable membrane and the vertical bone deficit with a connective tissue graft.

At the time of implant placement **(Fig 55)**, the buccal bone plate thickness was increased with particulate DBBM (Bio-Oss) **(Fig 56)** and a collagen membrane. In the same operation, a subepithelial connective tissue graft was harvested from the palate and placed in an L shape on the crest and buccally.

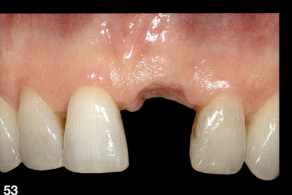
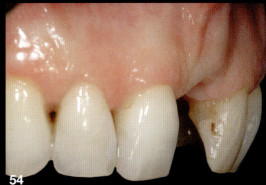
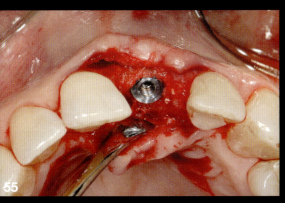
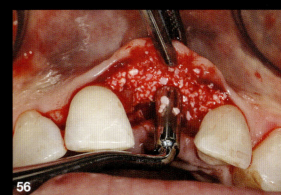

Fig 53 Alveolar ridge of a periodontal patient with an edentulous area in the site of the maxillary left central incisor. After full-mouth disinfection, the interproximal papillae of the adjacent teeth appear slightly atrophic. **Fig 54** Lateral view showing the slight vertical and horizontal bone deficiency. **Fig 55** An implant was placed without creating dehiscence, but with insufficient residual buccal bone thickness (< 2 mm). **Fig 56** Bone thickness was increased with a DBBM graft and a resorbable collagen membrane.

The graft was secured to the palate with a horizontal mattress suture **(Figs 57 and 58)**. The buccal flap was then released with a periosteal incision to achieve tension-free flap closure and was sutured to the palatal flap with a horizontal mattress suture and simple interrupted sutures **(Figs 19-59)**. After 4 months of healing, a mucosal soft tissue punch was performed, and a provisional was provided. After 6 months, the ceramic definitive restoration was placed **(Figs 19-60)**.

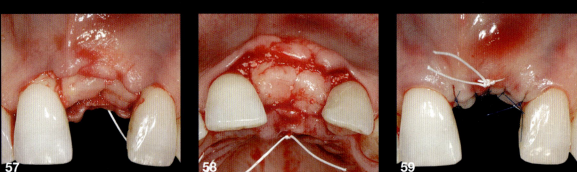

Fig 57 A connective tissue graft was harvested from the palate, placed in an L shape crestally and buccally and secured to the palatal flap with a mattress suture. **Fig 58** Occlusal view of the connective tissue graft. **Fig 59** The buccal flap was released with a periosteal incision and sutured with mattress and simple sutures

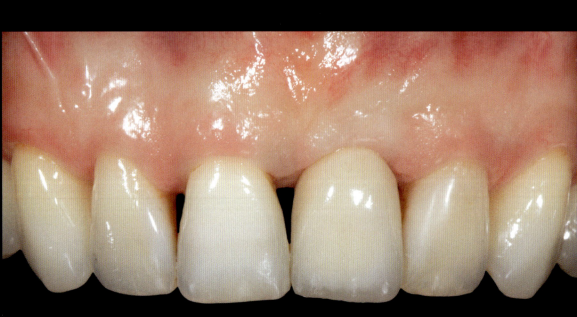

Fig 60 Final ceramic crown.

CLINICAL CASE 5

Connective tissue graft placed between the first and second surgical stages

A 46-year-old, nonsmoking patient presented with a complex clinical situation. Following a serious car accident involving the traumatic avulsion of the maxillary left central and lateral incisors and canine and loss of the buccal bone plate, the mucosa was left with deep palatal fissures and buccal scars **(Fig 61)**. Due to the poor condition of the mucosa, predisposing it to wound dehiscence, and the preeminent horizontal component of the defect, soft tissue regeneration with resorbable membranes was opted for.

Full-thickness buccal and palatal flaps were elevated with vertical incisions one tooth beyond the defect, both mesially and distally, one buccal crestal incision and two intrasulcular incisions. The buccal bone plate was perforated with a round bur to expose the trabecular bone, and a collagen membrane was secured palatally with four pins **(Fig 62)**. A particulate graft of 70% autologous bone and 30% DBBM (Bio-Oss) was placed over the defect, and the membrane was closed buccally with some tension **(Fig 64)**. The buccal flap was released and sutured to the palatal flap with mattress and simple sutures **(Fig 65)**.

After 8 months of healing, two hybrid implants were placed, and the regenerative procedure was repeated **(Figs 66 to 70)**. Prior to the second stage of implant surgery, after 4 months, the vertical bone volume deficiency was compensated for with a large connective tissue graft harvested from the palate **(Fig 71)**. A partial-thickness flap was prepared and elevated both palatally and buccally **(Fig 72)**, and an epithelial-connective tissue graft was harvested from the palate. The graft was completely deepithelialized and inserted in an L shape over the crest and buccally **(Fig 73)**. Because the flap was partial-thickness, a periosteal releasing incision was not necessary.

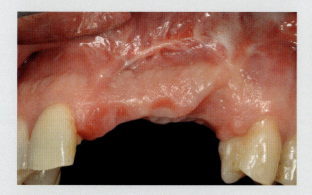

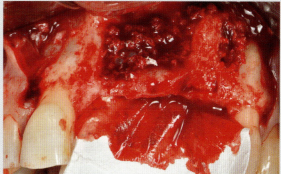

Fig 61 Posttraumatic alveolar ridge that is edentulous from the maxillary left central incisor to the left canine due to a car accident. Scarring is evident in the mucosa from both the trauma and the subsequent fracture reduction and stabilization surgery.

Fig 62 The horizontal component of the defect was corrected using a GBR technique with a resorbable collagen membrane. The buccal bone plate was extensively perforated.

The flaps were sutured with Laurell-Gottlow sutures and simple Prolene sutures (**Fig 74**), and a hyaluronic acid healing gel (Hobagel Plus) was applied (**Fig 75**). To avoid exerting any compression during the healing period, the provisional was not loaded (**Fig 76**). After the connection of the prosthetic abutments, the implant-supported provisional was maintained for another 6 months (**Fig 77**) before placement of the final ceramic prosthesis (**Figs 78 and 79**).

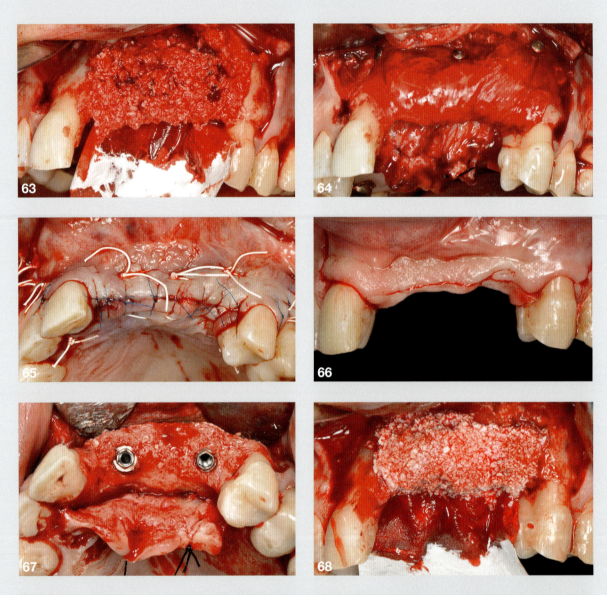

Fig 63 An autologous and heterologous particulate graft was placed in excess on the defect. **Fig 64** The membrane was adapted buccally and secured with three pins. **Fig 65** The periosteum at the base of the flap was incised, and the flaps were sutured with horizontal mattress and simple interrupted sutures. **Fig 66** After 7 months of healing, a new flap was elevated. **Fig 67** Two hybrid implants were placed in the sites of the maxillary left central incisor and canine. The bone ridge thickness appears adequate. **Fig 68** A second GBR technique was performed with a DBBM graft and a resorbable membrane.

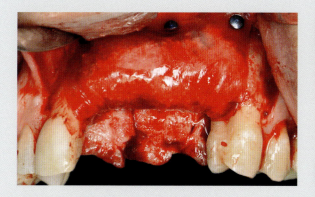

Fig 69 The membrane was secured with four titanium pins.

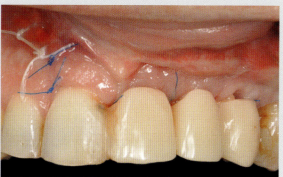

Fig 70 Healing occurred after 15 days without complications.

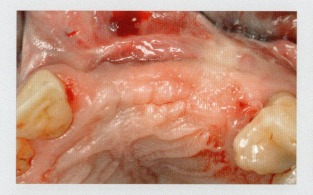

Fig 71 After 4 months, a connective tissue graft harvested from the palate was placed.

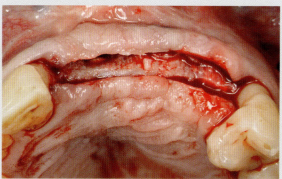

Fig 72 Split-thickness elevation of both the buccal and palatal flaps.

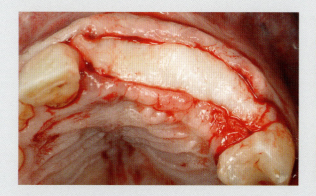

Fig 73 Epithelial-connective tissue graft harvested from the palate, completely deepithelialized, and inserted in an L shape over the crest and buccally.

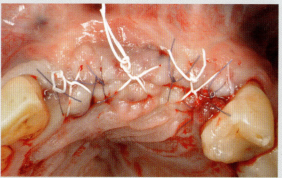

Fig 74 The flaps were sutured with Laurel-Gottlow and simple sutures.

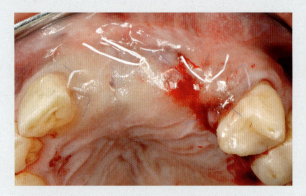

Fig 75 After suturing, a hyaluronic acid-based healing gel (Hobagel Plus) was applied.

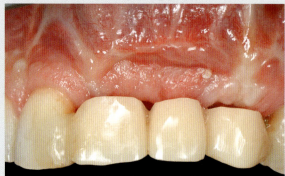

Fig 76 Healing after 1 month showed good vertical dimension of the hard and soft tissues.

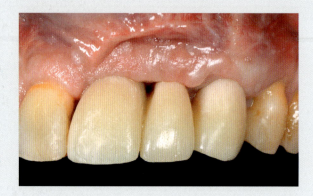

Fig 77 The implant-supported provisional was maintained for 6 months.

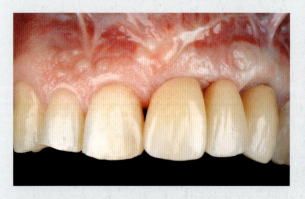

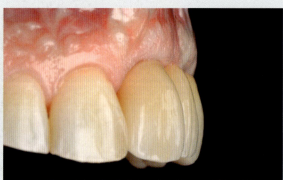

Figs 78, 79 Final ceramic prosthesis.

CLINICAL CASE 6

Placing a healing abutment with a mucosal punch during the second surgical stage

In this case, a single implant in the site of a maxillary first molar was uncovered. The keratinized mucosa of the edentulous ridge was abundant **(Fig 80)**, so it was possible to sacrifice some of it during uncovering. A free-hand no. 15C Bard-Parker blade or a soft tissue punch calibrated to the diameter of the implant platform can be used to uncover an implant **(Fig 81)**. The exact location of the hexagonal key of the implant cover screw can be found by perforating the mucosa with a periodontal probe so that it can be used as a reference point to center the soft tissue punch. The soft tissue punch is then pushed apically with rotary movements up to the bone crest. The mucosal cylinder is removed with a curette, the cover screw is removed, and the healing abutment is screwed into place **(Fig 82)**. No sutures are necessary, and the impression can generally be taken directly. In posterolateral areas, after 2 to 3 months of adaptation to the provisional, a definitive crown can be placed **(Fig 83)**.

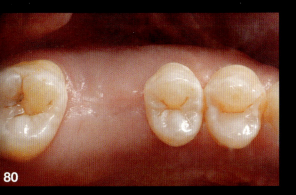
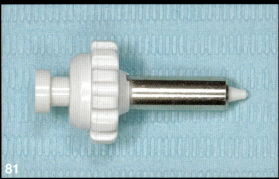
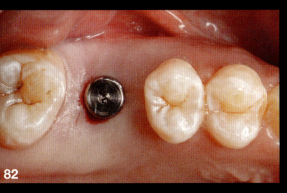
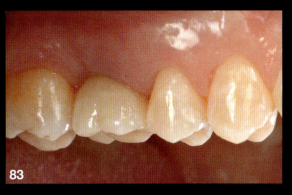

Fig 80 Wide ridge with abundant keratinized mucosa that is edentulous in the site of a maxillary first molar. **Fig 81** Manual circular soft tissue punch calibrated for the 5-mm-diameter implant. **Fig 82** The mucosal punch was performed, the cover screw was removed, and the healing abutment was screwed in place. **Fig 83** Final ceramic crown.

CLINICAL CASE 7

Second surgical stage to uncover multiple implants with an access flap

When reopening for multiple implants in the presence of abundant keratinized mucosa (**Fig 84**), the use of a soft tissue punch is not recommended due to the difficulty of finding the precise position of the implants, so it is advisable to make an access flap. Once the implants have been radiographically located, a slightly palatal incision is made, and only the buccal portion of the flap is partially detached. If the cover screws remain partially covered by the palatal flap or connective tissue, a gingivectomy at the not fully exposed portion can be performed. The cover screws are unscrewed, and the healing abutments are placed. The flap is generally closed with Laurell-Gottlow and simple sutures (**Fig 85**). Before an impression can be taken, it is necessary to wait for a minimum of 15 days for healing to take place because healing of the interproximal spaces occurs by secondary intention. Final crowns (**Fig 86**) can be placed after 3 months of tissue conditioning with a provisional.

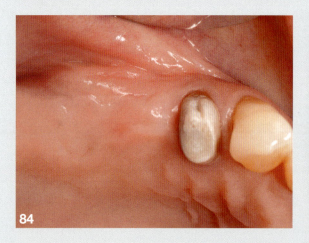

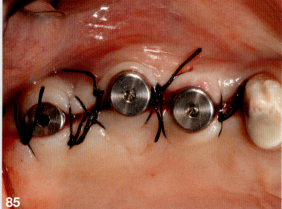

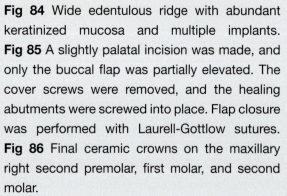

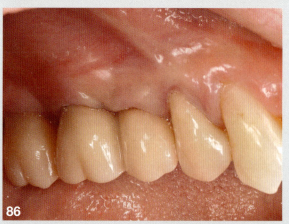

Fig 84 Wide edentulous ridge with abundant keratinized mucosa and multiple implants.
Fig 85 A slightly palatal incision was made, and only the buccal flap was partially elevated. The cover screws were removed, and the healing abutments were screwed into place. Flap closure was performed with Laurell-Gottlow sutures.
Fig 86 Final ceramic crowns on the maxillary right second premolar, first molar, and second molar.

CLINICAL CASE 8

Second surgical stage with a buccally and apically repositioned flap

In many cases of rehabilitation of completely edentulous maxillary ridges, the position of the implants is buccal to the boundary between the keratinized mucosa and the nonkeratinized alveolar mucosa (ie, the mucogingival junction). Using a soft tissue punch or an access flap at the cover screws would result in a total loss of keratinized mucosa buccal to the implants. In these cases, therefore, it is necessary to perform a partial-thickness flap with palatal access and then reposition it buccally and apically **(Fig 87)**.

Because the circumferential arc of the initial incision in the palate is narrower in diameter than that which the flap will assume once repositioned buccally, it is necessary to extend it at least 10 to 12 mm bilaterally beyond the most distal implants **(Fig 88)** to avoid being left with a flap that is too short at the time of suturing. It is also necessary to make distal vertical incisions at an inverted angle (ie, inclined with the apical part in a mesial direction) to allow for apical repositioning without tension.

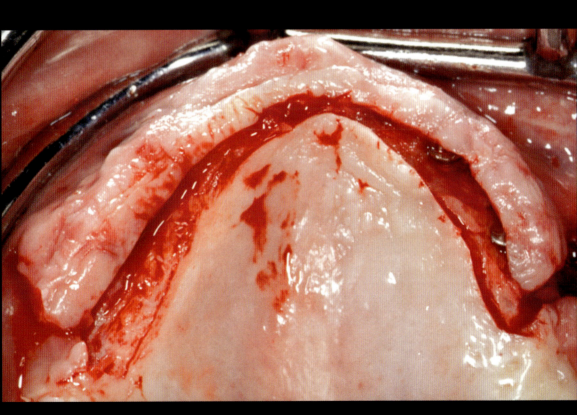

Fig 87 Completely edentulous patient with scarce buccal keratinized mucosa. A partial-thickness flap was performed with palatal access. The vertical releasing incisions are 12 mm more distal than the distal implants with a coronal to mesial inclination.

Excess connective tissue at the implants is removed with a soft tissue punch, and the cover screws are replaced with healing abutments. Suturing is performed with Laurell-Gottlow sutures anchored to the buccal periosteum to prevent coronal sliding of the flap **(Fig 89)**. Palatal healing will take place by secondary intention, so a minimum of 3 weeks must elapse before an impression is taken. The definitive prosthesis **(Fig 90)** is normally fitted after 3 months of using the provisional.

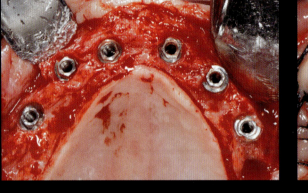

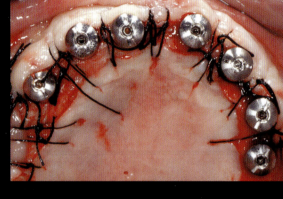

Fig 88 The connective tissue above the implants was removed with a soft tissue punch, and the cover screws were removed.

Fig 89 Healing abutments were screwed into place, and the buccal flap was secured with mattress sutures.

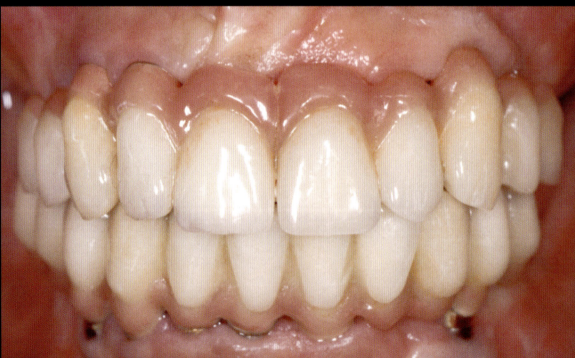

Fig 90 Full-arch implant-supported definitive ceramic prosthesis.

CLINICAL CASE 9

Epithelial-connective tissue graft surgery during the second surgical stage

A 43-year-old patient in good health with bilateral edentulism in the posterolateral sectors of the mandible was treated with vertical ridge elevation in the mandibular right sector. After 7 months, implants were placed in the sites of the mandibular left first and second premolars and first molar and the mandibular right second premolar and first molar. After another 3 months, the implants were uncovered, and the healing abutments were connected.

On both the right and left sides, the mucosa showed less than 1 mm of keratinized mucosa (**Figs 91 and 97**).

The initial incisions for the preparation of the recipient site were made along the buccal mucogingival lines, leaving all residual keratinized mucosa on the lingual aspect.

The buccal flaps were elevated partial thickness with a no. 15C Bard-Parker blade, leaving only the periosteum to cover the bone to obtain adherent mucosa (**Fig 92**). The residual keratinized component of the mucosa was moved lingually to allow for the removal of the implant cover screws and the placement of the healing abutments (**Figs 93 and 98**).

Epithelial-connective tissue grafts were harvested from the palate and shaped to fit the recipient sites, and semilunar incisions were made at the implants (**Figs 94 and 99**).

The grafts were sutured to the recipient sites with suspended sling sutures anchored to the buccal periosteum and with simple 6-0 Vicryl sutures (Ethicon) (**Figs 95 and 100**). Healing occurred within 15 days, with complete tissue maturation after 1 month (**Figs 96 and 101**).

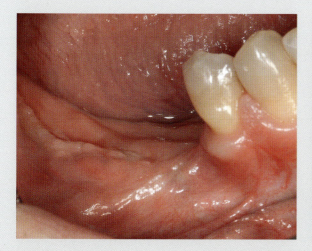

Fig 91 Edentulous span of the mandible after vertical ridge elevation. The keratinized mucosa is almost absent.

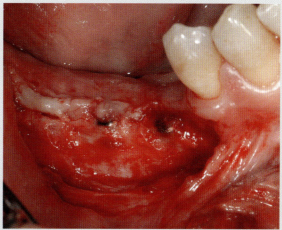

Fig 92 The recipient site was prepared with a partial-thickness incision from the buccal mucogingival line, leaving only the periosteum.

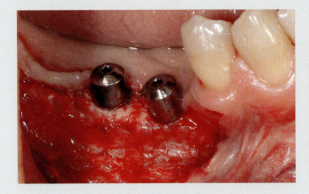

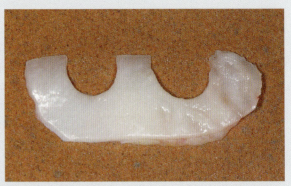

Fig 93 The residual keratinized mucosa was moved lingually, and the healing abutments were screwed into place. The buccal flap margin was regularized with Goldman-Fox scissors.

Fig 94 A 1-mm-thick epithelial-connective tissue graft was harvested from the palate, and two semilunar incisions were made at the implants.

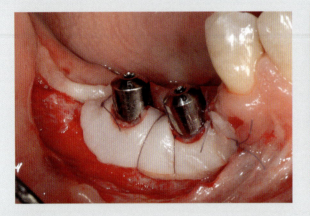

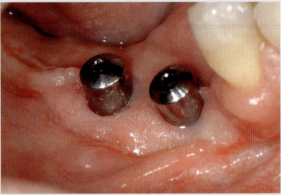

Fig 95 The graft was sutured with simple sutures to the lingual mucosa and with mattress sutures anchored to the buccal periosteum.

Fig 96 Healing after 1 month. The wide band of adherent keratinized mucosa is visible.

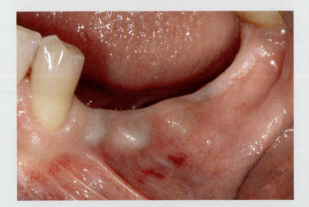

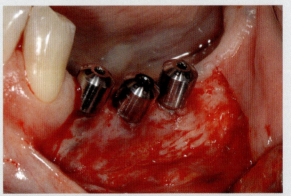

Fig 97 Contralateral side of the same patient. Extremely thin alveolar mucosa and a minimal amount of keratinized mucosa.

Fig 98 The recipient site was prepared, and the healing abutments were screwed into place.

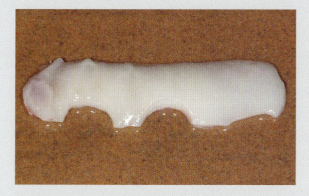

Fig 99 Epithelial-connective tissue graft harvest with semilunar incisions.

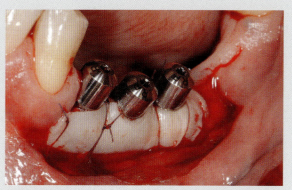

Fig 100 Graft secured with mattress and simple sutures.

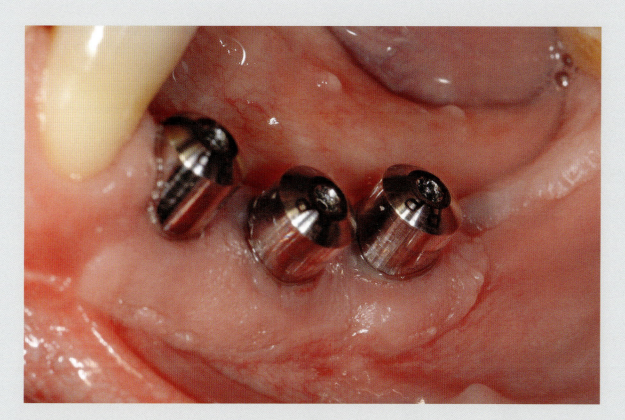

Fig 101 Healing after 1 month.

CLINICAL CASE 10

Treatment of peri-implant soft tissue dehiscence

This case involved peri-implant soft tissue dehiscence in the site of the maxillary left lateral incisor, which resulted in patient dissatisfaction with esthetics. The contralateral tooth was a conoid covered with a crown, with the altered passive eruption from which it was suffering undiagnosed and untreated. The patient's very high smile line made the esthetic resolution of the case very complex. The patient was offered maxillofacial surgical treatment to correct her gummy smile, but she rejected the idea, reporting that gingival exposure while smiling had never been a problem for her. What troubled her was the elongation of the prosthetic crown in the site of the maxillary left lateral incisor and the appearance of a dark area apical to the implant crown. It was difficult to convince the patient that the tooth in the position of the maxillary right lateral incisor was abnormally short because it suffered from altered passive eruption **(Fig 102)**. Determining the ideal position of the gingival margin of the right lateral incisor (0.5 to 1 mm coronal to the gingival margin of the central incisors) made it possible to determine the coverage that should occur of the peri-implant soft tissue dehiscence in the site of the left lateral incisor **(Fig 103)**. The presence of an overcontoured and buccally displaced implant crown and the presence of very thin papillae with a small apicocoronal dimension contraindicated the performance of any mucogingival coverage surgery directly on the implant crown and indicated a prosthetic-surgical approach. The combined approach involves a presurgical prosthetic phase aimed at quantitatively and qualitatively improving the buccal and interproximal soft tissue to

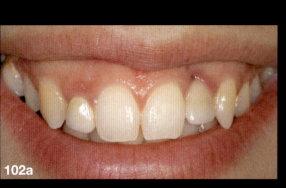
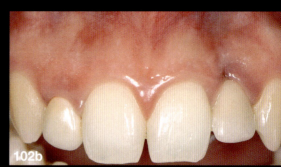
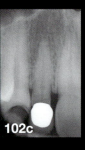
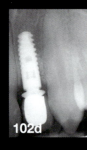
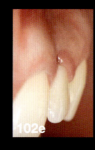
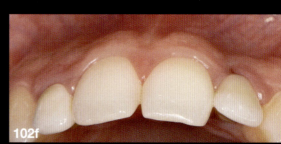

Fig 102 *(a to f)* The patient presented with uneven gingival margins between the implant crown in the position of the maxillary left lateral incisor, which was affected by soft tissue dehiscence, and the crown of the right lateral incisor, which was affected by altered passive eruption.

facilitate mucogingival coverage. This prosthetic phase consists of removing the buccally displaced crown, replacing the implant abutment with an abutment that is as narrow and thin as possible, and applying a short provisional crown that does not come into contact with the buccal and interproximal soft tissues (**Fig 104**). The duration of this phase varies from case to case but never lasts less than 2 months. The connective tissue graft (white areas in **Fig 19-105**) is placed approximately 1 mm coronal to the ideal position of the gingival margin of the implant crown. In this case, 2 months after removal of the crown and change of the abutment, large and deep papillae (red areas in **Fig 105**) remained despite the coronal position of the graft, which can be deepithelialized on the occlusal surface toward the palatal side. The absence of the crown allows for the formation of a soft tissue isthmus, which makes it possible to provide a larger vascular bed for the surgical papillae of the coronally advanced flap due to the deepithelialization of the anatomical papillae in the palatal direction (**Fig 105**).

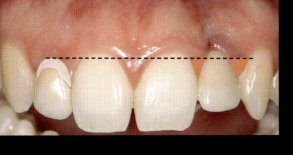

Fig 103 Ideal level of implant crown coverage dictated by correction of the altered passive eruption of the contralateral homologous tooth. The height of the peri-implant papillae is measured based on the ideal coverage level.

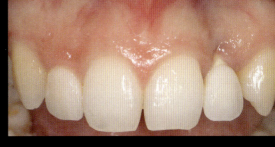

Fig 104 Small provisional crown to allow for peri-implant soft tissue growth.

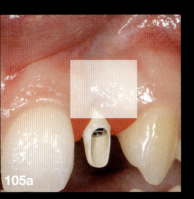
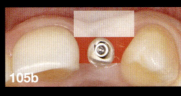
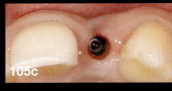
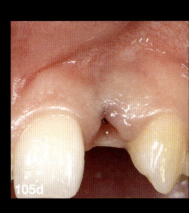

Fig 105 (a to d) Clinical situation 2 months after crown and abutment modification on the implant in the site of the left lateral incisor. The peri-implant papillae are wider and thicker and can be deepithelialized in the palatal direction to provide a greater vascular supply for the surgical papillae of the coronally advanced flap.

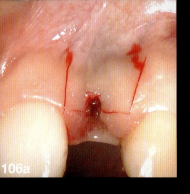
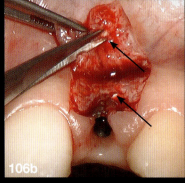
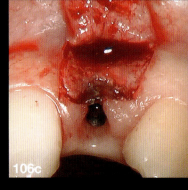

Fig 106 *(a to c)* Design of the trapezoidal flap that will be moved coronally. The arrows indicate the presence of nonosseointegrated biomaterial.

The surgery is performed by temporarily removing the abutment to facilitate execution of the incisions, especially at the level of the surgical papillae. The abutment is inserted again at the time of graft placement to give the graft a stable and convex firm surface.

The surgical technique consists of a coronally advanced trapezoidal flap with a connective tissue graft. The trapezoidal flap consists of two horizontal incisions approximately 3 mm wide and two slightly diverging vertical incisions that overcome the mucogingival junction. The flap is elevated with variable thicknesses, partial at the level of the surgical papillae, complete in the center until the buccal soft tissue is adherent to the underlying planes, then partial again apically to obtain coronal displacement of the flap.

This last partial-thickness portion of the flap consists of two incisions: one deep, split-thickness incision with the blade held parallel to the bone plane, separating the muscle insertions from the periosteum, and one superficial split-thickness incision with the blade parallel to the outer surface of the mucosa, removing the muscle insertions from the inner surface of the alveolar mucosa.

When raising the flap, it is common to find slow-resorbing biomaterial particles that are not osseointegrated. These must be removed because they can be colonized easily by bacteria in the event of infection.

The greatest challenge is removing the particles on the inner surface of the flap, which can result in excessive thinning or even perforation of the flap.

The most suitable instrument for removing these particles is microsurgical scissors used parallel to the inner surface of the flap (**Fig 106**). The soft tissue coronal and palatal to the horizontal incision lines forms the area of the anatomical papillae, which is deepithelialized with a blade and microsurgical scissors (**Fig 107**).

The connective tissue graft is derived from the extraoral deepithelialization of a free gingival graft, which is harvested from the most posterior areas of the palate to reduce patient discomfort and obtain the best quality connective tissue. In the harvesting technique, the horizontal coronal incision and the two vertical incisions are made first.

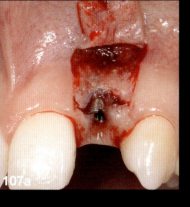
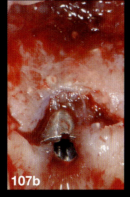
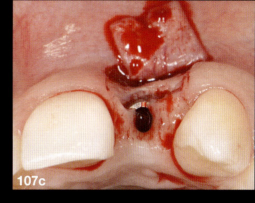

Fig 107 *(a to c)* Deepithelialized anatomical papillae also on the occlusal plane in the palatal direction.

The blade must be kept as parallel to the external surface as possible to give a uniform thickness to the graft without removing excessive palatal soft tissue, which must be maintained as much as possible to protect the palatal bone. Patient morbidity will be reduced if a greater thickness of submucosal tissue is maintained.

The horizontal apical incision connecting the vertical releasing incisions is made after all the graft has been separated from the deeper planes and is aimed at removing the graft. Proceeding in this way, the apical incision is deepened as little as possible, with the sole aim of obtaining release of the graft, thus reducing intraoperative bleeding and the risk of vascular complications **(Fig 108)**.

Deepithelialization of the free gingival graft is performed extraorally with magnification on a sterile surgical drape with a rough surface to avoid graft movement.

The scalpel blade is slightly angled so that an even layer of soft tissue is separated from the underlying tissue.

The layer that is being removed is the epithelium, with the blade cutting between the rougher, stiffer epithelium and the smoother, softer connective tissue. Once the tissue layer to be removed is determined, the blade is held parallel to the outer surface to remove a uniform layer. As soon as the layer is removed, differences in color, surface texture, and light reflection between the area where the epithelium has been removed and the area where the epithelium still needs to be removed become evident. It is these differences that guide the deepithelialization of the remaining part of the graft **(Fig 109)**.

The deepithelialized graft will have plasticity properties that allow it to easily adapt to the underlying structures. The mesiodistal dimension of the connective graft should be 5 to 6 mm greater than the diameter of the abutment. The apicocoronal dimension should be able to cover the distance from 1 mm coronal to the ideal position of the mucosal margin of the implant crown to 2 to 3 mm of buccal bone. It should be around 1 mm thick.

To place the graft in its correct position (ie, approximately 1 mm coronal to the ideal position of the implant crown), it is necessary to screw the abutment back into place to close the access hole with flowable composite.

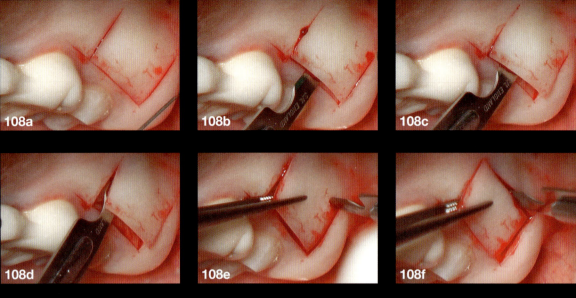

Fig 108 *(a to f)* Stages of epithelial-connective tissue graft harvesting in the palatal area. The thickness of the graft is calibrated at the level of the mesial releasing incision, and then the blade is held parallel to the outer surface of the palatal mucosa to give a uniform thickness to the graft. The apical incision is made at the end of debridement to complete the detachment of the graft.

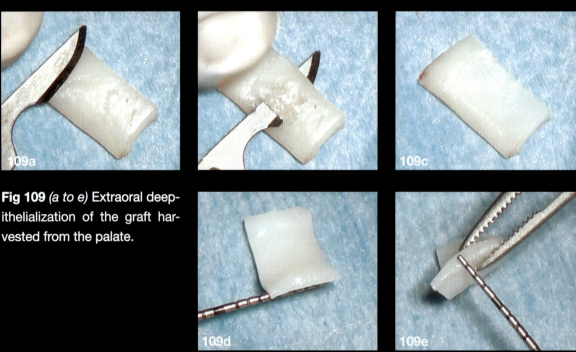

Fig 109 *(a to e)* Extraoral deep-ithelialization of the graft harvested from the palate.

The abutment provides a smooth, hard, convex surface on which the graft can be properly positioned **(Fig 110)**.

The composite makes it possible to give continuity to this surface where the screw access hole would be and serves as a stable surface for the flap that is positioned more coronally to completely cover the connective tissue graft.

The coronal fixation of the graft consists of two internal mattress sutures with palatal anchorage at the base of the anatomical deepithelialized papillae. The needle pierces the graft from the outside and runs inside the papilla, exiting at the level of the palatal mucosa. The needle reenters the palatal mucosa from the outside, horizontally with respect to the exit point, and sliding again within the thickness of the papilla to exit at the base of the papilla in a position slightly more coronal to the graft. The closure of the surgical knot on the graft allows it to be locked at the base of the anatomical deepithelialized papilla, leaving the latter free to receive the surgical papilla of the coronally advanced flap **(Fig 111)**.

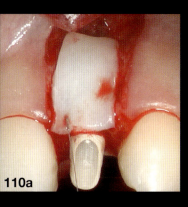 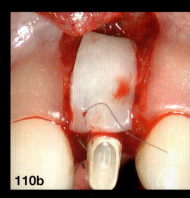 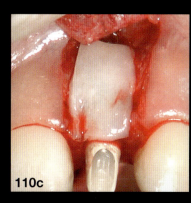

Fig 110 *(a to c)* Placement and suturing of the graft with internal mattress sutures anchored to the palatal soft tissue.

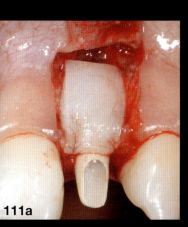 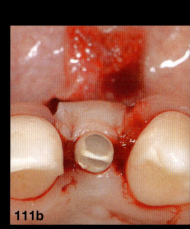 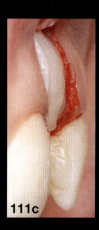 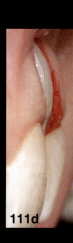

Fig 111 *(a to c)* The connective tissue graft covers the entire area of transparency and restores the loss of buccal volume.

If the plasticity of the graft allows it to adapt well to the underlying bone, no suturing is necessary. Otherwise, sutures anchored to the periosteum apical to the graft must be placed. The coronally advanced flap is sutured with simple interrupted sutures along the vertical releasing incisions and, at the level of the papillae, with two sutures suspended behind the palatal surface of the teeth adjacent to the implant site. In each suspended suture, the needle perforates the surgical papilla at the base, slides inside the anatomically deepithelialized papilla, and exits at the level of the palatal mucosa. From here, the needle reaches the buccal side again, passing under the point of contact between the adjacent teeth and taking anchorage in the papilla distal to the implant site.

The suture is finished with a surgical knot that compresses the surgical papilla above the deepithelialized anatomical papilla in a palatal direction. Suspended sutures allow for the optimal adaptation of the keratinized tissue of the flap with the buccal surface of the abutment and for healing between the surgical papillae and the corresponding deepithelialized anatomical papillae by primary intention (Figs 112 and 113). In addition, they allow for firm flap security that prevents clot leakage and guarantees stability. The provisional crown is shortened so that it does not touch the buccal and interproximal soft tissues and allows for undisturbed tissue healing (Fig 114).

At the time of suture removal after 14 days, the tissues appeared stable compared to their postsurgical position, and increased buccal soft tissue volume was already evident. The tissue is left undisturbed for a period of no less than 4 months to allow it to mature.

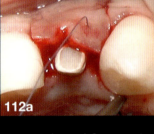
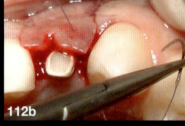
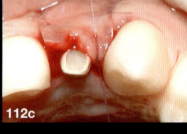

Fig 112 *(a to c)* Suspended sutures anchored to the palatal surface of teeth adjacent to the implant site.

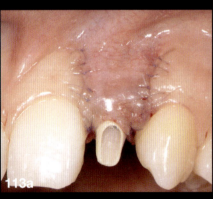
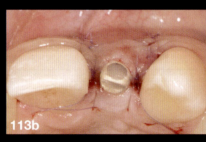
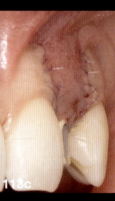

Fig 113 *(a to c)* Coronally displaced flap with simple interrupted sutures along the releasing incisions and coronal sling sutures.

During this period, the provisional is periodically removed and reduced to avoid tissue contact **(Fig 115)**. After 4 months, gingivectomy was performed around the contralateral homologous tooth in altered passive eruption, and the peri-implant soft tissue conditioning phase began **(Fig 116)**. Conditioning with a provisional serves the dual purpose of giving the buccal mucosal margin the esthetically ideal position and contour and achieving maximum coronal growth of the peri-implant papillae by modifying the emergence profiles and changing the position of the provisional contact points. Sometimes, a second set of provisional crowns is used to improve tissue conditioning **(Fig 117)**. The conditioning phase lasts approximately 3 to 4 months. When there is not significant change in the morphology and volume of the buccal soft tissues after conditioning compared to the last control, the definitive prosthesis can be delivered.

In this case, the comparison between the presurgical situation and that at the end of the soft tissue conditioning phase showed an increase in the volume and thickness of the buccal soft tissues, which allowed the prosthetic crown to have a correct emergence profile that was hygienically maintainable by the patient **(Fig 118)**.

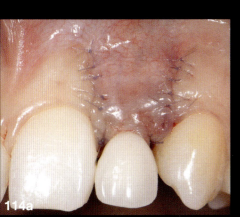
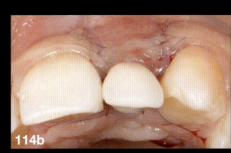
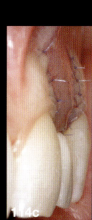

Fig 114 *(a to c)* Provisional crown repositioned and reduced at the buccal and interproximal level so as not to interfere with soft tissue healing.

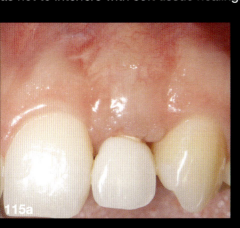
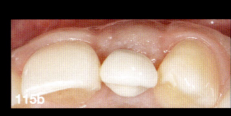
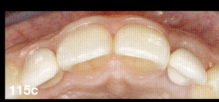
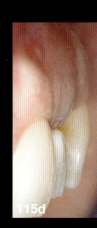

Fig 115 *(a to d)* Suture removal at 14 days.

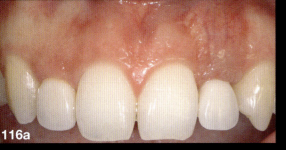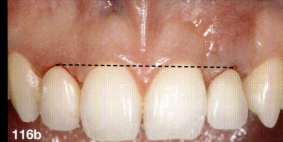

Fig 116 *(a and b)* Gingivectomy of the contralateral homologous tooth in the site of the maxillary right lateral incisor that is affected by altered passive eruption, and soft tissue conditioning with the provisional.

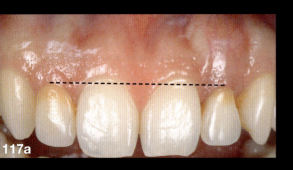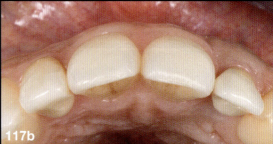

Fig 117 *(a and b)* A new set of provisional crowns is used to better condition the peri-implant soft tissue.

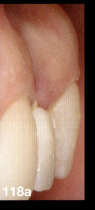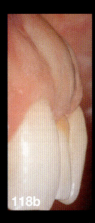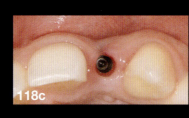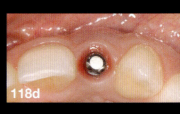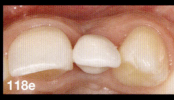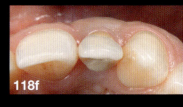

Fig 118 *(a to f)* Comparison between the presurgical situation and the final tissue conditioning phase. The increased soft tissue thicknesses due to the mucogingival technique allowed for a proper emergence profile of the implant crown and complete coverage of the underlying implant-prosthetic components.

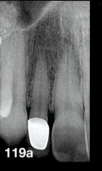
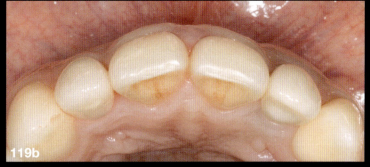
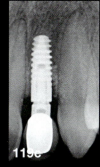

Fig 119 *(a to c)* Good stability of the peri-implant hard tissue.

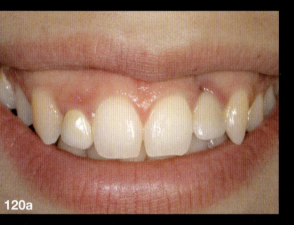
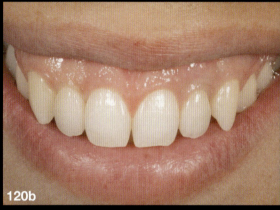

Fig 120 The patient's smile before *(a)* compared to 1 year after delivery of the final prosthesis *(b)*.

The implant prosthesis was well integrated into the buccal soft tissues—almost better than that on the natural homologous tooth, in which the soft tissues were not surgically augmented. Radiographs shows the good response of the hard tissues, with great stability of the peri-implant bone support **(Fig 119)**. The comparison between the initial situation and the situation 1 year after delivery of the definitive prosthesis highlights the esthetic improvements that fully met the patient's requirements **(Figs 120 and 121)**.

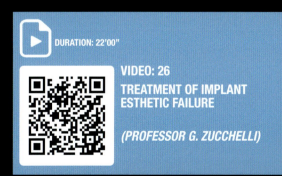

DURATION: 22'00"

VIDEO: 26
TREATMENT OF IMPLANT
ESTHETIC FAILURE

(PROFESSOR G. ZUCCHELLI)

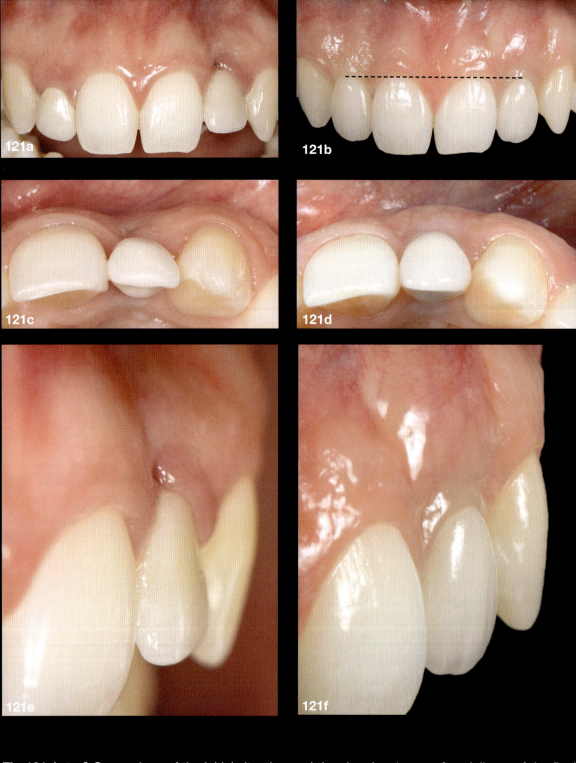

Fig 121 *(a to f)* Comparison of the initial situation and the situation 1 year after delivery of the final prosthesis. The buccal gingival margins of the lateral incisors are aligned, and the implant crown emerges quite naturally from the surgically augmented soft tissue.

HETEROLOGOUS GRAFTS

Replacing autologous connective tissue grafts with commercially available biomaterials is motivated by the desire to reduce the disadvantages of graft harvesting techniques. These disadvantages include the following:

- Relative difficulty of the technique, which requires manual dexterity, especially during harvesting and to manage hemostasis.
- Relative invasiveness, often leading to a painful postoperative period of 1 to 2 weeks at the donor site.
- Limited availability of connective tissue in patients with thin palatal mucosa and a limited tuberosity due to the presence of third molars.

Autologous soft tissue graft substitute biomaterials, however, are also not free of disadvantages. Substitutes cannot be used in all clinical situations, and autologous grafts are still the gold standard.[18]

The disadvantages of soft tissue substitutes include the following:

- Tissue specificity, which depends on the genetic message inherent in the native connective tissue, determines the degree of keratinization of the overlying epithelium. This is demonstrated in the studies by Karring et al.[9,10] Biomaterials are unable to transmit signals for determining the type of keratinization of the epithelium regenerating on them, so their effectiveness in keratinized mucosal augmentation techniques is very limited.
- Biomaterials, which are generally made of porcine-derived collagen, may undergo resorption over time, which limits their indication to cases requiring moderate increases in soft tissue thickness.

On the other hand, the advantages of these substitutes are considerable:

- Simplified and faster surgical technique
- Less invasive, with no need for a second surgical site
- Unlimited availability

Two types of biomaterials are available for use in implant indications: *(1)* biomaterials aimed at increasing the depth of the fornix and restoring the position of the mucogingival margin (for exposed applications) and *(2)* biomaterials for increasing the thickness of peri-implant mucosa or edentulous ridges.

Biomaterials aimed at increasing the depth of the fornix and restoring the position of the mucogingival margin

One of the most widely used heterologous biomaterials for increasing fornix depth and restoring the position of the mucogingival margin is a two-layer Type I/III collagen matrix of porcine origin that is not cross-linked (Mucograft, Geistlich Biomaterials). The outer layer is denser, and the inner layer is spongier. Rocchietta et al[19] investigated the biologic behavior of this material in a preclinical study. The collagen matrix was applied to an experimental animal as either a submerged graft to increases mucosal thickness or as an exposed graft to increase keratinized mucosa. Histologic analyses at 7, 15, and 30 days revealed excellent integration with native collagen without adverse inflammatory reactions **(Fig 122)**. After 30 days, the heterologous collagen appeared almost completely resorbed **(see Fig 122e)** and lost its dimensional characteristics. In addition to its uses in the periodontal field, this biomaterial is currently mainly used for alveolar ridge preservation techniques in combination with DBBM for mucosal closure of extraction sites and to reposition the mucogingival junction during horizontal and vertical ridge augmentations. It is indicated exclusively for exposed applications.

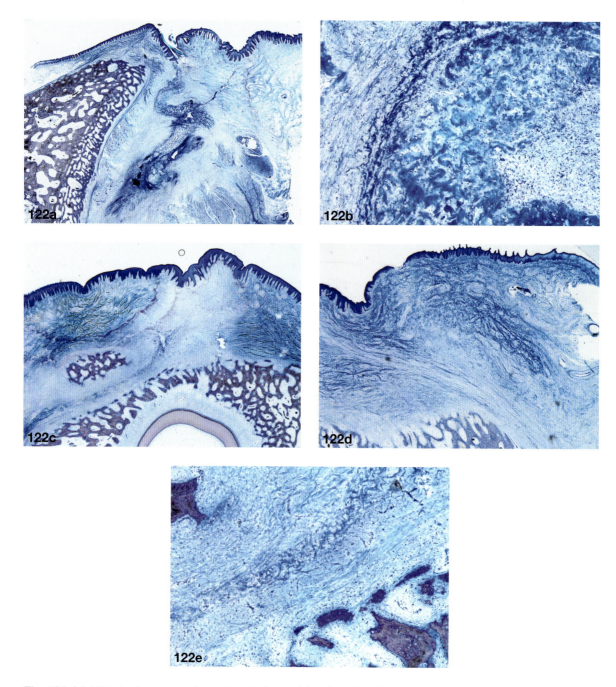

Fig 122 (a) *Histologic preparation after 7 days of healing. The Mucograft collagen matrix is still completely intact (Toluidine/Pyronine blue staining; ×10 magnification). (b) At higher magnification (×40), a modest inflammatory reaction can be seen (Toluidine/Pyronine blue staining). (c) After 15 days of healing, the collagen matrix is almost completely resorbed (Toluidine blue/Pyronine staining; ×10 magnification). (d) At higher magnification, there are no signs of inflammation. Instead, there is a complete integration of the matrix with the surrounding connective tissue (Toluidine/Pyronine blue staining; ×40 magnification). (e) After 1 month of healing, the matrix is completely resorbed (Toluidine/Pyronine blue staining; ×20 magnification). (Reprinted with permission from Int J Periodontics Restorative Dent 2012;32:e34–e40.)*

CLINICAL CASE 11

Repositioning of the mucogingival margin in a patient treated with osteogenic distraction

At the periodontology department of the University of Milan in the early 1990s, a 27-year-old, non-smoking patient in good health presented with partial edentulism in the sites of the maxillary left central and lateral incisors and canine, caused by motor vehicle trauma. The vertical dimension of the alveolar ridge appeared visibly deficient, whereas the horizontal dimension was within the normal range **(Fig 123a)**. In those years, osteogenic distraction according to the technique of G.A. Ilizarov[20] was met with great enthusiasm as an alternative to GBR for vertical ridge elevation. This patient, being in excellent health, a nonsmoker, and in need of a purely vertical elevation without a horizontal component, perfectly fulfilled all the inclusion criteria for this technique.

A full-thickness horizontal incision was made in the fornix, with a buccal flap only, with a U-shaped osteotomy to isolate a bone segment without dissecting it from the palatal mucosa. Then, an external distractor with four fixation screws was applied **(Figs 123b and Fig 123c)**, and suturing was performed. After 1 week of healing, distraction of the segment for 1 mm per day for 10 days was performed, followed by stabilization for 2 months, according to the protocol.

Healing occurred with a considerable vertical increase in bone but a reduction in ridge thickness, a considerable deviation of the mucogingival junction, and the development of a disfiguring scar in the mucosa **(Fig 124a)**.

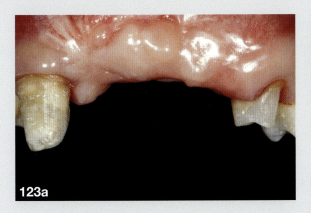

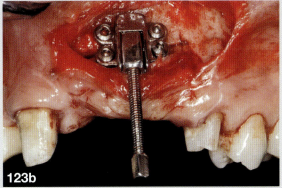

Fig 123 *(a)* Alveolar ridge with an edentulous span from the maxillary left central incisor to canine and vertical bone atrophy but sufficient horizontal bone thickness. *(b)* After performing a rectangular access osteotomy from the buccal side only, a bone distractor was placed. *(c)* Screwing the bone distractor showed that the bone segment was able to slide coronally.

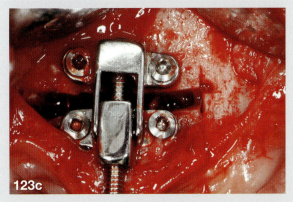

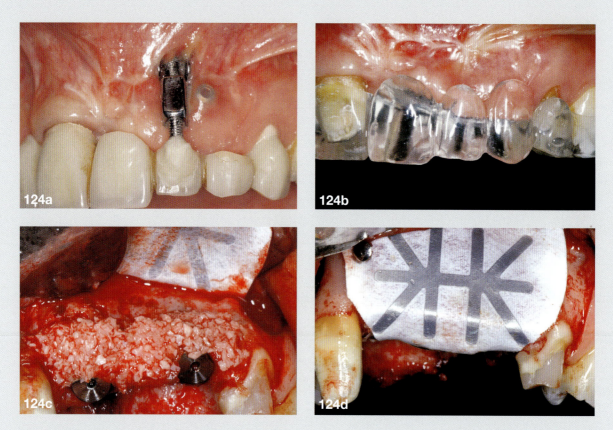

Fig 124 *(a)* After 1 week of healing and 10 days of segment distraction, the distractor was blocked for 2 months and then removed. *(b)* At the time of implant placement, the mucosa appeared scarred, with a deviated mucogingival junction. *(c)* Because the bone ridge had thinned, implant placement resulted in the formation of two areas of implant dehiscence, which were treated with an ePTFE membrane and autologous and heterologous particulate graft. *(d)* The membrane was closed buccally and secured with two pins.

The placement of implants resulted in the development of two areas of buccal dehiscence, which required correction with a GBR technique (**Figs 124b to 124d**).

After 7 months of healing, the ePTFE membrane was removed, the healing abutments were connected, and a provisional restoration with noncompressive emergence profiles was placed (**Figs 125a and 125b**). To restore the correct position of the mucogingival junction and eliminate the scar, a heterologous collagen graft was placed. The recipient site was prepared with a wide partial-thickness flap from a 1-mm incision within the keratinized mucosa. The flap was then sutured apically in the fornix (**Fig 125c**). The heterologous collagen matrix (Mucograft) was trimmed and secured with simple sutures and Vicryl 6-0 sling sutures (**Fig 125d**).

Healing resulted in the restoration of the original position of the mucogingival junction by the formation of a keratinized band of gingiva with the color and appearance of the surrounding gingiva. The provisional was modified several times over the next 6 months to reestablish the correct emergence profiles (**Fig 125e**), and finally, the final ceramic restoration was placed (**Fig 125f**).

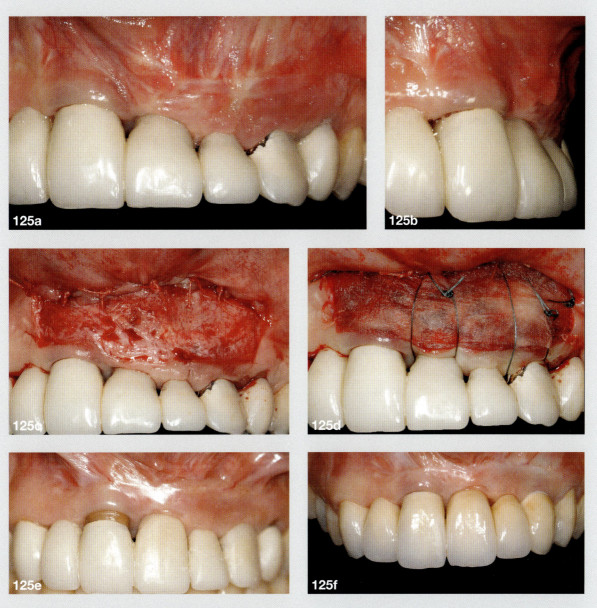

Fig 125 Healing occurred without complications, but with further deviation of the mucogingival margin. *(a)* Frontal view. *(b)* Lateral view. *(c)* The recipient site was prepared with a partial-thickness incision within the residual keratinized mucosa, leaving only the periosteum to cover the bone. The flap was sutured apically in the fornix with resorbable 6-0 Vicryl sutures. *(d)* The Mucograft collagen matrix was trimmed and secured to the site with simple resorbable sutures at the edges of the material and with sling sutures anchored to the periosteum. *(e)* Healing occurred with the restoration of the position of the mucogingival junction and the formation of a keratinized mucosa of the same origin and color as the surrounding mucosa. The provisional was relined for 6 months to establish the correct emergence profiles. (f) Definitive ceramic prosthesis.

M. Simion • G. Zucchelli

Biomaterials for the augmentation of peri-implant mucosa or edentulous ridge thickness

Recently, a weakly cross-linked porcine collagen matrix has been produced which slowly resorbs while maintaining biocompatibility (Fibro-Gide, Geistlich Biomaterials).

This material is used in a submerged position to increase soft tissue thickness in edentulous ridges in association with implant therapy. In addition to the preparation procedure, its special feature is that it expands when soaked in saline or blood. This allows it to withstand flap pressure without collapsing and differentiates it substantially from its predecessor, Mucograft. In preclinical studies, the biocompatibility, inflammatory response, vascularization process, resorption, and replacement with native connective tissue of this material were tested.[21,22] Remarkable dimensional stability was noted after 90 days of healing **(Figs 126a to 126f)**. A limited portion of collagen matrix was still present without causing any inflammatory response, but most of it had been reabsorbed by macrophage activity and replaced with native collagen **(Figs 126g and 126h)**.

The dimensional stability of this material was confirmed by additional clinical studies, which demonstrated behavior comparable to autologous connective grafts.[23–25]

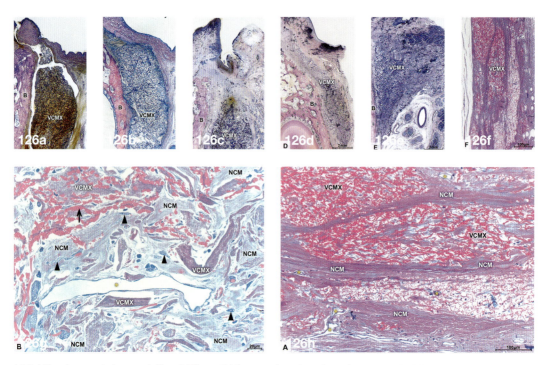

Fig 126 Histology of the stabilized Fibro-Gide matrix, showing the remarkable dimensional stability in the first 3 months of healing. (a) At insertion. (b) After 4 days. (c) After 7 days. (d) After 15 days. (e) After 30 days. (f) After 90 days. (g) Histologic section after 30 days at higher magnification showing the presence of newly formed collagen fibers (NCM) within the resorbed collagen matrix (VCMX). (h) Histologic section after 90 days showing complete integration of the matrix (VCMX) with the newly formed collagen fibrils (NCM) is evident. (Basic fuchsin and Toluidine blue staining). (Reprinted with permission from Int J Periodontics Restorative Dent 2012;32:e34–e40.)

CLINICAL CASE 12

Increase in soft tissue thickness

A 31-year-old patient presented with severe damage to the root structure of the maxillary left central and lateral incisors caused by numerous endodontic treatments and ill-fitting prostheses. The gingival tissues appeared inflamed, and CBCT showed vertical bone loss of 5 mm at the interproximal bone peak **(Figs 127 and 128)**. After extraction of the two teeth, two epithelial-connective tissue grafts were used to close the mucosa of the sockets without altering the mucogingival junction **(Fig 129)**. To restore the correct vertical dimension of the bone ridge, a GBR technique with titanium-reinforced ePTFE membrane (Neogen, Neoss) combined with 70% autologous and 30% heterologous particulate graft (Bio-Oss) was used.

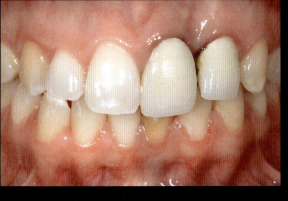

Fig 127 Left central and lateral incisor with compromised root structure and loss of the interdental bone peak caused by an ill-fitting prosthesis.

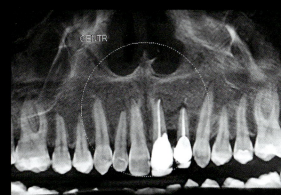

Fig 128 CBCT showing structural root impairment and interproximal bone loss.

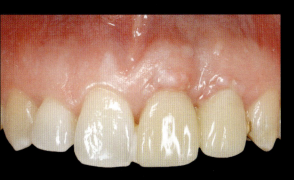

Fig 129 The teeth were extracted, and the sockets were treated with an alveolar preservation technique.

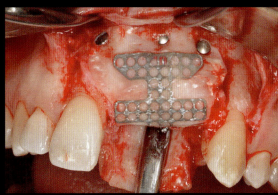

Fig 130 After 8 months, the ePTFE membrane was removed to expose the regenerated bone.

After 8 months of healing, the membrane was removed **(Figs 130 and 131)**, and two hybrid implants (iMAX, iRES) were inserted **(Fig 132)**. To increase the thickness of the soft tissue and allow for the development of adequate emergence profiles, a porcine collagen matrix (Fibro-Gide) was placed in an L shape crestally and buccally **(Fig 133)**. The buccal flap was released with a periosteal incision to avoid compression of the matrix during suturing, and horizontal ePTFE mattress and simple 6-0 Prolene sutures were placed **(Figs 134 to 136)**. After 4 months of healing, the volumetric increase of the mucosa was evident **(Figs 137 and 138)**. Implant uncovering was performed **(Fig 139)**, and the provisional was placed **(Figs 140 and 141)**. After an additional 6 months of tissue maturation, the final ceramic restoration was delivered **(Fig 142)**.

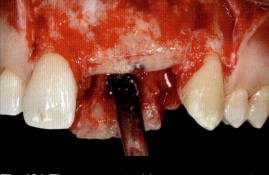

Fig 131 The regenerated bone appears to have the correct vertical and horizontal dimensions.

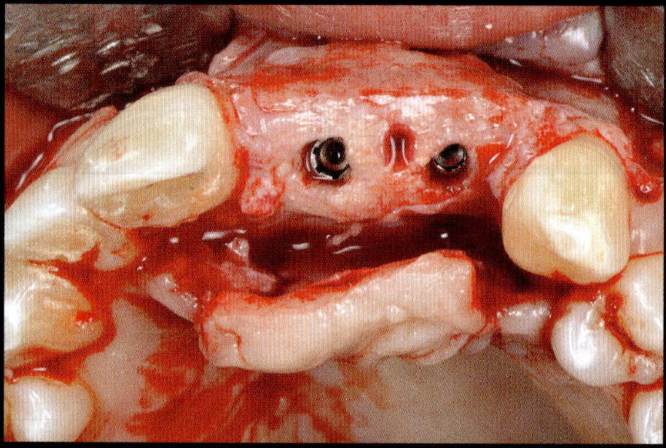

Fig 132 Two hybrid implants with diameters of 3.75 and 3.3 mm were inserted in the sites of the central incisor and lateral incisor, respectively.

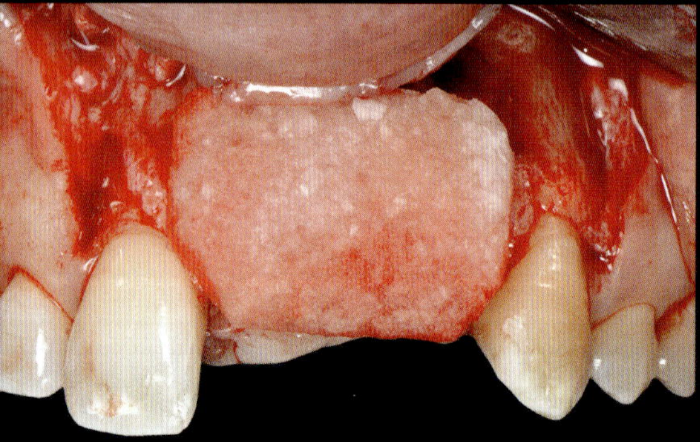

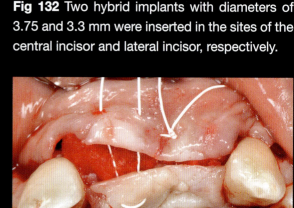

Fig 133 The buccal flap was released with a periosteal incision. A stabilized Fibro-Gide collagen matrix was trimmed, thinned to a thickness of 4 mm, and placed in an L shape over the crest and buccally.

Fig 134 The buccal flap was sutured with horizontal ePTFE mattress sutures and simple interrupted Prolene sutures.

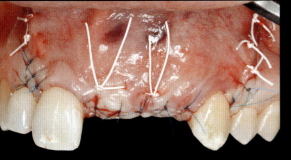

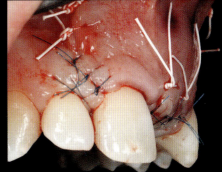

Fig 135 When suturing was completed, the matrix was completely covered by the mucosa so that healing by primary intention was achieved.

Fig 136 Lateral view of the matrix.

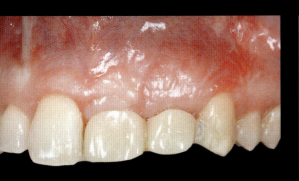

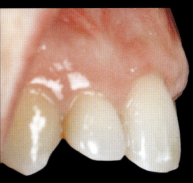

Fig 137 Mucosal healing after 4 months. From a frontal view, the considerable volumetric increase in the edentulous ridge is evident.

Fig 138 From a lateral view, the increased thickness in the buccal direction can be appreciated.

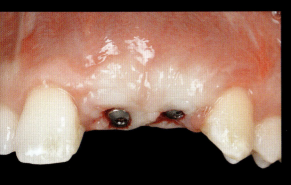

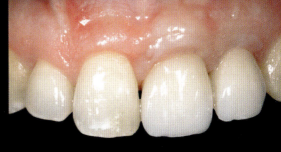

Fig 139 A soft tissue punch was used for the insertion of healing abutments.

Fig 140 The provisional crowns were retained for 6 months to achieve soft tissue maturation and the development of the correct emergence profiles.

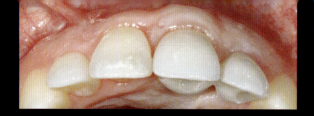

Fig 141 Occlusal view showing the considerable horizontal increase in the soft tissues.

DURATION: 27'38"

VIDEO: 27

PERI-IMPLANT HARD AND SOFT TISSUE AUGMENTATION WITH GBR AND A COLLAGEN MATRIX

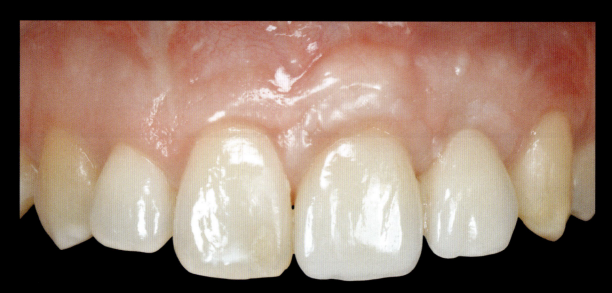

Fig 142 Final ceramic crowns. The interdental papillae appear well formed.

REFERENCES

1. Wennström JL, Bengazi F, Lekholm U. The influence of the masticatory mucosa on the peri-implant soft tissue condition. Clin Oral Implants Res 1994;5:1–8.

2. Strub JR, Gaberthüel TW, Grunder U. The role of attached gingiva in the health of peri-implant tissue in dogs. Clinical findings. Int J Periodontics Restorative Dent 1991;11:317–333.

3. Warrer K, Buser D, Lang NP, Karring T. Plaque-induced peri-implantitis in the presence or absence of keratinized mucosa. An experimental study in monkeys. Clin Oral Implants Res 1995;6:131–138.

4. Wennström JL, Derks J. Is there a need for keratinized mucosa around implants to maintain health and tissue stability? Clin Oral Implants Res 2012;23 (Suppl 6):136–146.

5. Roccuzzo M, Grasso G, Dalmasso P. Keratinized mucosa around implants in partially edentulous posterior mandible: 10-year results of a prospective comparative study. Clin Oral Implants Res 2016;27:491–496.

6. Canullo L, Peñarrocha-Oltra D, Covani U, Botticelli D, Serino G, Peñarrocha M. Clinical and microbiological findings in patients with peri-implantitis: A cross-sectional study. Clin Oral Implants Res 2016;27:376–382.

7. Linkevicius T, Apse P, Grybauskas S, Puisys A. The influence of soft tissue thickness on crestal bone changes around implants: A 1-year prospective controlled clinical trial. Int J Oral Maxillofac Implants 2009;24: 712–719.

8. Puisys A, Linkevicius T. The influence of mucosal tissue thickening on crestal bone stability around bone-level implants. A prospective controlled clinical trial. Clin Oral Implants Res 2015;26:123–129.

9. Karring T, Lang NP, Löe H. The role of gingival connective tissue in determining epithelial differentiation. J Periodontal Res 1975;10:1–11.

10. Karring T, Ostergaard E, Löe HJ. Conservation of tissue specificity after heterotopic transplantation of gingiva and alveolar mucosa. Periodontal Res 1971;6: 282–293.

11. Sullivan HC, Atkins JH. Free autogenous gingival grafts. Principles of successful grafting. Periodontics 1968;6:5–13.

12. Sullivan HC, Atkins JH. Free autogenous gingival grafts. 3. Utilization of grafts in the treatment of gingival recession. Periodontics 1968;6:152–160.

13. Edel A. Clinical evaluation of free connective tissue grafts used to increase the width of keratinized gingiva. J Clin Periodontol 1974;1:185–196.

14. Langer B, Langer L. Subepithelial connective tissue graft technique for root coverage. J Periodontol 1985;56:715–720.

15. Bruno JF. Connective tissue graft technique assuring wide root coverage. Int J Periodontics Restorative Dent 1994;14:126–137.

16. Chen ST, Dahlin C. Connective tissue grafting for primary closure of extraction sockets treated with an osteopromotive membrane technique: Surgical technique and clinical results. Int J Periodontics Restorative Dent 1996;16:348–355.

17. Triaca A, Minoretti R, Merli M, Merz B. Periosteoplasty for soft tissue closure and augmentation in preprosthetic surgery: A surgical report. Int J Oral Maxillofac Implants 2001;16:851–856.

18. Thoma DS, Benć GI, Zwahlen M, Hämmerle CH, Jung RE. A systematic review assessing soft tissue augmentation techniques. Clin Oral Implants Res 2009;20(Suppl 4):146–165.

19. Rocchietta I, Schupbach P, Ghezzi C, Maschera E, Simion M. Soft tissue integration of a porcine collagen membrane: An experimental study in pigs. Int J Periodontics Restorative Dent 2012;32:e34–e40.

20. Ilizarov GA. The principles of the Ilizarov method. Bull Hosp Jt Dis Orthop Inst 1988;48:1–11.

21. Ferrantino L, Bosshardt D, Nevins M, Santoro G, Simion M, Kim D. Tissue integration of a volume-stable collagen matrix in an experimental soft tissue augmentation model. Int J Periodontics Restorative Dent 2016;36:807–815.

22. Caballé-Serrano J, Zhang S, Ferrantino L, Simion M, Chappuis V, Bosshardt DD. Tissue response to a porous collagen matrix used for soft tissue augmentation. Materials 2019;12:3721.

23. Thoma DS, Zeltner M, Hilbe M, Hämmerle CH, Hüsler J, Jung RE. Randomized controlled clinical study evaluating effectiveness and safety of a volume-stable collagen matrix compared to autogenous connective tissue grafts for soft tissue augmentation at implant sites. J Clin Periodontol 2016;43:874–885.

24. Thoma DS, Naenni N, Benic GI, Hämmerle CH, Jung RE. Soft tissue volume augmentation at dental implant sites using a volume stable three-dimensional collagen matrix - histological outcomes of a preclinical study. J Clin Periodontol 2017;44:185–194.

25. Puisys A, Zukauskas S, Kubilius R, et al. Clinical and histologic evaluations of porcine-derived collagen matrix membrane used for vertical soft tissue augmentation: A case series. Int J Periodontics Restorative Dent 2019;39:341–347.

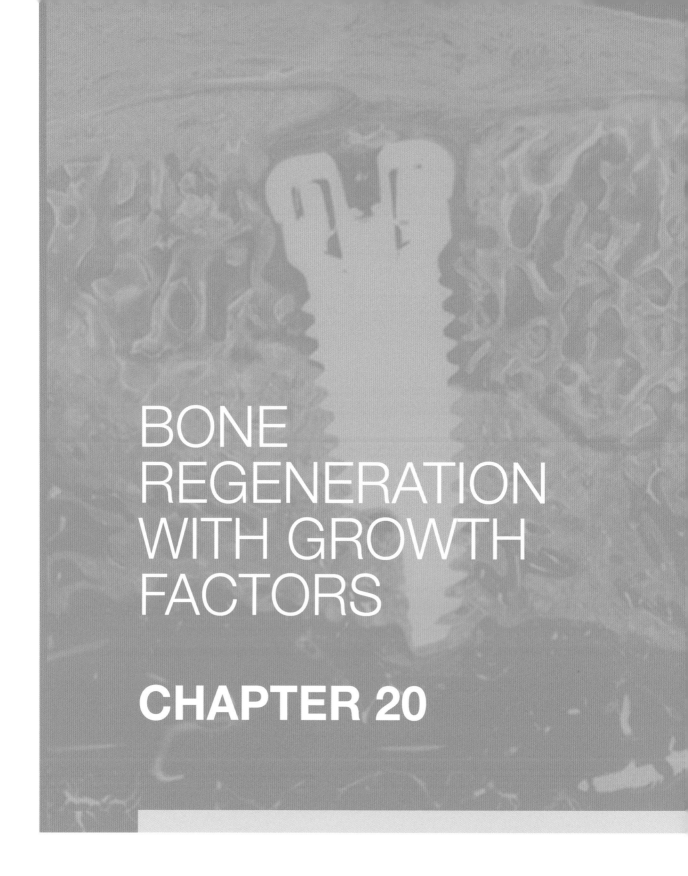

BONE REGENERATION WITH GROWTH FACTORS

CHAPTER 20

Edited by Myron Nevins, Marcelo Camelo, Massimo Simion,
Chia-Yu (Jennifer) Chen, David M. Kim

INTRODUCTION

One of the major challenges in implant dentistry is treating patients with severe bone atrophy caused by periodontal disease, congenital deformities, tumors, trauma, or bone resorption secondary to tooth loss. Bone regeneration requires complex interactions between cells, growth factors, and extracellular matrix components.[1] Whereas standard clinical approaches involve the use of autologous bone grafts with either intra- or extraoral graft harvesting, which can increase the morbidity of surgery, growth factors such as recombinant human bone morphogenetic protein 2 (rhBMP-2) and platelet-derived growth factor (rhPDGF-BB) can also be used to induce bone and periodontal regeneration with minimally invasive techniques.[2] Growth factors are natural proteins that regulate fundamental cellular functions, such as chemotactic attraction, differentiation, and proliferation.[3] Intracellular signals are activated after growth factors bind to specific receptors on the membranes of target cells, leading to the activation of genes that can alter cell activity and phenotype.

Growth factors are highly effective tools for stimulating bone regeneration. Unfortunately, their use in dentistry is still very limited due to both institutional problems and excessive cost.

Massimo Simion

M. Nevins • M. Camelo • M. Simion • C-Y. Chen • D.M. Kim

BONE MORPHOGENETIC PROTEINS

Osteoinduction is defined as the recruitment of totipotent mesenchymal cells located outside the bone (eg, in the muscle tissue) and their differentiation into chondrocytes and osteoblasts, resulting in the formation of an ossicle. The term bone morphogenetic protein (BMP) was first coined and presented to the scientific community by Urist and Strates in an article published in the Journal of Dental Research in 1971.[1] BMPs belong to the transforming growth factor beta (TGF-ß) family of cytokines. To date, 20 types of BMP have been recognized, and their importance in bone healing has been studied intensively.[4]

The characteristic property of BMPs is a cell differentiation factor. BMPs are capable of differentiating an undifferentiated mesenchymal cell into an osteoblast. PDGF, on the other hand, is a chemotactic and mitogenic factor in osteoblast precursors. BMPs, like PDGF, also play a key role in blood vessel formation by stimulating angiogenic peptides such as vascular endothelial growth factor (VEGF). BMPs can also bind to endothelial cells and stimulate their migration to promote blood vessel formation.[5]

Developing a technique to extract and purify BMPs from the bone matrix has taken many years. Wozney et al[6] cloned BMP-2 and BMP-4 in 1988, and in 1990, BMP-7 and BMP-8 were cloned by Ozkaynak et al.[7] Most rhBMPs have been produced on a large scale from the cellular system of mammals such as the Chinese hamster and the mouse.[8] The most studied of the recombinant BMPs is rhBMP-2 of human origin.

The first study to evaluate the ability of BMPs to induce bone neoformation in an experimental animal model involved performing a sinus elevation procedure in six adult goats, using collagen impregnated with rhBMP-2.[9] Collagen has been used as the delivery vehicle for bone regeneration because it has a biphasic release profile characterized by an immediate phase and a slow subsequent release. This feature makes rhBMP available to target cells throughout the healing phase.[3] The test side in the goats showed considerable bone neoformation, whereas the control side that did not use BMP was negative. Bone regeneration at the test sites occurred rapidly within 4 weeks **(Figs 1 and 2)**, and histologic examination at 4, 8, and 12 weeks showed the complete absence of immunologic, toxic, or adverse responses **(Figs 3 and 4)**.

The first clinical study on rhBMP-2 in humans included 12 patients treated with a sinus elevation procedure. The total dose of rhBMP-2 per patient ranged from 1.77 to 3.40 mg (mean 2.89 mg). Radiographic CT evaluation showed bone neoformation in all patients, and the clinical examination showed no signs of local or systemic side effects. The treated sites showed an average increase in vertical bone of 8.51 ± 4.13 mm. The amount and thickness of trabecular bone was moderate to large, with a variable component of woven bone. The data provided by this study supported the possibility of using rhBMP-2 with an absorbable collagen sponge (ACS) for sinus elevation procedures.

A second study aimed to evaluate two concentrations of rhBMP-2 for sinus elevation and subsequent treatment with endosseous implants.[10] In the study, 48 patients were treated with either an ACS impregnated with rhBMP-2 at a concentration of 0.75 mg/mL (n = 18) or a concentration of 1.50 mg/mL (n = 17), or with a bone graft (n = 13) **(Fig 5)**. The results showed no differences between the groups treated with the two different doses of rhBMP-2/ACS.

Biopsies performed at the time of implant placement after an average period of 6.9 months showed clear bone induction upon histologic examination **(Fig 6)**. A large amount of trabecular bone containing immature woven bone and lamellar bone had formed, and there were few to a moderate number of osteoblasts and few osteoclasts. No inflammatory cells were detected in any of the analyzed samples. The higher concentration of rhBMP-2/ACS was found to be the most effective, but implant success rates after 36 months of follow-up were the same in all three groups. In another randomized comparative study between rhBMP-2/ACS and autologous bone grafting for sinus elevation,[11] bone formation and implant integration and success were evaluated after 6 months and after 2 years of prosthetic loading **(Figs 7 to 9)**.

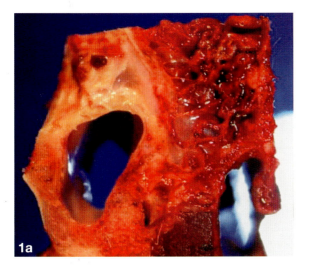
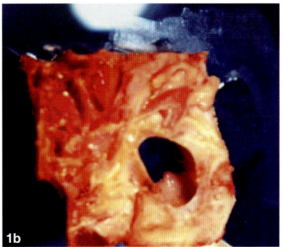

Fig 1 (a) *Section 12 weeks after elevation of the left sinus treated with an absorbable collagen sponge (ACS) alone.* (b) *Section 12 weeks after elevation of the right sinus treated with the ACS soaked in human rhBMP-2.*

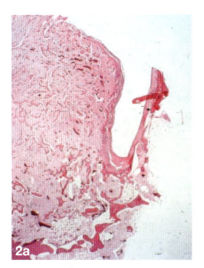
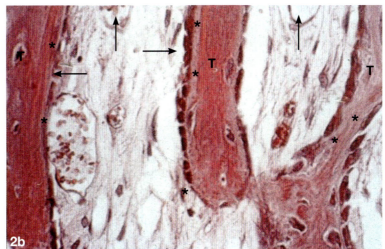

Fig 2 (a) *Hematoxylin/eosin- (H&E-) stained histologic section of the maxillary sinus treated with rhBMP-2 after 4 weeks of healing.* (b) *Higher magnification of the trabeculae. Cuboid osteoblasts (arrows) lie on a layer of osteoid tissue that has not yet mineralized. The Ts indicate blood vessels.*

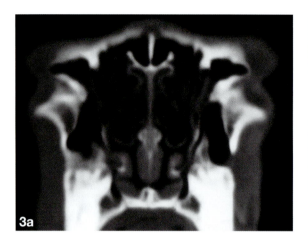
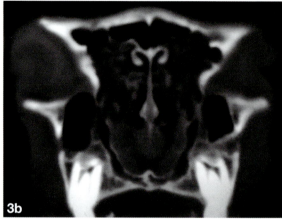

Fig 3 (a) *CT scan after 8 weeks showing greater radiopacity in the rhBMP-2/collagen-treated sinus compared to that treated with an ACS alone.* (b) *CT scan at 12 weeks.*

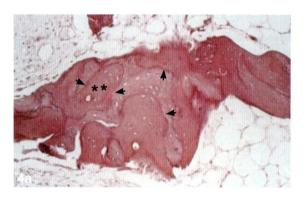
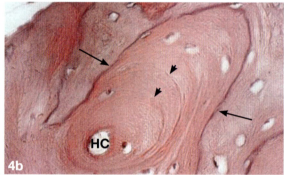

Fig 4 *H&E-stained section of a trabecula in yellow bone marrow at 12 weeks.* (a) *The cement lines (short arrows) separate the earliest deposited bone (dark pink) from the most recently deposited bone (light pink). The asterisks indicate the Haversian system.* (b) *Higher magnification of the same section showing the cement lines (arrows), the concentric rings of the Haversian system (short arrows), and the Havers canal (HC).*

A second randomized controlled trial was performed to evaluate bone regeneration in extraction sites with an rhBMP-2/ACS dose of 1.50 mg/mL without bone grafts.[12] That study demonstrated a significant loss of buccal bone plate in untreated sites. Examples of radiographs and clinical documentation before and after treatment are shown in **Figs 10 to 14**.

PDGF has also been intensively studied and is frequently used for periodontal and peri-implant regeneration. It is a polypeptide contained in platelet alpha granules and bone matrix. Four isomeric forms have been identified, PDGF-AA, PDGF-AB, PDGF-BB, and PDG-CC.[13–16]

RhPDGF-BB exerts a potent chemotactic and mitogenic effect on mesenchymal cells (including osteogenic cells), and it is also angiogenic, complementing the action of VEGF in vascular neoformation.[17–21]

It has been shown to stimulate the chemotactic and mitogenic activity of periodontal ligament (PDL) cells at a concentration of 1 mg/mL.[22]

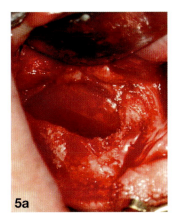
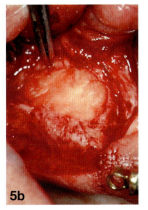
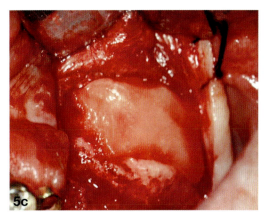

Fig 5 (a) *Elevation of the lateral sinus window was performed while maintaining the integrity of the sinus membrane. (b) The space within the sinus was filled with an ACS soaked in rhBMP-2. (c) A collagen membrane was placed before the flap was sutured, and no bone graft was inserted.*

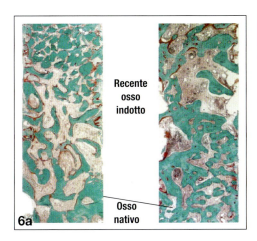
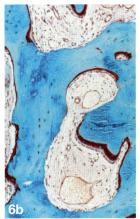

Fig 6 (a) *Trephine sampling demonstrates new bone regenerated with the ACS and rhBMP-2. (b) Higher magnification showing the regenerated bone.*

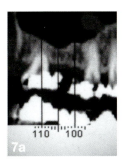
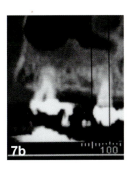
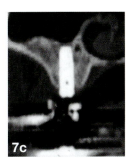
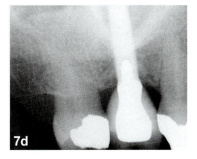

Fig 7 (a) *Presurgical CBCT showing minimal residual bone. (b) CBCT after 6 months. The sinus area was augmented with rhBMP-2/ACS. (c) The implant was placed after 6 months. (d) The implant prosthesis was placed.*

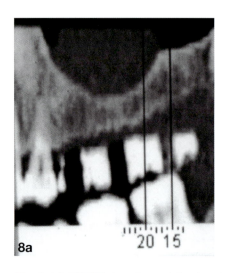
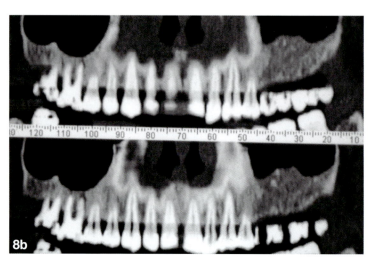

Fig 8 (a) *CBCT showing minimal residual bone in the areas of the maxillary left second premolar, first molar, and second molar. A resin stent was used to place three implants.* (b) *CBCT showing the significant increase in bone suitable for implant placement.* (c) *CBCT cross-section showing the correct position of the implants.*

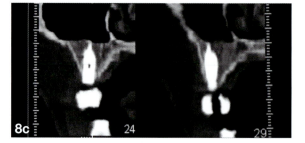

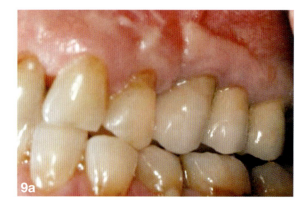
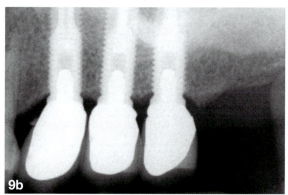

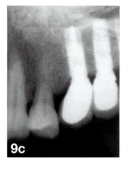
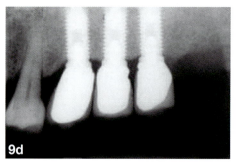
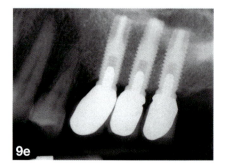

Fig 9 (a) *Final prosthetic rehabilitation (2002).* (b) *Final control radiograph.* (c) *After 1 year (2003).* (d) *After 6 years.* (e) *After 16 years.*

Delivered in a methylcellulose gel, rhPDGF-BB had a half-life of 4.2 hours and a clearance of over 96% in 96 hours in a canine model.[23] Thus, the powerful action of PDGF occurs soon after clinical application, when it triggers a cascade of biologic and cellular events that continue for weeks in the area of the surgical wound. This cascade is characterized by the recruitment and differentiation of mesenchymal cells and the formation of new vessels, ultimately promoting wound healing and regeneration.

In 2005, the FDA approved a new synthetic graft material, Gem 21S (Lynch Biologics), a combination of beta tricalcium phosphate (TCP-ß) and rhPDGF-BB (0.5 mL; 0.3 mg/mL) for the treatment of periodontal defects. FDA approval was based on efficacy data from preclinical and clinical studies, including those from a large-scale, prospective, randomized, controlled human trial. McGuire et al[24] demonstrated histologic regeneration of the buccal bone plate and new cementum and PDL in maxillary premolars intended for extraction for orthodontic therapy.[24]

ALVEOLAR BONE PRESERVATION IN EXTRACTION SITES

Alveolar preservation procedures have been developed to reduce the dimensional loss of bone following dental extractions to allow implants to be placed in a prosthetically correct position.[25] Clinical studies have shown a reduction in vertical alveolar bone size of 11% to 22% and an even greater reduction in thickness (29% to 63%) during the first 6 months after extraction.[26–31] Studies on the resorption of the alveolar bone plate after the extraction of prominent teeth have shown that alveolar preservation techniques are able to reduce the resorption of the buccal bone plate in a statistically significant way.

Current alveolar preservation techniques include the use of a variety of osteoconductive materials, sometimes associated with membranes. While numerous studies have reported clinical success, histologic evaluations have demonstrated a considerable amount of residual graft material. One clinical study evaluated the efficacy of a combination of 0.3 mg/mL rhPDGF-BB with a mineralized xenograft with collagen matrix in seven patients with biopsy samples after 4 or 6 months. Histomorphometric analysis with micro-CT and light microscopy showed signs of resorption of the xenograft with collagen matrix and replacement with new bone in contrast to numerous studies that showed minimal resorption of xenograft particles **(Fig 15)**. In another study,[32] to analyze healing of the buccal bone plate at extraction sites, 16 patients were randomized into four groups and treated with different grafting materials:

1. Xenograft with collagen matrix alone
2. Xenograft with collagen matrix and rhPDGF-BB 0.3 mg/mL
3. Xenograft with collagen matrix with an enamel matrix derivative (EMD)
4. EMD with hydroxyapatite

After 5 months, a trephine biopsy was performed for implant placement. The sites treated with rhPDGF showed the most favorable crestal morphology and greater bone neoformation at histomorphometric evaluation.

SINUS GRAFTS

Dental implants to replace teeth in the posterior regions of the maxilla have been validated with long-term studies.[33] Numerous materials for bone regeneration have been examined, and DBBM has been used extensively both alone and in combination with other matrices.[34–36]

In one study, ten patients with a vertical residual bone height of less than 6 mm were recruited. Sinus elevation procedures were performed with 0.3 mg/mL rhPDGF-BB.

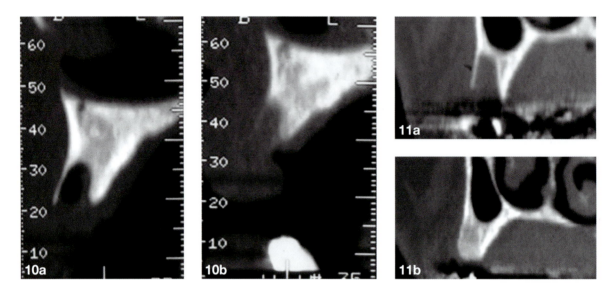

Fig 10 (a) *Extraction site with intact bone wall. No graft material was inserted because it was thought that the buccal wall was thick enough.* (b) *After healing, the buccal bone plate resorbed.* **Fig 11** (a) *CBCT showing the extraction site.* (b) *The site was treated with rhBMP-2/ACS. Note the bone regeneration compared to Fig 10b.*

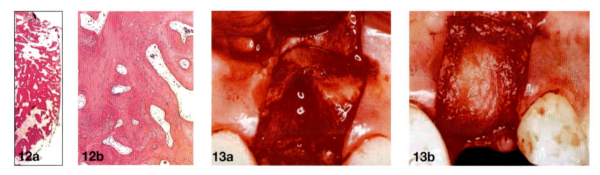

Fig 12 (a) *Bone core taken from an extraction site treated with rhBMP-2.* (b) *Magnification of regenerated bone.* **Fig.13** (a) *Extraction site with loss of the buccal bone wall.* (B) *The site was reopened 6 months after reconstruction with rhBMP-2 to insert an implant.*

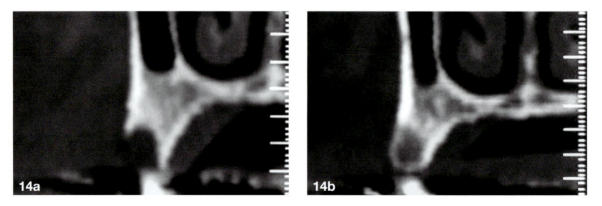

Fig 14 (a) *CBCT before bone reconstruction.* (b) *CBCT after bone reconstruction with rhBMP-2.*

The DBBM particles were saturated with 1 mL PDGF for a minimum of 15 minutes to allow for adequate impregnation of the graft particles.[37] The material was then placed in the sinus and covered with a resorbable collagen membrane. Biopsies were performed after 6 and 8 months. Histologic sections showed large areas of dense, well-shaped lamellar bone distributed throughout the specimens and numerous osteoblasts associated with osteoid tissue, a clear sign of ongoing bone formation. Residual particles of DBBM, normally slow to resorb, showed signs of resorption and replacement with new bone (Fig 16).

ATROPHIC ALVEOLAR RIDGE AUGMENTATION

Atrophic alveolar ridges with inadequate bone volume due to periodontal disease, traumatic extractions, or the excision of invasive neoformations require the performance of regenerative techniques. Various methods and materials are used for this purpose:

- Guided bone regeneration (GBR) with resorbable and nonresorbable membranes and particulate bone grafts (autologous, alloplastic, heterologous, and allogeneic)
- Block grafts of various kinds
- Growth factors and stem cells
- Osteogenic distraction
- Split crest and expansion techniques
- Combined methods

All these techniques have the potential to regenerate lost alveolar bone with varying degrees of success. Some techniques entail some morbidity, but their predictability is increasing due to new materials and new surgical procedures.[38–42] GBR uses barrier membranes to create and maintain space for bone regeneration while preventing soft tissue penetration. This technique requires excellent soft tissue management to avoid membrane exposure and subsequent bacterial contamination of the site. The use of stimulating molecules has been studied extensively in both preclinical models and in humans. Preclinical studies have shown that rhPDGF-BB combined with bone matrices can improve bone neoformation and wound healing in alveolar bone reconstructions and implant therapy. Simion et al[42] used rhPDGF-BB combined with DBBM blocks for vertical ridge elevations.[42] Six adult mastiffs underwent bilateral extraction of the mandibular premolars with the creation of a vertical bone defect. After 3 months, the defects were treated with one of three different block grafts and two implants:

1. Group A: Block with collagen membrane
2. Group B: Block infused with rhPDGF-BB
3. Group C: Block infused with rhPDGF-BB and covered with a collagen membrane

The histologic analysis of group B showed extensive bone regeneration and direct contact between the implants and regenerated bone. The results underscore the importance of the periosteum as a source of osteoprogenitor cells in growth factor–mediated regenerative techniques. The authors concluded that the membrane may have hindered the chemotactic activity of the growth factor. In a second dog study, blocks of equine bone (equine hydroxyapatite collagen [eHAC]) infused with rhPDGF-BB were used for vertical ridge augmentation.[43]

Bilateral vertical defects were surgically created in the posterior mandible of 12 adult mastiffs and allowed to heal for 2 months. The defects were then reconstructed with:

1. **Group A:** the eHAC block alone
2. **Group B:** the eHAC block covered with a collagen membrane
3. **Group C:** the eHAC block infused with rhPDGF-BB
4. **Group D:** the eHAC block infused with rhPDGF-BB covered with a collagen membrane

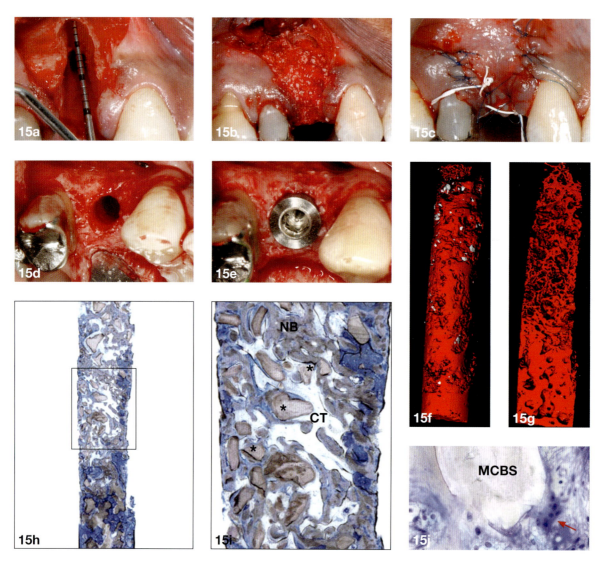

Fig 15 (a to c) *The extraction site was carefully curetted and treated with rhPDGF combined with a xenograft with collagen matrix.* (d and e) *After 4 months, a biopsy sample was taken with a trephine, and an implant was placed.* (f and g) *The micro-CT of the biopsy showed bone (in red) and xenograft with collagen matrix (in white).* (h and i) *Histologic sections showed bone neoformation (NB) around the xenograft particles.* (j) *Note the demineralization of a xenograft with collagen matrix particle by a giant multinucleated cell (arrow). (Reprinted with permission from Int J Periodontics Restorative Dent 2009;29:129–139.)*

Fig 16 (a) *A micro-CT of the biopsy taken at the time of implant placement showed almost 100% native bone (in red) and a minimal percentage of residual DBBM particles (in white).* (b) *Histologic examination confirmed significant bone neoformation over the entire specimen and few residual DBBM particles.* (c) *At higher magnification, osteoblasts secreting osteoid tissue, woven bone, and dense lamellar bone are visible.* (d) *Lower magnification showing some residual DBBM particles surrounded and interconnected with newly formed bone.* (e) *Preoperative periapical radiograph of the maxillary sinus to be treated.* (f) *Implant placement after sinus elevation. (Reprinted with permission from Int J Periodontics Restorative Dent 2009;29:583–591.)*

The equine block was malleable to allow for intimate contact between the block and the bone defect. After 5 months, excellent results were obtained in group C, where the membrane was not used. This extensive study once again highlighted the possibility that the membrane may hinder the chemotactic activity of rhPDGF-BB toward progenitor cells from the periosteum **(Figs 17 to 19)**. The application of this technique in two human subjects provided encouraging results.[44]

One patient was missing the mandibular premolars and molars due to periodontal disease. The residual alveolar ridge was grafted with a block of DBBM infused with rhPDGF-BB.

Clinical and radiographic images after 5 months of healing showed significant bone regeneration sufficient for the placement of three implants **(Figs 20 and 21)**.

The second patient presented with a vertical defect in a posterior mandibular sector.

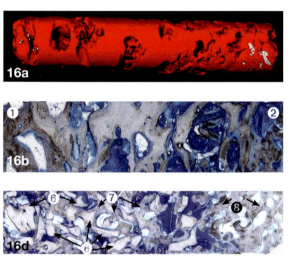

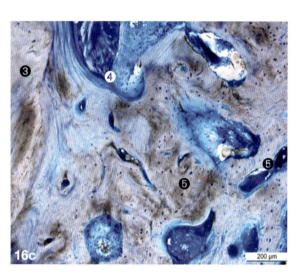

1. Coronal
2. Apical
3. Lamellar bone
4. Osteoid
5. Woven bone
6. DBBM
7. Newly formed bone
8. Native bone

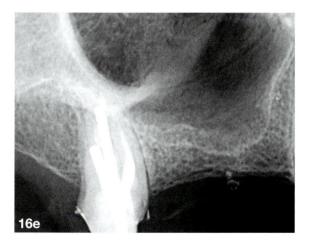

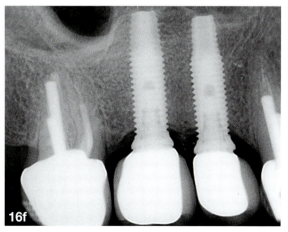

Bone regeneration was achieved with a technique similar to the previous one except for the use of a block of DBBM in a collagen matrix infused with rhPDGF-BB and fixed with an osteosynthesis screw **(Figs 22 to 24)**.

MINIMALLY INVASIVE HORIZONTAL RIDGE AUGMENTATION

In one study, a minimally invasive horizontal ridge augmentation (tunneling) technique with rhPDGF-BB in combination with different matrices was performed in 12 patients.[44] Patients were randomized into three groups:

1. **Group A:** 0.3 mg/mL rhPDGF-BB with lyophilized freeze-dried human bone allograft (FDBA)
2. **Group B:** 0.3 mg/mL rhPDGF-BB with DBBM
3. **Group C:** 0.3 mg/mL rhPDGF-BB DBBM in collagen matrix

Surgical reentry after 14 weeks showed sufficient bone regeneration for implant placement in all patients in groups A and B and in two out of four patients in group C. Biopsies with micro-CT, backscattered electron microscopy (BE-SEM), and light microscopy showed bone regeneration in all sites of groups A and B **(Figs 25 and 26)**.

TREATMENT OF LARGER EDENTULOUS RIDGE DEFECTS

The treatment of large defects in partially edentulous areas was performed with block allografts of bone infused with 0.3 mg/mL rhPDGF-BB.[45] Two patients scheduled for treatment with multiple implants consented to the removal of a nonstrategic implant to verify the healing process. After removal of the implant, the site was devoid of a buccal or lingual bone wall.
A block of FDBA was molded to fit the recipient site and hydrated with rhPDGF-BB for 15 minutes under vacuum in a syringe to allow for complete infusion.
Then the block was placed in the site and stabilized with an osteosynthesis screw **(Fig 27)**. After 11 months, a CBCT scan was performed to determine bone gain relative to bone volume. A reentry operation was also performed to remove the fixation screw and to assess healing and take a biopsy of the grafted area for histologic analysis **(Fig 28)**.

IMPROVED OSSEOINTEGRATION

In addition to regenerating bone defects, rhPDGF-BB can be applied directly to an implant surface to promote early osseointegration.[46] In a preclinical study, six beagle dogs were divided into three groups and treated with a total of 24 implants. The negative control group included 4 untreated implants, one test group included 10 mplants infused with commercially available rhPDGF-BB, and the other test group included 10 implants infused with a more intense prototype of rhPDGF-BB. In both test groups, the implant surface was left to infuse for a minimum of 10 minutes before implant insertion.
Histologic sections obtained after 3 weeks showed new bone formation between most of the implant threads in the test groups, whereas only a variable amount of new bone was present in the control group.
At 6 weeks, the test group with commercially available rhPDGF-BB showed a greater amount of trabecular bone and a higher percentage of bone-to-implant contact (BIC) than the other two groups **(Fig 29)**.

CONCLUSION

Great strides have been made in the field of periodontal regeneration thanks to the availability of rhPDGF.

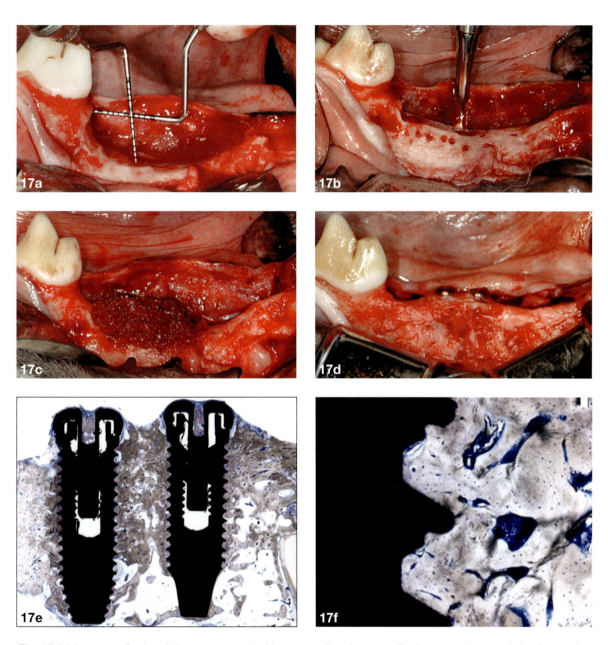

Fig 17 (a) *In group C, the defect was created by extracting the mandibular premolars and the first molar.* (b) *Perforations were made to the cortical of the defect.* (c) *An equine block infused with rhPDGF-BB was placed in the defect and stabilized with two implants.* (d) *The implants were completely surrounded by bone-like tissue 5 months later.* (e) *Examination under the light microscope showed excellent contact between the bone and implant. The newly formed bone can be distinguished from the native bone by its darker color, caused by its higher concentration of proteins.* (f) *At higher magnification, the bone-to-implant contact (BIC) and vascularization is visible. (Figures 17 to 19 reprinted with permission from Int J Periodontics Restorative Dent 2009;29:245–255.)*

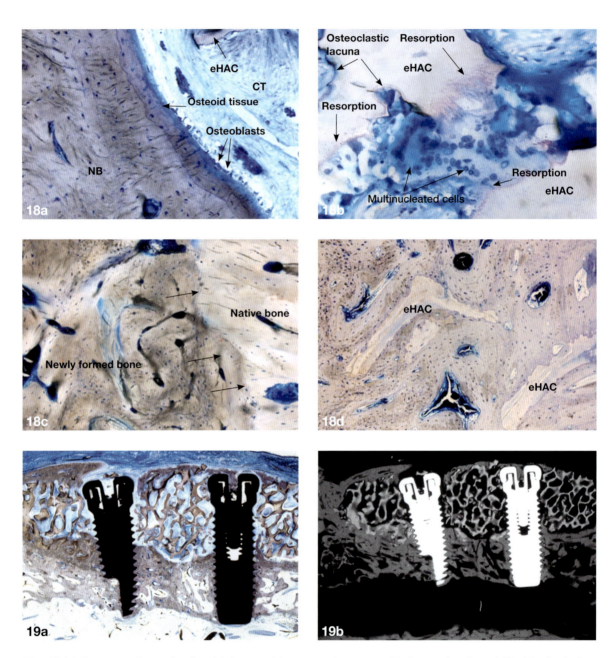

Fig 18 (a) *Bone neoformation in which osteoblasts produce osteoid tissue that is calcified by including collagen fibers. (b) Resorption process on the surface of the eHAC matrix. (c) The surface of the native bone is connected to the regenerated bone with intimate contact. (d) A magnification of ×100 is required to recognize the smallest amount of eHAC matrix. *Fig 19* In group D, the defect was treated with an eHAC block infused with rhPDGF-BB fixed with two implants and covered with a collagen membrane. The light microscope image (a) and the micro-CT (b) show that although some minimal bone regeneration has occurred, vertical regeneration remains incomplete, and a significant portion of the implant surface is surrounded by dense connective tissue.*

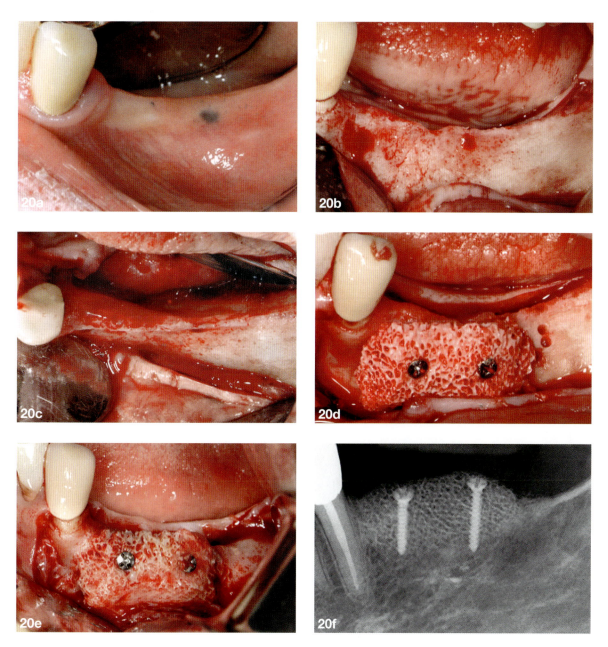

Fig 20 *Horizontal ridge augmentation using rhPDGF-BB–infused DBBM block. (a) Preoperative clinical image of the left mandibular atrophic edentulous alveolar ridge. (b) After elevation of a full-thickness flap, insufficient bone thickness was visible. (c) The blade-like ridge does not allow for the placement of implants. (d) A block of DBBM infused with rhPDGF-BB was secured to the buccal wall with two osteosynthesis screws. (e) After 5 months of submerged healing, the DBBM block appears well integrated with the native bone upon re-entry. (f) Control radiograph 5 months after grafting.*

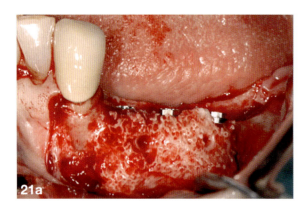
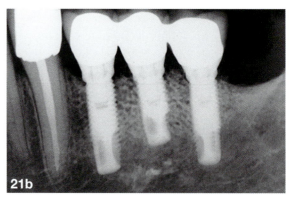

Fig 21 *Three implants were placed at the regenerated site* (a). *Periapical x-ray of the three implants (courtesy of: Int J Periodontics Restorative Dent. 2009;29:371–383)* (b).

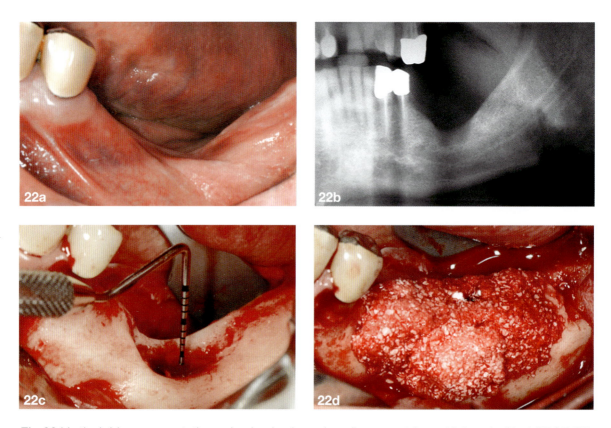

Fig 22 *Vertical ridge augmentation using bovine bone in collagen matrix and infused with rhPDGF-BB. (a) Preoperative view of the mandibular atrophic edentulous area on the right. (b) Panoramic radiograph of the vertical bone defect. (c) After elevation of a full-thickness flap, the vertical bone defect is evident. (d) Particles of DBBM immersed in collagen matrix infused with rhPDGF-BB were placed in the defect and stabilized with a fixation screw. (d) The site was reopened 5 months after surgery, and the defect appeared to be completely filled with clinically bone-like hard tissue.*

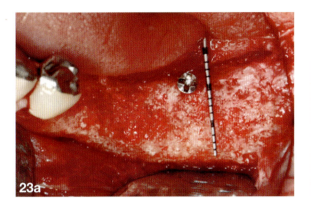
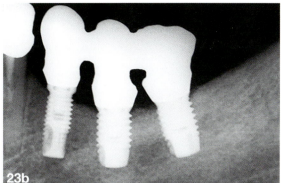

Fig 23 (a) *Vertical bone regeneration was approximately 8 mm.* (b) *Periapical radiograph 8 months after implant placement.*

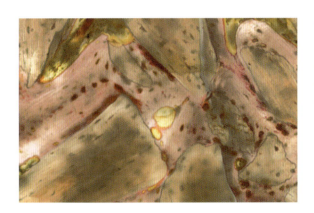

Fig 24 *Histologic image of the biopsy specimen showing mature lamellar regenerated bone in contact with the xenograft. (Figures 24 to 26 reprinted with permission from Int J Periodontics Restorative Dent 2009;29:371–383.)*

Clinicians and researchers are constantly searching for techniques to reduce the invasiveness of treatments, and the use of PDGF reduces complications and the morbidity of surgical procedures. PDGF increases the proliferation of gingival fibroblasts and the PDL, as well as the formation of new cementum on teeth with periodontal defects. Indications in which rhPDGF has been shown to improve healing of both bone and gingival tissue include alveolar preservation after dental extractions, bone augmentation in atrophic alveolar ridges, and sinus elevation procedures.

Numerous studies have demonstrated the safety and reliability of rhPDGF-BB in periodontal regeneration, and since rhPDGF-BB became commercially available for dental purposes in the United States in 2006 (Gem 21S), many scientific publications have demonstrated its predictability and efficacy in the treatment of bone defects. The results of preclinical studies, case reports, and practical experience have demonstrated the predictability and safety of using rhPDGF-BB in combination with various bone matrices for the treatment of alveolar defects. Only three adverse events have been reported in over a decade of use in patients. PDGF is a valuable tool for promoting bone and soft tissue healing in numerous clinical conditions.

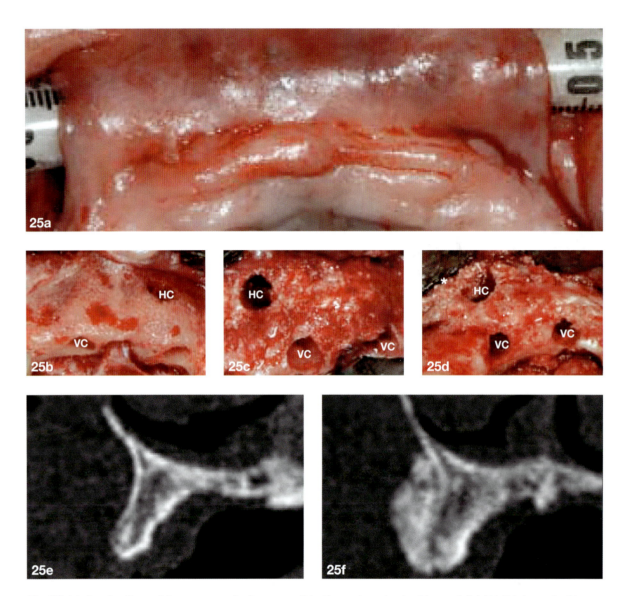

Fig 25 (a) *Application of the composite bone graft in the subperiosteal tunnel.* (b) *Well-integrated bone particles in group A sites.* (c) *Integrated particles of group B.* (d) *Integration deficiency (asterisk) of grafted particles in group C.* (e) *Preoperative CT scan of a patient from group A.* (f) *Postoperative CT scan of the same patient from group A. HC = horizontal biopsy sampling; VC = vertical biopsy sampling.*

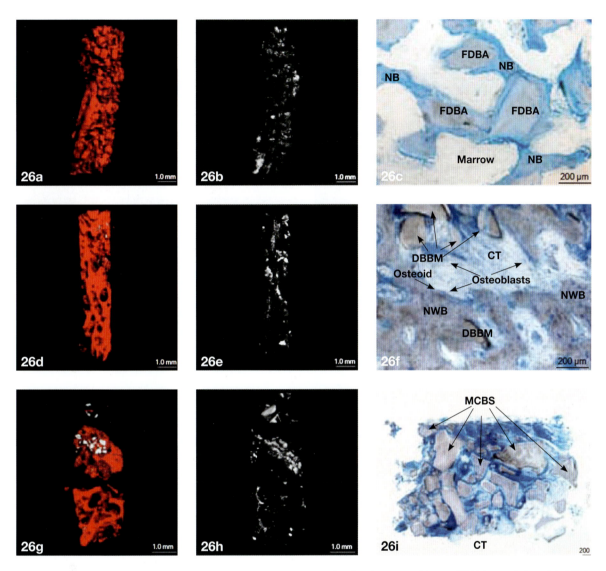

Fig 26 (a and b) *Micro-CT of a sample from group A. Red = bone; white = FDBA particles. (c) High magnification under light microscope showing FDBA particles surrounded by newly formed bone (NB). (d to f) Micro-CT of a sample from group B. Red = bone; white = DBBM particles. (g) High magnification light microscope showing DBBM particles surrounded by newly formed intertwined fiber bone (NWB). (h) Micro-CT of a group C sample. Red = bone; white = DBBM/DBBM with collagen matrix particles. (i) High magnification light microscope showing fibrous encapsulation of DBBM particles immersed in collagen matrix.*

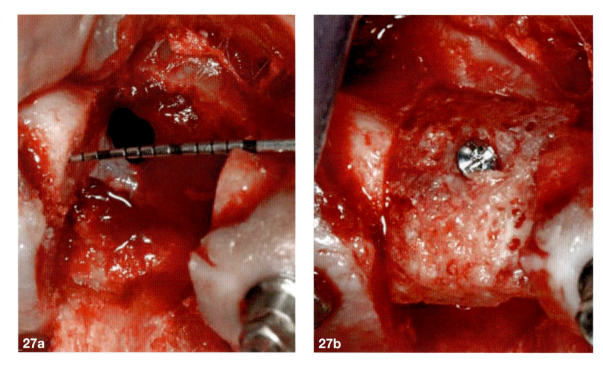

Fig 27 (a) *After implant removal, a two-walled defect remained.* (b) *A freeze-dried allogenic bone block was infused with rhPDGF-BB, placed in the defect, and secured with a fixation screw.*

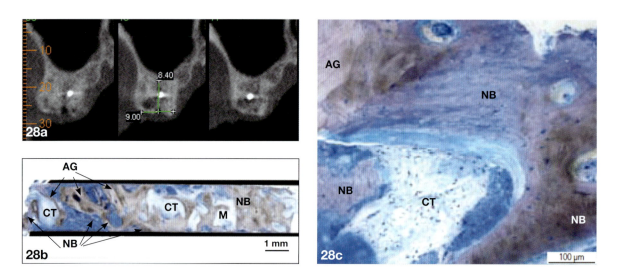

Fig 28 (a) *CBCT of the site after 11 months showed the restoration of the original morphology of the ridge, and surgical reentry showed a well-integrated block with a dense appearance and no signs of resorption.* (b and c) *On reentry, a biopsy was performed with histologic examination that showed the presence of allograft (AG), connective tissue (CT), medullary spaces (M), and newly formed bone (NB). (Reprinted with permission from Int J Periodontics Restorative Dent 2012;32:263–271.)*

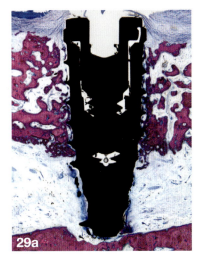
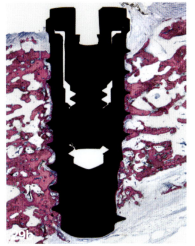
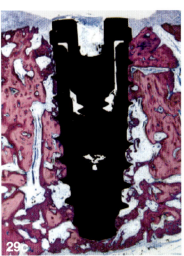
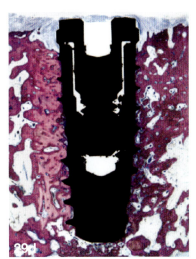
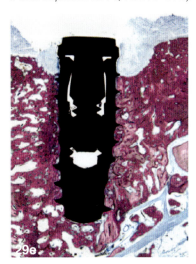

Fig 29 At 3 weeks, the control group (a) showed less trabecular bone and less BIC than the test group with commercially available rhPDGF-BB (b). At 6 weeks, the control group (c) still showed less trabecular bone and BIC than the test group with commercially available rhPDGF-BB (d), which also showed more trabecular bone and greater BIC than the other test group (e). (Reprinted with permission from J Oral Implantol 2014;40:543–348.)

REFERENCES

1. Urist MR, Strates BS. Bone morphogenetic protein. J Dent Res. 1971;50:1392–1406.

2. Chen D, Zhao M, Mundy GR. Bone morphogenetic proteins. Growth Factors. 2004;22:233–241.

3. Hoffmann A, Weich HA, Gross G, Hillmann G. Perspectives in the biological function, the technical and therapeutic application of bone morphogenetic proteins. Appl Microbiol Biotechnol. 2001;57:294–308.

4. Salazar VS, Gamer LW, Rosen V. BMP signalling in skeletal development, disease and repair. Nat Rev Endocrinol. 2016;12:203–221.

5. ten Dijke P, Fu J, Schaap P, Roelen BA. Signal transduction of bone morphogenetic proteins in osteoblast differentiation. J Bone Joint Surg Am. 2003;85-A Suppl 3:34– 38.

6. Wozney JM, Rosen V, Celeste AJ, Mitsock LM, Whitters MJ, Kriz RW, Hewick RM, Wang EA. Novel regulators of bone formation: molecular clones and activities. Science. 1988;242:1528–1534.

7. Ozkaynak E, Rueger DC, Drier EA, Corbett C, Ridge RJ, Sampath TK, Oppermann H. OP-1 cDNA encodes an osteogenic protein in the TGF-beta family. EMBO J. 1990;9:2085–2093.

8. Hammonds RG Jr, Schwall R, Dudley A, Berkemeier L, Lai C, Lee J, Cunningham N, Reddi AH, Wood WI, Mason AJ. Bone-inducing activity of mature BMP-2b produced from a hybrid BMP-2a/2b precursor. Mol Endocrinol. 1991;5:149–155.

9. Nevins M, Kirker-Head C, Nevins ML, Wozney JA, Palmer R, Graham D. Bone formation in the goat maxillary sinus induced by absorbable collagen sponge implants impregnated with recombinant human bone morphogenetic protein-2. Int J Periodont Rest Dent. 1996;16:8–19.

10. Boyne P, Lilly L, Marx R, Moy P, Nevins M, Spagnoli DB, Triplett RG. De novo bone induction by recombinant human bone morphogenetic protein-2 (rhBMP-2) in maxillary sinus floor augmentation. J Oral Maxillofac Surg. 2005;63:1693–1707.

11. Triplett G, Nevins M, Marx R, Spagnoli D, Oates TW, Moy PK, Boyne PJ. Pivotal, randomized, parallel evaluation of recombinant human bone morphogenetic protein-2/absorbable collagen sponge and autogenous bone graft for maxillary sinus floor augmentation. J Oral Maxillofac Surg. 2009;67:1947–1960.

12. Fiorellini JP, Howell TH, Cochran D, Malquist J, Lilly LC, Spagnoli D, Tolijanic J, Jones A, Nevins M. Randomized study evaluating recombinant human bone morphogenetic protein-2 for extraction socket augmentation. J Periodontol. 2005;76:605–613.

13. Hammacher A, Hellman U, Johnsson A, Ostman A, Gunnarsson K, Westermark B, Wasteson A, Heldin CH. A major part of platelet-derived growth factor purified from human platelets is a heterodimer of one A and one B chain. J Biol Chem. 1988;263:16493–16498.

14. Hart CE, Bailey M, Curtis DA, Osborn S, Raines E, Ross R, Forstrom JW. Purification of PDGF-AB and PDGF-BB from human platelet extracts and identification of all three PDGF dimers in human platelets. Biochemistry 1990;29:166–172.

15. Fang L, Yan Y, Komuves LG, Yonkovich S, Sullivan CM, Stringer B, Galbraith S, Loker NA, Hwang SS, Nurden P, Phillips DR, Giese NA. PDGF C is a selective alpha platelet-derived growth factor receptor agonist that is highly expressed in platelet alpha granules and vascular smooth muscle. Arterioscler Thromb Vasc Biol. 2004;24:787–792.

16. Alvarez RH, Kantarjian HM, Cortes JE. Biology of platelet-derived growth factor and its involvement in disease. Mayo Clin Proc. 2006;81:1241-1257.

17. Heldin CH, Westermark B. Mechanism of action and in vivo role of platelet-derived growth factor. Physiol Rev. 1999;79:1283–1316.

18. Betsholtz C. Insight into the physiological functions of PDGF through genetic studies in mice. Cytokine Growth Factor Rev. 2004;15:215–228.

19. Fredriksson L, Li H, Eriksson U. The PDGF family: four gene products form five dimeric isoforms. Cytokine Growth Factor Rev. 2004;15:197–204.

20. Bouletreau PJ, Warren SM, Spector JA, Steinbrech DS, Mehrara BJ, Longaker MT. Factors in the fracture microenvironment induce primary osteoblast angiogenic cytokine production. Plast Reconstr Surg. 2002;110: 139–148.

21. Sato N, Beitz JG, Kato J, Yamamoto M, Clark JW, Calabresi P, Raymond A, Frackelton AR Jr. Platelet-derived growth factor indirectly stimulates angiogenesis in vitro. Am J Pathol. 1993;142:1119–1130.

22. Oates TW, Rouse CA, Cochran DL. Mitogenic effects of growth factors on human periodontal ligament cells in vitro. J Periodontol. 1993;64:142–148.

23. Lynch SE, de Castilla GR, Williams RC, Kiritsy CP, Howell TH, Reddy MS, Antoniades HN. The effects of short-term application of a combination of platelet-derived and insulin-like growth factors on periodontal wound healing. J Periodontol. 1991;62:458–467.

24. McGuire MK, Scheyer ET, Schupbach P. Growth factor-mediated treatment of recession defects: a randomized controlled trial and histologic and microcomputed tomography examination. J Periodontol. 2009;80:550–564.

25. Nevins ML, Camelo M, Schupbach P, Nevins M, Kim SW, Kim DM. Human buccal plate extraction socket regeneration with recombinant human platelet-derived growth factor BB or enamel matrix derivative. Int J Periodontics Restorative Dent. 2011;31:481–492.

26. Nevins M, Camelo M, De Paoli S, Friedland B, Schenk RK, Parma-Benfenati S, Simion M, Tinti C, Wagenberg B. A study of the fate of the buccal wall of extraction sockets of teeth with prominent roots. Int J Periodontics Restorative Dent. 2006;26:19–29.

27. Schropp L, Wenzel A, Kostopoulos L, Karring T. Bone healing and soft tissue contour changes following single-tooth extraction: a clinical and radiographic 12-month prospective study. Int J Periodontics Restorative Dent. 2003;23:313–323.

28. Froum S, Cho SC, Rosenberg E, Rohrer M, Tarnow D. Histological comparison of healing extraction sockets implanted with bioactive glass or demineralized freeze-dried bone allograft: a pilot study. J Periodontol. 2002;73: 94–102.

29. Artzi Z, Tal H, Dayan D. Porous bovine bone mineral in healing of human extraction sockets. Part 1: histomorphometric evaluations at 9 months. J Periodontol. 2000;71:1015–1023.

30. Nevins ML, Camelo M, Schupbach P, Kim DM, Camelo JM, Nevins M. Human histologic evaluation of mineralized collagen bone substitute and recombinant platelet-derived growth factor-BB to create bone for implant placement in extraction socket defects at 4 and 6 months: a case series. Int J Periodontics Restorative Dent. 2009;29:129–139.

31. Araujo M, Linder E, Wennstrom J, Lindhe J. The influence of Bio-Oss Collagen on healing of an extraction socket: an experimental study in the dog. Int J Periodontics Restorative Dent. 2008;28:123–135.

32. Nevins M, Hanratty J, Lynch SE. Clinical results using recombinant human platelet-derived growth factor and mineralized freeze-dried bone allograft in periodontal defects. Int J Periodontics Restorative Dent. 2007;27: 421–427.

33. Nevins M, Langer B. The successful application of osseointegrated implants to the posterior jaw: a long-term retrospective study. Int J Oral Maxillofac Implants. 1993;8:428–432.

34. Froum SJ, Wallace SS, Elian N, Cho SC, Tarnow DP. Comparison of mineralized cancellous bone allograft (Puros) and anorganic bovine bone matrix (Bio-Oss) for sinus augmentation: histomorphometry at 26 to 32 weeks after grafting. Int J Periodontics Restorative Dent. 2006;26: 543–551.

35. Gapski R, Neiva R, Oh TJ, Wang HL. Histologic analyses of human mineralized bone grafting material in sinus elevation procedures: a case series. Int J Periodontics Restorative Dent. 2006;26:59–69.

36. Wallace SS, Froum SJ, Cho SC, Elian N, Monteiro D, Kim BS, Tarnow DP. Sinus augmentation utilizing anorganic bovine bone (Bio-Oss) with absorbable and nonabsorbable membranes placed over the lateral window: histomorphometric and clinical analyses. Int J Periodontics Restorative Dent. 2005;25:551–559.

37. Nevins M, Garber D, Hanratty JJ, McAllister BS, Nevins ML, Salama M, Schupbach P, Wallace S, Bernstein SM, Kim DM. Human histologic evaluation of anorganic bovine bone mineral combined with recombinant human platelet-derived growth factor BB in maxillary sinus augmentation: case series study. Int J Periodontics Restorative Dent. 2009;29:583–591.

38. Milinkovic I, Cordaro L. Are there specific indications for the different alveolar bone augmentation procedures for implant placement? A systematic review. Int J Oral Maxillofac Surg. 2014;43:606–625.

39. Aloy-Prosper A, Penarrocha-Oltra D, Penarrocha-Diago M, Hernandez-Alfaro F, Penarrocha-Diago M. Peri-implant Tissues and Patient Satisfaction After Treatment of Vertically Augmented Atrophic Posterior Mandibles with Intraoral Onlay Block Bone Grafts: A Retrospective 3-Year Case Series Follow-up Study. Int J Oral Maxillofac Implants. 2018;33:137–144.

40. Carpio L, Loza J, Lynch S, Genco R. Guided bone regeneration around endosseous implants with anorganic bovine bone mineral. A randomized controlled trial comparing bioabsorbable versus non-resorbable barriers. J Periodontol.2000;71:1743–1749.

41. Fontana F, Maschera E, Rocchietta I, Simion M. Clinical classification of complications in guided bone regeneration procedures by means of a nonresorbable membrane. Int J Periodontics Restorative Dent. 2011;31:265–273.

42. Simion M, Rocchietta I, Kim D, Nevins M, Fiorellini J. Vertical ridge augmentation by means of deproteinized bovine bone block and recombinant human platelet-derived growth factor-BB: a histologic study in a dog model. Int J Periodontics Restorative Dent. 2006;26: 415–423.

43. Simion M, Nevins M, Rocchietta I, Fontana F, Maschera E, Schupbach P, Kim DM. Vertical ridge augmentation using an equine block infused with recombinant human platelet-derived growth factor-BB: a histologic study in a canine model. Int J Periodontics Restorative Dent. 2009;29:245–255.

44. Nevins ML, Camelo M, Nevins M, Schupbach P, Friedland B, Camelo JM, Kim DM. Minimally invasive alveolar ridge augmentation procedure (tunneling technique) using rhPDGF-BB in combination with three matrices: a case series. Int J Periodontics Restorative Dent. 2009;29: 371–383.

45. Nevins M, Camelo M, Nevins ML, Ho DK, Schupbach P, Kim DM. Growth factor-mediated combination therapy to treat large local human alveolar ridge defects. Int J Periodontics Restorative Dent. 2012;32:263–271.

46. Al-Hezaimi K, Nevins M, Kim SW, Fateh A, Kim DM. Efficacy of growth factor in promoting early osseointegration. J Oral Implantol. 2014;40:543–548.

SINUS FLOOR ELEVATION

CHAPTER 21

Edited by Fabio Bernardello, Paolo Bozzoli, Luca Ferrantino e Massimo Simion

INTRODUCTION

The alveolar ridge undergoes constant change. Many factors may contribute to its progressive resorption, including periodontal disease, endodontic pathologies, destructive carious lesions, and sometimes traumatic events.[1] Tooth extraction also leads to a progressive loss of bone volume in the extraction site area. Horizontal bone atrophy is characterized by loss of the buccal component of bone, which is greater than the palatal/lingual component.[2] In the posterolateral areas, at the maxillary sinuses, horizontal resorption rarely results in insufficient crestal width for implant placement. Physiologic vertical resorption, however, leads to progressive pneumatization of the maxillary sinuses, which often results in insufficient residual bone height. In these cases, sinus floor elevation, sometimes associated with vertical ridge augmentation, is the technique of choice.

Sinus floor elevation can be performed with a crestal or lateral approach.

Crestal ("blind") techniques involve raising the floor of the sinus directly with a crestal osteotomy. Crestal techniques are divided into expansive-compaction techniques, based on the use of manual osteotomes that expand the ridge and raise the sinus floor, and ablative-subtractive techniques, in which sequential burs or inserts for ultrasonic or sonic systems are used to progressively remove the subantral portion of bone without damaging the sinus membrane.

Sinus floor elevation is now a routine procedure. In most cases, it is characterized by medium levels of difficulty and low complication rates, but some cases involve hidden pitfalls.

Massimo Simion

A graft is then inserted, which lifts the sinus membrane. Lateral approach techniques involve the detachment of a flap, an osteotomy in the lateral sinus wall, detachment of the sinus membrane, and insertion of a graft material. Crestal and lateral sinus elevation techniques can be performed as either a single-stage procedure, with the simultaneous insertion of one or more implants, or as a two-stage procedure, in which only the elevation is performed and implant placement is deferred for 6 to 9 months. The choice is made based on the height of the residual bone and the possibility of obtaining sufficient primary implant stability.

PREOPERATIVE ANATOMICAL CONSIDERATIONS

To assess the anatomical parameters that may influence the choice of a technique, a 3D radiographic (CBCT) evaluation is required to assess specific structures and conditions.

Osteomeatal complex

It is essential to assess the patency of the osteomeatal complex, a structure that ensures the adequate drainage of fluids from the sinus cavity into the nasal cavities (Fig 1). Surgical trauma during sinus elevation can result in the accumulation of blood or serous effusions, which if not drained effectively, can trigger acute postoperative sinusitis. Therefore, if the osteomeatal complex is not pervious, the patient must be referred to an ear, nose, and throat (ENT) specialist for case evaluation and possible endoscopic treatment before proceeding with sinus elevation surgery.

Sinus pathology

The sinuses should be assessed with a careful patient history, objective examination, and CBCT to identify potential thickening of the sinus membrane and any sinus pathology, such as sinusitis, pseudocysts, mucoceles, osteomas, mycetoma, and dislocated teeth or implants.

Sinus membrane thickening up to 2 mm occurs in 50% of patients, and even up to 3 to 4 mm of thickening is not a contraindication to either crestal or lateral sinus elevation procedures. Greater thickening require more in-depth investigation.

Acute sinusitis is always symptomatic and is associated with dull, diffuse pain and mucopurulent rhinorrhea lasting less than 3 to 4 weeks. With CBCT, regular thickening of the sinus membrane along the sinus walls is usually observed. Acute sinusitis is of bacterial or viral origin, and it is treated with antibiotic therapy.

Initially, amoxicillin and clavulanic acid (1 g every 8 hours for at least 8–10 days) is administered. However, bacteria that sustain acute forms of sinusitis are usually particularly sensitive to treatment with fluoroquinolones (levofloxacin), which are effective on both aerobic gram-positive and gram-negative bacteria, combined with a nasal aerosol lincosamide (lincomycin) that is active on anaerobic strains. In many cases, it is also useful to combine a mucolytic and a corticosteroid in decreasing doses.

Chronic sinusitis lasts for more than 3 months and is of bacterial or fungal origin. If chronic sinusitis is being maintained by an odontogenic, endodontic, or periodontal problem, endodontic treatment or tooth extraction is performed. Nasal cortisone sprays are also useful.

The patient is then reassessed after at least 2 months. If the chronic sinusitis is not of odontogenic origin (antral pseudocyst, polyp, mucocele, mycetoma), the patient should be referred to an ENT specialist for endoscopic fibroscopy.

Antral pseudocysts, often described as "rising sun cysts" (and erroneously referred to as mucoceles), are asymptomatic, nonexpansive, and radiologically well-defined structures. They originate from mucus- or serum-secreting glandular structures and are generally not an absolute contraindication to sinus augmentation.

During lateral sinus elevations, it is sometimes possible to insert a syringe needle to aspirate their contents. If the pseudocyst is serous, the procedure will be effective, leaving the pseudocyst almost completely empty **(Figs 2 and 3)**. In the case of mucinous contents, this maneuver will be almost impossible.

A particular form of chronic sinusitis, which is actually a fungal infection during preexisting sinusitis, is characterized by a mass of fungal hyphae growing inside the sinus and forming a sinus mycetoma (ie, a fungus ball).

The etiologic agent most often responsible for this pathology is aspergillus.

Diagnosis via CBCT is based on diffuse radiopacity of the sinus with hyperdense ovoid areas with a metallic appearance **(Fig 4)**. Clinically, mycetoma manifests itself with sometimes intense facial pain, purulent discharge, and cacosmia (a sensation of malodorous discharge in the nose).

The treatment of mycetoma is of otorhinolaryngologic relevance.

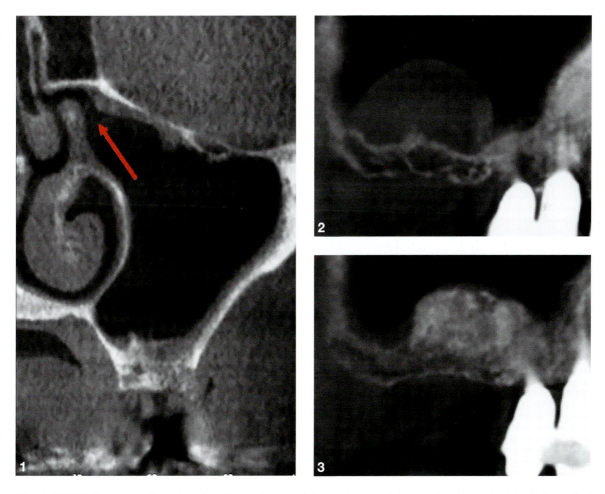

Fig 1 CBCT Cross-section showing the patency of the osteomeatal complex (arrow). *Fig 2* An antral pseudocyst (ie, "rising sun cyst"). *Fig 3* Newly performed lateral sinus elevation with simultaneous aspiration of the serous contents of the antral pseudocyst.

Maxillary sinus septa

Careful CBCT evaluation of the sinuses allows clinicians to locate any bony septa, sometimes called Underwood's septa. Septa may be single or multiple and follow either a buccomedial **(Fig 5)** or mesiodistal **(Fig 6)** course. They are present in about 30% of cases, with an average height of about 8 mm. They are most frequently located in the anterior part of the sinus.[3]

In some cases, an extended, transverse, and complete buccomedial septum compartmentalizes the sinus into two or more distinct cavities **(Figs 7)**. When performing a lateral sinus elevation

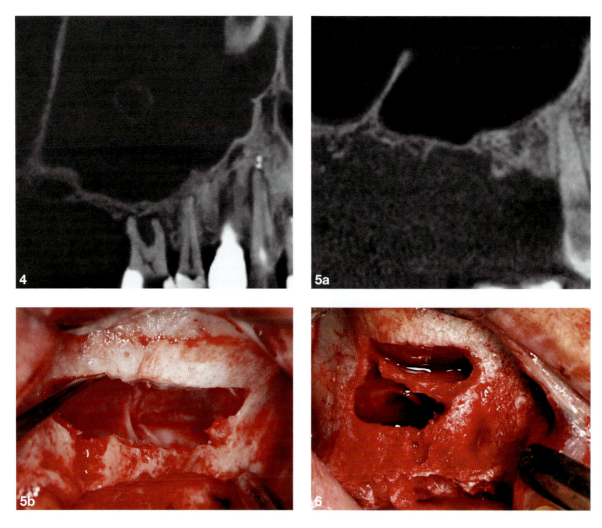

Fig 4 *Diffuse opacity of the right maxillary sinus. In the center is a rounded, more radiopaque structure, suggestive of chronic sinusitis with a fungal superinfection.* **Fig 5** *(a) A septa in the right maxillary sinus. (b) A buccomedial septa.* **Fig 6** *A septa parallel to the sinus floor in the mesiodistal direction.*

procedure in these cases, two separate bony windows must be created, and the two cavities must be treated as if they were single maxillary sinuses of reduced size.

The presence of incomplete septa can make elevation of the membrane very tortuous, increasing the risk of tears. Septa must also be assessed carefully in cases of sinus elevation via a crestal approach. A septa that is located exactly at the point where the crestal osteotomy is to be prepared may result in the formation of two separate small osteotomies and difficulties in lifting the membrane with the graft. The septum will, however, contribute to primary implant stability.

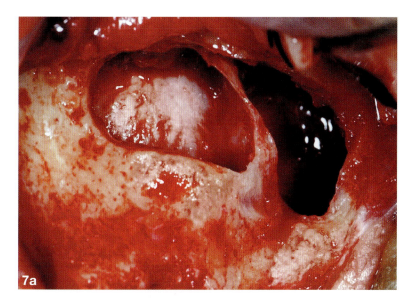

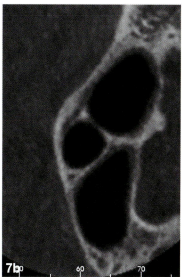

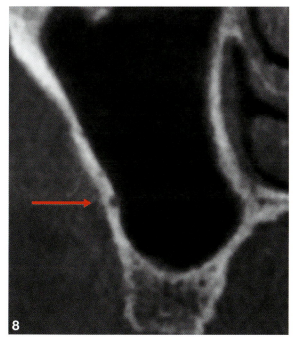

Fig 7 (a) *A single complete septum dividing the sinus cavity into two compartments.* (b) *Axial CBCT image showing the presence of multiple septa compartmentalizing the right sinus into multiple cavities.* *Fig 8* *Cross-section of a CBCT showing a small vascular structure on the lateral wall of the sinus: the alveolar antral artery (arrow).*

Alveolar antral artery

CBCT examination must also be used to assess for the presence of an arterial vessel on the lateral wall of the sinus—the alveolar antral artery, which is formed by anastomosis between the dental branch of the posterosuperior maxillary artery and the circumflex artery, itself a branch of the infraorbital artery (see chapter 2). The alveolar antral artery normally runs about 20 mm from the crestal plane, but this distance can be significantly affected by crestal atrophy. It may run extraosseously, attached to the sinus membrane, or intraosseously. It is generally single and of small caliber **(Fig 8)**, but in rare cases, it may have a large caliber **(Fig 9)** or be multiple **(Fig 10)**. In most cases, the caliber of this vessel is minimal and, if severed, will not result in excessive bleeding.

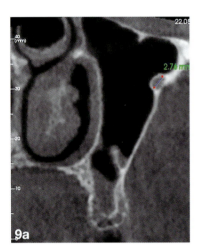
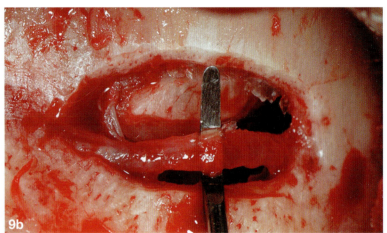

Fig 9 (a) *Cross-section of a CBCT showing an alveolar antral artery of considerable caliber on the lateral sinus wall.* (b) *An alveolar antral artery of considerable diameter isolated from the bone window.*

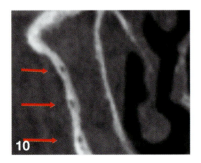
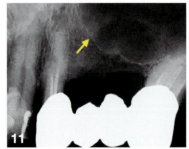
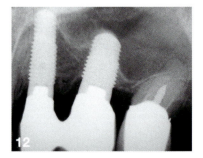

Fig 10 Cross-section of a CBCT showing the unusual presence of three alveolar antral arteries on the lateral sinus wall (arrows). *Fig 11* Failure of the mesial abutment of this prosthesis required implant rehabilitation. In the edentulous zone, the maxillary sinus had a strong inclination, greater than 45 degrees (yellow arrow). *Fig 12* Control radiograph 3 years after implant therapy showing crestal elevation that resulted in a sufficient amount of bone.

INDICATIONS FOR CHOOSING A CRESTAL OR LATERAL TECHNIQUE

The lateral and crestal approaches for sinus elevation are two alternative procedures, and in many cases, the selection of a procedure is left to clinician preference.

There are, however, specific conditions in which one technique is preferable to the other. The main factors to consider when deciding which technique to use are described here.[4]

Residual alveolar ridge height

In the presence of at least 3.5 to 4 mm of residual alveolar ridge height, data from the literature report a higher survival rate (96.3%) of implants that are placed at the same time as crestal elevation with osteotomes.[5,6] In cases of reduced vertical bone height, such that primary implant stability would be compromised, a two-stage technique (a first stage for the elevation procedure and a second stage for implant placement) with a lateral approach is preferable.

Inclination of the sinus floor

Inclined sinus floors are far from rare and are encountered mainly in the area of the mesial recess. An especially oblique sinus floor is not an absolute contraindication to sinus elevation, and a useful trick is to slightly tilt the osteotomy preparation axis so as to approach the sinus floor as perpendicularly as possible (**Figs 11 and 12**).

Multiple implants

When several implants must be placed in the same sector, the crestal technique can be unnecessarily time-consuming and complex, with the procedure being repeated for each surgical site. It is therefore more practical to opt for a lateral approach.

Sinus width

Until very recently, the height of the residual alveolar ridge was considered the only useful parameter for the choice of technique. However, it has recently been shown that sinus width also plays a very important role. A sinus can be classified as either narrow or wide by using CT imaging to measure the distance between the buccal wall and the medial wall of the sinus 10 mm apical to the alveolar crest (**Fig 13**). If the width is less than 12 mm, the sinus is considered narrow. A measurement between 12 and 15 mm denotes a medium sinus, and a measurement greater than 15 mm denotes a wide sinus.

It has been pointed out that the crestal approach is more predictable with more viable bone formation in narrow sinuses rather than in wide sinues.[7] Another study confirmed this observation by demonstrating histologically that 6 months after crestal elevation, in the presence of less than 5 mm of native bone, the proportion of viable bone was no more than 3% in wide sinuses, whereas in narrow sinuses, the proportion of viable bone was 36%.

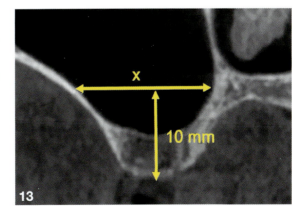

Fig 13 *In accordance with the literature, the sinus width is measured as the distance between the buccal and medial walls of the sinus at a height of 10 mm, including the height of the residual ridge.*

Thus, in the presence of atrophic ridges (< 5 mm) and a wide sinus, a crestal approach is contra-indicated.[8]

In cases of extremely atrophic ridges and narrow sinus anatomy, a two-stage crestal approach may be a viable option as an alternative to the lateral approach.

In light of these observations, a very recent publication proposes the use of a decision tree to guide the choice of either a crestal or lateral approach and whether to perform the procedure in one or two steps.

This is dependant on the height of the residual bone and the width of the maxillary sinus: "narrow" if < 12 mm, and "wide" if > 12 mm **(Fig 14)**.[9]

CRESTAL APPROACH TO SINUS ELEVATION

The crestal approach to sinus elevation is less invasive than the lateral window technique, but does not allow for direct visualization, meaning the clinicians must rely on tactile sensation to confirm the correct progress of the procedure.

The crestal technique involves performing an osteotomy through the residual bone ridge to the sinus membrane without damaging or perforating the membrane.

The membrane is lifted by gently inserting a well-hydrated graft material. A single-stage procedure can be performed if the height of the residual

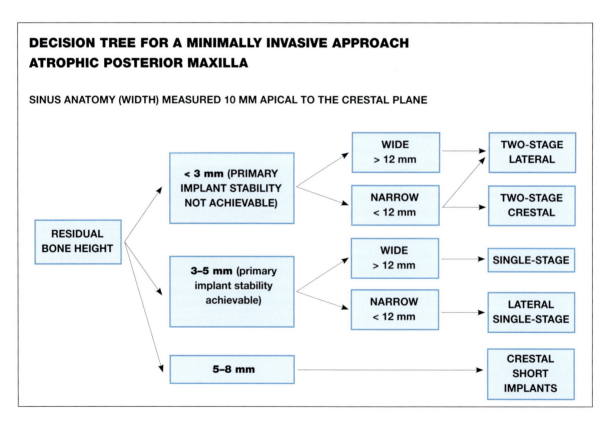

DECISION TREE FOR A MINIMALLY INVASIVE APPROACH ATROPHIC POSTERIOR MAXILLA

SINUS ANATOMY (WIDTH) MEASURED 10 MM APICAL TO THE CRESTAL PLANE

RESIDUAL BONE HEIGHT

< 3 mm (PRIMARY IMPLANT STABILITY NOT ACHIEVABLE) → WIDE > 12 mm → TWO-STAGE LATERAL
NARROW < 12 mm → TWO-STAGE CRESTAL

3–5 mm (primary implant stability achievable) → WIDE > 12 mm → SINGLE-STAGE
NARROW < 12 mm → LATERAL SINGLE-STAGE

5–8 mm → CRESTAL SHORT IMPLANTS

Fig 14 *Decision tree for selecting a sinus elevation technique according to the height of the residual bone and the width of the maxillary sinus.*

bone (3–4 mm) allows for sufficient primary implant stability (30 Ncm), or a two-stage technique can be performed by postponing implant placement until 6 months after grafting.

History of the crestal technique

The first publication documenting a crestal sinus elevation technique belongs to Summers, who in 1994, described the possibility of raising the sinus membrane with osteotomes to create a greenstick fracture in the cortical of the sinus floor coinciding with the future implant site.[10]

Then, by pushing the fractured piece of bone apically, the sinus membrane can be progressively raised, obtaining a space for bone regeneration to take place.

In later years, this expansive-compaction technique based on the use of osteotomes was supplanted by ablative-subtractive techniques, based on the use of either special drills used sequentially[6] or dedicated inserts for ultrasonic or sonic systems. Because these latter techniques do not require percussion instruments, they are perceived by the patient to be less traumatic and invasive.[11]

Surgical procedure with sequential drills

Devised by Dr Cosci in the 1980s, the technique described in this section is based on the sequential use of burs equipped with depth stops and was the first sequential method for crestal elevation. It is an erosive technique that allows for the progressive and complete preparation of the bone up to the sinus cortical without damaging the sinus membrane.

The technique can be divided into four stages:
1. Sinus access
2. Detachment of the sinus membrane
3. Grafting the biomaterial
4. Positioning the implant

Sinus access

After a full-thickness flap is performed, an initial osteotomy is created with a pilot drill in the area where the implant is to be inserted, then the site is enlarged with an intermediate drill until a diameter of 3 mm is obtained.

These first two sharp burs, equipped with depth stops, have a length of 3 mm, so there is no risk of perforating the membrane at this stage (the technique being limited to ridges with at least 5 mm of residual native bone).

Burs with a flat apex are then used to progressively erode the remaining bone.

The cutting angles are suitably rounded so that the bone is slowly removed without the risk of tearing the membrane if there is direct contact with it. These drills are also equipped with depth stops. The burs are used in a progressive sequence, increasing the working depth at each pass by 1 mm without ever losing control of the instrument in the apical direction until the sinus membrane is exposed.

Once the sequential osteotomy phase has been completed, the integrity of the membrane can be confirmed with a rounded probe to gently feel its elastic resistance. In some cases, it is also possible to visually verify the integrity of the membrane (Fig 15).

Detachment of the sinus membrane

Before inserting the grafting biomaterial, it is useful to insert a few fragments of collagen sponge well soaked in saline into the osteotomy, which will allow for uniform pressure on the membrane and reduce the risk of tearing. By pushing the collagen sponges apically with a rounded instrument, the sinus membrane will begin to peel away from the bony cortical, facilitating the creation of a space for the insertion of the biomaterial. This creates a kind of airbag that protects the membrane from subsequent contact with biomaterial particles that could cause small perforations.

An interesting alternative is the use of highly colla- genized, reduced-grain gel grafts, which are inject- ed directly through the osteotomy and dislodge the membrane safely and effectively **(Figs 16)**.

Grafting the biomaterial

The biomaterial is inserted through the osteotomy with a rounded instrument in limited increments to gently and progressively elevate the membrane.

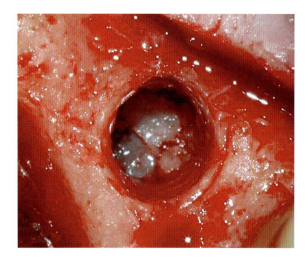

Fig 15 *Occlusal view of a crestal elevation proce- dure in which the intact sinus membrane is directly visible.*

The material of choice is deproteinized bovine bone (DBBM). Abundant hydration is important because it allows the membrane to be lifted with evenly distributed pressure, according to Pascal's law. After the first injections of biomaterial, an intra- operative radiograph is recommended to confirm the formation of a regular dome-shaped elevation with sinus membrane integrity **(Fig 17)**.

In the case of membrane perforation, the biomat- erial will appear irregularly distributed and partially dispersed in the sinus **(Fig 18)**.

Membrane perforation necessitates the interrup- tion of the procedure to avoid further intrasinus dispersion of biomaterial, which could lead to for- eign body sinusitis. It is highly recommended to use a grafting biomaterial with a small grain size (0.25–1 mm) because, in the event of accidental dispersion into the sinus, the particles can be more easily drained and eliminated by the physiologic ciliary movement of the sinus epithelium through the osteomeatal complex.

Positioning the implant

Implants with a diameter of 3.75 to 4 mm can be inserted directly into the osteotomy created with crestal elevation drills that have a diameter of 3.1 mm.

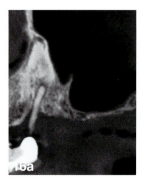 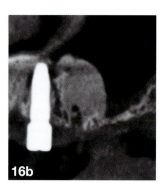 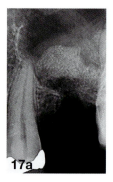 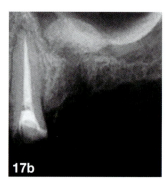

Fig 16 *Crestal elevation performed with a preheated gel graft. (a) Preoperative image. (b) Postoper- ative image. Note how the fluid material passed through the present septum without any problems.*
Fig 17 *Intraoperative radiographs showing the raising of the sinus membrane with the biomaterial. The regular dome shape indicates the integrity of the membrane.*

Underpreparation is essential to achieve adequate primary implant stability. If the procedure was performed correctly, radiography will show an implant surrounded by a regular dome of biomaterial in the apical portion **(Figs 19 to 21)**.

Graft remodeling and waiting times

Once the crestal sinus elevation has been performed, regardless of whether a one- or two-stage procedure is being performed, it is necessary to determine the waiting time for allowing the graft to integrate with the newly formed bone. In the case of a minimal crestal elevation (3–4 mm) when the basal bone proportion is 5 to 6 mm, the waiting time is slightly longer than that for physiologic osseointegration—6 months maximum. After major crestal elevations with reduced residual basal bone, waiting time must allow for the osseointegration of the implant in both the minimal residual native bone and the newly formed bone—7 to 9 months. Even in the two-stage approach, the waiting time before placing the implants should not be less than 7 months.

A radiographic sign of successful sinus elevation is the disappearance of the previous sinus floor cortical and the formation of a new one apical to the implant. The absence of new bone and a new cortical indicates that the elevation procedure was unsuccessful.

Complications

Complications with crestal elevation surgery are generally less common than with a lateral elevation. The survival of implants placed at the same time as crestal elevation is comparable to that reported for implants placed in native bone (about 95%).[20] This is true even in the presence of less than 5 mm of residual bone.[6–12] The main complications include perforation of the sinus membrane **(Fig 22)** with consequent leakage of graft biomaterial within the sinus and insufficient primary implant stability, which can lead to penetration of the implant within the sinus.

In the event of a membrane perforation, if there is less than 4 to 5 mm of residual bone height, the procedure should be aborted and repeated after approximately 2 months. Alternatively, a lateral sinus elevation procedure can be performed immediately if care is taken to start by elevating the membrane in an area away from the perforation. In this way, the membrane loses tension, and the perforation tends to collapse spontaneously. In these cases, it is necessary to close the perforation with a collagen membrane before inserting the biomaterial to avoid the risk of biomaterial leakage into the sinus.

In the presence of at least 5 to 6 mm of residual bone height, an implant of the same length or just exceeding it can still be inserted. In fact, it has been shown that it is possible to insert an implant that penetrates no more than 1 to 2 mm into the sinus in the presence of a perforated membrane because the portion of the implant that protrudes into the sinus is then regularly covered by both the membrane and a thin layer of bone.[13] A very recent study has shown that implant survival in these cases is comparable to that in which the crestal elevation procedure has been performed correctly.[14]

A lack of primary implant stability does not necessarily entail failure of the procedure, but a larger diameter implant must be inserted. If an implant becomes accidentally dislodged inside the sinus, it is essential to extract it immediately with a Cadwell-Luc-type lateral window.

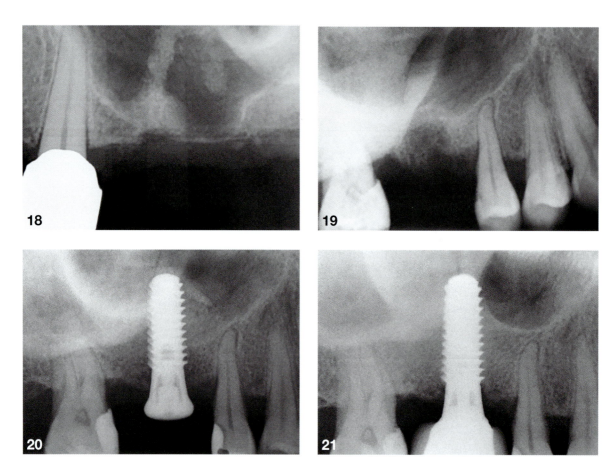

Fig 18 Intraoperative radiograph revealing a perforation of the sinus membrane. Elevation of the membrane by the biomaterial appears irregular, and dispersion of the biomaterial within the sinus is noticeable. The procedure must be aborted in this case. **Fig 19** Preoperative radiograph. **Fig 20** Postoperative radiograph showing the biomaterial around the apical portion of the implant. **Fig 21** Radiograph 8 years after implant insertion, showing the new sinus cortical, including the regenerated bone volume.

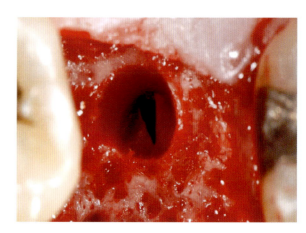

Fig 22 Membrane perforation that occurred during a crestal sinus elevation.

CLINICAL CASE 1

Single-stage crestal sinus elevation in the site of the maxillary left first and second molars

This case illustrates a frequent clinical situation in which limited residual bone height (4–5 mm) poses a problem between selecting either a crestal or lateral approach to sinus elevation. In these cases, careful evaluation of the sinus anatomy is important to verify whether one is dealing with a narrow or wide sinus[7–9] **(see Figs 13 and 14)**. A 67-year-old patient presented with an abscess in the maxillary left first molar caused by a root fracture **(Fig 23)**. The second molar had been extracted many years earlier. After antibiotic treatment, the first molar was extracted, and an alveolar ridge preservation procedure was performed to maintain bone volume **(Fig 24)**. About 6 months later, CBCT showed good bone volume maintenance in the extraction area, with a residual bone height of about 5 mm in the sites of the first and second molars, as well as narrow sinus anatomy **(Fig 25)**, which led to the decision to perform sinus elevation with a crestal approach.

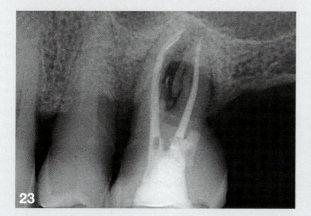
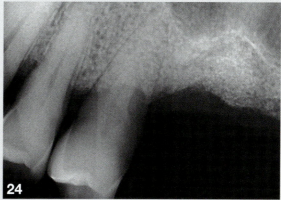

Fig 23 Following an abscess episode, a root fracture is evident. **Fig 24** Alveolar ridge preservation performed with nanocrystalline hydroxyapatite (HA) (control at 3 months).

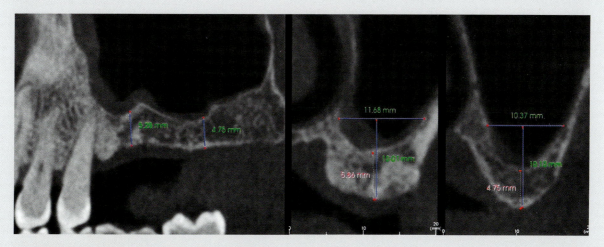

Fig 25 Preoperative CBCT showing a residual bone height of 4 to 5 mm and narrow sinus anatomy (< 12 mm) at the sites of the maxillary left first and second molars.

Both osteotomies were performed with dedicated sequential drills according to Cosci's technique, and once the integrity of the sinus membrane was verified with a Valsalva maneuver, collagen sponges were placed first to protect the membrane and then synthetic nanohydroxyapatite biomaterial was inserted (**Fig 26**). Next, the two implants were inserted into the residual bone of about 5 mm, which allowed for sufficient primary stability (**Fig 27**).

Postoperative CBCT confirmed the integrity of the sinus membrane around both implant apices, which appeared to be surrounded by a sufficient amount of biomaterial (**Fig 28**). Implant uncovering was performed after approximately 5 months of submerged healing. After 1 month, the implants were restored with two zirconium-ceramic crowns. The follow-up CBCT about 3 years after loading confirmed the stability of the bone levels and the regeneration obtained with the sinus elevation, revealing the formation of a new cortical above the implant apices (**Fig 29**).

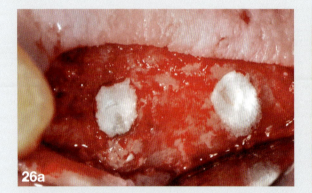
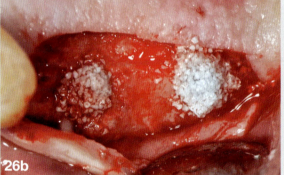

Fig 26 Sinus elevation, performed through crestal osteotomies, with the placement of collagen sponges *(a)*, followed by nanocrystalline HA *(b)*.

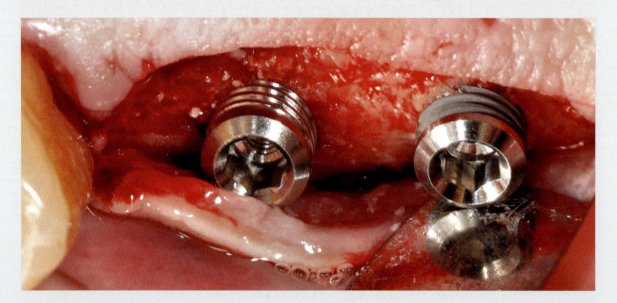

Fig 27 The two implants almost completely inserted.

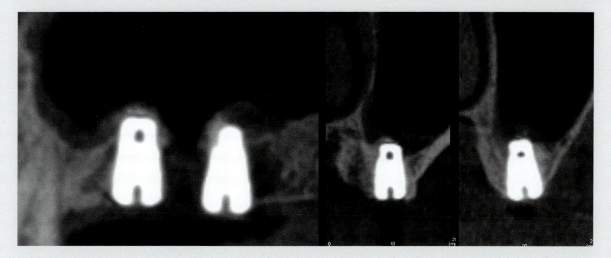

Fig 28 Postoperative CBCT showing that the sinus membrane has been correctly raised and is intact at both sites.

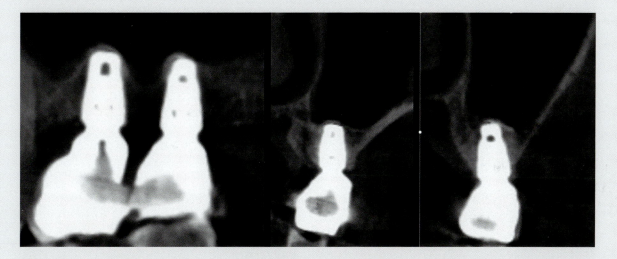

Fig 29 The control CBCT about 3 years after loading shows good bone regeneration in the crestal rise area and the formation of a new cortical above the implant apices.

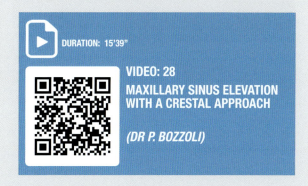

DURATION: 15'39"

VIDEO: 28
MAXILLARY SINUS ELEVATION WITH A CRESTAL APPROACH

(DR P. BOZZOLI)

SINUS ELEVATION WITH A LATERAL APPROACH

This technique was introduced into clinical practice in the 1980s by Boyne and James[15] and by Tatum[16] as a modification of Caldwell-Luc's sinus revision surgery, with the difference being that the lateral approach is performed without damaging the sinus membrane.

Surgical technique
Locoregional anesthesia

The area is anaesthetized locally (articaine 4%, with adrenalin 1:100,000) by slowly infiltrating subperiosteally at the level of the fornix on both the buccal and palatal sides. To ensure a deeper action of the anesthetic, it may be useful to infiltrate deeply into the buccal area distal to the tuber to block the posterosuperior alveolar nerve and in the area of the second premolar to block the infraorbital nerve.

Flap design

The flap is designed by making a crestal incision in the keratinized mucosa and two divergent vertical incisions: one mesial incision, which will vary according to the extent of the sinus, and one distal incision at the level of the maxillary tuberosity. In the presence of natural teeth, a paramarginal incision is recommended. The flap is elevated to full thickness while maintaining the integrity of the periosteum as much as possible **(Figs 30 and 31)**.

Performing the bone window

Remaining natural teeth can be very useful as a reference point for calculating the appropriate measurements on radiographs. In the presence of a thin buccal wall, the sinus area can be identified by its bluish color, due to the underlying membrane. Another useful feature is the thick convex profile of the lateral sinus wall **(Fig 32)**.

The shape of the bone window must be adapted to the shape of the sinus floor and not have sharp

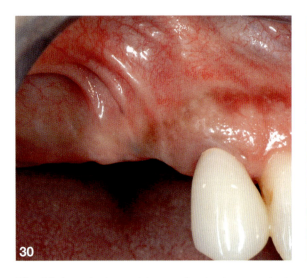
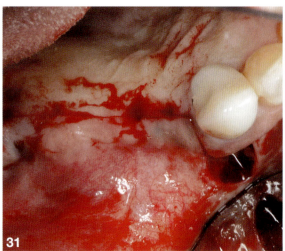

Fig 30 *A patient requiring an implant-supported restoration for the first sextant in the presence of an expanded maxillary sinus.* **Fig 31** *Crestal incision with vertical divergent incisions. The mesial incision is paramarginal, and the distal incision is at the level of the tuberosity.*

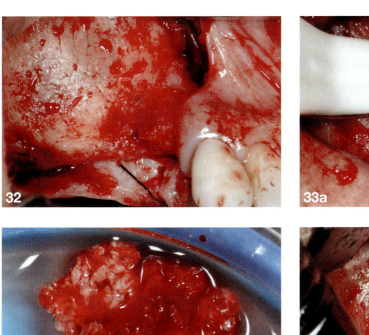
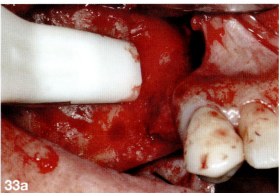
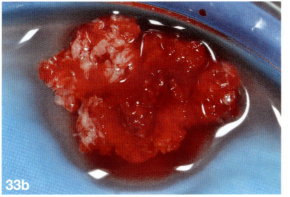
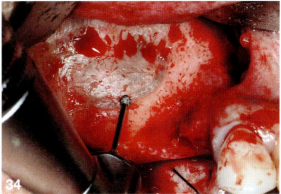

Fig 32 After elevation of the full-thickness flap, the convexity and bluish transparency at the maxillary sinus is evident. *Fig 33* The lateral wall of the sinus is thinned with a bone scraper (a) to collect autologous particulate bone (b). *Fig 34* The antrostomy is performed with a 1.4-mm-diameter diamond bur, adapting it to the shape of the sinus floor.

edges. It must also be of adequate size, extending up to the mesial recess, to reduce the risk of tearing the membrane due to difficult access. If the thickness of the lateral sinus wall is considerable (> 2 mm), it can be thinned to make the osteotomy easier.

Thinning can be performed with manual bone scrapers **(Fig 33a)**, making it possible to harvest a good quantity of autologous bone **(Fig 33b)** to be mixed with DBBM. The antrostomy can be performed with rotary, ultrasonic, or sonic instruments.

In case of the former, a straight handpiece or a multiplier contra-angle with diamond burs, 1.4 to 2 mm in diameter **(Fig 34)**, is used under copious irrigation with saline solution.

Burs that are too small should be avoided to have a good bearing surface and to avoid falling inside the sinus and perforating the membrane. In ablative, sonic or ultrasonic systems, even small-diameter diamond ball inserts can be used.

The choice of the type of instrument to be used is clinician-dependent.

However, the literature shows a double incidence of perforations in cases where rotary instruments are used compared to piezoelectric or manual bone scraper systems.[17]

Bone window size

The size of the bone window may vary depending on the number and length of the planned implants, the presence of septa, the course of the alveolar antral artery, and the experience of the clinician. As clinicians gain confidence, they can reduce the size of the window to ensure a better vascular supply to the graft.

The window is usually about 20 mm in the mesio-distal direction and about 10 mm in the cranio-caudal direction. The lower profile of the window should match the profile of the sinus floor, remaining approximately 3 mm apical to it to have a containing shape for the graft.

Sinus membrane elevation

Once the bone window is complete, the sinus membrane can be visualized, and its integrity and characteristics can be assessed (Fig 35). If it appears grayish-white, it is usually thick and strong, whereas if it is bluish-gray, it is likely to be very thin

and more at risk for tearing. Clinical studies confirm that membranes with thicknesses < 1.5 mm are much more likely to be perforated.[18]

Before proceeding with membrane elevation, it is important to smooth any rough or sharp osteotomy edges. The sinus membrane elevation phase begins with gentle percussion at the bone window to dislodge it inward by fracturing the last remnants of circumferential bone.

The cleavage plane between the membrane and the inner sinus wall is then found with a Kramer-Nevins curette **(Fig 36)**. The bone window can be retained and displaced within the sinus or removed. A fundamental requirement to avoid tearing the membrane is that any instrument that is used should be kept firmly in contact with the bone plane to avoid putting pressure on the membrane where it is not adhered to the bone. As a rule, four blunt manual periosteal elevators are used.

Generally, the partial elevation at the floor of the sinus is done first, proceeding with mesiodistal movements until reaching the medial wall **(Fig 37a)**. In this way, the area of the mesial recess is reached with the membrane already free of tension, reducing the risk of tearing. Subsequently, elevation is continued with mesiodistal

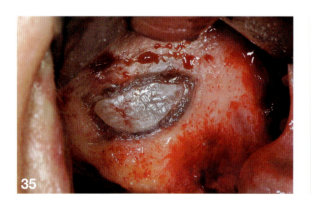
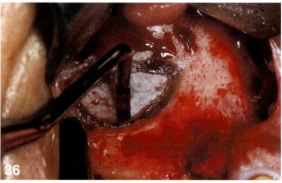

Fig 35 The bone window has been completed, and the sinus membrane appears perfectly intact.
Fig 36 With a Kramer-Nevins curette, the bone window is pushed inward, and the cleavage plane between the mucosa and the inner sinus wall is found.

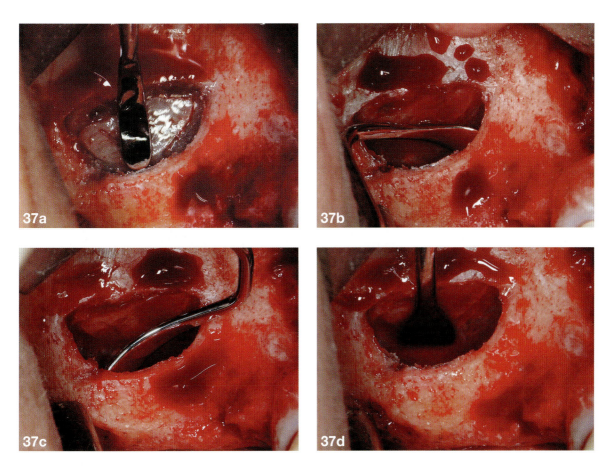

Fig 37 (a) *With a blunt instrument, the floor of the sinus is elevated in the medial direction with mesiodistal movements. The mucosa is elevated with blunt instruments in the mesial (b), distal (c), and medial (d) directions.*

movements **(Figs 37b and 37c)** in the cranial direction of the medial or palatal wall **(Fig 37d)**. Correct exposure of this wall will result in a very wide surface exposure that will ensure good vascularization of the graft. In the event that the palatal wall is not sufficiently exposed, a cul-de-sac membrane recess may form, which may lead to incomplete bone regeneration and partial re-pneumatization of the sinus.

During elevation, it is useful to check the movement of the membrane with the patient breathing, although this sign is not an absolute guarantee of its integrity.

Preparation of the implant sites

Each implant site must be prepared before inserting the graft. Dedicated piezoelectric drills or inserts can be used, with a Pritchard periosteal elevator used to protect the membrane from accidental contact with the preparation drills. To achieve adequate primary implant stability, considerable underpreparation (at least 1 mm) is always necessary. For example, preparation with 2.8-mm-diameter drills is performed for 3.75- to 4-mm-diameter implants. Slightly conical implant designs with self-tapping apices are recommended to facilitate insertion in heavily underprepared sites, and a hybrid surface to facilitate bone apposition apically, in the graft area.[19] When preparing the site, it is advisable to leave sufficient buccal thickness to avoid fracturing the ridge during implant insertion **(Fig 38)**.

Insertion of grafting material

After being hydrated with saline, the graft material should be placed in the subantral space created by elevation of the membrane.

The first areas to be grafted are the least accessible, so it is advisable to start by placing the material in the mesial recess, in the distal recess, and in the palatal wall area, making sure to bring the graft into contact with the bone wall. If no implant placement is planned at the same time, the material is then inserted in the floor area until reaching the buccal wall **(Fig 39)**.

In the case of single-stage surgery, after placing the graft material mesially, distally, and medially, the implants are inserted, and lastly, the filling is completed buccal to the implants themselves until the lateral wall is reached **(Fig 40)**.

Choosing a grafting material

Based on systematic reviews of the literature, two important data emerge. The first relates to the quality of the newly formed bone. Autologous bone provides the highest percentage of viable bone and the lowest proportion of residual graft,[20] which does not, however, translate into a higher

percentage of implant survival. On the contrary, studies show that implants placed using only heterologous grafting material (DBBM) show the highest long-term survival rates (96%) compared to cases where only autologous graft was used (85%). Mixing autologous bone with heterologous grafts does not seem to improve the results.[21] The studies also show that after 4.5 months of healing, the percentage of newly formed bone is still very low, so it is advisable to wait at least 7 to 8 months for augmentations performed in situations of extreme atrophy.[20]

Suturing

Once the grafting has been completed, the bone flap is repositioned if it had been removed, and the window area is protected with a resorbable collagen membrane **(Fig 41)**. Although the usefulness of the membrane is still unclear, some studies show higher rates of vital bone and better implant survival when it is used.[22]

The sutures must reposition the flap passively, but release incisions to the periosteum are generally not necessary unless horizontal or vertical regeneration techniques have been performed simultaneously.

The first suture repositions the mesial angle formed by the union of the crestal incision with the mesial vertical incision.

Then suturing at the crest is continued with horizontal mattress sutures interspersed with simple interrupted sutures, completing the closure of the releasing incisions with other simple interrupted sutures **(Fig 42)**. Sutures are usually removed after 10 to 12 days.

Healing times

In the case of a two-stage lateral sinus elevation, the waiting time before placing the implants should never be less than 7 to 8 months to allow time for the graft to integrate into the newly formed bone.

DURATION: 34'38"

VIDEO: 29
MAXILLARY SINUS ELEVATION WITH THE SUCTION OF CYSTIC FLUID

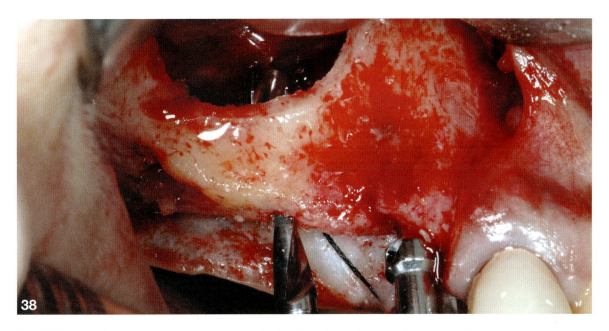

Fig 38 The implant sites are prepared prior to the insertion of the particulate graft.

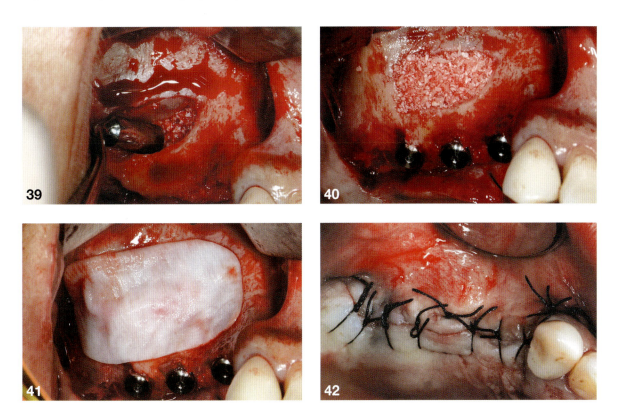

Fig 39 The graft material is first gently placed in the mesial, medial, and distal recesses with a special obturator. *Fig 40* The implants were inserted and graft material was added up to the lateral sinus wall. *Fig 41* The bone window is protected with a resorbable collagen membrane. *Fig 42* Suturing was executed with 4-0 horizontal mattress silk sutures interspersed with simple sutures.

Because they are largely inserted into newly formed bone, which is often of poor quality and vitality, implants should be left submerged and unloaded for at least 4 months.

In the case of sinus elevation with simultaneous implant placement, waiting times are related to the amount of residual bone and graft material but must never be less than 7 to 8 months. In the case of totally or partially edentulous patients, removable prostheses should not be used in the presence of sutures to avoid the risk of wound dehiscence.

Prostheses that have been properly unloaded and relined with soft materials can be returned to the patients after 2 weeks.

Complications

Both intraoperative and postoperative complications can occur after a sinus elevation procedure with lateral access.

Intraoperative complications

The most frequent complication (15.7% of cases)[17] of sinus elevation with lateral access is perforation/laceration of the sinus membrane. Generally, the procedure should not be aborted when the membrane is perforated.

Instead, once the perforation has been identified, it is recommended to close it immediately with a resorbable collagen patch and to continue to elevate the membrane along the surrounding areas to reduce tension. In this way, perforations and small tears tend to resolve spontaneously **(Figs 43)**. In the case of larger lacerations, an attempt can be made to suture the laceration with very fine resorbable material or to suture the membrane to the lateral bone wall by drilling a series of small holes **(Fig 44)**.

Both of these solutions are far from simple and are dependent on the skills of the clinician. An alternative is to harvest an autologous bone block from the mandibular ramus to be fixed with transcrestal osteosynthesis screws to the sinus floor **(Fig 45)**. This procedure avoids the dispersion of particulate material within the sinus but involves increased morbidity due to the opening of a second operation site for bone harvesting.

Another intraoperative complication, albeit rare (0.4% of cases) and rarely serious, is bleeding caused by accidental severance of the alveolar antral artery during window preparation. Generally, crushing the bone canal with a Klemmer or using a bipolar electrocoagulator or bone wax is sufficient to achieve hemostasis. Another possibility, in the rare case of a particularly large artery, is to isolate the severed vessel by gently removing the bone upstream of the area of interruption and ligating it with resorbable suture **(vd Fig 9b)**.

A third intraoperative complication may be the dispersion of the particulate graft within the sinus cavity.

This may occur as a consequence of unidentified perforations during membrane elevation or very vigorous compaction that tears the membrane. Generally, the dispersed biomaterial is eliminated via the osteomeatal complex without further consequences, and intervention is necessary only in cases of massive biomaterial dispersion or subsequent infectious complications.

Early postoperative complications

Early postoperative complications include suture dehiscence with the consequent leakage of biomaterial and contamination of the graft through the bone window.

In these cases, the patient must be carefully monitored, and if the clinical and radiographic evaluation indicate infection, treatment for acute sinusitis must be performed. The most serious early complication is the onset of acute sinusitis in the first few days after surgery, even if the immediate postoperative CBCT showed no abnormalities **(Fig 46a)**.

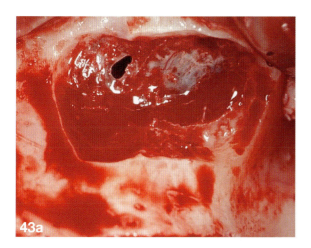

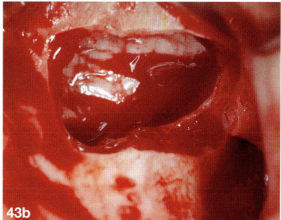

Fig 43 (A) *Small perforation of the sinus membrane that occurred during an osteotomy of the lateral sinus wall.* (b) *The perforation was protected with a resorbable collagen membrane before debridement was continued.*

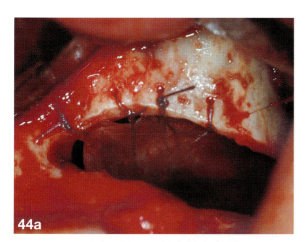

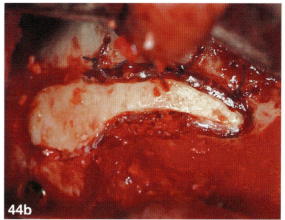

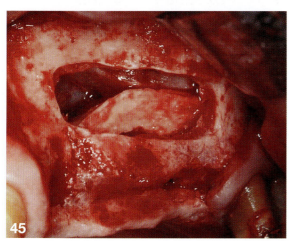

Fig 44 (a) *Significant tear in the sinus membrane during the elevation phase. Small holes were drilled into the lateral sinus wall, and the membrane margin was sutured.* (b) *Autologous and heterologous graft material were gently inserted, and the original bone flap was repositioned to close the antrostomy.* *Fig 45* *Due to a major tear in the sinus membrane, a block of autologous bone harvested from the mandibular ascending ramus was secured to the sinus floor with two osteosynthesis screws.*

F. Bernardello • P. Bozzoli • L. Ferrantino • M. Simion

The diagnosis is made on the basis of dull and diffuse pain symptoms, the presence of mucopurulent discharge from the ipsilateral nostril, and obvious signs of inflammation or fistulae in the buccal mucosa **(Fig 46b)**. CBCT always shows opacification of the ipsilateral sinus cavity **(Figs 46c and 46d)**. Therapy consists of immediate antibiotic prescription and sinus revision surgery. A full-thickness flap is elevated and, with several rinses with hydrogen peroxide and antibiotics, all granulation tissue outside and inside the sinus is removed **(Fig 47)**. All

previously inserted graft material must also be removed with an alveolar spoon without injuring the sinus membrane, which is usually thickened. Finally, a prolonged wash with hydrogen peroxide is performed while simultaneously aspirating the inside of the sinus **(Fig 48)**, and sutures are applied **(Fig 49)**. Successful healing is evidenced by the disappearance of pain symptoms, the absence of signs of inflammation, and the radiographic finding of a drastic reduction of the opacification of the sinus cavity after 3 months **(Fig 50)**.

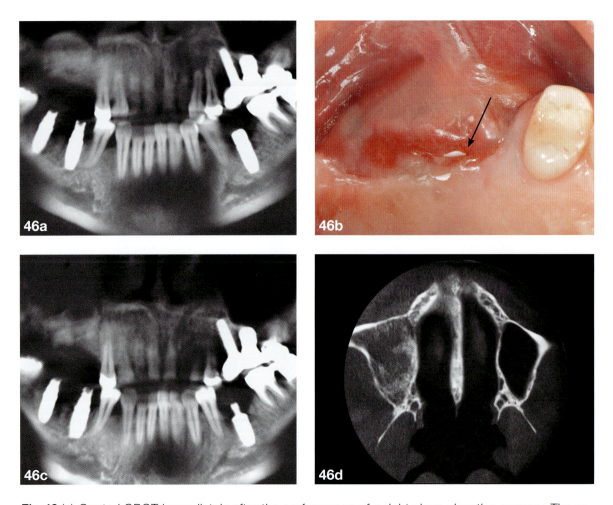

Fig 46 (a) *Control CBCT immediately after the performance of a right sinus elevation surgery. The operation was free of intraoperative complications, the mucosa appeared normal, and the sinus cavity seemed completely pervious. (b) After 20 days of healing, the mucosa appears inflamed and a fistula (arrow) with serum-purulent exudate is present. (c) CBCT shows complete opacification of the right sinus. (d) Axial view.*

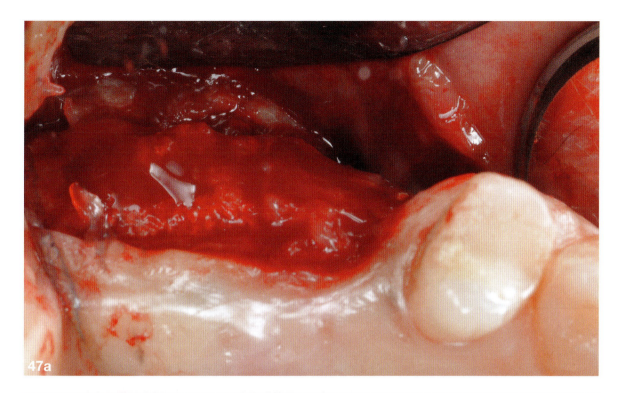

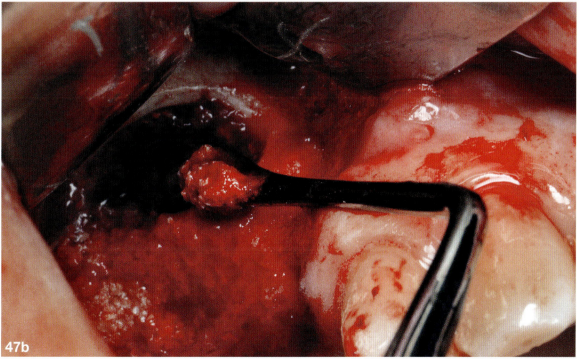

Fig 47 (a) *A full-thickness flap was peeled back to perform a complete sinus revision procedure. Abundant inflammatory tissue is evident.* (b) *All granulation tissue was removed, and the sinus cavity was gently debrided of all biomaterial with an alveolar spoon and copious rinsing with hydrogen peroxide and saline.*

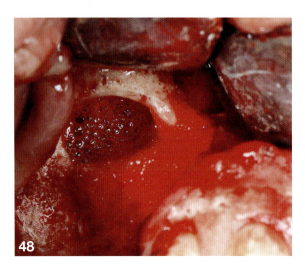

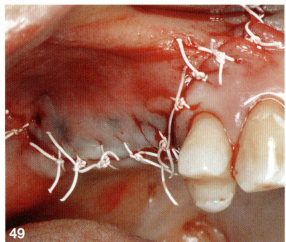

Fig 48 *A final wash is performed, alternating a bacteriostatic (tetracycline) and hydrogen peroxide while simultaneously aspirating fluid from inside the sinus.* **Fig 49** *Finally, the flap is sutured with simple sutures.*

Fig 50 *After 3 months, a significant reduction in the sinus infiltrate is evident, a sign that, combined with the absence of symptoms, indicates ongoing healing. (a) Panoramic image. (b) Cross-sectional image.*

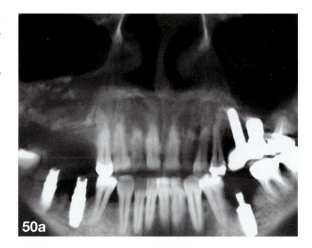

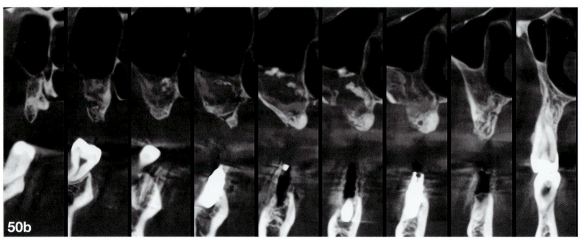

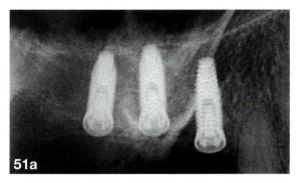

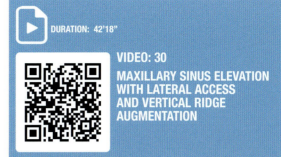

DURATION: 42'18"

VIDEO: 30
MAXILLARY SINUS ELEVATION
WITH LATERAL ACCESS
AND VERTICAL RIDGE
AUGMENTATION

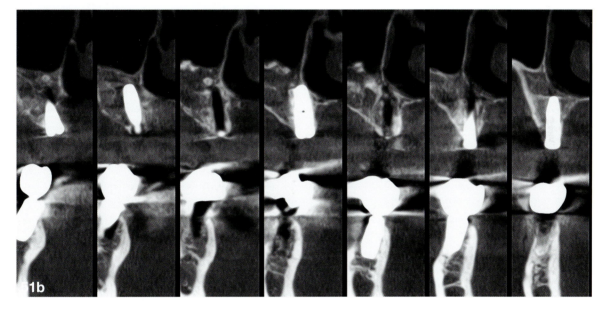

Fig 51 (a) *It was still possible to insert three hybrid implants with additional crestal access 7 months after the first operation.* (b) *CBCT 4 months after implant placement before the second surgical step. The peri-implant bone tissue appears sufficiently mature.*

In many cases, it is still possible to place implants with a crestal augmentation technique after 7 to 8 months because a certain amount of new bone forms even without grafting, thanks to the action of the blood clot **(Fig 51)**.

Late postoperative complications

A rare late complication that only becomes apparent at the time of implant placement after 6 to 9 months is the failure of the bone regeneration process in the absence of infectious complications. This is caused by poor-quality grafting biomaterial, which is why it is always advisable to use products with extensive scientific documentation supporting their efficacy.

In these cases, the grafting material appears encased in a kind of fibrous tissue, and the only solution is to remove it completely and then perform a new sinus elevation procedure after 2 months.

REFERENCES

1. Van der Weijden F, Dell'acqua F, Slot DE. Alveolar bone dimensional changes of post-extraction sockets in humans: A systematic review. J Clin Periodontol 2009;36:1048–1058.

2. Cardaropoli G, Araùjo M, Lindhe J. Dynamics of bone tissue formation in tooth extraction sites an experimental study in dogs. J Clin Periodontol 2003;30:809–818.

3. Krennmair G, Ulm CW, Lugmayr H, Solar P. The incidence, location, and height of maxillary sinus septa in the edentulous and dentate maxilla. J Oral Maxillofac Surg 1999;57:667–671.

4. Starch-Jensen T, Jensen JD. Maxillary sinus floor augmentation: A review of selected treatment modalities. J Oral Maxillofac Res 2017;8:e3.

5. Pjetursson BE, Rast C, Brägger U, Schmidlin K, Zwahlen M, Lang NP. Maxillary sinus floor elevation using the (transalveolar) osteotome technique with or without grafting material. Part I: Implant survival and patients' perception. Clin Oral Implants Res 2009;20:667–676.

6. Bernardello F, Righi D, Cosci F, Bozzoli P, Soardi CM, Spinato S. Crestal sinus lift with sequential drills and simultaneous implant placement in sites with <5 mm of native bone: A multicenter retrospective study. Implant Dent 2011;20:439–444.

7. Spinato S, Bernardello F, Galindo-Moreno P, Zaffe D. Maxillary sinus augmentation by crestal access: A retrospective study on cavity size and outcome correlation. Clin Oral Implants Res 2015;26: 1375–1382.

8. Stacchi C, Lombardi T, Ottonelli R, Berton F, Perinetti G, Traini T. New bone formation after transcrestal sinus floor elevation was influenced by sinus cavity dimensions: A prospective histologic and histomorphometric study. Clin Oral Implants Res 2018;29:465-479.

9. Stacchi C, Spinato S, Lombardi T, et al. Minimally invasive management of implant-supported rehabilitation in the posterior maxilla. Part II. Surgical techniques and decision tree. Int J Periodontics Restorative 2020;40:e95–e102.

10. Summers RB. A new concept in maxillary implant surgery: The osteotome technique. Compend Contin Educ Dent 1994;15:152–160.

11. Esposito M, Cannizzaro G, Barausse C, Cosci F, Soardi E, Felice P. Cosci versus summers technique for crestal sinus lift: 3-year results from a randomised controlled trial. Eur J Oral Implantol 2014;7:129–137.

12. Soardi E, Cosci F, Checchi V, Pellegrino G, Bozzoli P, Felice P. Radiographic analysis of a transalveolar sinus-lift technique: A multipractice retrospective study with a mean follow-up of 5 years. J Periodontol 2013;84:1039–1047.

13. Schwarz L, Schiebel V, Hof M, Ulm C, Watzek G, Pommer B. Risk factors of membrane perforation and postoperative complications in sinus floor elevation surgery: Review of 407 augmentation procedures. J Oral Maxillofac Surg 2015;73:1275–1282.

14. Ragucci GM, Elnayef B, Suárez-López del Amo F, Wang H-L, Hernández-Alfaro F, Gargallo-Albiol, J. Influence of exposing dental implants into the sinus cavity on survival and complications rate: A systematic review. Int J Implant Dent 2019;5:1–9.

15. Boyne P, James RA. Grafting of the maxillary sinus floor with autogenous marrow and bone. J Oral Surg 1980;38:613–616.

16. Tatum H Jr. Maxillary and sinus implant reconstructions. Dent Clin North Am 1986;30:207–229.

17. Stacchi C, Andolsek F, Berton F, Perinetti G, Navarra CO, Di Lenarda R. Intraoperative complications during sinus floor elevation with lateral approach: A systematic review. Int J Oral Maxillofac Implants 2017;32: 107–118.

18. Cho SC, Wallace SS, Froum SJ, Tarnow DP. Influence of anatomy on schneiderian membrane perforations during sinus elevation surgery: Three-dimensional analysis. Pract Proced Aesthet Dent 2001;13:160–163.

19. Trisi P, Marcato C, Todisco M. Bone-to-implant apposition with machined and MTX microtextured implant surfaces in human sinus grafts. Int J Periodontics Restorative Dent 2003;23:427–437.

20. Danesh-Sani SA, Engebretson SP, Janal MN. Histomorphometric results of different grafting materials and effect of healing time on bone maturation after sinus floor augmentation: A systematic review and meta-analysis. J Periodontal Res 2017;52:301–312.

21. Del Fabbro M, Wallace SS, Testori T. Long-term implant survival in the grafted maxillary sinus: A systematic review. Int J Periodontics Restorative Dent 2013;33:773–783.

22. Tawil G, Mawla M. Sinus floor elevation using a bovine bone mineral (Bio-Oss) with or without the concomitant use of a bilayered collagen barrier (Bio-Gide): A clinical report of immediate and delayed implant placement. Int J Oral Maxillofac Implants 2001;16:713–721.

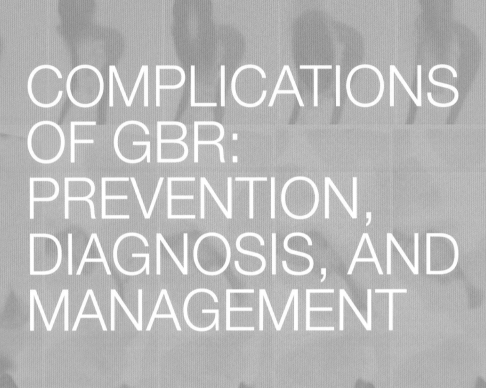

COMPLICATIONS OF GBR: PREVENTION, DIAGNOSIS, AND MANAGEMENT

CHAPTER 22

Edited by Massimo Simion e Filippo Fontana

INTRODUCTION

Today, guided bone regeneration (GBR) remains the most effective tool for treating atrophic alveolar ridges and peri-implant defects. The results of GBR, however, have the disadvantage of being extremely sensitive to the skill and experience of the clinician. The surgical protocol for GBR was established after countless studies in the early 1990s,[1-4] and the slightest deviation from these standards inevitably leads to the development of complications that may partially or totally prevent bone regeneration.

Numerous studies have shown that nonresorbable polytetrafluorethylene (PTFE) membranes must remain submerged beneath the mucosa for a minimum period of 6 months, and in some cases up to 9 months, to allow time for osteogenic cells to migrate into the defect.[5-6] If a membrane is exposed to the oral cavity early, the amount of bone regeneration is drastically reduced, as has been demonstrated by both experimental studies on animals[7-8] and clinical investigations in humans.[6,9-12] The consequences of wound dehiscence resulting in membrane exposure may be minor (such as removal of the membrane and reduced bone regeneration) or major (such as the development of abscesses, total failure of the regenerative procedure, loss of implants, and patient suffering).[9-12]

The incidence of complications with nonresorbable membranes varies considerably depending on the studies considered, the techniques used, and clinician experience. A systematic review of the literature on vertical ridge augmentations with GBR

GBR techniques are not very difficult to perform, but they do not forgive even the slightest clinician error. Surgical steps fine-tuned over a period of 30 years must be performed scrupulously to avoid complications that are disastrous to the success of the operation.

Massimo Simion

by Rocchietta et al[2] considered a range of complications with incidences between 0 and 45.5%. In clinical cases treated in the 1990s, Buser et al[13] reported a 2.5% incidence of early membrane exposure in horizontal augmentation procedures, whereas Tinti et al[14] and Simion et al[15] reported complication incidences of 16 and 17%, respectively, in vertical augmentations.

Further along the learning curve, complications decreased but still remained at around 10% for early membrane exposures and postoperative infections.[4,16–17]

CLASSIFICATION OF GBR COMPLICATIONS

In 2007, Verardi and Simion[18] presented a proposal for the management of GBR complications, but the definitive classification with treatment modalities was published by Fontana et al[19] in 2011, which proposes a classification with treatment modalities based on more than 20 years of clinical experience. Complications can be related to surgery (flap damage, neurologic complications, vascular complications) or occur during the healing period.

Surgical complications

Periosteal releasing incisions at the buccal and lingual flaps to achieve tension-free flap closure are fundamental for all GBR techniques. As reported in numerous studies,[1,4,11–14] the release of the buccal flap is performed by means of a superficial and continuous incision of the periosteum, whereas the lingual flap is released by simply reflecting it slightly beyond the insertion of the mylohyoid muscle. These maneuvers can lead to both flap and neurologic/vascular damage (see chapter 9).

Flap damage

An incision that is too deep or too coronal can compromise the integrity of the flap. Excessive thinning or perforation of the flap compromises vascularization and causes marginal flap necrosis. The resulting early exposure of the membrane can result in failure of the regenerative procedure.

Neurologic complications

Neurologic complications involve injury to the mental nerve in the mandible and the infraorbital nerve in the maxilla. Injuries may be direct, from incision or incorrect use of the scalpel, or indirect, from stretching of the nerve with periosteal elevators or retractors.

Vascular complications

The most serious vascular complications are edema or hemorrhages in the sublingual space. This is a very delicate area between the mylohyoid muscle, the mandibular body, and the geniohyoid and genioglossus muscles, and it contains important anatomical structures, including the sublingual artery (a branch of the lingual artery), the mylohyoid artery (a branch of the inferior lingual artery), the lingual nerve, the submandibular duct, the sublingual gland, and some extrinsic muscle fibers of the tongue (see chapter 2). Injury to these structures can cause very serious complications, so it is imperative to be fully aware of the topographic anatomy of the area and the correct flap elevation and releasing procedures.

Complications during the healing period

Four classes of complications can occur during the healing period:
- **Class I:** small membrane exposures (< 3 mm) without purulent exudate
- **Class II:** large membrane exposures (> 3 mm) without purulent exudate
- **Class II:** membrane exposure with purulent exudate
- **Class IV:** abscess without exposure of the membrane

Class I membrane exposure

Class I membrane exposure consists of a small soft tissue fenestration that usually occurs within the first few days of healing and shows no exudate secretion upon gentle digital compression of the surrounding area. Little information exists on the treatment of this complication. An in vitro study[19] showed that when exposed to semipermeable expanded PTFE (ePTFE) membranes, bacteria take about 3 to 4 weeks to cross the membrane tissue and infect regenerating tissue. In dense PTFE (dPTFE) membranes, which are not permeable, bacteria take approximately the same amount of time to make their way along the membrane surface and infect deep tissue.

Based on this information and clinical experience, the exposed membrane should not be removed immediately, but left in place for up to 1 month to allow for some maturation of the regenerating tissue. Nevertheless, it is essential to establish a strict disinfection regimen, with cleansing of the exposed area twice a day with single-tuft brushes soaked in 0.2% chlorhexidine gel for 1 minute. The patient should be monitored at least once a week to identify any purulent exudate or initial infectious processes at an early stage. In rare cases, small, noninfected fenestrations can be closed by removing the exposed portion of membrane and placing a connective tissue graft harvested from the palate. In cases of late exposures, the membrane can be removed with a traditional or flapless technique.

Class II membrane exposure

Class II membrane exposure is a clinical situation in which more than 3 mm of the membrane is exposed without purulent exudate. Despite the absence of infection, the membrane must be removed immediately due to the high risk of bacterial contamination of the tissue that is being regenerated. In these cases, the bone graft is not yet infected with bacteria, so it must not be touched. After removal of the membrane, the site must be disinfected with antibiotics (eg, tetracycline), and the flaps must be sutured with complete coverage of the underlying tissue to achieve healing by primary intention.

Class III membrane exposure

Any form of membrane exposure, whether it is small or large, is categorized as a class III exposure if it is associated with serous or purulent exudate. The infected membrane must be removed immediately because every day that it remains in situ further compromises the possibility of regeneration. In such cases, infected graft particles and inflammatory tissue should also be removed gently with curettes, and the site should be disinfected with 10% hydrogen peroxide and antibiotics. If this adverse event occurs within the first month of healing after the GBR procedure, the chances of retaining part of the graft are slim, and generally, bone regeneration is virtually nil. Before planning a second regenerative intervention, it is necessary to wait at least 2 to 3 months for the soft tissue to heal and mature completely.

CLINICAL CASE 1

Treatment of early class I membranes exposure

A 43-year-old, nonsmoking patient underwent vertical GBR surgery at the sites of the maxillary right central and lateral incisors. After 1 month of healing, the operation site showed a small membrane exposure along the suture line **(Fig 1a)**. The margins of the exposure showed no signs of inflammation, and no serous or purulent discharge was evident with two-finger palpation.

A small flap was elevated without vertical incisions to expose the crestal surface of the membrane **(Fig 1b)**. A portion of the membrane extending 3 mm beyond the exposed portion was incised and removed with a periosteal elevator **(Fig 1c)**. To protect the tissue that was being regenerated and to compensate for any lack of vertical dimension, a connective tissue graft was harvested from the palate and placed in an L shape on the crestal surface **(Fig 1d)**. After releasing the buccal flap with a periosteal incision, a horizontal mattress suture and simple sutures were applied **(Fig 1e)**.

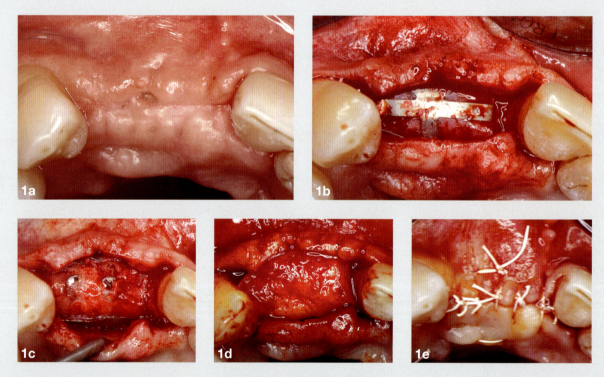

Fig 1 *(a)* A small exposure of the ePTFE membrane 1 month after a regenerative procedure. *(b)* A full-thickness flap is used to isolate the PTFE membrane. *(c)* The portion of the membrane exposed to the oral cavity, along with a few extra millimeters, are cut and removed. *(d)* A connective tissue graft is harvested from the palate and placed as a barrier to protect the underlying regenerating tissue. *(e)* The buccal and palatal flaps are closed with a double suture line.

CLINICAL CASE 2

Treatment of early class II membrane exposure

A 35-year-old, nonsmoking patient was treated with vertical ridge elevation with a nonresorbable, titanium-reinforced membrane in the sites of the maxillary right central and lateral incisors. Healing occurred without any adverse events, but after 5 months, exposure of a membrane margin occurred (**Fig 2a**). The margins of the dehiscence showed moderate inflammation but no serous secretion. However, exposure of the membrane margins results in rapid bacterial colonization of its deep surface and impairment of the regenerated bone.

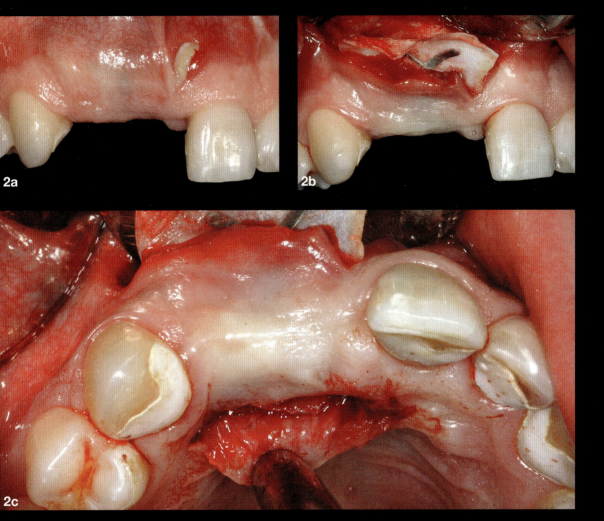

Fig 2 *(a)* Small Class II membrane exposure after 5 months of submerged healing. Because this is an esthetic area, removal of the membrane using a flapless tunnel technique is indicated. *(b)* Horizontal incisions were made in the fornix and palate at the level of the fixation pins. *(c)* The pins were removed, and the membrane was separated from the surrounding tissues with a periosteum elevator and pulled out in one piece from the buccal side.

Given the long submergence time, it was decided to completely remove the membrane without opening a flap to avoid exposing the regenerated tissue. Two horizontal incisions were made: one in the vestibular fornix and one in the palate (**Fig 2b**), the fixation screws were removed, and the membrane was removed in one piece with help of a periosteal elevator (**Fig 2c**). The regenerated tissue was not touched because it appeared mature and free of inflammation (**Fig 3a**). The wound was sutured with simple silk sutures (**Fig 3b**), and healing occurred without any additional adverse events (**Fig 3c**). After another 2 months of healing, the prosthetic abutments were connected. The periapical radiograph showed complete regeneration of the crestal bone (**Fig 3d**).

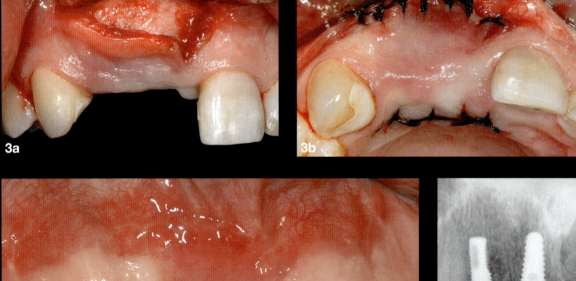

Fig 3 *(a)* The regenerated tissue under the membrane appears mature and free of inflammation. *(b)* The buccal and palatal incisions are closed with simple sutures. *(c)* Healing occurred without complications. After 2 months, the healing abutments will be connected. *(d)* Radiograph after connection of the healing abutments. Bone regeneration was not affected.

CLINICAL CASE 3

Treatment of early class III membranes exposure

A 34-year-old, nonsmoking patient in good health suffered a serious car accident that resulted in fracture of the viscerocranium and the loss of the maxillary right lateral incisor, left central incisor, left lateral incisor, and left canine. An autologous bone block graft harvested from the mandibular ascending ramus had been used to reconstruct the alveolar process to reduce and stabilize the fracture. The patient presented with a severe vertical and horizontal bone deficit in the span from the maxillary left central incisor to left canine, fibrotic mucosa with diffuse scarring, epithelial invaginations, and palatine fissures **(Fig 4a)**. CBCT showed two large vertical bone defects, with the distal one extending almost to the base of the left pyriform opening. The block graft appeared to be almost completely resorbed **(Figs 4b to 4d)**.

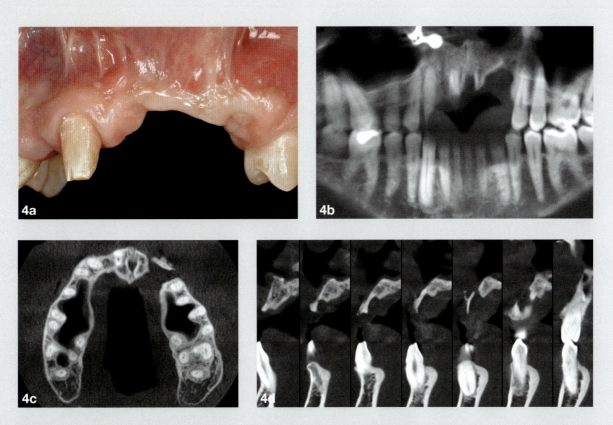

Fig 4 *(a)* Clinical image showing the severe vertical and horizontal bone defect from the site of the maxillary left central incisor to the site of the left canine. The mucosa appears disfigured by scarring and epithelial invaginations. *(b)* CBCT showing a severe vertical bone defect approaching the left nasal cavity. *(c)* Axial view showing the extent of the defect, which appears complete in the buccopalatal direction. A residue of the block bone graft appears almost completely resorbed. *(d)* Cross-sectional view of the same area.

After making a full-thickness crestal incision with two vertical incisions distal to the adjacent elements, full-thickness flaps were reflected buccally and palatally to expose the defect (**Figs 5a and 5b**). Two support screws were placed vertically, and then a titanium-reinforced ePTFE membrane was placed to protect a particulate graft containing 70% autologous bone and 30% deproteinized bovine bone (DBBM) (**Fig 5c**).

The membrane was secured with four titanium pins (**Fig 5d**). The release of the buccal flap was particularly complex because the mucosa was extremely fibrotic and rigid throughout. Traditional closure with horizontal mattress and simple interrupted sutures presented a considerable challenge due to the excessive stiffness of the tissues and the presence of palatine fissures with epithelial invaginations (**Fig 6a**).

After 15 days of healing there was extensive wound dehiscence with class III exposure of the membrane. Palpation caused serous discharge from the edges of the exposure, a clear sign of infection (**Fig 6b**).

After the administration of a systemic antibiotic, a flap was immediately elevated, and the membrane was removed. The most superficial graft particles appeared yellowish, were mobile, and were

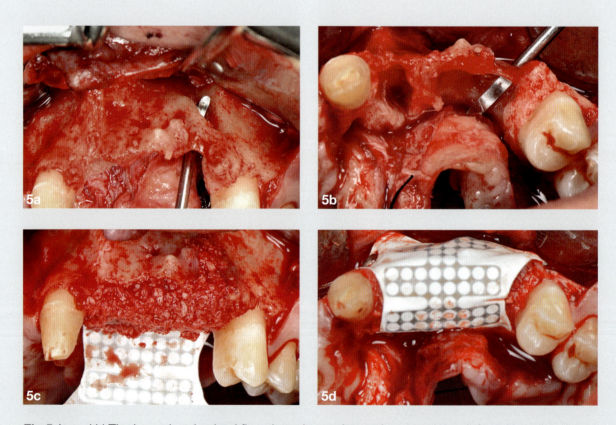

Fig 5 *(a and b)* The buccal and palatal flaps have been elevated to reveal the defect. Note the almost complete resorption of the previous block graft. *(c)* An ePTFE membrane was secured palatally, and a particulate graft of 70% autologous bone and 30% DBBM was placed. *(d)* The membrane was secured buccally with titanium pins.

evidently contaminated **(Fig 6c)**, so they were removed to a depth of about 3 mm, until an area with a more compact and bleeding fibrin clot was revealed. The area was then disinfected with 5% hydrogen peroxide and a tetracycline solution. The buccal flap was released again with a periosteal incision, a resorbable collagen membrane was placed **(Fig 6d),** and the flap was sutured **(Fig 6e)**. After 3 months of healing, the site showed a very large vertical residual defect, a sign of total failure of the regenerative technique **(Fig 6f)**.

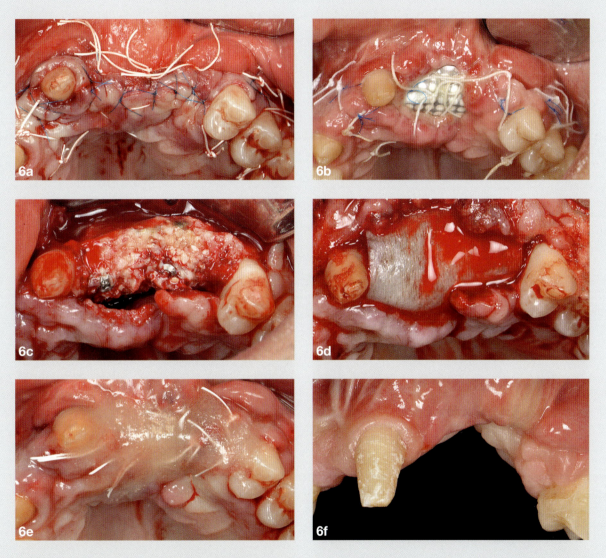

Fig 6 *(a)* After flap release, horizontal mattress and simple sutures were applied. *(b)* Extensive class III membrane exposure after 15 days. A serous exudate can be seen at the edges of the dehiscence. *(c)* After removal of the membrane, bacterial contamination of the graft is evident. *(d)* After removal of the infected particles and disinfection of the site, a resorbable collagen membrane was placed. *(e)* The flaps were sutured, and an antiseptic gel with hyaluronic acid was applied. *(f)* Deep vertical defect remaining 3 months after removal of the infected membrane.

Two full-thickness flaps were elevated again, revealing a vertical defect similar to the one at baseline and minimal horizontal regeneration (**Fig 7a**). The regenerative technique was then repeated with a resorbable porcine collagen membrane to reduce the risk of further exposure. The membrane was secured over an autologous and heterologous (70%/30%) particulate graft, with numerous palatal and buccal titanium pins (**Figs 7b and 7c**). Healing occurred without further complications, but numerous scars remained in the mucosa (**Fig 7d**).

After 3 months, an epithelial-connective tissue graft harvested from the palate was placed (**Figs 8 and 9**), significantly improving the quality of the mucosa (**Fig 10**).

After another 3 months, a full-thickness flap was elevated. The bone ridge appeared significantly improved in terms of horizontal dimension, but a modest vertical bone deficit remained (**Figs 11 and 12**). Therefore, two implants were placed in the sites of the maxillary left central incisor and canine (**Fig 13a**), and a GBR technique with a resorbable membrane was repeated (**Figs 13 and 14**). The postoperative CBCT showed adequate filling with graft material and correct implant positioning (**Figs 15 and 16**).

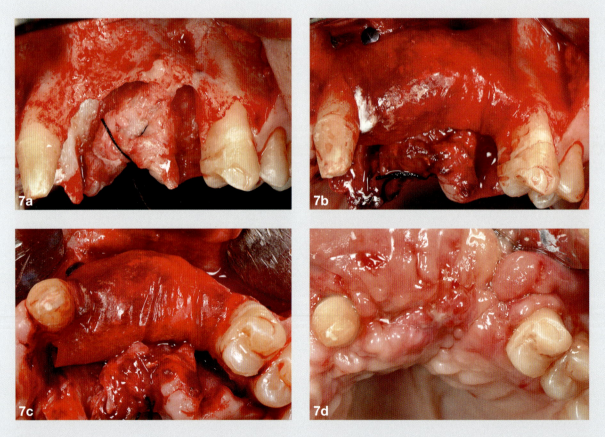

Fig 7 *(a)* Buccal view of the bone ridge. *(b)* A resorbable collagen membrane was placed to protect an autologous and heterologous (70% / 30%) particulate graft. *(c)* Occlusal view. *(d)* Healing after 15 days. At the time of suture removal, deep scars are visible.

The submergence period of the implants lasted 4 months (**Fig 17**), then a soft tissue punch was used to connect the provisional abutments (**Fig 18**). After 1 week, a new implant-supported provisional was placed (**Fig 19**). Due to the severe lack of keratinized mucosa, it was decided to again prepare a partial-thickness recipient site to receive a free gingival graft harvested from the palate (**Fig 20**). The epithelial-connective tissue graft was sutured with simple and sling sutures anchored to the periosteum (Vicryl 6-0 [Ethicon]) (**Fig 21**). After 15 days of healing, the sutures were removed, and the superficial epithelial layers of the graft were gently excised (**Fig 22**). After 6 months, the final ceramic prosthesis was placed (**Fig 23**).

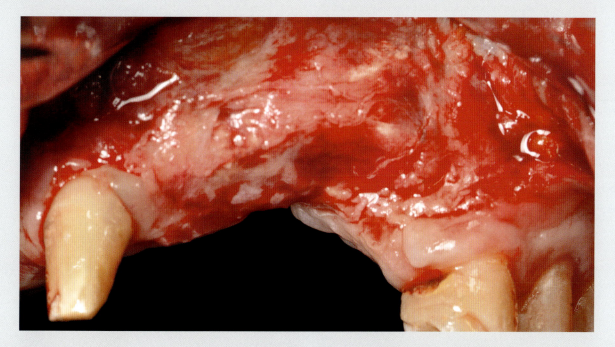

Fig 8 Preparation of the partial-thickness recipient site for an epithelial-connective tissue graft.

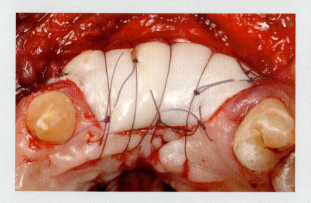

Fig 9 The graft was positioned and stabilized with simple and suspended sutures.

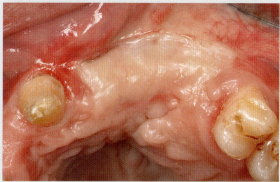

Fig 10 Graft healing after 3 months.

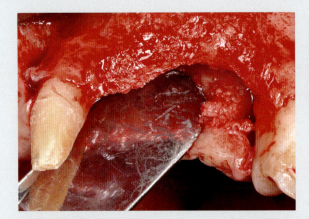

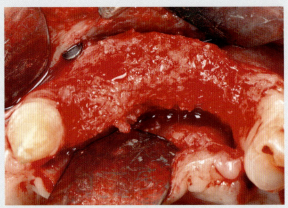

Fig 11 The alveolar ridge after 6 months of healing. Sufficient horizontal bone regeneration can be observed.

Fig 12 Buccal view showing a residual vertical bone deficit.

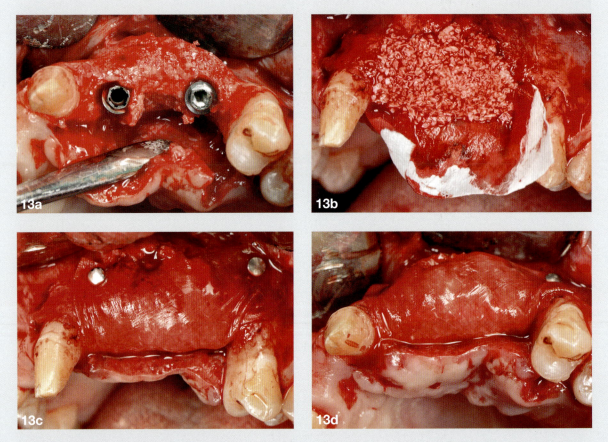

Fig 13 *(a)* Two hybrid implants were placed in the sites of the maxillary left central incisor and canine. *(b)* An additional 70%/30% composite particle graft was placed and covered with a resorbable collagen membrane. *(c)* Buccal view. *(d)* Palatal view.

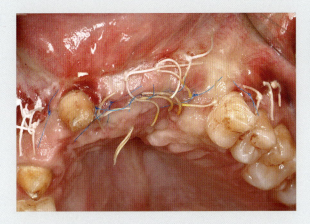

Fig 14 The site was sutured, and healing occurred without further complications.

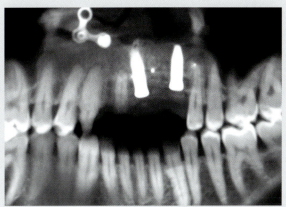

Fig 15 CBCT showing correct implant positioning.

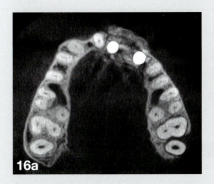

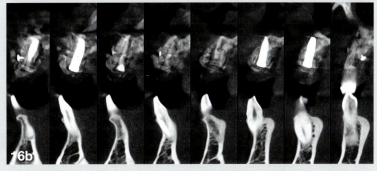

Fig 16 *(a)* Axial image showing a sufficient amount of graft buccal and palatal to the implants. *(b)* Cross-sectional view.

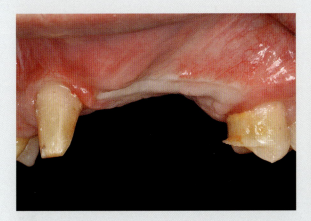

Fig 17 Tissue healing after 4 months. Notice the lack of keratinized mucosa and adherent gingiva on the right central incisor.

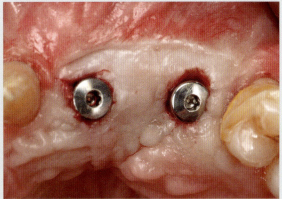

Fig 18 Connection of the healing abutments after use of a soft tissue punch.

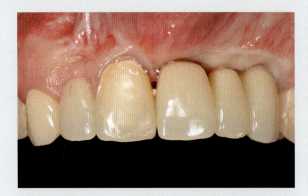

Fig 19 Provisional implant-supported prosthesis.

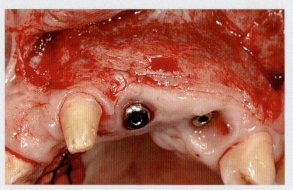

Fig 20 Preparation of the recipient site for a free gingival graft using a partial-thickness flap.

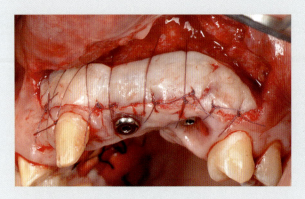

Fig 21 Epithelial-connective tissue graft harvested from the palate and sutured with sling and simple interrupted sutures in Vicryl 6-0.

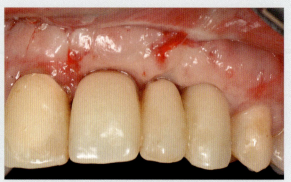

Fig 22 The sutures were removed, as well as the superficial epithelial layers.

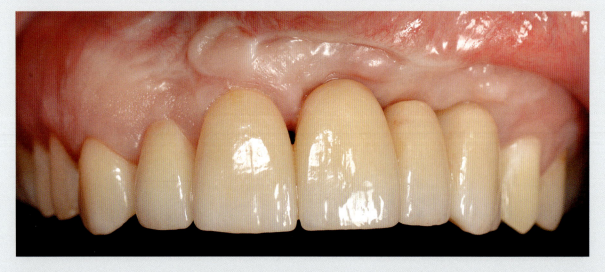

Fig 23 Definitive ceramic prosthesis delivered 6 months later. The epithelial-connective tissue graft has acquired a keratinization and color similar to the harvest site in the palate.

Class IV abscess infection

Class IV abscess infection is perhaps the most serious complication and is characterized by the development of an abscess without exposure of the membrane. It usually occurs during the first month of healing.

A biphasic course of the swelling is characteristic. The surgical site regularly deflates 10 to 15 days after surgery, but after an additional 10 to 15 days, it swells due to purulent collection.

Draining fistulas may be present. Infection is due to either contamination of the graft during harvesting or contamination of the PTFE membrane during handling.

Infected adjacent dental elements, such as mesially inclined third molars or ill-fitting prosthetic crowns also predispose the regenerating area to infection.

After antibiotic therapy is administered to the patient, the site must be reopened immediately, with the membrane and graft completely removed and the area disinfected with 5% to 10% hydrogen peroxide and antibiotics (**Fig 24**). If the removal of the infected membrane is delayed by even a few days, there is a risk of losing not only the graft but also part of the native basal bone.

COMPLICATION PREVENTION

Complications with GBR techniques can be very frequent if proper patient selection and preparation protocols are not strictly followed. The treatment of complications is often difficult, with incomplete regeneration of bone tissue, so prevention is crucial to the success of therapy.

Complications can be traced back to well-known factors associated with the following aspects of treatment:

- Patient preparation
- Quality of the soft tissue
- Surgical technique
- Provisional prosthesis management

Patient preparation

Infectious complications are caused by contamination of the membrane or graft material during surgery, so it is essential to reduce the bacterial load in the patient's oral cavity as much as possible. Prior to surgery, patients must undergo intensive causal therapy, whether or not periodontal pathology is present. Rinses with 0.2% chlorhexidine should be prescribed starting 3 days before surgery, along with antibiotic therapy with amoxicillin and clavulanic acid (1 g twice a day) starting 1 hour before surgery and continuing for 7 days after surgery. Mesially inclined third molars adjacent to the treatment area must be extracted before surgery, and any ill-fitting prostheses with overhanging margins must be replaced. In the case of periodontal patients, periodontitis must be treated prior to regenerative surgery.

Surgery must take place under aseptic conditions with sterile drapes, gloves, and instruments. The perioral skin must be cleansed with gauze soaked in disinfectant, and immediately before surgery, the patient must perform a 1-minute rinse with 0.2% chlorhexidine. During surgery, the surgeon and assistant must change their gloves for new, sterile ones before handling the membrane and grafts.

Soft tissue quality

Many early membrane exposures are caused by the presence of scarring or clefts in the mucosa that are secondary to trauma or tooth avulsions. After an avulsion, it is essential to wait for a healing period of at least 2 months to achieve sufficient soft tissue maturation before proceeding with surgery. An incompletely healed extraction site is a sure cause of marginal flap necrosis and consequent membrane exposure.

Compressive pontic elements, whether they are part of the provisional or permanent prosthesis, also create decubitus in the mucosa that predisposes a site to marginal necrosis in the immediate postoperative period. Thus, prosthetic elements must be reduced at least 15 days before surgery so that they do not touch the mucosal surface.

Surgical technique

It is important to release the flap with periosteal incisions to achieve tension-free closure. Most early membrane exposures are caused by flaps that are too rigid and sutures that are too tight and strangle the flaps, causing necrosis of the margins. Correct suture removal is also crucial and should be performed only after thorough cleaning of sutures with gauze soaked in 0.2% chlorhexidine gel for 3 minutes. Mattress sutures must be removed completely by cutting only one of the two ends inside the knot and pulling out all the thread running

inside the flaps. Residual sutures below the flaps, and in contact with the membrane, are a sure source of infection.

Provisional prosthesis management

Flap necrosis frequently occurs due to compression caused by provisional prostheses during the early stages of healing. Mucosal-supported prostheses should not be used because it is impossible to effectively control their resilience and they tend to compress the soft tissue above the membrane, causing dehiscence. Only fixed, resin-bonded provisionals should be used, with shortened pontic elements that they do not touch the mucosal surface. Provisionals should be delivered after 1 week, when the postoperative edema, which peaks on the third or fourth day, tends to recede.

CLINICAL CASE 4

Treatment of class IV abscess infection

A 50-year-old patient who smoked 10 cigarettes per day was treated for an atrophic distal alveolar ridge. Healing occurred without early exposure of the nonresorbable, titanium-reinforced membrane, but after 30 days, the patient presented with swelling at the surgical site and a fistula in the site of the mandibular right third molar. The mucosa was inflamed and edematous, and on palpation, a floating abscess collection was evident **(Fig 24a)**.

A mucoperiosteal flap was reflected, and the ePTFE membrane appeared to be nonintegrated and mobile **(Fig 24b)**. The membrane was removed, revealing contaminated yellowish and mobile graft material **(Fig 24c)**. Disinfection of the site was performed by aspirating all the mobile graft material, gently curetting the site until denser, more stable tissue was found, and irrigating with hydrogen peroxide and tetracycline **(Fig 24d)**. The flaps were then sutured, and after 3 months of healing, the operation had to be repeated. The cause of the infection was the presence of a post and core with ill-fitting and infected margins in the site of the mandibular right first premolar.

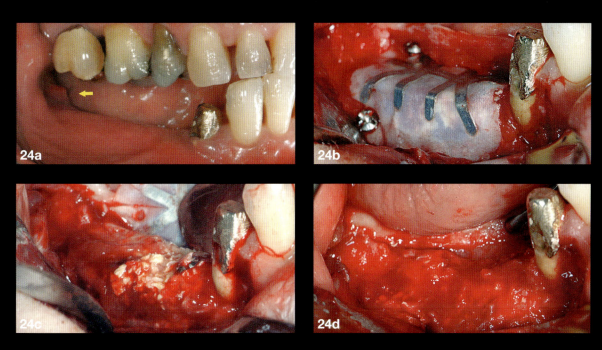

Fig 24 *(a)* Postoperative infection about 1 month after regeneration surgery with GBR. There is no exposure of the membrane, but a fistula (arrow) is present in the site of the mandibular right third molar. *(b)* A mucoperiosteal flap is elevated to remove the PTFE membrane. Note the purulent material transpiring from beneath the membrane. *(c)* After removal of the barrier membrane, infection of the bone graft is evident. It is necessary to remove most of the graft material by suction, gentle curettage, and irrigation with hydrogen peroxide and antibiotics. The membrane support screws must also be removed. *(d)* The infected material is removed until more compact tissue organized into a stable fibrin clot is reached.

REFERENCES

1. Simion M, Jovanovic SA, Tinti C, Benfenati SP. Long-term evaluation of osseointegrated implants inserted at the time or after vertical ridge augmentation. A retrospective study on 123 implants with 1-5 year follow-up. Clin Oral Implants Res 2001;12:35–45.

2. Rocchietta I, Fontana F, Simion M. Clinical outcomes of vertical bone augmentation to enable dental implant placement. A systematic review. J Clin Periodontol 2008;35(8 Suppl):203–215.

3. Esposito M, Grusovin MG, Kwan S, Worthington HV, Coulthard P. Interventions for replacing missing teeth: Bone augmentation techniques for dental implant treatment. Cochrane Database Syst Rev 2008;(3):CD003607.

4. Fontana F, Santoro F, Maiorana C, Iezzi G, Piattelli A, Simion M. Clinical and histological evaluation of allogenous bone matrix versus autogenous bone chips associated with titanium reinforced e-ptfe membrane for vertical ridge augmentation: A prospective pilot study in the human. Int J Oral Maxillofac Implants 2008;23:1003–1012.

5. Becker W, Becker BE. Guided tissue regeneration for implants placed into extraction sockets and for implant dehiscences: Surgical techniques and case report. Int J Periodontics Restorative Dent 1990;10:376–391.

6. Becker W, Dahlin C, Becker BE, et al. The use of e-PTFE barrier membranes for bone promotion around titanium implants placed into extraction sockets: A prospective multicenter study. Int J Oral Maxillofac Implants 1994;9:31–40.

7. Kohal RJ, Trejo PM, Wirsching C, Hürzeler MB, Caffesse RG. Comparison of bioabsorbable and bioinert membranes for guided bone regeneration around non-submerged implants. An experimental study in the mongrel dog. Clin Oral Implants Res 1999;10:226–237.

8. Lekholm U, Becker W, Dahlin C, Becker B, Donath K, Morrison E. The role of early versus late removal of GTAM membranes on bone formation at oral implants placed into immediate extraction sockets. An experimental study in dogs. Clin Oral Implants Res 1993;4:121–129.

9. Buser D, Brägger U, Lang NP, Nyman S. Regeneration and enlargement of jaw bone using guided tissue regeneration. Clin Oral Implants Res 1990;1:22–32.

10. Buser D, Dula K, Belser U, Hirt HP, Berthold H. Localized ridge augmentation using guided bone regeneration. Surgical procedure in the maxilla. Int J Periodontics Restorative Dent 1993;13:29–45.

11. Simion M, Trisi P, Piattelli A. Vertical ridge augmentation using a membrane technique associated with osseointegrated implants. Int J Periodontics Restorative Dent 1994;14:496–511.

12. Jovanovic SA, Spiekermann H, Richter EJ. Bone regeneration around titanium dental implants in dehisced defect sites: A clinical study. Int J Oral Maxillofac Implants 1992;7:233–245.

13. Buser D, Dula K, Hirt HP, Schenk RK. Lateral ridge augmentation using autografts and barrier membranes: A clinical study with 40 partially edentulous patients. J Oral Maxillofac Surg 1996;54:420–432.

14. Tinti C, Parma-Benfenati S, Polizzi G. Vertical ridge augmentation: What is the limit? Int J Periodontics Restorative Dent 1996;16:221–229.

15. Simion M, Jovanovic SA, Trisi P, Scarano A, Piattelli A. Vertical ridge augmentation around dental implants using a membrane technique and autogenous bone or allografts in humans. Int J Periodontics Restorative Dent 1998;18:8–23.

16. Simion M, Fontana F, Rasperini G, Maiorana C. Vertical ridge augmentation by expanded-polytetrafluoroethylene membrane and a combination of intraoral autogenous bone graft and deproteinized anorganic bovine bone (bio-oss). Clin Oral Implants Res 2007;18:620–629.

17. Merli M, Migani M, Esposito M. Vertical ridge augmentation with autogenous bone grafts: Resorbable barriers supported by ostheosynthesis plates versus titanium-reinforced barriers. A preliminary report of a blinded, randomized controlled clinical trial. Int J Oral Maxillofac Implants 2007;22:373–282.

18. Verardi S, Simion M. Management of the exposure of e-PTFE membranes in guided bone regeneration. Pract Proced Aesthet Dent 2007;19:111–117.

19. Fontana F, Maschera E, Rocchietta I, Simion M. Clinical classification of complications in guided bone regeneration procedures by means of a nonresorbable membrane. Int J Periodontics Restorative Dent 2011;31:265–273.